MAGNETIC RESONANCE
SPECTROSCOPY

MAGNETIC RESONANCE SPECTROSCOPY

Tools for Neuroscience Research and Emerging Clinical Applications

Edited by

CHARLOTTE STAGG

Oxford Centre for Functional MRI of the Brain (FMRIB),
Department of Clinical Neurosciences, University of Oxford

DOUGLAS ROTHMAN

Departments of Diagnostic Radiology, Magnetic Resonance Research Center,
Yale University School of Medicine

AMSTERDAM • BOSTON • HEIDELBERG • LONDON
NEW YORK • OXFORD • PARIS • SAN DIEGO
SAN FRANCISCO • SINGAPORE • SYDNEY • TOKYO
Academic Press is an imprint of Elsevier

Academic Press is an imprint of Elsevier
32 Jamestown Road, London NW1 7BY, UK
225 Wyman Street, Waltham, MA 02451, USA
525 B Street, Suite 1800, San Diego, CA 92101-4495, USA

British Library Cataloguing-in-Publication Data
A catalogue record for this book is available from the British Library

Library of Congress Cataloging-in-Publication Data
A catalog record for this book is available from the Library of Congress

ISBN: 978-0-12-401688-0

For information on all Academic Press publications
visit our website at elsevierdirect.com

Typeset by MPS Limited, Chennai, India
www.adi-mps.com

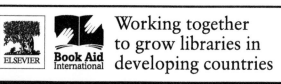

Contents

3

APPLICATIONS OF PROTON-MRS

Acknowledgements

The editors would like to thank April Graham and Mica Haley for expertly steering this book from conception to production with constant good humor and seemingly endless patience. Thanks also go to our many colleagues around the globe who generously gave up so much of their time to contribute such excellent chapters to the volume. CJS would like to thank Heidi Johansen-Berg, as always, for her generosity and support in allowing this book to be started and Emily Aspden for arriving just late enough to ensure it could be completed.

Contributors

Prasanth Ariyannur Uniformed Services University of the Health Sciences, Bethesda, MD

Peethambaran Arun Uniformed Services University of the Health Sciences, Bethesda, MD

Carles Arús Centro de Investigación Biomédica en Red en Bioingeniería, Biomateriales y Nanomedicina and Institut de Biotecnologia i de Biomedicina, Universitat Autònoma de Barcelona, Cerdanyola del Vallès, Spain

Ian C. Atkinson Center for Magnetic Resonance Research, University of Illinois at Chicago, Chicago, IL

Velicia Bachtiar Oxford Centre for Functional MRI of the Brain, University of Oxford, United Kingdom

Kevin L. Behar Yale University School of Medicine, New Haven, CT

Jonathan G. Best Oxford Centre for Functional MRI of the Brain, University of Oxford, United Kingdom

Andrew Bivard University of Melbourne, Melbourne Brain Centre, Melbourne, Australia

Vincent O. Boer University Medical Center Utrecht, Utrecht, The Netherlands

Jennifer Brawn Functional Magnetic Resonance Imaging of the Brain Centre, University of Oxford, United Kingdom

Dallas Card Hospital for Sick Children, Toronto, Ontario, Canada

Kim C. Cecil Cincinnati Children's Hospital Medical Center at the University of Cincinnati College of Medicine, Cincinnati, OH

Olga Ciccarelli University College London Institute of Neurology, London, United Kingdom; National Institute for Health Research University College London Hospitals Biomedical Research Centre, London, United Kingdom

Henk M. De Feyter Magnetic Resonance Research Center, Yale University School of Medicine, New Haven, CT

Robin A. de Graaf Magnetic Resonance Research Center, Yale University, School of Medicine, New Haven, CT

Nicola De Stefano University of Siena, Italy

Andrea Dennis Oxford Centre for Functional MRI of the Brain, University of Oxford, United Kingdom

Nicholas Gant Centre for Brain Research, The University of Auckland, New Zealand

Antonio Giorgio University of Siena, Italy

Rolf Gruetter University of Geneva, Switzerland; Center for Biomedical Imaging and Laboratory of Functional and Metabolic Imaging, Ecole Polytechnique Federale de Lausanne, Switzerland; University of Lausanne, Switzerland

Hoby Hetherington University of Pittsburgh Medical Center, Pittsburgh, PA

Amber Michelle Hill University College London Institute of Neurology, London, United Kingdom

Christoph Juchem Magnetic Research Center, Yale University School of Medicine, New Haven CT

Margarida Julià-Sapé Centro de Investigación Biomédica en Red en Bioingeniería, Biomateriales y Nanomedicina and Institut de Biotecnologia i de Biomedicina, Universitat Autònoma de Barcelona, Cerdanyola del Vallès, Spain

Dennis W.J. Klomp University Medical Center Utrecht, Utrecht, The Netherlands

Hongxia Lei University of Geneva, Switzerland; Center for Biomedical Imaging, Ecole Polytechnique Federale de Lausanne, Switzerland

Joanne C. Lin Centre for Brain Research, The University of Auckland, New Zealand

Carles Majós L'Hospitalet de Llobregat, Barcelona, Spain; Centro de Investigación Biomédica en Red en Bioingeniería, Biomateriales y Nanomedicina, Cerdanyola del Vallès, Spain

Vladimír Mlynárik Center for Biomedical Imaging, Ecole Polytechnique Federale de Lausanne, Switzerland

John R. Moffett Uniformed Services University of the Health Sciences, Bethesda, MD

Aryan M.A. Namboodiri Uniformed Services University of the Health Sciences, Bethesda, MD

Jamie Near McGill University and Centre d'Imagerie du Cerveau, Douglas Mental Health University Institute, Montreal, Quebec, Canada

Jullie Pan University of Pittsburgh Medical Center, Pittsburgh, PA

Mark Parsons University of Newcastle, Newcastle, United Kingdom

Brian D. Ross Huntington Medical Research Institutes, Magnetic Resonance Spectroscopy Unit, Pasadena, CA

Douglas L. Rothman Magnetic Research Center, Yale University School of Medicine, New Haven, CT

Jun Shen Molecular Imaging Branch, National Institute of Mental Health, Bethesda, MD

Nicola R. Sibson CR-UK/MRC Gray Institute for Radiation Oncology and Biology, University of Oxford, Oxford, United Kingdom

John G. Sled Research Institute, Hospital for Sick Children, Toronto, Ontario Canada; University of Toronto, Toronto, Ontario Canada

Charlotte J. Stagg Oxford Centre for Functional MRI of the Brain, University of Oxford, United Kingdom

Peter Stanwell University of Newcastle, Newcastle, United Kingdom

Margot J. Taylor Hospital for Sick Children and Medical Imaging, Toronto, Ontario Canada; University of Toronto, Toronto, Ontario, Canada

Matthew Taylor Institute of Psychiatry, London, United Kingdom

Keith R. Thulborn Center for Magnetic Resonance Research, University of Illinois at Chicago, Chicago, IL

Clare E. Turner Centre for Brain Research, The University of Auckland, New Zealand

Katy Vincent Functional Magnetic Resonance Imaging of the Brain Centre, University of Oxford, United Kingdom

Lijing Xin University of Lausanne, Switzerland; Laboratory of Functional and Metabolic Imaging, Ecole Polytechnique Federale de Lausanne, Switzerland

Introduction

Magnetic resonance spectroscopy (MRS) is a noninvasive technique that uses the same physics principles and detection methods as magnetic resonance imaging (MRI) of H_2O, but adds an additional dimension of information by also detecting the resonance frequencies of metabolites. From the resonance frequencies (referred to as chemical shift) and other properties of these resonances the identity, concentration, and stable isotope enrichment of biochemicals can be determined. ^{1}H MRS, which is the most widely used, was first performed on the brain by Behar and coworkers in the lab of Professor Robert G Shulman in 1983 (Behar et al., 1983). In this pioneering study, performed on a rat in a vertical bore magnet, resonances of N-acetylaspartate (NAA), glutamate, glutamine, choline, creatine, and lactate were assigned. These remain the only major metabolites studied using *in vivo*[1] H MRS. Within several years after this study the first high-field (1.5 T and above) human magnets were built by Oxford Instruments and in 1985 Bottomley and coworkers at General Electric published the first localized human brain ^{1}H MRS spectra (Bottomley et al., 1985). The first applications to human disease were presented at the meeting of the Society of Magnetic Resonance in Medicine in 1986 by den Hollander and colleagues working at Philips, and these were soon followed by several groups who performed pioneering studies in stroke, tumors, and other clinical conditions.

Following these and other pioneering studies ^{1}H MRS has been used for many years in clinical neuroscience as a method for investigating brain neurochemistry, critical to understanding neurological and psychiatric disease. However, a relatively low signal-to-noise (SNR) ratio has limited its use on standard clinical scanners. Over recent years, with the increasing availability of high and ultrahigh field scanners, as well as a much increased understanding of how metabolism plays a critical role in neuroenergetics and neurotransmission, MRS has undergone something of a renaissance and gained traction within the MR community for translational and clinical neuroscience. Improved acquisition and analysis approaches have increased interest in its use both for traditional clinical applications and also for neuroscience research. However, although excellent books exist covering the technical aspects of MRS for physicists, there is currently no book targeted at clinicians and neuroscientists that covers all aspects of the technique. In this book we attempt to address this need. It is organized as a reference text that is aimed not at physicists but at experts in the *application* of MRS such as neurologists, psychiatrists, radiologists, and neuroscientists. However, we hope that the coverage of applications and basic methodologies is complete enough that physicists entering the field may benefit and even experienced MR physicists working in other areas could use it to determine the state-of-the-art methodology used in the field.

To achieve these goals we have divided the book into three sections, which we outline below.

SECTION 1: HOW MRS IS ACQUIRED

In this section we have enlisted experts in the field of MRS data acquisition and processing to provide an introduction to the field and an overview of state-of-the-art methodology in these areas. Even though the mathematics is kept at a minimum, enough technical detail is included to allow readers to understand the principles and relative strengths and weaknesses of the different methods. In Chapter 1.1 Drs. Christoph Juchem and Douglas Rothman describe the basis of Magnetic Resonance focusing on basic principles but also give an overview of some of the most common methods used in MRS and chemicals measured. In Chapter 1.2 Drs. Hongxia Lei, Lijing Xin, Rolf Gruetter, and Vladimír Mlynárik describe the state of the art of single-volume ^{1}H MRS as well as novel recent approaches such as ultra short TE MRS. This chapter describes the methods needed to meet the stringent requirements for volume localization with MRS due to large resonances from water and scalp lipids. The critical importance and optimal methods for improving field homogeneity and suppressing intravoxel water are also described in detail as well as artifacts that may occur if adequate criteria are not met. MRS can both be obtained as information from a single volume (or several) in the brain or as a metabolic image. In Chapter 1.3 Drs. Vincent Boer and Dennis Klomp provide an introduction to magnetic resonance spectroscopic imaging (MRSI) including its application at ultrahigh fields such as 7 T. This chapter demonstrates the great potential of MRSI but also reviews its limitations, many of which relate to the need to establish adequate static and radiofrequency magnetic field homogeneity throughout the volume imaged (as compared to single-volume MRS where optimization is only required in a small region of the brain). With optimal B_0 homogeneity and higher B_0 fields more and more metabolites can be distinguished based on their resonance frequencies (chemical shift), but lower concentration metabolites such as γ-amino butyric acid (GABA) still cannot be resolved at clinical 3 T fields. To overcome these spectral overlap limitations MRS methods that separate resonances based not just upon resonance frequency but also upon quantum J-coupling between resonances within a single molecule have been developed. These methods are often referred to as "spectral editing" because they edit out resonances from specific chemicals from overlapping resonances from other chemicals. In Chapter 1.4 Dr. Robin de Graaf provides a guide to modern editing and related 2D MRS methods. While these methods have largely been limited to specialized research MR systems recent developments in clinical 3 T systems have greatly expanded their applicability. Even with the best data acquisition methodology the analysis and calibration methods used in MRS play a critical role in the accuracy and precision of the results obtained. In Chapter 1.5 Dr. Jamie Near covers in detail methods used to analyze and quantitate the *in vivo* MRS spectrum as well as the advantages and pitfalls of each.

SECTION 2: BIOCHEMISTRY—WHAT UNDERLIES THE SIGNAL?

This section covers the biochemistry of the major neurochemicals, and what we can infer from increased or decreased levels of these in the brain and what cannot be elucidated provide a description of modern strategies for interpreting MRS results. In Chapter 2.1 Drs. John Moffett, Prasanth Ariyannur, Peethambaran Arun, and Aryan Namboodiri cover *N*-acetylaspartate (NAA) and *N*-acetylaspartylglutamate (NAAG) in central nervous system (CNS) health and disease. NAA was identified in the very first *in vivo*[1] H MRS brain study performed and due to its high concentration and the presence of a singlet methyl group (which increases sensitivity by 3 × due to proton multiplicity) has been the major biochemical studied in clinical MRS. Despite its wide use there is considerable uncertainty about the function of NAA in the CNS and how to interpret changes seen in the MRS spectrum. In this chapter evidence for our present understanding of the roles of NAA and NAG and their underlying biochemistry are covered in detail along with implications for clinical MRS studies. In Chapter 2.2 Drs. Clare Turner and Nicholas Gant cover creatine, another

major metabolite measured in the MRS spectrum, again due to its high concentration and the presence of a methyl group. Creatine is often used as a concentration reference in the MRS spectrum (as described in Chapter 1.5) so that it is important to understand conditions where its concentration may change. Metabolites that have often been used in clinical MRS studies are the combined resonances of choline-containing compounds. In Chapter 2.3 Drs. Nicholas Gant and Joanne Lin cover in detail the biochemistry and functional roles of choline in the brain and how choline levels may reflect pathologies. Changes in choline, creatine, and NAA tend to be relatively slow, with the time for biosynthetic replacement of the pools (turnover time) on the order of days. However, MRS can also look at metabolites that are dynamically turning over through their involvement in energy metabolism and neurotransmission. In Chapter 2.4 Dr Jun Shen describes the role of glutamate in brain energy metabolism and neurotransmission and how these roles can be studied using ^{1}H MRS and ^{13}C MRS (which is followed up in more detail in Sections 3 and 4). This chapter also provides additional background on the MRS measurement of glutamate. In Chapter 2.5 Drs. Jonathan Best, Charlotte Stagg, and Andrea Dennis cover the biochemistry and functional roles of myo-inositol, GABA, glutamine, and lactate. GABA and glutamine provide, respectively, a measure of metabolism in GABAergic neurons and glial cells, which along with glutamatergic neurons (they contain the majority of the glutamate signal) account for the large majority of cells in the brain. The GABA signal measured by ^{1}H MRS is also related to tonic GABAergic inhibition, which opens up ^{1}H MRS to be applied to a variety of neuroscience-related applications as described in Section 3. Due to its production by nonoxidative glycolysis, lactate levels are highly sensitive to the oxygenation status of brain tissue and, as further described in Section 3, can be diagnostic for necrotic tumors and other conditions such as brain ischemia. Myo-inositol appears to be primarily localized to glial cells and the resonance is highly sensitive to the presence of neurodegenerative disease as well as alterations in brain osmotic levels like those found in ketoacidotic hyperglycemia and hyperammonemia.

SECTION 3: APPLICATIONS OF PROTON MRS

MRS is theoretically feasible on any nucleus that possesses a magnetic moment; however, by far the most common nucleus for study is the proton. Protons have the greatest gyromagnetic ration of any nuclei seen *in vivo* and are also by far the most abundant nucleus in the brain. These two factors mean that ^{1}H MRS has a relatively high SNR and, because protons are found in all metabolically interesting compounds, there is great potential for the study of the brain. In addition, MRI is performed on H_2O, meaning that clinical MR scanners can be used for ^{1}H MRS without buying expensive additional hardware, theoretically opening up its use to a wide range of users.

This section discusses the undoubted potential of ^{1}H MRS for both clinical and neuroscientific applications, as well as raising the limitations of the technique in the context of the conditions in which they have been applied. In Chapter 3.1 Drs. Carles Majós, Margarida Julià-Sapé, and Carles Arús discuss the clinical applications of MRS in tumor detection and management—exploring the application of MRS most commonly seen in clinical practice. MRS can be used to distinguish between tumors and non-tumors, can help the clinician to determine the nature of a tumor before pathology can be acquired, and can monitor the sequelae of treatment by distinguishing between tumor regrowth and post-treatment changes. In Chapter 3.2 Drs. Nicola De Stefano and Antonio Giorgio discuss the potential of MRS to determine pathology and monitor progression in inflammatory conditions, particularly in multiple sclerosis. Although MRS has undoubted potential to provide informative biomarkers for the development of potential treatments for MS, these are currently limited by the difficulty of acquiring reproducible data between different scanners, and possible solutions to this problem are discussed.

Chapter 3.3 focuses on epilepsy, a common neurological condition and one in which, as Drs. Julie Pan and Hoby Hetherington discuss, the ability of MRS to quantify neuroenergetics means that ^{1}H MRS is invaluable in allowing underlying pathologies to be studied. They also describe complementary work using ^{31}P and ^{13}C MRS, nuclei covered in more detail in Section 4, to further assess altered energetics in epileptogenic tissue. In Chapter 3.4 Drs. Andrew Bivard, Peter Stanwell, and Mark Parsons review the potential of MRS to study the metabolic events in the hyperacute phases of stroke recovery and its developing use as a window into the changes underlying the recovery of function in the months that follow. As with all neurological conditions, however, there are significant challenges in acquiring and interpreting ^{1}H MRS data from these patients, particularly data acquired from within and surrounding the lesioned region where the tissue inhomogeneity leads to greatly broadened linewidths. Some potential solutions are discussed as well as the potential pitfalls associated with interpreting these data.

In Chapter 3.5 Dr. Kim Cecil discusses the unique potential of MRS in the study of pediatric conditions, where the acquisition of diagnostic information noninvasively (e.g., with no injected radioactive tracers) is perhaps of heightened importance. The study of inborn errors of metabolism such as the leukodystrophies and Canavan's disease in particular has shed considerable light on the pathology of these conditions. Chapter 3.6 highlights the potential of ^{1}H MRS to improve our understanding of psychiatric conditions. Dr. Matthew Taylor focuses particularly on psychotic conditions and mood disorders, where a range of abnormalities in neural metabolism and glutamatergic signaling have been identified. The final clinical MRS application to be considered is that of spinal MRS in Chapter 3.7, where Drs. Amber Hill and Olga Ciccarelli discuss the potential of this technologically challenging approach. Despite the difficulties of acquiring spectra of adequate quality from the cord, given its relatively small size and intrinsic movement, several preclinical and clinical studies have been performed, the results of which suggest that this may well become a much more widely used approach in the future.

Chapter 3.8 moves toward the application of ^{1}H MRS for neuroscientific questions. Drs. Velicia Bachtiar and Charlotte Stagg provide an overview of the potential of MRS studies focusing on GABA and glutamate in particular to increase our understanding of how differences in behavior between people may be driven by underlying physiology. In Chapter 3.9 Drs. Dallas Card, Margot Taylor, and John Sled discuss the use of MRS to study natural aging, where studies have been targeted in particular both at the rapid development occurring in the brains of infants during development *in utero* and in the elderly. The importance of these data, and the challenges of longitudinal studies, particularly in infants, are discussed.

In Chapter 3.10 Drs. Jennifer Brawn and Katy Vincent discuss the role of MRS in the study of hormonal influences in the brain. Until relatively recently the substantial effects of hormones on brain activity were not recognized, but there is now increasing evidence that hormones, their precursors, and their derivatives all have striking effects on neuronal metabolism and cell signaling. In particular, the role of the menstrual cycle is discussed in some detail, as this may be important to take into account when interpreting the results of MRS studies in other contexts. Finally, in Chapter 3.11, Drs. Nicola Sibson and Kevin Behar discuss the use of ^{13}C MRS to study brain biochemistry. Although not as widely available as ^{1}H MRS, ^{13}C MRS has a unique potential to study brain energetics and metabolism *in vivo*. ^{13}C MRS has already provided many insights into brain function in animal models and, with the ongoing improvements in the technique, its potential for the study of brain function in humans is beginning to be realized, a topic covered in more detail in Section 4.

SECTION 4: APPLICATIONS OF NON-PROTON MRS

Although the majority of *in vivo* MRS studies of the CNS have used the ^{1}H nucleus there is a large amount of complimentary information that can be obtained using other nuclei, including ^{13}C, sodium (^{23}Na), oxygen (^{17}O), phosphorus (^{31}P), and potassium (^{39}K). Considerable insights into brain energetics and function have been obtained in research studies using these nuclei, several of which are described in Sections 2 and 3. Because these nuclei gain in sensitivity with field to a greater degree than the ^{1}H nucleus they may become standard as ultrahigh field systems such as 7 T become more common. In this section we cover present and potential uses of these nuclei and how they can add information to both clinical diagnosis and basic understanding of brain metabolism and function. In Chapter 4.1 Drs. Keith Thulborn and Ian Atkinson provide an introduction to state-of-the-art sodium, oxygen, and phosphorous MRS, MRSI, and MRI and show how at ultrahigh fields even imaging of potassium is possible. MRI of sodium and potassium has great potential for detecting clinical imbalances that may profoundly impact brain function as well as even a more direct form of functional imaging. Further, the authors introduce the concept of bioscales in the clinical applications of these measurements making a strong argument for going beyond standard MRI and ^{1}H MRS. In Chapter 4.2 Drs. Henk De Feyter and Douglas Rothman cover the methodology and applications of ^{13}C MRS in combination with ^{13}C-labeled brain substrates such as glucose and acetate. While this is one of the most challenging areas of MRS due to the need for stable isotope infusion, metabolic modeling and modified MR hardware, it has already provided novel insight into brain function and disease and has shown high sensitivity to a variety of clinical conditions including Alzheimer's disease and healthy aging, cancer, developmental disorders, diabetes, depression, and stroke. It is also the only method that can be used to study cell type-specific metabolism and glutamate and GABA neurotransmission in humans.

An additional limitation of using ^{13}C MRS is its low sensitivity relative to ^{1}H MRS, which results in relatively course spatial resolution. While this can be recovered using inverse ^{1}H-[^{13}C] MRS, particularly at high fields, the overall achievable spatial resolution is still well below PET scanning and other metabolic imaging methods. However, this limitation has been overcome recently through the development of hyperpolarized ^{13}C MRS. The MRS signal is proportional to the difference in the number of nuclear spins pointing parallel versus antiparallel to the main magnetic field. Normally the excess is a small fraction of the total nuclei, but in hyperpolarized ^{13}C MRS the sensitivity of detection (and in principle spatial resolution) can be improved by over 10,000-fold due to prepolarization of the ^{13}C-labeled precursor prior to injection. In Chapter 4.3 Dr. Brian Ross describes the state of the art of the use of hyperpolarized ^{13}C MRS to study the brain. This application has been very challenging due to both the difficulties involved in performing conventional MRS and the additional challenges of delivering the hyperpolarized compound to the brain before it reverts through relaxation back to normal levels of polarization (losing the enhancement). However, recent breakthroughs described in this chapter make the prospects of performing these scans in patients much more promising.

References

Behar, K. L., den Hollander, J. A., Stromski, M. E., Ogino, T., Shulman, R. G., Petroff, O. A., & Prichard, J. W. (1983). High resolution ^{1}H nuclear magnetic resonance study of cerebral hypoxia in vivo. *Proceedings of the National Academy of Sciences USA, 80*(16), 4945–4948.

Bottomley, P. A., Edelstein, W. A., Foster, T. H., & Adams, W. A. (1985). *In vivo* solvent suppressed localized hydrogen nuclear magnetic resonance spectroscopy: a window to metabolism? *Proceedings of the National Academy of Sciences USA, 82*, 2148–2152.

TECHNICAL ASPECTS— HOW MRS IS ACQUIRED

Basis of Magnetic Resonance

Christoph Juchem[1,2] and Douglas L. Rothman[1]

[1]Department of Diagnostic Radiology [2]Department of Neurology, Yale School of Medicine, Massachussetts, USA

INTRODUCTION

Magnetic resonance spectroscopy (MRS) allows the detection and quantification of chemical compounds from localized portions of the living tissue, e.g., the brain, in a noninvasive fashion. It thereby provides a powerful tool to assess key aspects of brain metabolism and function. In the clinics, the repertoire of measurable compounds along with the quantitative character of the derived information makes MRS a versatile tool for the identification of clinical conditions, for longitudinal patient monitoring and for treatment control. The goal of this chapter is to summarize the basic concepts of commonly applied *in vivo* MRS methods. These concepts will be developed more in subsequent chapters as well as more advanced MRS methods such as spectroscopic imaging and J-editing, and measurement of specific chemicals and metabolic pathways. The descriptions in this chapter will be kept at a relatively basic level. For a more advanced but still very accessible treatment of basic MRS spin physics as well as MRS methodology we recommend de Graaf (2008).

In Vivo Spectroscopy

Atomic nuclei with a magnetic moment (or "spin") can exhibit resonance behavior in a magnetic field. This magnetic resonance effect is governed by the Larmor equation as a simple linear relationship between the magnetic field B perceived by the nucleus and the resultant resonance frequency ω.

$$\omega = -\gamma B \tag{1}$$

The relative scaling γ, the so-called gyromagnetic ratio, is a nucleus-specific constant. The hydrogen nucleus ^1H (i.e., a proton) is the prime example for an MR-sensitive isotope as ^1H resonance signals from hydrogen nuclei bound in tissue water provide the basis for MR imaging (MRI) of the human body. Nuclear spins can be thought of as microscopic magnets. When placed in a magnetic field these magnetic moments become polarized, and are either parallel or antiparallel to the field. The spins that are polarized parallel to the field are in a lower energy state, so slightly more are present in this alignment than antiparallel to the field. When radiofrequency (RF) energy is applied to spins in a magnet at the Larmor frequency, the spins will absorb energy and undergo a transition from the antiparallel to the parallel state as with optical and other forms of resonance spectroscopy. MRS, however, differs in that in the process of absorption the spins will become polarized with the RF field such that when the RF field is shut off the spins will effectively rotate along the axis of the magnet (by convention the z-axis in MRS). This phenomenon creates a rotating magnetic field at the Larmor frequency. When an RF receiver coil is used the rotating magnetization induces an oscillating voltage by induction, which is then detected by the MR spectrometer (which is essentially a large RF transmitter and receiver). At field strengths available for clinical MRS the Larmor frequency will vary from $\sim$60 to 300 MHz corresponding to magnet field strengths of 1.5 and 7.0 T, respectively. The low resonance frequency (6 to 7 orders of magnitude lower than optical resonances) is disadvantageous from a sensitivity standpoint, because the energy per absorption or emission is proportional to frequency. However, unlike optical spectroscopy or imaging, the human body is relatively transparent to RF at the MHz range and therefore is completely accessible to measurement by MRS.

3

When a human subject is placed in the scanner of a given field strength, one could assume that all of the body's ^{1}H nuclei exhibit the same resonance frequency. In reality, however, minute frequency variations are observed depending on the molecular structure the atomic nucleus is embedded in. The field variations to cause these frequency shifts are based on two different effects. The electronic, i.e., the chemical, environment around the atomic nucleus at hand results in a so-called "chemical shift" and the correlation of different nuclei of the same molecule mediated through their binding electrons is referred to as dipolar or J-coupling. Chemical shift and J-coupling critically rely on the molecules' chemical and geometric composition. As such, their measurement provides a wealth of intra-molecular, microscopic information from a relatively simple, "macroscopic" MRS experiment. Notably, chemical shift and J-coupling are the basis for the key role MRS is playing in structural and analytical chemistry. Although chemical shift and J-coupling were discovered in the 1950s, it was not until 20 years later that MRS was applied to identify and quantify biochemicals in living cells (Shulman et al., 1979) and eventually *in vivo* (Ackerman et al., 1980). With this paradigm shift, the goal was no longer to study the physicochemical properties of substances, but to use the knowledge on the substance-specific spectroscopic patterns, i.e., their spectroscopic fingerprint, to separate and quantify these substances *in vivo* to infer the concentrations of metabolites and the fluxes of metabolic pathways.

MRS allows the noninvasive quantification of neurochemicals that contain MR-sensitive isotopes (e.g., ^{1}H). Hydrogen is prevalent in most metabolites of the human brain and the ^{1}H nucleus is the most relevant isotope for *in vivo* MRS. The gyromagnetic ratio of ^{1}H is highest for all stable isotopes; therefore, its sensitivity in MR experiments is higher than for any other nucleus. Furthermore, the natural abundance of the ^{1}H nucleus is almost 100%. The first *in vivo* MRS measurements of the living brain were in 1982 on a small-bore high-field MR system (Behar et al., 1983). With the subsequent rapid development of large-bore high-field magnets and volume localization by the mid-1980s, the first ^{1}H MR spectra of human brain were obtained (Bottomley et al., 1983; Frahm et al., 1989) and today ^{1}H MR spectra can be somewhat routinely obtained on all clinical MRI systems of 1.5 T and higher in field strength.

Although a series of brain metabolites can be identified with ^{1}H MRS (Govindaraju et al., 2000), the number of substances that are assessable under *in vivo* conditions does not exceed 15–20 (Mekle et al., 2009; Tkac et al., 2009; Emir et al., 2011a) and is typically well below. Further MR-visible isotopes with biochemical relevance have been shown to provide valuable information on tissue physiology and biochemistry.

Phosphorus (^{31}P) MRS, for instance, allows the quantification of key components of the tissues' energy metabolism (ATP, ADP, and phosphocreatine) and to study, for example, bioenergetic deficits in response to disease (Befroy & Shulman, 2011). MRS employing the ^{13}C isotope enables the study of Krebs (TCA) cycle intermediates, and the predictable transfer of infused ^{13}C-label between specific positions of the carbon chains of these intermediates stands out by providing turnover rates and metabolic fluxes (Rothman et al., 2011). Today's clinical MRS, however, mostly relies on ^{1}H whereas other nuclei are predominantly used in basic and preclinical research. The need for nonstandard hardware and specialized MRS methods for non-^{1}H MRS might be reasons why these applications have yet to prevail in clinical practice. This chapter therefore focuses on the basic principles of ^{1}H MRS, although where appropriate extensions to other nuclei will be discussed (for more detail on this topic see Chapters 4.1–4.3.).

MRS METHODS

Basics of MRS

The goal of *in vivo* ^{1}H MRS is to quantify biochemical substances in a noninvasive fashion. In general, the signal amplitudes of an MRS acquisition and the resultant peaks in the reconstructed spectrum directly scale with the number of resonating nuclei and the substance amount seen by the MRS experiment. As such, spectral peaks and patterns provide a direct measure for the concentration of the metabolite at hand. Water is by far the most prevalent [1]H-containing compound in human tissue; therefore it contributes the largest part of the MR signal (Fig. 1.1.1A). Since the water concentration itself is of little clinical relevance, its signal is typically minimized in MRS experiments to better reveal the metabolites of interest (Fig. 1.1.1B). A prominent limitation of ^{1}H MRS of brain metabolites is the small frequency spread between spectral peaks. This limited spectral dispersion leads to severe spectral overlap of the observed patterns and poses a significant challenge for the identification and separation of the individual compounds. Notably, the problem of spectral overlap is further complicated *in vivo* by limited magnetic field homogeneity and the resultant broadening of spectral lines. The strongest limitation for the quantification of tissue metabolites, however, arises from the inherently poor sensitivity of MR methods. Metabolite concentrations in the millimolar range are therefore necessary with ^{1}H MRS to achieve signal amplitudes that sufficiently exceed the inevitable measurement noise. Moreover, adequate signal-to-noise ratio (SNR) is particularly relevant when partially

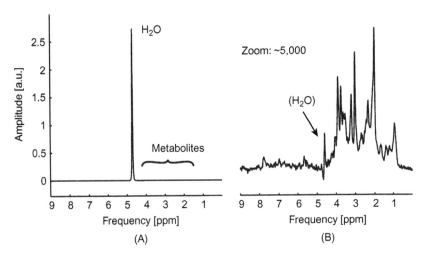

FIGURE 1.1.1 The role of water suppression for *in vivo* ^{1}H MRS of the human brain. (A) The water content in human brain tissue largely exceeds the concentrations of other observable substances and therefore dominates the appearance of the spectrum. (B) Suppression of the water signal allows an unobstructed view of the neurochemicals of interest.

overlapping spectral structures are to be disentangled, as is typically the case for ^{1}H MRS.

Fortunately, the selection of accessible brain metabolites includes many key neurochemicals involved in brain energetics and neurotransmission as well as other critical neurochemical pathways. The majority of chemical compounds present in the brain, however, have concentrations well below the detection limit. Dopamine levels in human brain tissue, for instance, are in the micromolar range, which precludes the quantification of this important neurotransmitter with MRS methods. Stronger scanner B_0 fields increase the available MR sensitivity and SNR, and can somewhat improve the detection limit (Ugurbil et al., 2003). Within an experiment, the attainable SNR can be increased when larger volumes are considered as the available signals scale with the number of covered spins and, therefore, the amount of tissue exhibiting a given substance. The concomitant reduction of spatial (and therefore anatomic/functional) specificity, however, is an obvious caveat to this approach. Alternatively, SNR improvements can be realized by combining the data from various repetitions of an identical experiment, since the summation signal grows linearly with the number of repetitions, whereas the noise contribution only increases with its square root. As such, SNR gains of the square root of the number of repeats are achieved. In practice, however, the applicability of this approach is limited by the progressively larger time penalty per additional SNR gain. For instance, the SNR of a single acquisition is doubled when four identical scans are summed together. An SNR gain of f4, however, requires 16 averages, i.e., an additional 12 scans are necessary to double the SNR from 2 to 4, while 4 scans were enough to double it from 1 to 2. Most MRS applications apply data summation for SNR/sensitivity improvement, but the number of repeats rarely exceeds 128 or 256 averages. Although the discussed approaches can alleviate some of the burdens of low MR sensitivity, in reality, they all have obvious limitations and are not able to fundamentally overcome the millimolar detection limit of ^{1}H MRS.

Chemical Shift

Based on the Larmor condition, the resonance frequency of a nucleus is determined by its gyromagnetic ratio and the magnetic field to which it is exposed. If the nucleus is not free but part of a chemical compound, (in most cases) a shielding of the external field B_0 by the surrounding electrons is observed. The change of the nucleus' MR frequency due to this screening is called chemical shift and provides the main concept of MRS. The effect of electronic shielding is field dependent and so are the resultant absolute frequency shifts in Hertz. When resonance frequencies ω are assigned relative to a reference frequency ω_{ref}, the derived chemical shift δ becomes independent of the applied external magnetic field, which facilitates the comparison of spectra that have been acquired at different scanner B_0 field strengths.

$$\delta = \frac{\omega - \omega_{ref}}{\omega_{ref}} \qquad (2)$$

^{1}H chemical shifts observed *in vivo* are in the order of parts per million (ppm) and typically referenced using internal standards such as the 2.02 ppm methyl singlet of *N*-acetylaspartate (NAA). Several ^{1}H downfield resonances (found at higher ppm values) have been reported (Arus et al., 1985; Rothman et al., 1997); however, clinical MRS largely relies upon the upfield resonances covering the 1−4 ppm range. For ^{13}C MRS and 31P MRS there are much larger chemical shift ranges of ~200 and 30 ppm, respectively (see Chapters 4.1 and 4.2).

Scalar Coupling

The electronic shielding of a nucleus depends on both the chemical bonding and the perturbation of this chemical bonding by the spins of neighboring nuclei. Nuclei in a molecule may not only couple directly, but also indirectly via their chemical bindings. Since the linkage of these nuclear spins is provided by their binding electrons, the interaction has been named J-coupling. Coupling constants of this weak scalar interaction are in the range of 1–15 Hz for ^{1}H–^{1}H couplings, and the corresponding shifts split the individual resonances into characteristic multiplet structures. If the chemical shift differences of a compound are big compared to its J-coupling constants, the spectrum is considered to be of first order. Spectra, for which the J-couplings and the differences in chemical shift are of the same order of magnitude, are considered second order. While absolute values of the chemical shift depend on the magnetic field strength, J-couplings do not, which leads to a strong field dependence of the overall MR spectrum. Many ^{1}H brain metabolites exhibit J-couplings and, along with SNR gains, strong scanner B_0 fields are therefore also advantageous to improve their spectral dispersion and to simplify spectral patterns by reduction of second-order coupling effects. The use of scalar coupling to perform spectral editing is described in Chapter 1.4.

Quantification of MR Spectra

The goal of *in vivo* MRS is the noninvasive quantification of chemical compounds in living tissue. The signal of an MRS resonance, corresponding to the area of its spectral peak, is proportional to the abundance of the resonating nucleus; thereby it allows the quantification of its host compound. If the chemical has more than one resonating nucleus, more than one peak is observed in the spectrum and the concomitant redundancy in information can be used to improve the accuracy of the substance quantification. The metabolite-specific combination of chemical shifts and J-couplings gives rise to unique spectral patterns similar to a human finger print. ^{1}H MR spectra acquired from the human brain *in vivo*, however, contain the combined information from all observable metabolites as sum of their individual spectroscopic patterns (Fig. 1.1.1), which need to be disentangled to derive the individual metabolite concentrations. The limited spectral dispersion (i.e., the spread of the observed resonance peaks) for ^{1}H MRS (Govindaraju et al., 2000) and the limited (broad) line-widths achievable *in vivo* (Tkac et al., 2001) lead to severe spectral overlap. In practice, the reliable identification of individual metabolites proves difficult despite the principle specificity of their spectral patterns. The simple integration of spectral peaks, i.e., the summation of their shape, is typically not possible and statistical methods are required. Different ways have been proposed to assess spectral composites of *in vivo* ^{1}H MR spectra of brain metabolites and to achieve a reliable

quantification either in the time (or measurement) domain (Vanhamme et al., 2001) or, equivalently, in the spectral domain (Mierisova & Ala-Korpela, 2001). Since the experimentally measured spectrum is considered the sum of the individual metabolite contributions, any quantification method aims at reproducing the overall spectrum by an appropriately scaled linear combination of the potential individual metabolite contributions (Provencher, 1993, 2001). The necessary scalings then correspond to the metabolite concentrations (Fig. 1.1.2). Deconvolution and therefore quantification errors are typically estimated as Cramér-Rao lower bounds, which describe the lowest possible standard deviations of all unbiased model parameter estimates (Cavassila et al., 1999). The analysis requires prior knowledge of the basis spectra, i.e., the specific spectral patterns of the potentially detected metabolites. This information can be derived experimentally by MRS measurements of metabolite solutions or by numerical simulation based

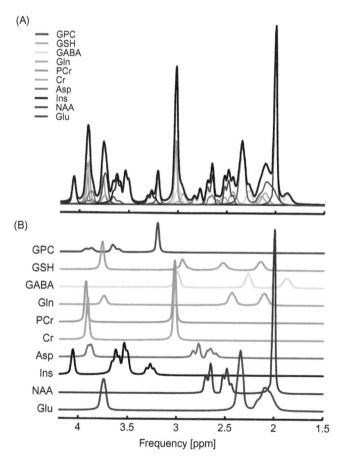

FIGURE 1.1.2   Quantification of ^{1}H MR spectra as a linear combination of model spectra (LCModel). (A) *In vivo* ^{1}H spectra consist of a sum of signals from the apparent neurochemical profile. (B) The quantification therefore aims at reproducing the spectrum at hand as a scaled combination of the spectral patterns from individual metabolites. For each substance, the necessary scaling corresponds to the apparent concentration.

on the spectroscopic characteristics of the metabolites, such as the chemical shifts, the J-couplings, and the number and type of nuclei. Notably, basis spectra are specific for the MRS experiment at hand, since their appearance relies on the scanner B_0 field strength and details of the MRS experiment such as RF pulses, gradient scheme, or sequence timing. The exact magnitude of the spectral metabolite signals depends on experimental parameters like RF coil performance, the voxel geometry, the B_0 field strength, the receive channel characteristics, and the MR sequence including the adjustment quality. The overall correction factor to compensate for these effects can be expected to be identical for all metabolites. Therefore, if this correction can be derived from a quantitative standard, i.e., if the concentration of at least one of the observed substances is known, it can be applied to all other metabolites to derive absolute tissue concentrations. Mostly, the concentrations from NAA, total creatine (Cr + PCr), or water are used for this purpose as they are easy to detect, to quantify, and known to be reasonably stable under regular physiological conditions (Kreis et al., 1993; Danielsen & Henriksen, 1994). Although MRS, in principle, is a quantitative method, the reliable and reproducible quantification of neurochemicals with MRS remains challenging in clinical practice (Chard et al., 2002). Potential error sources include methodological and technical aspects, but can also be of a physiological or clinical nature. For instance, metabolite relaxation times have been reported to be affected by disease (Brief et al., 2010) and the use of water as a quantitative reference can be prohibitive when its concentration is pathologically altered, such as in inflamed tissue of acute MS lesions (for more detail on quantitation, see Chapter 1.5).

Single-Voxel Spectroscopy

Brain metabolism consists of complex mechanisms not only at the gross anatomical scale, but also with an extensive cellular heterogeneity (Rothman, 1994). It is therefore desirable to derive metabolic information selectively from a specific anatomical, functional, or clinical target area (e.g., a tumor or an MS lesion). A variety of pulse sequences has been developed to obtain metabolic information from single, rectangular voxel volumes, or so-called single-voxel MRS techniques. They mainly differ by the way the excitation pulses are used (slice selective vs. global) and by the number of acquisitions required to achieve volume selection. In practice, the methods of Point RESolved Spectroscopy (PRESS; Bottomley, 1984) and STimulated Echo Acquisition Mode (STEAM; Frahm et al., 1987) have largely prevailed due to their single-shot character, i.e., full 3D volume selection is achieved in a single acquisition. Their susceptibility to movement artifacts is inherently lower compared to multishot techniques

where several acquisitions need to be combined (e.g., ISIS; Ordidge et al., 1986). The PRESS sequence is based on a double-spin echo experiment consisting of a 90 degree RF pulse for excitation and two 180 degree refocusing pulses. Each of the RF pulses is applied in a frequency-selective fashion in the presence of a magnetic field gradient to extract a planar slice (Fig. 1.1.3). With the use of orthogonal slice orientations, the voxel volume for MRS is extracted as the intersection of the three slices (Fig. 1.1.4). Localization with STEAM relies on the same geometric principle; however, three 90 degree RF pulses are used to obtain the spectroscopic information in the form of a stimulated echo. With STEAM, T_2 relaxation is apparent only during part of the MR sequence and echo times as short as 1 ms can be realized (Tkac et al., 1999), which is considered an advantage over PRESS. However, in recent years, short echo times have also been demonstrated for PRESS and PRESS-like methods under certain conditions (Zhong & Ernst, 2004; Mekle et al., 2009). On the downside, the theoretically achievable signal for STEAM is only one-half of the spin-echo method PRESS (and can be further reduced; de Graaf, 2008). Fully or partially adiabatic versions of PRESS called Localization by Adiabatic SElective refocusing (LASER; Garwood & DelaBarre, 2001) and semi-LASER (Scheenen et al., 2008), respectively, stand out by their robustness against RF amplitude variations (e.g., with the use of surface coils) and their improved volume localization (Kaiser et al., 2008). The necessary application of pairs of adiabatic RF pulses with LASER-type sequences can be prohibitive, however, due to the increased concomitant RF power

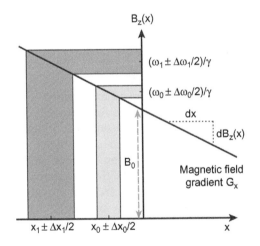

FIGURE 1.1.3 Magnetic field gradient: Slice selection and CSD. The application of a band-limited RF pulse in the presence of a linear magnetic field gradient (here G_x) allows the selection of a planar slice, since the Larmor condition is only fulfilled for the spins within this area. Slice position x and slice thickness Δx are hereby defined by the center frequency of the RF pulse ω and the width of the RF pulse $\Delta\omega$, respectively, relative to the strength of the applied gradient field $G_x = dB_z(x)/dx$.

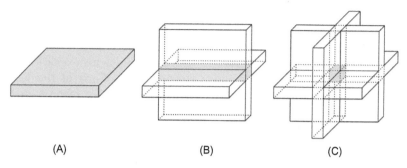

(A)   (B)   (C)

FIGURE 1.1.4   Concept of gradient-based localization for single-voxel MRS methods such as STEAM and PRESS. The combination of three slice-selective RF pulses (compare with Fig. 1.1.3) reduces the sensitive volume to a slice (A), a column (B), and ultimately a voxel (C) as intersection of the three slices. The method allows region-specific MRS, since the acquired spectral signals stem from the selected volume only. Magnetization that it is located outside the selected voxel and therefore has not been excited by all three RF pulses is eliminated by additional "spoiler" gradients (not shown).

deposition (specific absorption rate). In practice, the best technique for the problem at hand depends on study design parameters such as the targeted metabolites (which define the echo time to be used) along with the technical capabilities of the available MR system including RF peak power, maximum gradient strength, and gradient slew rate.

Optimal MRS performance relies on the accurate implementation of the MR sequence. Along with the obvious such as the interplay of RF pulses and slice-selection gradients used for spatial localization or the sequence timing, it also includes the not so obvious. Examples for the latter include the proper integration and dimensioning of crusher gradients to eliminate unwanted signals via gradient spoiling or the cycling of transmit and receive phases to cancel out spurious signals from outside the region of interest (ROI). The reader interested in this level of methodological detail is referred to the literature (Kreis, 1997; de Graaf, 2008) as well as Chapter 1.2.

MR Spectroscopic Imaging

Spectroscopic findings need to be put in a meaningful frame of reference for the study of metabolic alterations or abnormalities as a consequence of disease. This can be achieved by statistical comparison of neurochemical information between patient and control cohorts in a group analysis. With this approach, potential intrasubject abnormalities are convoluted with regular intersubject variability, a problem that does not exist if reference information is provided from the same subject. Such metabolic information from various regions of the same brain can either be achieved by multiple (subsequent or interleaved), single-voxel MRS acquisitions or by MRS in which the volume of interest (VOI) is further subdivided using MRI techniques, so-called MR spectroscopic imaging (MRSI). Two-dimensional MRSI, for instance, is typically achieved by (pre)selecting a slice-shaped volume with STEAM

or PRESS, before the metabolite signals from that slice are mapped by an additional phase-encoding scheme along two spatial dimensions. Data reconstruction then reveals a spatially resolved array of MR spectra from the considered 2D slice (Brown et al., 1982; Maudsley et al., 1983). As such, MRSI provides intrasubject reference information (e.g., from neighboring or contralateral areas) and thereby allows the mapping of the brain's regional metabolite distribution in an unbiased fashion. Notably, pixels can be shifted with MRSI or summed together postacquisition as long as the ROI has been covered, whereas with single-voxel MRS, the ROI has to be chosen for the experiment at hand. The SNR achievable with MRSI shares the same dependency on field-of-view (FOV) and spatial resolution with regular MRI, i.e., it is proportional to the MRSI voxel volume, and (for homogeneous k-space coverage) increases with the square root of the acquisition time (Macovski, 1996). On the downside, optimal experiment conditions, e.g., with respect to RF pulse power or magnetic field homogeneity, are more difficult to achieve over large MRSI volumes compared to single-voxel MRS.

The correct spatial representation of spectral information is essential for meaningful MRSI. Since the MRSI data reconstruction is based on spatial Fourier transformations, it relies on the same principles as the corresponding MRI methods and faces the same limitations with respect to spatial accuracy. For MRI, image matrix sizes are typically large (≥ 128), and the signal bleeding from the true spatial position to neighboring image voxels appears to be small. Long MRS repetition times, however, mandate significantly smaller matrix sizes (≤ 16) for MRSI due to total acquisition time constraints. The spatial reconstruction of such small matrix dimensions via Fourier transform leads to significant spatial misregistration. The spatial response function (SRF) describes the signal contributions of the entire FOV to the center voxel position and provides a

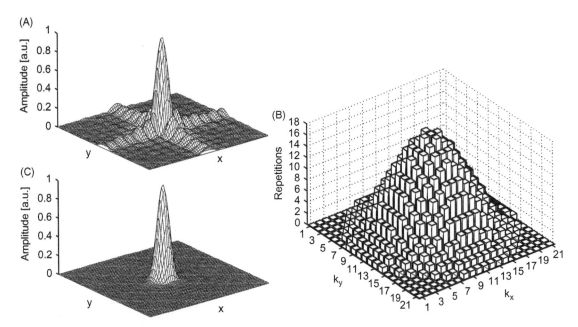

FIGURE 1.1.5 Benefits of acquisition weighting for MRSI. Accurate spatial representation is of paramount importance for meaningful MRSI; however, acquisition time constraints limit the size of k-space encoding schemes that can be realized *in vivo*. Consequences of limited k-space size and homogenous sampling include significant sidebands of the SRF, i.e., spatial misregistration (A). A weighted acquisition scheme that focuses on the central k-space positions by sampling them more often (B) can alleviate artificial SRF sidebands and provide largely improved spatial accuracy without penalty in experiment sensitivity. (C) The weighted sampling distribution in k-space.

measure for the registration accuracy of an imaging method (Pohmann & von Kienlin, 2001). A reduction of spatial contaminations, corresponding to a minimization of the SRF's sidebands, can be achieved by spatial low-pass filtering. This filtering should not be done by postprocessing, but should be realized by a weighted acquisition of the sampled k-space during the experiment for improved SNR (Fig. 1.1.5). The loss in spatial resolution concomitant to such filtering can be compensated for by increasing the imaging matrix size without time penalty (Pohmann & von Kienlin, 2001).

The substitution of one phase-encoding direction with an echo-planar imaging (EPI) readout considerably reduces the minimal acquisition time (Mansfield, 1984; Macovski, 1985) and other fast MRSI techniques with different types of EPI gradient waveforms (Adalsteinsson et al., 1995; Posse et al., 1997) or SPIRAL readout trajectories (Adalsteinsson et al., 1998) have been presented. Conventional phase encoding and the fast MRSI techniques, however, share the same dependency on the acquired SNR per time (Adalsteinsson et al., 1995; de Graaf, 2008). In other words, there is no net gain in sensitivity with the use of fast MRSI techniques and more data averaging is required to match the sensitivity of conventional MRSI. As such, fast techniques allow significant scan time reductions if SNR is not limited, but should be avoided otherwise. Higher demands on gradient performance, increased susceptibility to artifacts, and the need for nonstandard MR

sequences and data analysis with fast MRSI techniques might be reasons why conventional phase encoding remains the method of choice for most clinical MRSI applications. For more detail on MRSI see Chapter 1.3.

Water Suppression

The largest part of the human body consists of water with contents of at least two-thirds in all types of tissue, except fatty tissue and bone. The exact values are in the range of 50 M, but depend on anatomy, sex, age, and health status. In the healthy human brain, water concentrations of 83 and 70% were reported for the gray and white matter, respectively (McIlwain, 1985). Concentrations of the detectable brain metabolites are, in contrast, 10^3-10^4 times smaller and therefore much harder to detect. A two-step subtraction scheme has been presented recently to remove water signals from MR spectra by frequency-selective inversion of the metabolite signals in one of the MRS acquisitions (Dreher and Leibfritz, 2005; de Graaf et al., 2006). The direct suppression of the water signal, however, remains the most widely applied solution to the problem. To this end, differences in the chemical shifts of water and the brain metabolites are used to selectively excite the water resonance by a frequency-selective RF pulse. The water signal is then minimized (i.e., spoiled) by phase-spoiling gradients, while the metabolite signals remain unaffected. This CHEmical Shift-Selective (CHESS; Haase, 1986) method for water suppression is typically repeated several times to improve the suppression factor. Since there is no interaction with the metabolite signals with CHESS, water suppression can be performed prior to (and for STEAM even during) the MRS acquisition.

Outer Volume Suppression

MRS relies on the assumption that the observed biochemical information indeed originates from the targeted brain area, i.e., its proper spatial registration. Combinations of slice-selective RF pulses are used with single-voxel MRS methods to define the VOI. The inevitable sidebands of spatial selection RF pulses, i.e., deviations from an ideal boxcar profile, however, cause some excitation of signals from outside the addressed volume for each of the three slice selections. The resultant contributions to the acquired ^{1}H MR spectrum cannot be distinguished from signals of the targeted brain area and therefore falsify the quantitative results. The more prominent problem for ^{1}H MRS arises from lipid and fat resonances that originate from the cranial bone at signal strengths 100–1000 times stronger than those of the detectable brain metabolites (Rothman, 1994). Even low-amplitude sidebands from the target voxel selection within the brain lead to strong and broad artificial resonances in the 0.9–1.9 ppm range in the obtained spectra (Seeger et al., 1999, 2003) and strongly hamper the spectrum quantification (Rothman, 1994). If the magnetization from outside the selected volume is actively spoiled before the MRS acquisition, the risk of artificial signal contributions is minimized. The most commonly applied method for outer volume suppression (OVS) employs a frequency-selective RF pulse in the presence of a magnetic field gradient to excite the unwanted magnetization from the spatial slice (outside the ROI) before it is erased by phase spoiling (Fig. 1.1.6; Duyn et al., 1993). Since T_2 relaxation times of brain metabolites are longer than those for water or fat, OVS is particularly important for MRS at a short echo time of 10 ms or below.

Magnetic Field Homogeneity and Shimming

MRS, like any other MR method, relies on the Larmor equation (Eq. 1), i.e., the linear relation of the magnetic field B_0 experienced by the spin and its resonance frequency. If the magnetic field varies over the VOI, e.g., an MRS voxel, a distribution of Larmor frequencies is observed rather than a single frequency and spectral peaks appear broadened on top of the natural linewidth. In MRS, line broadening leads to loss of sensitivity and spectral resolution; therefore, excellent spatial homogeneity of the magnetic field over the target volume is essential for optimal results. Materials differ in their permeability to magnetic

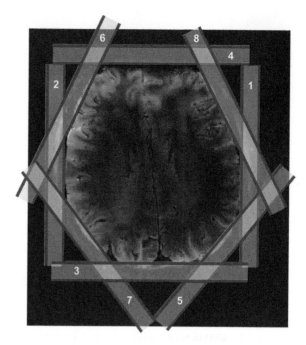

FIGURE 1.1.6 OVS for MRSI of the human brain. Signals from cranial lipids can be minimized by their selective excitation (compare with Fig. 1.1.3) followed by phase spoiling gradients to eliminate them. The oval shape of the skull in an axial section through the human head is hereby typically approximated by a series of planar OVS slices. This figure is reproduced in color in the color plate section.

fields, an effect governed by the material's magnetic susceptibility. The placement of a human head in a magnetic field therefore generates magnetic field distortions due to the susceptibility differences between tissue and the surrounding air. Spectral line broadening based on magnetic field inhomogeneity cannot be corrected for by postprocessing; therefore, it needs to be minimized experimentally before or throughout the MRS experiment. The importance of magnetic field homogeneity for MRS cannot be overstated and various correction (so-called "shimming") methods have been developed in recent years (Gruetter, 1993; Shen et al., 1999b; Juchem et al., 2010, 2011). Their discussion, however, exceeds the focus of this chapter and the interested reader is referred to the literature.

Chemical Shift Displacement

The dependence of the Larmor frequency on chemical shift and J-coupling is the basis of MRS and used to identify metabolites based on their spectral pattern. Spatial localization for MRS and MRSI is achieved by magnetic field gradients via the spatial frequency dependency they create. This ambiguity of spectroscopic and spatial frequency encoding is the origin of an artifact called chemical shift displacement (CSD),

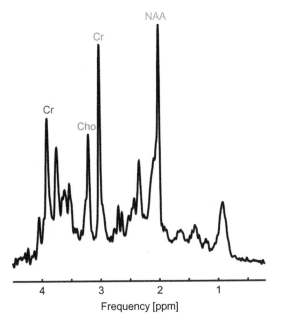
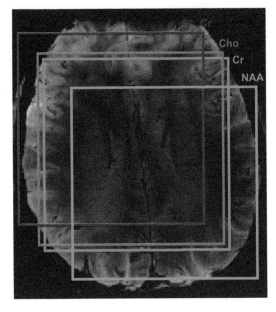

FIGURE 1.1.7 CSD in MRSI. Spatial encoding for MRSI is achieved by magnetic field gradients via the spatial frequency dependency they create (compare with Fig. 1.1.3). A spectroscopic frequency difference due to J-coupling or chemical shift, however, is misinterpreted with gradient-based encoding as spatial shift. In MRSI, this so-called CSD leads to metabolite contributions that originate from partially differing spatial positions and metabolic maps of different resonances happen to be shifted with respect to each. This figure is reproduced in color in the color plate section.

i.e., differences in spatial encoding based on the particular metabolic chemical shift. For MRS, CSD leads to metabolite contributions that originate from partially differing spatial positions, whereas metabolic maps of different resonances happen to be shifted with respect to each other with MRSI (Fig. 1.1.7). This effect is inherent to the use of magnetic field gradients for spatial encoding and cannot be avoided completely. It can be minimized, however, when gradients are large compared to the spectral dispersion of the MR isotope at hand and by optimized RF pulse selection (Kaiser et al., 2008; Scheenen et al., 2008).

Sequence Imperfections and Eddy Currents

The fast switching of magnetic field gradients is known to induce currents in the conducting structures of its close environment. These so-called eddy currents result in secondary, artificial magnetic fields throughout the scanner bore that alter the original gradient field spatially and temporally. The field artifacts that originate from eddy currents of the scanner's cold-conducting structures can extend over hundreds of milliseconds and reach into the MRS sequence and acquisition window. The resultant, temporally varying phase modulations lead to spectral baseline artifacts in the MRS spectrum that can easily mask the targeted metabolite signals, thereby rendering the experiment useless. If the phase modulation is known, however, it

can be rewound and removed from the data. Metabolite MRS should therefore always be accompanied by the acquisition of an identical dataset without water suppression as the resultant high SNR water signal contains the phase behavior from the eddy current-induced field terms and can be used to correct the lineshape artifacts of the metabolite signals (Klose, 1990). For a comprehensive review of artifacts and pitfalls associated to MRS/MRSI, the reader is referred to the literature (Kreis, 2004; de Graaf, 2008).

Advanced Techniques

Although many neurochemicals can be measured with basic STEAM- and PRESS-based MRS or MRSI, specific techniques have been developed to improve the quantification accuracy of selected metabolites or to access additional ones. The refocusing of an individual J-coupled resonance, for instance, allows its selective inversion, while the rest of the spectrum remains unaffected. The subtraction of two spectra with and one without this inversion then cancels all but the selected resonance. While a large part of the spectroscopic information is compromised with this so-called J-difference editing, a specific metabolite resonance and therefore the metabolite of interest itself can be quantified at higher precision. GABA quantification is the prime example for J-difference editing (Rothman et al., 1993), and reliable *in vivo* quantification of GABA has been demonstrated throughout the brain (Oz et al., 2006; Morgan et al., 2012). Similarly, glutathione and vitamin C (ascorbate) quantification has been demonstrated (Kaiser et al., 2010; Emir et al., 2011b). These methods are described in more detail in Chapter 1.4.

Alternate Nuclei

A variety of substances with biochemical relevance contain MR-detectable nuclei other than ^1H thereby allowing complementary insights in the brain's pathoneurochemistry. MRS of substances containing phosphorus (and therefore the MR-sensitive isotope ^{31}P) provides access to the brain's energy metabolism and related disorders. ^{13}C MRS has been proven beneficial for the study of clinical conditions such as Alzheimer's disease, Canavan's disease, or epilepsy; however, its use remains largely limited to preclinical research and ^{13}C MRS only slowly finds its way into the clinical routine (Ross et al., 2003). ^{23}Na, ^{19}F, and ^{17}O MRS are less often applied (Zhu et al., 2005; de Graaf et al., 2008; McIntyre et al., 2011) but still have been used in a variety of applications, particularly ^{23}Na (see Chapter 4.1). The combination of information derived from multinuclear MRS, i.e., MRS employing various isotopes, proves powerful to assess multiple aspects of a disease. Current examples include the combination of ^1H and ^{31}P in multiple sclerosis (Hattingen et al., 2011), or the study of liver tumors with ^1H, ^{31}P, and ^{13}C MRS (Ter Voert et al., 2011). More examples and details on the methods are given in Chapters 1.4, 3.3, 4.1, and 4.2.

Other advanced MRS methods aim to increase the measurement sensitivity by polarization transfer, spin decoupling, or the infusion of enriched substrates, i.e., metabolites that exhibit the considered isotope at concentrations beyond its natural abundance. As described in Chapter 4.2 the infusion of ^{13}C-labeled acetate or glucose, for instance, allows the determination of TCA cycle intermediates (and fluxes) and the glutamate/glutamine cycling at largely increased sensitivities compared to signals purely based on the low natural abundance of ^{13}C of only 1% (Badar-Goffer et al., 1990; Shen et al., 1999a; Rothman et al., 2011). Similarly, increased spin polarization that exceeds regular values, so-called hyperpolarization, has been used to increase the MRS signal strength and therefore its detection sensitivity.

Advanced MRS techniques provide powerful and elegant tools for biomedical research. The need for sophisticated methodology and (in many cases) specific hardware, however, might be the reasons why their application has been mostly limited to basic and preclinical research (de Graaf, 2008).

CONCLUSIONS

In this chapter we have reviewed the methods for performing localized MRS measurements with a focus on the basic MR principles involved. Since the initial studies in intact animals and humans there have been continuous improvements in MR technology and advances in pulse sequences and data analysis. However, the present limitations and potential future advances in MRS methods can still be understood from the basic physics and engineering principles that underlie it. In the later chapters in this book more practical information and experimental examples are provided of the implementation and application of these methods to both basic neuroscience and clinical research as well as to patient diagnosis.

References

Ackerman, J. J. H., Grove, T. H., Wong, G. G., Gadian, D. G., & Radda, G. K. (1980). Mapping of metabolites in whole animals by 31P NMR using surface coils. *Nature, 283*(5743), 167–170.
Adalsteinsson, E., Irarrazabal, P., Spielman, D. M., & Macovski, A. (1995). Three-dimensional spectroscopic imaging with time-varying gradients. *Magnetic Resonance in Medicine, 33*(4), 461–466.
Adalsteinsson, E., Irarrazabal, P., Topp, S., Meyer, C., Macovski, A., & Spielman, D. M. (1998). Volumetric spectroscopic imaging with spiral-based k-space trajectories. *Magnetic Resonance in Medicine, 39*(6), 889–898.
Arus, C., Yen, C., & Barany, M. (1985). Proton nuclear magnetic resonance spectra of excised rat brain. Assignment of resonances. *Physiological Chemistry & Physics & Medical NMR, 17*(1), 23–33.
Badar-Goffer, R. S., Bachelard, H. S., & Morris, P. G. (1990). Cerebral metabolism of acetate and glucose studied by 13C-n.m.r. spectroscopy. A technique for investigating metabolic compartmentation in the brain. *Biochemical Journal, 266*(1), 133–139.
Befroy, D. E., & Shulman, G. I. (2011). Magnetic resonance spectroscopy studies of human metabolism. *Diabetes, 60*(5), 1361–1369.
Behar, K. L., den Hollander, J. A., Stromski, M. E., Ogino, T., Shulman, R. G., Petroff, O. A., et al. (1983). High-resolution 1H nuclear magnetic resonance study of cerebral hypoxia in vivo. *Proceedings of the National Academy of Sciences USA, 80*(16), 4945–4948.
Bottomley, P. A. (1984). Selective volume method for performing localized NMR spectroscopy. U.S. patent No. 4480228 A.
Bottomley, P. A., Hart, H. R., Edelstein, W. A., Schenck, J. F., Smith, L. S., Leue, W. M., et al. (1983). NMR imaging/spectroscopy system to study both anatomy and metabolism. *Lancet, 2*(8344), 273–274.
Brief, E. E., Vavasour, I. M., Laule, C., Li, D. K., & Mackay, A. L. (2010). Proton MRS of large multiple sclerosis lesions reveals subtle changes in metabolite T(1) and area. *NMR in Biomedicine, 23*(9), 1033–1037.
Brown, T. R., Kincaid, B. M., & Ugurbil, K. (1982). NMR chemical shift imaging in three dimensions. *Proceedings of the National Academy of Sciences USA, 79*(11), 3523–3526.
Cavassila, S., Deval, S., Huegen, C., Van Ormondt, D., & Graveron-Demilly, D. (1999). The beneficial influence of prior knowledge on the quantitation of in vivo magnetic resonance spectroscopy signals. *Investigative Radiology, 34*(3), 242–246.

Chard, D. T., Griffin, C. M., McLean, M. A., Kapeller, P., Kapoor, R., Thompson, A. J., et al. (2002). Brain metabolite changes in cortical grey and normal-appearing white matter in clinically early relapsing-remitting multiple sclerosis. *Brain, 125*(Pt 10), 2342–2352.

Danielsen, E. R., & Henriksen, O. (1994). Absolute quantitative proton NMR spectroscopy based on the amplitude of the local water suppression pulse. Quantification of brain water and metabolites. *NMR in Biomedicine, 7*(7), 311–318.

de Graaf, R. A. (2008). *In Vivo NMR Spectroscopy: Principles and Techniques* (2nd ed.). London: John Wiley and Sons.

de Graaf, R. A., Brown, P. B., Rothman, D. L., & Behar, K. L. (2008). Natural abundance (17)O NMR spectroscopy of rat brain *in vivo*. *Journal of Magnetic Resonance, 193*(1), 63–67.

de Graaf, R. A., Sacolick, L. I., & Rothman, D. L. (2006). *Water and metabolite-modulated MR spectroscopy and spectroscopic imaging*. Paper presented at the ISMRM, Annual Meeting, Seattle, Washington.

Dreher, W., & Leibfritz, D. (2005). New method for the simultaneous detection of metabolites and water in localized *in vivo* ¹H nuclear magnetic resonance spectroscopy. *Magnetic Resonance in Medicine, 54*(1), 190–195.

Duyn, J. H., Gillen, J., Sobering, G., van Zijl, P. C., & Moonen, C. T. (1993). Multisection proton MR spectroscopic imaging of the brain. *Radiology, 188*(1), 277–282.

Emir, U. E., Auerbach, E. J., Van De Moortele, P. F., Marjanska, M., Ugurbil, K., Terpstra, M., et al. (2011a). Regional neurochemical profiles in the human brain measured by (1) H MRS at 7T using local B(1) shimming. *NMR in Biomedicine, 25*(1), 152–160.

Emir, U. E., Raatz, S., McPherson, S., Hodges, J. S., Torkelson, C., Tawfik, P., et al. (2011b). Noninvasive quantification of ascorbate and glutathione concentration in the elderly human brain. *NMR in Biomedicine, 24*(7), 888–894.

Frahm, J., Bruhn, H., Gyngell, M. L., Merboldt, K. D., Hanicke, W., & Sauter, R. (1989). Localized high-resolution proton NMR spectroscopy using stimulated echoes: initial applications to human brain in vivo. *Magnetic Resonance in Medicine, 9*(1), 79–93.

Frahm, J., Merboldt, K. D., & Hanicke, W. (1987). Localized proton spectroscopy using stimulated echoes. *Journal of Magnetic Resonance, 72*, 502–508.

Garwood, M., & DelaBarre, L. (2001). The return of the frequency sweep: designing adiabatic pulses for contemporary NMR. *Journal of Magnetic Resonance, 153*(2), 155–177.

Govindaraju, V., Young, K., & Maudsley, A. A. (2000). Proton NMR chemical shifts and coupling constants for brain metabolites. *NMR in Biomedicine, 13*(3), 129–153.

Gruetter, R. (1993). Automatic, localized in vivo adjustment of all first- and second-order shim coils. *Magnetic Resonance in Medicine, 29*(6), 804–811.

Haase, A. (1986). Localization of unaffected spins in NMR imaging and spectroscopy (LOCUS spectroscopy). *Magnetic Resonance in Medicine, 3*(6), 963–969.

Hattingen, E., Magerkurth, J., Pilatus, U., Hubers, A., Wahl, M., & Ziemann, U. (2011). Combined (1)H and (31)P spectroscopy provides new insights into the pathobiochemistry of brain damage in multiple sclerosis. *NMR in Biomedicine, 24*(5), 536–546.

Juchem, C., Nixon, T. W., Diduch, P., Rothman, D. L., Starewicz, P., & de Graaf, R. A. (2010). Dynamic shimming of the human brain at 7 Tesla. *Concepts in Magnetic Resonance, 37B*(3), 116–128.

Juchem, C., Nixon, T. W., McIntyre, S., Boer, V. O., Rothman, D. L., & de Graaf, R. A. (2011). Dynamic multi-coil shimming of the human brain at 7 Tesla. *Journal of Magnetic Resonance, 212*, 280–288.

Kaiser, L. G., Marjanska, M., Matson, G. B., Iltis, I., Bush, S. D., Soher, B. J., et al. (2010). (1)H MRS detection of glycine residue of reduced glutathione *in vivo*. *Journal of Magnetic Resonance, 202*(2), 259–266.

Kaiser, L. G., Young, K., & Matson, G. B. (2008). Numerical simulations of localized high field 1H MR spectroscopy. *Journal Magnetic Resonance, 195*(1), 67–75.

Klose, U. (1990). In vivo proton spectroscopy in presence of eddy currents. *Magnetic Resonance in Medicine, 14*(1), 26–30.

Kreis, R. (1997). Quantitative localized 1H MR spectroscopy for clinical use. *Progress in NMR Spectroscopy, 31*, 155–195.

Kreis, R. (2004). Issues of spectral quality in clinical 1H-magnetic resonance spectroscopy and a gallery of artifacts. *NMR in Biomedicine, 17*(6), 361–381.

Kreis, R., Ernst, T., & Ross, B. D. (1993). Absolute quantitation of water and metabolites in the human brain. II. metabolite concentrations. *Journal of Magnetic Resonance B, 102*, 9–19.

Macovski, A. (1985). Volumetric NMR imaging with time-varying gradients. *Magnetic Resonance in Medicine, 2*(1), 29–40.

Macovski, A. (1996). Noise in MRI. *Magnetic Resonance in Medicine, 36* (3), 494–497.

Mansfield, P. (1984). Spatial mapping of the chemical shift in NMR. *Magnetic Resonance in Medicine, 1*(3), 370–386.

Maudsley, A. A., Hilal, S. K., Perman, W. H., & Simon, H. E. (1983). Spatially resolved high resolution spectroscopy by "four-dimensional" NMR. *Journal of Magnetic Resonance, 51*, 147–152.

McIlwain, H. (1985). *Biochemistry and the Central Nervous System* (5th ed.). Edinburgh: Churchill Livingstone.

McIntyre, D. J., Howe, F. A., Ladroue, C., Lofts, F., Stubbs, M., & Griffiths, J. R. (2011). Can localised (19)F magnetic resonance spectroscopy pharmacokinetics of 5FU in colorectal metastases predict clinical response? *Cancer Chemotherapy and Pharmacology, 68*(1), 29–36.

Mekle, R., Mlynarik, V., Gambarota, G., Hergt, M., Krueger, G., & Gruetter, R. (2009). MR spectroscopy of the human brain with enhanced signal intensity at ultrashort echo times on a clinical platform at 3T and 7T. *Magnetic Resonance in Medicine, 61*(6), 1279–1285.

Mierisova, S., & Ala-Korpela, M. (2001). MR spectroscopy quantitation: a review of frequency domain methods. *NMR in Biomedicine, 14*(4), 247–259.

Morgan, P. T., Pace-Schott, E. F., Mason, G. F., Forselius, E., Fasula, M., Valentine, G. W., et al. (2012). Cortical GABA levels in primary insomnia. *Sleep, 35*(6), 807–814.

Ordidge, R. J., Connelly, A., & Lohman, J. A. B. (1986). Image-selected in vivo spectroscopy (ISIS). A new technique for spatially selective NMR spectroscopy. *Journal of Magnetic Resonance, 66*, 283–294.

Oz, G., Terpstra, M., Tkac, I., Aia, P., Lowary, J., Tuite, P. J., et al. (2006). Proton MRS of the unilateral substantia nigra in the human brain at 4 tesla: detection of high GABA concentrations. *Magnetic Resonance in Medicine, 55*(2), 296–301.

Pohmann, R., & von Kienlin, M. (2001). Accurate phosphorus metabolite images of the human heart by 3D acquisition-weighted CSI. *Magnetic Resonance in Medicine, 45*(5), 817–826.

Posse, S., Dager, S. R., Richards, T. L., Yuan, C., Ogg, R., Artru, A. A., et al. (1997). *In vivo* measurement of regional brain metabolic response to hyperventilation using magnetic resonance: proton echo planar spectroscopic imaging (PEPSI). *Magnetic Resonance in Medicine, 37*(6), 858–865.

Provencher, S. W. (1993). Estimation of metabolite concentrations from localized in vivo proton NMR spectra. *Magnetic Resonance in Medicine, 30*(6), 672–679.

Provencher, S. W. (2001). Automatic quantitation of localized in vivo ¹H spectra with LCModel. *NMR in Biomedicine, 14*(4), 260–264.

Ross, B., Lin, A., Harris, K., Bhattacharya, P., & Schweinsburg, B. (2003). Clinical experience with 13C MRS *in vivo*. *NMR in Biomedicine, 16*(6-7), 358–369.

Rothman, D. L. (1994). *1H NMR Studies of Human Brain Metabolism and Physiology*. San Diego: Elsevier Science and Technology Books.

Rothman, D. L., Behar, K. L., Prichard, J. W., & Petroff, O. A. (1997). Homocarnosine and the measurement of neuronal pH in patients with epilepsy. *Magnetic Resonance in Medicine, 38*(6), 924–929.

Rothman, D. L., De Feyter, H. M., de Graaf, R. A., Mason, G. F., & Behar, K. L. (2011). 13C MRS studies of neuroenergetics and neurotransmitter cycling in humans. *NMR in Biomedicine, 24*(8), 943–957.

Rothman, D. L., Petroff, O. A., Behar, K. L., & Mattson, R. H. (1993). Localized 1H NMR measurements of gamma-aminobutyric acid in human brain *in vivo. Proceedings of the National Academy of Sciences USA, 90*(12), 5662–5666.

Scheenen, T. W., Klomp, D. W., Wijnen, J. P., & Heerschap, A. (2008). Short echo time 1H-MRSI of the human brain at 3T with minimal chemical shift displacement errors using adiabatic refocusing pulses. *Magnetic Resonance in Medicine, 59*(1), 1–6.

Seeger, U., Klose, U., Lutz, O., & Grodd, W. (1999). Elimination of residual lipid contamination in single volume proton MR spectra of human brain. *Magnetic Resonance Imaging, 17*(8), 1219–1226.

Seeger, U., Klose, U., Mader, I., Grodd, W., & Nagele, T. (2003). Parameterized evaluation of macromolecules and lipids in proton MR spectroscopy of brain diseases. *Magnetic Resonance in Medicine, 49*(1), 19–28.

Shen, J., Petersen, K. F., Behar, K. L., Brown, P., Nixon, T. W., Mason, G. F., et al. (1999a). Determination of the rate of the glutamate/glutamine cycle in the human brain by in vivo 13C NMR. *Proceedings of the National Academy of Sciences USA, 96*(14), 8235–8240.

Shen, J., Rothman, D. L., Hetherington, H. P., & Pan, J. W. (1999). Linear projection method for automatic slice shimming. *Magnetic Resonance Medicine, 42*(6), 1082–1088.

Shulman, R. G., Brown, T. R., Ugurbil, K., Ogawa, S., Cohen, S. M., & den Hollander, J. A. (1979). Cellular applications of 31P and 13C nuclear magnetic resonance. *Science, 205*(4402), 160–166.

Ter Voert, E., Heijmen, L., van Laarhoven, H., & Heerschap, A. (2011). In vivo magnetic resonance spectroscopy of liver tumors and metastases. *World Journal of Gastroenterology, 17*(47), 5133–5149.

Tkac, I., Andersen, P., Adriany, G., Merkle, H., Ugurbil, K., & Gruetter, R. (2001). In vivo ^{1}H NMR spectroscopy of the human brain at 7T. *Magnetic Resonance in Medicine, 46*(3), 451–456.

Tkac, I., Oz, G., Adriany, G., Ugurbil, K., & Gruetter, R. (2009). *In vivo* 1H NMR spectroscopy of the human brain at high magnetic fields: metabolite quantification at 4T vs. 7T. *Magnetic Resonance in Medicine, 62*(4), 868–879.

Tkac, I., Starcuk, Z., Choi, I. Y., & Gruetter, R. (1999). In vivo ^{1}H NMR spectroscopy of rat brain at 1 ms echo time. *Magnetic Resonance in Medicine, 41*(4), 649–656.

Ugurbil, K., Adriany, G., Andersen, P., Chen, W., Garwood, M., Gruetter, R., et al. (2003). Ultrahigh field magnetic resonance imaging and spectroscopy. *Magnetic Resonance Imaging, 21*(10), 1263–1281.

Vanhamme, L., Sundin, T., Hecke, P. V., & Huffel, S. V. (2001). MR spectroscopy quantitation: a review of time-domain methods. *NMR in Biomedicine, 14*(4), 233–246.

Zhong, K., & Ernst, T. (2004). Localized *in vivo* human 1H MRS at very short echo times. *Magnetic Resonance in Medicine, 52*(4), 898–901.

Zhu, X. H., Zhang, N., Zhang, Y., Zhang, X., Ugurbil, K., & Chen, W. (2005). *In vivo* 17O NMR approaches for brain study at high field. *NMR in Biomedicine, 18*(2), 83–103.

1.2

Localized Single-Voxel Magnetic Resonance Spectroscopy, Water Suppression, and Novel Approaches for Ultrashort Echo-Time Measurements

Hongxia Lei[1,2], Lijing Xin[3,4], Rolf Gruetter[1,2,3,4] and Vladimír Mlynárik[2]

[1]University of Geneva, Switzerland [2]Center for Biomedical Imaging (CIBM), Ecole Polytechnique Federale de Lausanne, Switzerland [3]University of Lausanne, Switzerland [4]Laboratory of Functional and Metabolic Imaging (LIFMET), Ecole Polytechnique Federale de Lausanne, Switzerland

INTRODUCTION

In localized spectroscopy, the magnetic resonance (MR) signal is acquired from a volume of interest (VOI) prescribed in a human or animal organ. In contrast to MR imaging (MRI), which utilizes frequency and phase encoding, the shape and position of the desired volume is defined only by a combination of band-selective radiofrequency (RF) pulses and magnetic field gradients. Since only three orthogonal gradients are usually available in clinical or research MR systems, the excited VOIs usually have a cuboid shape. Therefore, we will focus on basic principles of single-voxel ^{1}H MR spectroscopy (MRS) providing spectra from cuboid volumes of interest.

Principles of Localization for Proton MRS

In localized proton MRS, three different concepts of localization are available. The first uses slice-selective or slab-selective pulses (band-selective pulses and gradients) to excite proton nuclei or to refocus transverse magnetization in the selected VOI (Fig. 1.2.1). The protons around the VOI are either not excited or the transverse magnetization created by the slice-selective pulses outside the VOI is dephased by spoiler gradients. Using this concept, the localized spectrum can be obtained in one acquisition.

The second concept is based on slice-selective inversion of the longitudinal magnetization and nonselective excitation of the whole volume. The slice-selective inversion pulse is applied to alternate scans, and the acquired signals from scans without and with inversion are subtracted; then, only the MR signal coming from the target slice is accumulated. However, this concept requires at least two scans to achieve 1D localization (image-selected *in vivo* spectroscopy; ISIS) (Ordidge et al. 1986).

In the third concept called outer volume saturation (OVS), the magnetization around the VOI is saturated by slice-selective excitation pulses followed by spoiling field gradients. Afterwards, the longitudinal magnetization left in the VOI is excited and the corresponding MR signal is acquired.

All three concepts are used for spatial localization in proton MRS. Depending on how they are combined, the resulting pulse sequence has more or less favorable properties regarding the length of echo time, chemical shift displacement (CSD) errors, amount of signal available during acquisition, and contamination by the signals from surrounding tissues. To minimize contamination in localized proton spectroscopy, a combination of the selective excitation with OVS is

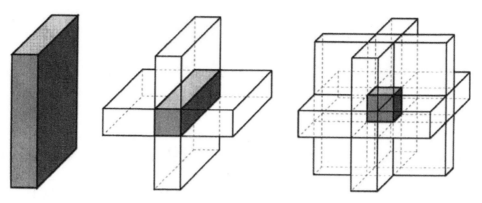

FIGURE 1.2.1   The principle of volume determination using three slices.

commonly used. Specific pulse sequences are described below.

Challenges in Acquiring Quality Single-Voxel Proton MR Spectra

The performance of localization sequences is never ideal. Hence, the VOI cannot be overly small compared to the volume of the surrounding tissue in the vicinity of the RF coil, since real band-selective RF pulses always create a small amount of transverse magnetization outside the nominal bandwidth. In addition, dephasing transverse magnetization created by the slice-selective pulses outside the VOI is never complete (Moonen et al., 1992). Both factors lead to the contamination of localized spectra by signals coming from outside the VOI.

Compared with MRS of other nuclei, localized hydrogen (proton) MRS has several particular features. First of all, soft tissues contain considerably large amounts of water and some also contain a large amount of free lipids. The concentrations of water and lipids (in mol/kg of wet tissue) are much higher than those of other metabolites of interest (in mmol/kg of wet tissue and lower). Except special cases when a ratio of water and lipid concentration is of interest, the huge water and lipid peaks complicate acquisition and quantification of the spectra of other metabolites. Thus, a localization technique must be highly efficient to eliminate contamination by MR signals of lipids and water coming from adjacent tissues.

We will now describe basic instrumental features affecting the quality of volume definition in localized MRS. In the next section, fundamental factors influencing spectral quality are summarized. The last section gives a description of basic localization pulse sequences suitable for short echo-time proton MRS.

INSTRUMENTAL IMPACTS ON VOLUME DEFINITION

The spatial position of the target volume is determined by applying band-selective RF pulses in the presence of magnetic field gradients; the performance of applied RF pulses and gradients affect the accuracy with which the volume is determined. The excitation profiles of the RF pulses influence not only the sharpness of volumetric edges, but also the CSD errors when the available gradients become limited (maximum gradient strength). In addition, the applied RF pulses can be limiting factors because of the specific absorption rate (SAR) in humans.

RF Pulses

Since nearly all relevant band-selective pulses in localized ^{1}H MRS methods are 90 and 180°, we will focus on these two types. A 90° pulse flips the spins from the longitudinal axis (M_Z) to the transverse plane, where the MR signals (M_{XY}) can be detected. A 180° pulse is used to invert or to refocus magnetization, e.g., to generate a spin echo. Optimally designed excitation, inversion, or refocusing pulses allow us to define precise volumes with sharp edges. Frequency profiles of band-selective RF pulses can be simulated using the Bloch equation, or approximated as a Fourier transform of pulses from the time domain to the frequency domain, as shown in Fig. 1.2.2.

Slice-Selective 90° Pulses

Slice-selective RF excitation pulses must be played concurrently with a corresponding slice-selection gradient. For localized ^{1}H MRS, excitation pulses should produce a uniform flip angle (e.g., 90°) within the desired slice. A band-selective RF pulse is prepared by multiplying the pulse envelope by a carrier signal. The

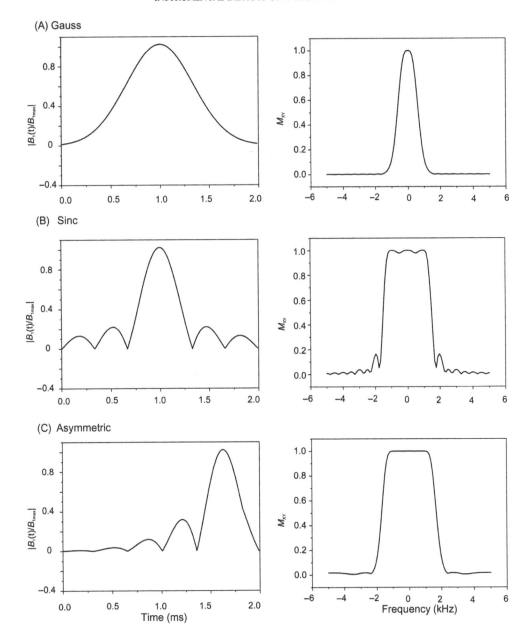

FIGURE 1.2.2 (A–C) Gauss, sinc and asymmetric (Tkáč et al., 1999) band-selective RF pulses (2 ms, 90°), in time domain (left column) and frequency domain (right column).

carrier is a sinusoidal waveform oscillating at precisely the desired frequency (e.g., the proton resonance frequency at a specific magnetic field strength).

Fig. 1.2.2 illustrates three excitation pulses: gauss, sinc, and asymmetric (Tkáč et al., 1999). Note that both sinc and asymmetric pulses give better slice profiles than the gauss pulse when all pulse amplitudes are adjusted to a flip angle of 90° on resonance (Table 1.2.1). Each pulse requires its own peak amplitude ($\gamma B_1/2\pi$ in Hz) to produce the desired flip angle.

Here, both the asymmetric and the sinc pulse (five-lobe) require higher power, but provide a broader bandwidth and a more uniform excitation profile than the gauss pulse. It also clearly shows that the peak RF amplitude ($B_1(t)$) of the asymmetric pulse lies in the last quarter of the entire pulse length (Fig. 1.2.1c and Table 1.2.1). Consequently, only a small portion of the entire pulse length contributes to the echo time (TE); hence, it is shorter (see the section, Basic localization ^{1}H MRS methods).

TABLE 1.2.1   Comparison of Three 90° RF Pulses

RF pulse (2 ms)	90° flip angle amplitude ($\gamma B_1/2\pi$, Hz)	Bandwidth (kHz)	% of pulse length to TE
Gauss	300	1.25	50
Sinc	700	3.0	50
Asymmetric	830	3.0	20–30

Unlike the sinc pulse, the slice profile of the asymmetric pulse consistently presents positive sidebands along the excitation direction. Thus, a signal outside the excitation band is not partially canceled out and OVS is recommended to eliminate contamination (see the section, Factors affecting spectral quality).

Slice-Selective 180° Pulses for Inversion and Refocusing

RF pulses (180°) must be applied before the excitation to invert slices, or after the excitation to form spin echoes. Slice profiles of inversion and refocusing pulses should meet similar requirements as the excitation pulses.

As shown in Fig. 1.2.3, sinc, asymmetric, and hyperbolic secant (sech) pulses can produce satisfactory slice profiles. Similarly to the asymmetric pulse used for excitation (Fig. 1.2.2c and Table 1.2.1), approximately 20–30% of the entire asymmetric pulse duration contributes to TE (Table 1.2.2) and greatly reduces crusher gradients (see section, Gradients). The sech pulse has indeed the largest bandwidth for a given peak power (amplitude). The broad bandwidth pulse helps minimize the chemical shift error, which will be described at the end of this section.

Gradients

In general, three orthogonal gradients are available in commercial MR systems. The gradient coils are a key element that ensures spins at different locations resonate at frequencies unique to their own location. In other words, field gradients allow the identification of the spatial position by adding a spatially dependent magnetic field (G, gauss/cm or mT/m) to the static magnetic field (B_0), giving a total magnetic field $B(r) = B_0 + rG$ at a position r relative to the center of the magnet. As a result, the resonance frequency ($\omega(r) = 2\pi f(r)$) becomes linearly dependent on position r and can be described using the following equation:

$$\omega(r) = \gamma B_0 + rG = 2\pi f_0 + rG \tag{1}$$

The available gradient strengths limit the minimum slice thickness for a given RF pulse. Fig. 1.2.4 shows the slice profile achieved by a single RF pulse, applied under two different field gradient strengths producing two distinct slices, i.e., r_1 and r_2. It is evident that for a given RF pulse, the stronger the applied magnetic field gradient is, the thinner the slice will be. For instance, the slice r_2 was selected with $G_2 > G_1$ and is therefore thinner than r_1.

To generate magnetic field gradients, the electric current in the gradient coils must be switched on and off. When the gradients switch, eddy currents are induced in surrounding electrical components and conductors, which may potentially distort the signal during acquisition and induce localization errors. Eddy currents increase with the strength of the field gradient and with the gradient duration. Commercially available MR systems minimize the eddy current effects using electronic and/or digitally controlled compensation techniques.

Chemical Shift Displacement

Protons of various metabolites resonate at slightly different frequencies due to their chemical structure, known as chemical shifts (usually expressed in parts per million (ppm) of the reference resonance frequency). For an RF pulse with a given bandwidth at a frequency f_0, a metabolite at a chemical shift, i.e., $\Delta f = \Delta\omega/2\pi$ Hz from the carrier frequency (Fig. 1.2.5a), is measured from its own VOI. The shifted VOI is Δcm away from that corresponding to the carrier frequency (Fig. 1.2.5a). In Equation 1, the Larmor frequency difference ($\Delta\omega$), slice-selective gradient strength (G), and gyromagnetic ratio (γ) will define the displacement of the target slice. This is the so-called CSD error $\Delta = \Delta\omega/\gamma G$. With increased bandwidth of the RF pulse and gradient strength, a slice with identical thickness can be selected, as shown in Fig. 1.2.5; however, the CSD error will be smaller.

With increased field strength, spectral dispersion becomes larger and causes problems achieving sufficient pulse bandwidth without exceeding SAR limits. When the bandwidth of the RF pulses (BW_{max}) is limited, e.g., by the maximum available peak power, the displacement error can be calculated as $L \times \Delta\omega/BW_{max}$, where L is the size of VOI in the direction of the gradient.

The displacement errors can also cause complications for spectra of homonuclear scalar-coupled spin systems at long echo times (Jung et al., 2001).

FACTORS AFFECTING SPECTRAL QUALITY

Several instrumental and methodological factors may affect the quality of the measured spectral

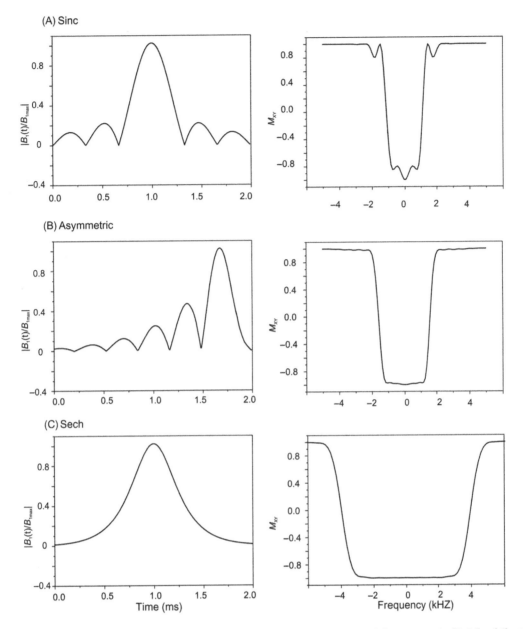

FIGURE 1.2.3 Shapes and profiles of slice-selective 2 ms 180° RF pulses, including sinc (A), asymmetric (B; Mlynárik et al., 2006), and sech (C) displayed in the time domain (left column) and frequency domain (right column), with the peak amplitude adjusted for a flip angle of 180° on resonance (Table 1.2.2).

pattern, i.e., the signal-to-noise ratio (SNR), resolution, the absence of spurious peaks, and the flatness of the baseline.

TABLE 1.2.2 Comparison of Three 180° RF Pulses

RF pulse (2 ms)	180° flip angle amplitude ($\gamma B_1/2\pi$, Hz)	Bandwidth (kHz)	% of pulse length to TE
Sinc	1400	2.3	50
Asymmetric	2500	3.2	20–30
Sech	3200	8.0	50

Sensitivity

One of the most dominating factors affecting spectral quality is the sensitivity of the nucleus of interest, i.e., hydrogen (proton). The signal increases not only with the main magnetic field strength, it also critically depends on the RF coil performance.

Magnetic Field Strength

Sensitivity rises with increasing magnetic field strength, i.e., the SNR is nearly proportional to the magnetic field strength B_0 (Hoult & Richards, 1976). Theoretically, the signal increases with the square of the main magnetic field strength, B_0^2, when the achievable sensitivity is exclusively due to the increase in B_0. However, taking into account the electrical components, the RF coil and the sample as major sources of noise, the increased sensitivity with B_0 becomes close to linear.

Resonance linewidths and relaxation times, which were assumed to be the same at different field strengths in the prior discussion, can also influence signal intensity. Longitudinal relaxation times increase with B_0, which leads to increased signal saturation at shorter repetition times. However, recent studies at high magnetic fields (i.e., above 9.4 T) reported T_1 of metabolites increased only slightly (de Graaf et al.,

2006; Cudalbu et al., 2009). Thus, the decrease in sensitivity due to T_1 is unlikely to be substantial. In contrast, T_2* decreases considerably with increasing B_0 due to an amplified effect of the magnetic susceptibility, which leads to line broadening and decreased peak height (see section, Field homogeneity and shimming). Despite this fact, SNR per unit of acquisition time increases at high magnetic fields.

RF Coil Performance

Localized ^{1}H MRS requires RF coils that deliver homogenous RF fields (B_1) to the target region and detect signals with the highest possible sensitivity. Among numerous coil designs, volume coils deliver homogenous RF fields and, when used as a receiver, provide homogeneous sensitivity over the whole field of view (FOV). However, as a consequence of the large FOV, the coil is also sensitive to noise from the whole sample. Unlike the MR signal, noise is not localized by field gradients; the only way to reduce noise detected by the RF coil (and hence increase SNR) is to reduce the coil's sensitive volume. This is the approach taken when using surface coils, which have a very restricted FOV, producing a much higher transmit efficiency and receive sensitivity rather than volume coils. However, they also produce a highly inhomogeneous RF field.

Consider, for example, acquiring data from a voxel in a mouse brain. The brain occupies a relatively small proportion of the head but a volume coil detects signal, and hence noise, from the whole head (Fig. 1.2.6a). A surface coil, designed to be sensitive only to the brain region, reduces the detected noise and so improves the SNR (Fig. 1.2.6b).

Two coil arrangements are commonly used for MRS. One is to use a surface coil as both transmitter and receiver, offering high transmit efficiency and high sensitivity over a small VOI. However, the inhomogeneous transmit field may be problematic, requiring the use of adiabatic RF pulses, which are able to

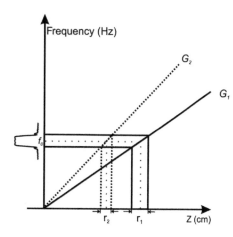

FIGURE 1.2.4 A frequency-selective scheme with two different gradient strengths. Having an RF pulse with a bandwidth at frequency f_0 with two gradient strengths (G_1 and G_2) along Z, two different slices can be selected: r_1 (straight line) and r_2 (dashed line). This figure is reproduced in color in the color plate section.

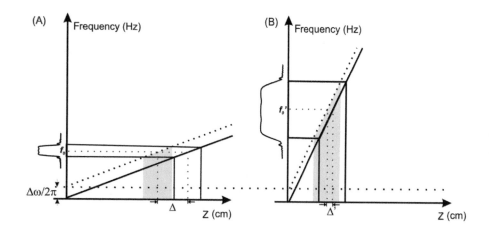

FIGURE 1.2.5 Comparison of CSD errors (Δ, Δ') for two RF pulses with different bandwidths. The slice selected for a chemical shift $\Delta\omega$ will be excited in a distance (Δ) away (dashed line and slice in gray) from the nominal slice position (A). The CSD error can be reduced using an RF pulse with a larger bandwidth and a stronger field gradient (Δ', in B). This figure is reproduced in color in the color plate section.

generate a homogenous excitation with an inhomogeneous B_1 field (Tannus & Garwood, 1997). The second approach is to use a volume transmit coil to provide homogeneous excitation, in combination with a surface receive coil for high detection SNR.

Field Homogeneity and Shimming

Dispersion of resonance frequencies in proton spectra is small with the peaks used for the quantification of most metabolites lying in the chemical shift range from 0 to 5 ppm. Since most resonance lines are multiplets, due to indirect spin–spin coupling (J-coupling), the proton resonance lines often overlap. Thus, spectral linewidth, which is a function of the B_0 field homogeneity over the measured VOI, is the most critical parameter affecting precision and accuracy of metabolite quantification.

The B_0 field homogeneity in a selected VOI *in vivo* is mainly affected by the presence of paramagnetic species in the vicinity of the VOI; the main source is oxygen in the air at the tissue–air interface. Thus, shimming VOIs located deeper in an organ, e.g., in brain, is easier than that close to the brain surface. Decreased blood perfusion increases the amount of paramagnetic deoxyhemoglobin in the tissue, which also leads to an increase in spectral linewidth. Shimming relatively small volumes for localized spectroscopy, where a function describing spatial distribution of B_0 field inhomogeneity is not too complex, is feasible by passing electric currents through first-order (linear) and second-order (quadratic) shimming coils. For larger VOIs, such as those for spectroscopic imaging, higher order shimming coils might be necessary. Before applying any shimming method, mapping the B_0 magnetic field distribution is necessary, which is based either on 3D field mapping or on field projections.

In single-voxel localized spectroscopy, localized B_0 shimming improves field homogeneity over the VOI. At the same time, localized shimming leads to increased variability of B_0 outside the VOI (Carlssonet al., 2011). Thus, chemical shift-selective saturation of the water signal might not be sufficient, and a combination with OVS can improve spectra quality (Fig. 1.2.7; Tkáč et al., 1999; Öz & Tkáč, 2011).

Water Suppression

Among the proton signals, water presents the dominating peak because of its high concentration *in vivo*, e.g., about 80% of wet weight in brain. Water protons in soft tissues *in vivo* resonate at 4.65 ppm. When unsuppressed, the huge water peak overlaps almost all relevant metabolite peaks and distorts the spectral baseline. Additionally, the bottom part of the water signal is not smooth and contains a lot of spurious peaks due to mechanical vibrations of the gradient system. These artifacts overlap real peaks and make the quantification of spectral lines of metabolites impossible. On the other hand, water suppression (WS) may affect peak intensities close to the water signal and can cause magnetization transfer effects due to saturation of bound protons (Leibfritz & Dreher, 2001). The unsuppressed water signal can be used as an internal reference for absolute quantification, and for motion and lineshape corrections. Thus, attempts to measure water-unsuppressed spectra have also been reported (van der Veen et al., 2000; Serrai et al., 2002; Dong et al, 2006). However, in most cases saturation of the water peak is used since it substantially facilitates spectra processing (Fig. 1.2.8).

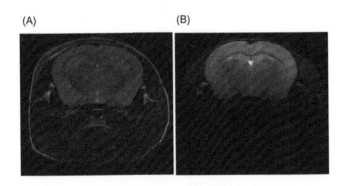

(A)　　　　　　　　(B)

FIGURE 1.2.6 Fast spin-echo images demonstrating coverage of a mouse head using (A) a volume coil (35 mm diameter) and (B) a quadrature surface coil (two physically decoupled 10 mm diameter loops). Identical imaging parameters were used for both images.

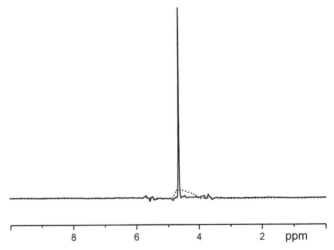

FIGURE 1.2.7 A typical localized water signal measured from a $3 \times 3 \times 3\,mm^3$ volume of a saline phantom without shimming (dashed line) and with optimized field homogeneity (solid line) at 14.1 T.

In general, a peak due to a molecule (e.g., water) can be suppressed by utilizing particular physical properties specific to this molecule. Several suppression methods are available for water peak suppression, such as frequency-selective saturation and/or refocusing, employing specific relaxation properties, and

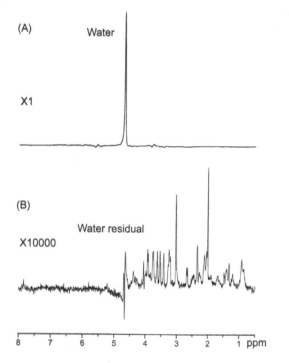

FIGURE 1.2.8   *In vivo* ^{1}H NMR spectra of rat brain before (A) and after (B) the WS (SPECIAL sequence; Mlynárik et al., 2006) with VAPOR water suppression, TE = 2.8 ms, TR = 4000 ms, VOI = 2 × 1.5 × 2.5 mm^3, 160 averages).

spectral editing. Water has a unique chemical shift different from peaks of most metabolites. Thus, the most common WS for short echo-time ^{1}H MRS relies on frequency-selective pulses. Seven chemical shift-selective pulses with optimized flip angles and timing (VAriable Pulse power and Optimized Relaxation delays, VAPOR; Tkáč et al., 1999) exhibit efficient WS in *in vivo* brain studies because of its insensitivity to the applied RF power.

Saturation with Frequency-Selective (Band-Selective) Pulse Excitation

Taking advantage of the difference in chemical shift between water resonance and metabolite resonances, a common technique is to use a 90° (or slightly bigger) frequency-selective RF pulse with a narrowband to excite the water resonance, and then to dephase the transverse water magnetization using a subsequent dephasing (spoiler) magnetic field gradient (Fig. 1.2.9a). This method is called CHEmical Shift-Selective (CHESS) water suppression (Hasse et al., 1985), and achieves zero longitudinal (M_z) magnetization of the water prior to the start of the excitation pulse in the localization sequence with minimal perturbation of the longitudinal magnetization of metabolites of interest. Therefore, a CHESS element is commonly used prior to any localization sequence. To avoid the recovery of water magnetization due to T_1 relaxation, the delay between CHESS pulse and excitation pulse should be kept short.

Ideal B_0 and B_1 magnetic field homogeneity allows efficient WS by using one CHESS element. However,

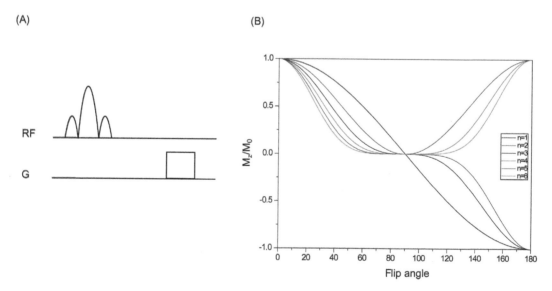

FIGURE 1.2.9   (A) A basic CHESS element for WS consists of one frequency-selective excitation pulse (i.e., a three-lobe sinc pulse here) followed by a dephasing magnetic field gradient. (B) With an increasing number of the CHESS elements ($n = 1-6$), the efficiency of WS becomes less sensitive to the flip angle variation of the frequency-selective pulse. This figure is reproduced in color in the color plate section.

this is not the case in reality where B_0 and B_1 inhomogeneity does cause imperfect excitation of water. As a result, the residual longitudinal magnetization of water remains, which leads to incomplete WS. Therefore, multiple CHESS elements are commonly employed to achieve broader excitation profiles with a larger range of flip angles (Fig. 1.2.9b) and insensitivity to B_0 and B_1 inhomogeneity. For instance, three CHESS elements lead to a suppression factor of ~2000 with 10% B_1 variation (Ogg et al., 1994). When using multiple CHESS elements, one should keep in mind that the water-suppression RF pulses could create unwanted echoes. To eliminate those unwanted signals, spoiler gradients should be carefully adjusted to avoid refocusing of the spoiled transverse water magnetization by the gradients in the localization sequence (Moonen & Vanzijl, 1990).

In addition to water signal presaturation, a CHESS element can also be applied during the localization sequence, when the useful magnetization is stored along the longitudinal axis, such as the mixing time TM period of a stimulated echo sequence (STimulated Echo Acquisition Mode, STEAM; see section, STEAM localization). In this way, further suppression of partially recovered water magnetization due to T_1 relaxation may enhance the efficiency of the water suppression (Moonen & Vanzijl, 1990).

Methods Based on T_1 Relaxation Time

Another WS technique takes advantage of the difference between T_1 relaxation times of water and metabolites. A representative example is the water-eliminated Fourier transform (WEFT) method (Patt & Sykes, 1972). It uses a nonselective 180° pulse followed by a delay $d = T_{1water} \ln(2)$ to achieve zero longitudinal magnetization of water. However, this method is usually more time-consuming than CHESS, due to the waiting time necessary to null longitudinal magnetization of water. Furthermore, it intrinsically leads to a partial suppression of metabolites, due to the small difference in T_1 of water and metabolites (Xin et al., 2012). However, using selective inversion pulse at water resonance frequency, the partial metabolite peak suppression can be avoided. Moreover, WEFT is optimized for one T_1 relaxation time, and the heterogeneity of T_1 of water in vivo (white matter, gray matter, and cerebrospinal fluid) (Marques et al., 2010) leads to incomplete suppression of the signal originating from these different tissues.

To achieve high WS efficiency in the presence of an inhomogeneous B_1 field (e.g., when using a surface coil as a transmitter) and heterogeneity of water T_1 relaxation times, WS techniques were optimized based on the optimal T_1 recovery time and the combination of inversion pulses with CHESS elements using optimized pulse flip angles (WS enhanced through T_1

effects; WET; Ogg et al., 1994) and VAPOR (Tkáč et al., 1999). Among them, the VAPOR pulse sequence provides excellent suppression of the water signal using seven CHESS elements with optimized interpulse delays (Fig. 1.2.10). Compared to three CHESS elements, VAPOR demonstrates suppression of water for a large range of flip angles. It is also insensitive to T_1 variation; the residual longitudinal water magnetization is below 2% for T_1 of 1–2 s when the flip angle varies from 55 to 125°.

Frequency-Selective Refocusing

In contrast to presaturation using frequency-selective excitation pulse and magnetic field gradients, other WS methods such as WATER suppression by GrAdient Tailored Excitation (WATERGATE; Piotto, 1992), excitation sculpting (Hwang & Shaka, 1995), and a MEscher–GArwood (MEGA) frequency-selective refocusing technique (Mescher et al., 1996) are available. During the localization sequence, one or more band-selective pulses are integrated into this sequence together with magnetic field gradients, which selectively defocus (destroy) water magnetization and refocus the magnetization of metabolites of interest. As an example, the combination of the MEGA scheme with a single spin-echo sequence is demonstrated in Fig. 1.2.11. After a nonselective 90° pulse, all magnetization (water and metabolites) is flipped into the transverse plane. Two pairs of field gradients, G_1 and G_2, are applied in the delays between 180° pulses, as shown in Fig. 1.2.11. The transverse magnetization of water is inverted three times by one nonselective and two selective 180° pulses and is dephased by the G_1 and G_2 magnetic field gradients; however, the transverse magnetization of metabolites is inverted only once with a nonselective 180° pulse and is not affected by the G_1 and G_2 field gradient pairs. The theoretical description of the methods can be found in the literature (Hwang & Shaka, 1995; Mescher et al., 1996). Such methods offer WS without any risk of recovery of the water magnetization due to T_1 relaxation. On the other hand, insertion of the RF pulses and magnetic field gradients prolongs the echo time (TE), which leads to a signal loss due to T_2 relaxation and multiplet distortion due to J-modulations. The MEGA method does not affect the performance of spectral editing sequences at long TE. Compared to WATERGATE and excitation sculpting, it inherits the merit of excitation sculpting, which is less sensitive to the flip angle imperfection relative to WATERGATE, and provides an additional advantage of refocusing metabolite signals with a single spin echo, which in turn allows the use of a shorter TE (Mescher et al., 1996).

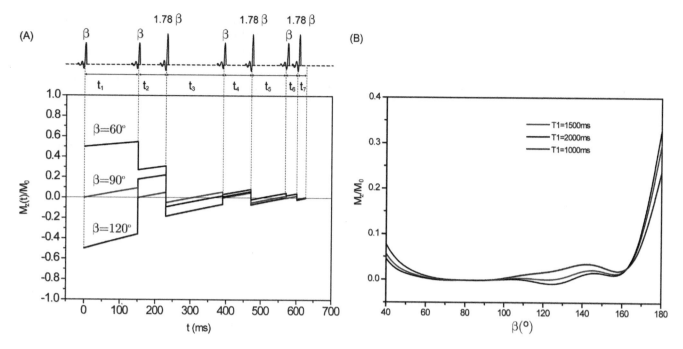

FIGURE 1.2.10   (A) A pulse sequence diagram of VAPOR and simulated time evolution of the longitudinal magnetization of water during the VAPOR module with three different flip angles (β = 60, 90, and 120°), assuming that the T_1 of water is 1.5 s. Using optimized time delays (the respective values of t_1 to t_7 are 150, 80, 160, 80, 100, 30, 26 ms), the residual longitudinal magnetization (M_Z) reaches zero at the end of t_7, when an excitation pulse for the localization pulse sequence is applied. (B) The dependence of the residual longitudinal water magnetization M_z on the flip angle β at T_1 of water = 1–2 s indicates that the VAPOR sequence is insensitive to the flip angle and water T_1 variations over a wide range. This figure is reproduced in color in the color plate section.

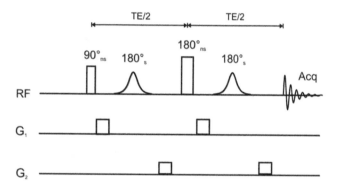

FIGURE 1.2.11   MEGA WS combined with a single spin-echo sequence. Two selective refocusing pulses for water and two pairs of magnetic field gradients (G_1 and G_2) are used to dephase transverse magnetization of water. The magnetization of metabolites experiences only one nonselective refocusing pulse, and is then refocused by the field gradients before signal acquisition.

OVS

Slice-selective pulses can be applied to eliminate signals outside the VOI, so-called OVS (Connelly et al., 1988). OVS is useful for large VOIs because it generates suppression slices with sufficient thickness without exceeding RF limitations, and is widely used for proton spectroscopic imaging of brain. This technique eliminates the contamination of spectra with signals

from extracranial water and lipid, in particular in ultrashort echo-time spectroscopy when asymmetric pulses are used (Tkáč et al., 1999; Öz & Tkáč, 2011).

Numerous RF pulses (Figs. 2.2 and 2.3) can be used for OVS. Among them, sech pulses and other modified adiabatic pulses are useful because they provide large excitation frequency bandwidths with sharp edges, which do not change with varying pulse power. Therefore, these pulses are excellent candidates for OVS. For more detailed information, see section, OVS localization.

Benefits of Short Echo Time

The ultimate aim of *in vivo* localized proton spectroscopy is to determine absolute or relative concentrations of as many metabolites as possible. To do so, the localized MR spectra should be measured under quantitative conditions, so that signal intensities will not be substantially affected by T_1 and T_2 relaxation. Thus, it is necessary to use sufficiently long repetition times while keeping echo times as short as possible.

At a short echo time (TE = 1–2 ms for animal scanners and TE = 6–20 ms for human scanners), singlets and coupled resonances are in pure absorption mode, the loss of signal intensity due to transverse relaxation is minimal, and minimal signal modulation is induced

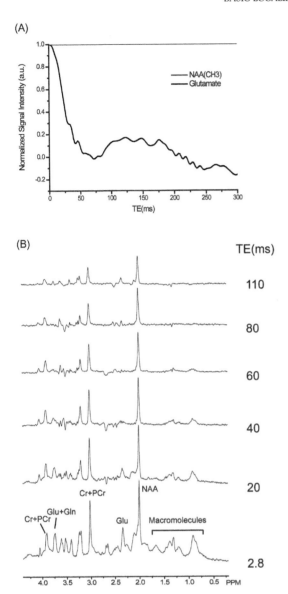

FIGURE 1.2.12 (A) The effect of TE on simulated integral intensity of glutamate J-coupled multiplets and the NAA methyl group (a singlet). T_2 relaxation effect is not included in the simulation. At long TE, the maximum signal occurs at TE values in the range of 130–160 ms (TE ∼ 1/J), and the first minimum at TE values 60–80 ms (TE ∼ 1/2J). (B) *In vivo* water-suppressed ^{1}H MR spectra of the rat brain measured using SPECIAL (Mlynárik et al., 2006) at TE ranging from 2.8 to 110 ms (VOI = 2.5 × 5 × 5 mm^3, TR = 4 s, 160 scans). This figure is reproduced in color in the color plate section.

by J-coupling of multiplet resonances of coupled spin systems (Fig. 1.2.12). As TE increases, signal intensity decreases due to transverse relaxation, but the lineshape of singlets [such as *N*-acetylaspartate (NAA) CH$_3$ protons at 2.01 ppm, the total creatine (tCr) CH$_3$ protons at 3.03 ppm, or CH$_2$ protons at 3.92 ppm] remains unchanged. However, for J-coupled resonances, both signal intensity and multiplet shapes change with TE, because of the combined effect of transverse relaxation

and J-modulation (Fig. 1.2.12). Therefore, MRS performed at short TE can minimize J-modulation and signal losses, which in turn allows higher quantification precision compared to that at a long TE. On the other hand, in short TE MR spectra, the presence of broad macromolecule resonances is a confounding factor for quantification and should be taken into account (Cudalbu et al., 2007). Macromolecular resonance signals decay almost completely after 60–80 ms due to their short T_2 relaxation time. Therefore, if only NAA, tCr, total choline, and lactate need to be quantified, ^{1}H MRS studies can be performed at long TE, to avoid the confounding effect of macromolecular signals on metabolite quantification. Most ^{1}H MRS editing techniques are typically performed at moderate to long TE (Terpstra et al., 2002, 2003) by taking advantage of specific J-evolution of multiplets of interest. For the quantification of MRS spectra at long TE, accurate spectral patterns of metabolites at specific TE and T_2 relaxation times are required (Xin et al., 2008).

BASIC LOCALIZATION ^{1}H MRS METHODS

Localization Based on Slice-Selective Inversion

ISIS Localization

This method exploits the slice-selective principle of MRI techniques for localizing proton MR signals from a specific volume, as suggested by Ordidge et al. (1986). The technique is based on a slice-selective inversion of spins prior to their excitation and signal acquisition. More specifically, to obtain an MR signal from a slice (Fig. 1.2.13, 1D ISIS) two scans are required. In the first, the free induction decay (FID) is obtained with all the spins in the volume having the same phase (Fig. 1.2.13, #1); in the second, the FID is acquired in the same way except that spins in the target slice are first inverted using a slice-selective 180° pulse (Fig. 1.2.13, #2). When the two FIDs are subtracted, only signal from the target slice remains (Fig. 1.2.13, S).

A 3D volume can be localized using linear combinations of three pairs of such scans (Fig. 1.2.13, 3D ISIS), which cancels out unwanted signals from outside the target volume.

The advantage of this method is the absence of any T_2 weighting and J-evolution, since there is no echo time in this pulse sequence. The ISIS technique can be used for proton localization, but is also extremely useful for other nuclei.

However, ISIS relies on inverting spins in the region of interest, which can result in signal loss due to T_1 relaxation and imperfect slice profiles for metabolites

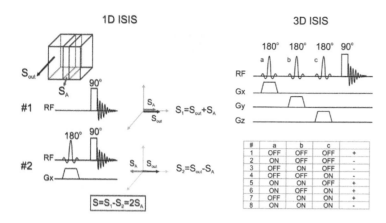

FIGURE 1.2.13 Schematic diagrams and add–subtract schemes of 1D ISIS (left column) and 3D ISIS (right column). S_A indicates a signal from the inverted slice and S_{out} stands for a signal from the surrounding volume. G_X denotes a specific slice-selective gradient. #1 and #2 are the scans without (S_1) and with inverted magnetization (S_2) in the slice, respectively. 1D ISIS is achieved and the target signal S is then calculated. Three slice-selective inversion modules (a–c) are combined to achieve localization of the desired volume in 3D ISIS.

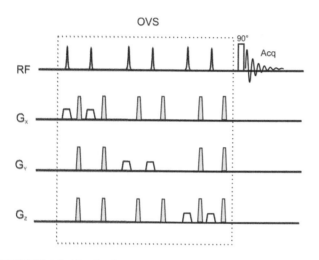

FIGURE 1.2.14 A schematic drawing of OVS acquisition. In one OVS module (in a dashed square), three pairs of 90° slice-selective RF pulses with the corresponding gradients (G_X, G_Y, and G_Z nonshaded trapezoids) are applied to flip the spins outside the VOI. Immediately after the OVS module(s), a non-slice-selective pulse is applied before acquisition (Acq). The spoiler gradients (shaded trapezoids) are applied to dephase unwanted signals.

with short relaxation times. Additionally, a minimum number of eight scans is necessary for the volume localization, and the signal addition and subtraction scheme makes localization vulnerable to any subtraction errors related to motion, RF pulse imperfections, etc.

OVS Localization

Instead of exciting the spins in the target VOI, slice-selective schemes can be applied to destroy magnetization outside the target VOI by flipping it into the transverse plane and dephasing it with spoiler gradients, so that no net magnetization outside the VOI remains.

To localize 1D, two suppression slices must be placed at both sides of the target slice. As shown in Fig. 1.2.14, a volume may be defined using three pairs of OVS pulses. The frequencies of the paired slice-selective pulses are placed in the center of the suppression slices

instead of the center of the target VOI. Once six suppression slices are properly positioned and the pulses are applied, a localized ^{1}H MR spectrum can be acquired by using a simple nonselective excitation RF pulse. The selected pair or the entire OVS module can be repeated several times, to ensure a robust suppression of the surrounding magnetization.

The OVS module (Fig. 1.2.14) can achieve localization in one scan and is, therefore, resistant to subject motion and system instability. In addition, OVS allows data acquisition immediately after the nonselective RF pulse and has advantages for obtaining short T_2 metabolites.

It is clear that suppression is the key element to ensure localization and must be extremely efficient to avoid unwanted signals. Therefore, adjustment of OVS can be difficult. Suppression slices should cover the whole part of the body that contributes to the signal acquired by the receiver coil. Thus, the thicknesses of the suppression slices depend on the location of the target volume in the organ and are not necessarily identical. With increasing subject size and reducing size of the VOI, OVS can be very challenging because strong signals from the outer volume need to be suppressed, which requires RF pulses with large bandwidths and high amplitudes. The OVS *per se* is usually not efficient enough to obtain clean proton MR spectra and is, therefore, used in combination with other localization techniques.

Localization Based on Echo Formation

The nature of echo formation in MRS allows refocusing only those spins that experienced all RF pulses, and dephasing all other spins in the vicinity of the VOI. By applying 90 and 180° RF pulses separated by delays TE/2, TM, and τ, the following echoes can be formed: a stimulated echo (STE, 90°-TE/2-90°-TM-90°-TE/2-Acq), a spin echo (SE, 90°-TE/2-180°-TE/2-Acq), and multiple (Carr–Purcell–Meiboom–Gill) echoes

(CPMG-SE, 90°-[-τ-180°-τ-]n − Acq, $n > 1$, TE = $n \times$ 2τ), etc. These echoes can be formed by slice-selective RF pulses (the band-selective RF pulses in the presence of corresponding field gradients) to achieve the desired 3D localization in one scan. In this section, we will focus on the most useful sequences for clinical and research platforms.

STEAM Localization

As mentioned previously, three 90° RF pulses generate a simulated echo after the last 90° pulse with an

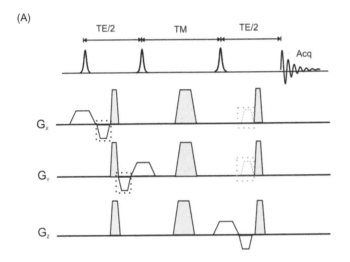

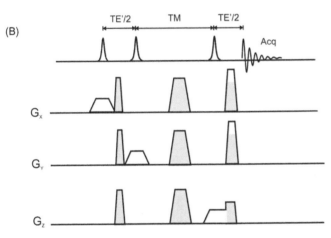

FIGURE 1.2.15 An example of shortening echo time for a standard STEAM sequence. (A) TE is long enough so that all slice-selective gradients (open trapezoids) and crusher gradients (shaded trapezoids) can be organized without overlapping. The slice refocusing gradients (in dashed black squares) can be placed at alternative positions, i.e., in the second echo period (in dashed gray squares). (B) A shorter TE is achievable if the newly arranged gradients fulfill the identical gradient conditions as in (A). For example, the second half area (shaded area) of the last G_z gradient is equivalent to the gradient difference between the positive crusher gradient and the negative slice-selective refocus gradient, as shown in (A). The order in which the slice-selective pulses are applied is arbitrary.

identical delay to that between the first two 90° pulses (Fig. 1.2.15). With the applied gradients, only signals undergoing three slice-selective pulses are refocused to create a desired stimulated echo from the VOI.

Typically, commercial STEAM sequences only offer three slice gradients and crusher gradients, as shown in Fig. 1.2.15a.

To reduce echo time, the gradients can be rearranged. For example, one slice-rephasing gradient is combined with the following crusher gradient to form another arbitrary gradient (Fig. 1.2.15b). The particular STEAM sequence (Fig. 1.2.16) looks very different from commercial sequences (Fig. 1.2.15a), mainly due to the gradients.

The use of only 90° pulses allows increased bandwidth at a given RF power. This intrinsically minimizes CSD errors (see section, Instrumental impacts on volume definition). Another advantage of this method is that the mixing time (TM) (Figs. 2.15 and 2.16) does not contribute to the entire echo time. This period can be used to apply strong crusher gradients and additional WS without affecting the length of TE, as shown in Fig. 1.2.16.

TE can be shortened when three RF pulses are replaced by asymmetric pulses such as those described by Tkáč et al. (1999). These pulses contribute only ~20% of their length to the entire echo time (Fig. 1.2.16). In this case, the echo time only starts from the shifted center of RF pulse (see Fig. 1.2.2c) and ends at the center of another RF pulse shifted in an opposite way.

The stimulated echo has only 50% of signal intensity relative to that of a spin echo. This is because the second 90° pulse only rotates half of the excited spins from the transverse plane to the longitudinal axis, while the other half is dephased by the crushers in TM. When using the asymmetric pulses (Tkáč et al.,

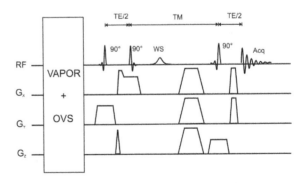

FIGURE 1.2.16 A schematic drawing of one representative STEAM sequence. The STEAM sequence can achieve ultrashort echo-time ^{1}H MRS (Tkáč et al., 1999). Three asymmetric RF pulses are placed in a manner to shorten TE. For instance, the maximum amplitudes of the RF pulses are arranged toward the TE/2 periods. The additional WS (VAPOR) and OVS are also applied. One additional WS can be inserted in the mixing time (TM) period.

1999), OVS is highly recommended because of the specific excitation profiles of these RF pulses (Fig. 1.2.2c).

PRESS Localization

A spin echo followed by an additional 180° pulse generates another echo with a time delay identical to that from the spin echo and the last 180° pulse, a so-called double-spin echo. This spin phenomenon was adapted to perform the 3D localization scheme by Bottomley (1984). Here, localization is achieved by a slice-selective 90° pulse in one plane, followed by two slice-selective 180° pulses in the remaining two planes. For ideal RF pulses, only spins that experienced all three pulses form the desired echo at acquisition. To suppress unwanted coherences due to non-ideal RF pulses, spoiler gradients are necessary; in combination with the slice-selective gradients they can have a "butterfly" shape (Fig. 1.2.17).

PRESS achieves 3D localization with the entire magnetization in one scan, and is relatively insensitive to motion and instability of the system. However, two slice-selective 180° pulses produce a lot of transverse magnetization and false echoes. Thus, strong spoiler gradients are necessary, as shown in Fig. 1.2.17. The TE can be minimized when both pulse lengths and gradients are shortened without exceeding the limits of both SAR and the maximum gradient strength. However, compared with other localization sequences, the minimum TE achievable by PRESS is relatively long.

Localization by Adiabatic SElective Refocusing (LASER)

This sequence applies an adiabatic multiple spin-echo scheme (CPMG) to achieve 3D localization. Instead of using three 180° slice-selective pulses in three directions, three pairs of adiabatic full passage (AFP; e.g., sech) pulses are used after a nonselective excitation by a 90° adiabatic BIR-4 pulse to acquire localized MR signals independent of the RF amplitude and with a low CSD error (Garwood & DelaBarre, 2001).

This sequence is completely adiabatic when using one nonselective adiabatic excitation pulse (Fig. 1.2.18, BIR-4), and the applied broad bandwidth AFP pulses help to improve localization because of the minimal CSD and sharpness of the localization edges (see section, Instrumental impacts on volume definition).

Unlike other inversion pulses (e.g., sinc), the adiabatic pulses generate a nonlinear phase variation across the slice and must be applied in pairs to obtain a slice-selective spin echo (Conolly et al., 1989). Since three pairs of AFP pulses are used, strong crusher gradients to dephase all unwanted coherences are necessary. Taking the number of pulses and gradients (Fig. 1.2.18) into account, the minimum TE would inherently increase.

Slice-Selective Localization by Adiabatic Selective Refocusing (Semi-LASER)

In this sequence, a slice-selective excitation module is applied instead of the BIR-4 90° pulse in LASER (Fig. 1.2.17). Therefore, a 3D localization scheme is

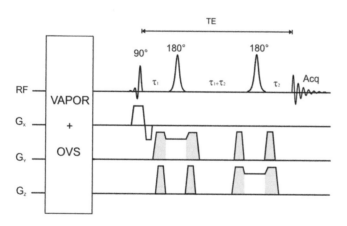

FIGURE 1.2.17 A diagram of the PRESS pulse sequence based on Bottomley (1984). An excitation 90° pulse was applied with a gradient in the X direction (G_X), followed by two slice-selective 180° pulses along Y (G_Y) and Z (G_Z) directions. To satisfy the double-spin echo scheme, the time delays $\tau 1$ and $\tau 2$ between the RF pulses and the acquisition should be kept as indicated in the figure. Besides slice-selective gradients at two 180° pulses, strong crusher gradients (shaded areas) are applied. Note the "butterfly" shape of the first G_Y and the last G_Z gradients. The localized signal was acquired (Acq) at a time delay (TE) after the first excitation 90° pulse. Both WS (VAPOR) and OVS (in a solid square) are applied before the double-spin echo sequence. The order in which the slice-selective pulses are applied is arbitrary.

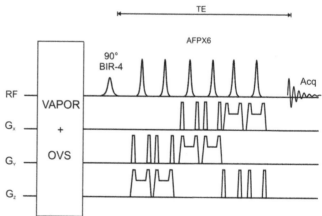

FIGURE 1.2.18 Pulse sequence diagram for LASER. A nonselective excitation is applied using an adiabatic pulse, i.e., BIR-4. Each pair of AFP pulses along with the corresponding gradients refocus magnetization in one slice. Here, slice selection by a pair of slice-selective refocusing pulses along Z is followed by pairs of slice-selective pulses along Y and X, respectively. Three pairs of AFP pulses (AFP ×6) define a 3D volume. Both WS (i.e., VAPOR) and OVS can be placed at the beginning of the pulse sequence.

accomplished with only two pairs of frequency-selective AFP refocusing pulses (Fig. 1.2.19; Öz and Tkáč, 2011) instead of three pairs in LASER (Fig. 1.2.18).

This particular scheme is designed for use with a surface coil. As a surface coil produces an RF field, which is relatively homogeneous in the direction parallel to the plane of the coil, the slice-selective excitation is applied along this direction. For better suppression of unwanted magnetization, the two frequency-selective pairs of adiabatic pulses, along Z and Y directions, may be played in an interleaved manner.

As mentioned previously (see section, OVS localization), the dephasing (spoiler) gradients should be carefully adjusted to eliminate unwanted FIDs or echoes.

Hybrid Sequence: SPin ECho Full Intensity Acquired Localized Localized (SPECIAL) Spectroscopy

This sequence combines 1D ISIS (described in Fig. 1.2.13) and a spin-echo sequence in the other two directions to localize a VOI (Mlynárik et al., 2006). It is optimized for a surface coil used as both transmitter and receiver that is placed horizontally, with the 1D ISIS applied along the axis with the strongest RF field gradient, i.e., along Y.

The method preserves the full signal intensity from the target VOI while keeping certain advantages of the STEAM sequence. Only one slice-selective 180° pulse is employed, which allows TE to be shortened almost as much as in STEAM. The time between ISIS and SE modules can be used for crusher gradients without increasing TE (Fig. 1.2.20). The adiabatic pulse in ISIS

reduces B_1 dependence of the acquired signals compared to STEAM (Fig. 1.2.17).

Since the SPECIAL sequence includes 1D ISIS, the inherent problems from ISIS remain in this scheme, i.e., sensitivity to motion between two subsequent scans.

Pros and Cons of Different Localization Schemes

Selection of the optimal localization sequence depends on the subject studied (animal or human), hardware performance, and specific aims and requirements of the study. As mentioned earlier, 3D ISIS and localization using only OVS are not usually efficient enough to obtain good quality short TE proton spectra. PRESS is generally less useful for short TE studies, due to its relatively large CSD error and complications in eliminating spurious FIDs and echoes that contaminate signals at short echo times.

Compared to animal scanners, human MR systems have strict limits regarding the maximum field gradient amplitudes and the minimum time delays to reach such amplitudes (rise times), as well as the maximum number of RF pulses, and their length and power. Hence, methods with a reduced CSD error (STEAM, LASER, and semi-LASER) are preferable for short TE human studies. STEAM offers intrinsically lower signal intensity; LASER methods give full signal intensity, but the minimum TE is longer, which can introduce more T_2 weighting of signal intensities. All these techniques are also less sensitive to the RF field (B_1) inhomogeneities and can be used with an RF surface coil as transmitter. Alternatively, SPECIAL can combine full

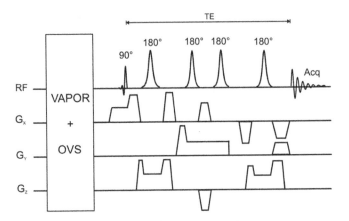

FIGURE 1.2.19 A layout of a semi-LASER pulse sequence (Öz & Tkáč, 2011). This sequence applies slice excitation along X, followed by an adiabatic slice-selective pair along Z. In between this adiabatic frequency-selective pair, another two adiabatic frequency-selective pulses along Y are applied. The additional WS (VAPOR) and OVS module can be applied before the localization sequence.

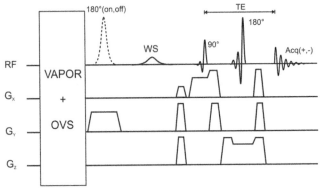

FIGURE 1.2.20 A SPECIAL pulse sequence. A 1D ISIS scheme is applied along Y (180° pulse in dashed line) and a spin echo is then created with two other slice-selective asymmetric pulses along X and Z. Two scans must be acquired with the first 180° pulse on and off, respectively, and the two scans are then subtracted. In addition, both WS (VAPOR) and OVS are applied before 1D ISIS. Another water-suppression pulse is applied before the 90° excitation pulse.

signal intensity with short TE; however, OVS must be carefully adjusted to avoid spectra contamination.

In short TE animal studies, STEAM is useful for larger VOIs and high RF coil sensitivities. For experiments using a surface RF coil as a transceiver, SPECIAL can provide the same spectra quality with increased SNR, which can be traded off for smaller VOIs or shorter measurement time.

Acknowledgments

We would like to thank Dr. Nicole Detzer for copyediting this chapter and Dr. Arthur W. Magill for discussions relating to hardware details.

References

Bottomley, P.A. (1984). Selective volume method for performing localized NMR spectroscopy. U.S. Patent 4480228.

Carlsson, Å., Ljungberg, M., Starck, G., & Forssell-Aronsson, E. (2011). Degraded water suppression in small volume ^{1}H MRS due to localised shimming. *Magnetic Resonance Materials in Physics Biology and Medicine, 24*(2), 97–107.

Connelly, A., Counsell, C., Lohman, J. A., & Ordidge, R. J. (1988). Outer volume suppressed image related in vivo spectroscopy (OSIRIS), a high-sensitivity localization technique. Journal of Magnetic Resonance (1969), 78 519–525.

Conolly, S., Nishimura, D., & Macovski, A. (1989). A selective adiabatic spin-echo pulse. *Journal of Magnetic Resonance (1969), 83*(2), 324–334.

Cudalbu, C., Bucur, A., Graveron-Demilly, D., Beuf, O., Cavassila, S. (2007). Comparison of two strategies of background-accommodation: Influence on the metabolite concentration estimation from in vivo Magnetic Resonance Spectroscopy data. Paper presented at the Engineering in Medicine and Biology Society, August 22-26, 2007. EMBS 2007. 29th Annual International Conference of the IEEE.

Cudalbu, C., Mlynarik, V., Xin, L., & Gruetter, R. (2009). Comparison of T_1 relaxation times of the neurochemical profile in rat brain at 9.4 tesla and 14.1 tesla. *Magnetic Resonance in Medicine, 62*(4), 862–867.

de Graaf, R. A., Brown, P. B., McIntyre, S., Nixon, T. W., Behar, K. L., & Rothman, D. L. (2006). High magnetic field water and metabolite proton T_1 and T_2 relaxation in rat brain in vivo. *Magnetic Resonance in Medicine, 56*(2), 386–394.

Dong, Z., Dreher, W., & Leibfritz, D. (2006). Toward quantitative short-echo-time in vivo proton MR spectroscopy without water suppression. *Magnetic Resonance in Medicine, 55*(6), 1441–1446.

Garwood, M., & DelaBarre, L. (2001). The return of the frequency sweep: designing adiabatic pulses for contemporary NMR. *Journal of Magnetic Resonance, 153*(2), 155–177.

Hasse, S., Frank, J. A., Hanicke, W., & Matthaei, D. (1985). ^{1}H NMR chemical shift selective (CHESS) imaging. *Physics in Medicine and Biology, 30*(4), 341–344.

Hoult, D. I., & Richards, R. E. (1976). The signal-to-noise ratio of the nuclear magnetic resonance experiment. *Journal of Magnetic Resonance, 24*(1), 71–85.

Hwang, T. L., & Shaka, A. J. (1995). Water suppression that works. Excitation sculpting using arbitrary wave-forms and pulsed-field gradients. *Journal of Magnetic Resonance, Series A, 112*(2), 275–279.

Jung, W. I., Bunse, M., & Lutz, O. (2001). Quantitative evaluation of the lactate signal loss and its spatial dependence in press

localized ^{1}H NMR spectroscopy. *Journal of Magnetic Resonance, 152*(2), 203–213.

Leibfritz, D., & Dreher, W. (2001). Magnetization transfer MRS. *NMR in Biomedicine, 14*(2), 65–76.

Marques, J. P., Kober, T., Krueger, G., van der Zwaag, W., Van de Moortele, P. -F., & Gruetter, R. (2010). MP2RAGE, a self bias-field corrected sequence for improved segmentation and T1-mapping at high field. *NeuroImage, 49*(2), 1271–1281.

Mescher, M., Tannus, A., Johnson, M. O. N., & Garwood, M. (1996). Solvent suppression using selective echo dephasing. *Journal of Magnetic Resonance, Series A, 123*(2), 226–229.

Mlynárik, V., Gambarota, G., Frenkel, H., & Gruetter, R. (2006). Localized short-echo-time proton MR spectroscopy with full signal-intensity acquisition. *Magnetic Resonance in Medicine, 56*(5), 965–970.

Moonen, C. T. W., Sobering, G., Van Zijl, P. C. M., Gillen, J., Von Kienlin, M., & Bizzi, A. (1992). Proton spectroscopic imaging of human brain. *Journal of Magnetic Resonance (1969), 98*(3), 556–575.

Moonen, C. T. W., & Vanzijl, P. C. M. (1990). Highly effective water suppression for in vivo proton NMR-spectroscopy (drysteam). *Journal of Magnetic Resonance, 88*(1), 28–41.

Ogg, R. J., Kingsley, P. B., & Taylor, J. S. (1994). WET, a T_1- and B_1-insensitive water-suppression method for in vivo localized ^{1}H NMR spectroscopy. *Journal of Magnetic Resonance, Series B, 104*(1), 1–10.

Ordidge, R. J., Connelly, A., & Lohman, J. A. B. (1986). Image-selected in vivo spectroscopy (ISIS). A new technique for spatially selective NMR spectroscopy. *Journal of Magnetic Resonance (1969), 66*(2), 283–294.

Öz, G., & Tkáč, I. (2011). Short-echo, single-shot, full-intensity proton magnetic resonance spectroscopy for neurochemical profiling at 4 T: Validation in the cerebellum and brainstem. *Magnetic Resonance in Medicine, 65*(4), 901–910.

Patt, S. L., & Sykes, B. D. (1972). Water eliminated Fourier transform NMR spectroscopy. *The Journal of Chemical Physics, 56*(6), 3182–3184.

Piotto, M., Saudek, V., & Sklenář, V. (1992). Gradient-tailored excitation for single-quantum NMR spectroscopy of aqueous solutions. *Journal of Biomolecular NMR, 2*(6), 661–665.

Serrai, H., Clayton, D. B., Senhadji, L., Zuo, C., & Lenkinski, R. E. (2002). Localized proton spectroscopy without water suppression: removal of gradient induced frequency modulations by modulus signal selection. *Journal of Magnetic Resonance, 154*(1), 53–59.

Tannus, A., & Garwood, M. (1997). Adiabatic pulses. *NMR in Biomedicine, 10*(8), 423–434.

Terpstra, M., Henry, P. -G., & Gruetter, R. (2003). Measurement of reduced glutathione (GSH) in human brain using LCModel analysis of difference-edited spectra. *Magnetic Resonance in Medicine, 50*(1), 19–23.

Terpstra, M., Ugurbil, K., & Gruetter, R. (2002). Direct in vivo measurement of human cerebral GABA concentration using MEGA-editing at 7 Tesla. *Magnetic Resonance in Medicine, 47*(5), 1009–1012.

Tkáč, I., Starčuk, Z., Choi, I. Y., & Gruetter, R. (1999). In vivo ^{1}H NMR spectroscopy of rat brain at 1 ms echo time. *Magnetic Resonance in Medicine, 41*(4), 649–656.

van der Veen, J. W. C., Weinberger, D. R., Tedeschi, G., Frank, J. A., & Duyn, J. H. (2000). Proton MR spectroscopic imaging without water suppression. *Radiology, 217*(1), 296–300.

Xin, L., Gambarota, G., Mlynárik, V., & Gruetter, R. (2008). Proton T_2 relaxation time of J-coupled cerebral metabolites in rat brain at 9.4 T. *NMR in Biomedicine, 21*(4), 396–401.

Xin, L., Schaller, B., Mlynarik, V., Lu, H., & Gruetter, R. (2012). Proton T_1 relaxation times of metabolites in human occipital white and gray matter at 7 T. *Magnetic Resonance in Medicine, 69*(4), 931–936.

1.3

Technical Considerations for Multivoxel Approaches and Magnetic Resonance Spectroscopic Imaging

Vincent O. Boer and Dennis W.J. Klomp

Department of Radiology, University Medical Center Utrecht, Utrecht, The Netherlands

INTRODUCTION

In single-voxel magnetic resonance spectroscopy (MRS) localization techniques are applied to acquire metabolic information from a prescribed location of interest, where the location is guided by acquired MR images. Unfortunately, it can be difficult to precisely define such a region of interest if the pathology is not clearly seen with imaging techniques, therefore the area of interest may be missed. Furthermore, it might be interesting to study the spatial heterogeneity of metabolism. In these cases it will be advantageous to run MR spectroscopic imaging (MRSI) where information is obtained from multiple voxels in the same acquisition. However, MRSI requires optimization of its sequence for a larger region of interest compared to a small single voxel acquisition. This places different requirements on the quality of B_0 shimming, flip angle homogeneity, and water and lipid suppression of the MRSI compared to single-voxel MRS and can lead to increased scan times and more complex data processing. In this chapter an overview of the possibilities and challenges for different types of MRSI are given. A more technical description can be found in other textbooks, for example: *In Vivo NMR Spectroscopy* (de Graaf, 2008).

MULTIVOLUME SELECTION

The most direct way of performing multivoxel MRS is the acquisition of multiple voxels in one repetition time (TR). During the T_1 recovery time after a single voxel acquisition, a spectrum from another voxel can be acquired. In this way, multiple voxels can be defined and interleaved in a single scan, very similar to multislice acquisitions in MR imaging (Fig. 1.3.1). However, since three orthogonal slice-selective radio-frequency (RF) pulses are used for the selection of a volume, care should be taken in the planning of the voxels, not to place it on any of the slices used to select the other voxels, since this would lead to partial saturation of the signal (Ernst & Hennig, 1991). Similarly, care should be taken to prevent overlap with possible outer volume saturation (OVS) pulses. An advantage of multivoxel MRS is that it is possible to perform location-specific flip angle calibration and optimize water suppression for every location individually. Where dynamic B_0 shim updating is available, the B_0 homogeneity (shimming) can also be optimized for every individual voxel (Koch et al., 2007), resulting in similar spectral quality to that which can be obtained with separate single-voxel acquisition in the time of only a single acquisition. In contrast to most other MRSI methods, where a compromise is required to allow for optimization of the whole region of interest that incorporates all acquired voxels, the multivoxel approach can be optimized for each voxel independently. Furthermore, phase/frequency alignment in postprocessing is still possible with this method; this is more complex with methods where the signal from multiple locations is encoded in the acquisition.

SPATIAL ENCODING

Distinct from multivoxel acquisitions, other MRSI methods are available where the signal from one large voxel is subdivided into smaller voxels to acquire spatially distributed metabolic information. Basically a division separating the signal from a large voxel into multiple smaller voxels can be made in one of two ways: RF-based encoding or gradient-based encoding. Of these, gradient-based encoding is the most widely used. Currently, RF encoding is not implemented on most clinical MR systems.

RF Encoding

In RF encoding, or Hadamard encoding (Bolinger & Leigh, 1988), RF pulses are used to invert the spins in parts of a larger voxel. In the simplest case, two

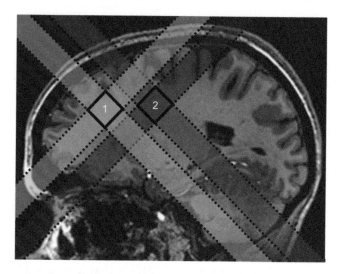

FIGURE 1.3.1 Multivoxel MRS. Two voxels can be interleaved in the same repetition time, as long as the slices of the RF pulses used for voxel selection do not overlap. In this way, spectroscopic information can be acquired for multiple locations in the same scan time.

acquisitions are performed. In the second acquisition a part of the volume (part A) is inverted with an additional inversion RF pulse. The other half (part B) remains unaffected. The first acquisition now contains the sum of both signals A + B and the signal of the second acquisition is $(-A) + B$ due to the inversion pulse. Subtraction of the two acquisitions now results in a spectrum originating from location A, whilst a summation of the two acquisitions results in a signal from volume B (Fig. 1.3.2). More complicated matrices can be used for selection of more voxels in 1D, 2D, or 3D. Scan time increases with the number of voxels that are to be acquired, since all voxels have to be encoded. The minimally required number of signal acquisitions is equal to the number of voxels that are to be reconstructed. Although in theory Hadamard encoding results in a good localization and sharp voxel edges, addition and subtraction of multiple scans makes the method sensitive to patient motion, and requires a long TR for full T_1 relaxation. Also the additional inversion pulses increase RF power deposition and interfere with water-suppression schemes.

Gradient-Based Encoding

Gradient encoding is the most widely used technique for MRSI. Gradient encoding is based on the excitation of a larger volume, where encoding B_0 field gradients are applied before or during the signal readout. The signal from multiple acquisitions with varying encoding gradients can afterward be combined and reconstructed into separate voxels, mostly with a Fourier reconstruction in a similar way to phase encoding in 2D or 3D MR imaging. The main difference with MR imaging is that in MRSI frequency information has to stay intact and can therefore not be used for spatial encoding. The simplest case is 1D chemical shift imaging (CSI; Brown et al., 1982), which is based on phase encoding (Fig. 1.3.3, right). For 1D CSI, a number of acquisitions (Nx) from a

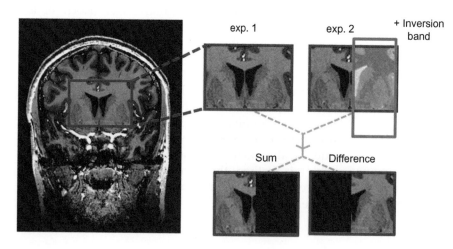

FIGURE 1.3.2 This is an illustration of Hadamard encoding. In multiple experiments, parts of a large voxel are inverted with additional inversion RF pulses. Here it is shown how a voxel can be subdivided into two parts, by performing two experiments. In the second experiment an inversion band is placed on part of the voxel. By summing or subtracting the signal of the two experiments, either the left or the right part of the voxel can be selected. This figure is reproduced in color in the color plate section.

large voxel are required resulting in a time domain signal of *t* points in every acquisition. Phase-encoding gradients of varying strength are applied in one gradient direction and every acquisition is stored in a k-space of dimension *t* by *Nx*. After a Fourier transform this results in *Nx* spatially resolved spectra where every point is filled with a spectrum from that location (Fig. 1.3.3, left). The same procedure can be similarly applied for 2D or 3D encoding of a volume, where the resulting scan time increases by the required number of phase-encoding steps to fill the k-space; $TR*Nx*Ny*Nz$. This can be reduced by not acquiring a full cubic volume, but replacing the encoding scheme by either circular (in 2D) or spherical sampling (in 3D) to reduce the required number of phase-encoding steps to fill the k-space.

Since the reconstruction of a spectrum on a location is based on a Fourier reconstruction of all acquisitions, the reconstructed signal in a voxel can also be contaminated by signals from all locations. This is an inherent consequence of the limited spatial resolution, and the resulting so-called point spread function of the Fourier transform, but can also be due to incoherence between the acquisitions due to patient motion or other sources of signal instability. The limited resolution leads to a truncation in the k-space, which leads to effects where the signal from one location leaks into neighboring voxels (Fig. 1.3.4). The resulting voxel shape shows a severe ripple resulting in a mixing of signals from different locations. The use of a suitable filter can reduce this ripple, but will increase the voxels' size, and thereby reduces the effective spatial resolution. However, by incorporating the shape of the filter into the acquisition, and by sampling the center of k-space more often than the outskirts, most negative effects of such a filter can be reduced (Pohmann & von Kienlin, 2001). The downside of using acquisition weighting is an even longer scan time, since the k-space has to be acquired several times.

FAST GRADIENT-ENCODING METHODS

Conventional MRSI with gradient encoding as described above is most widely used for MRSI, and implemented in most clinical MR systems. However, encoding of the whole k-space in 2D or 3D can take a long time, since only one point in k-space is acquired every TR (one to several seconds). For example, the total scan time for a $32 \times 32 \times 8$ acquisition with a TR of 1 s already takes more than 1 h. To reduce the total encoding time, several acceleration approaches exist, and new techniques are still being developed. Unfortunately most of these methods are not available as standard on most commercial MR systems. Still, a short overview of the currently developed methodologies is given.

A straightforward approach is to sample multiple spin echoes after an excitation to fill multiple points of a k-space in one TR (Duyn & Moonen, 1993). This increases the RF power deposition of the sequence due to the additional refocusing pulses. Also, since all echoes will have different T_2 weighting, the point spread function is influenced. Generally, the later echoes are placed at the outer parts of k-space to predominantly cause spatial voxel broadening only.

Other MRSI acceleration techniques rely on gradient encoding. With conventional MRS, no gradients are applied during signal readout in order to be able to observe the different resonance frequencies of the metabolic compounds. For acceleration, however, readout gradients can be applied during signal acquisition. This mixes the frequency information from chemical shift and spatial offset, and with multiple readouts of the signal at different evolution times, both the resonance frequencies and spatial locations can be reconstructed. The duration of each successive readout defines the resulting spectral bandwidth, which is limited by the gradient performance of the MR system. A variety of different flavors for the specific readout trajectory exists. The two most basic ones are the echo-planar readout (Mansfield, 1984) and the spiral readout (Adalsteinsson et al., 1998), where in the first case spatial information is encoded in one direction with gradient switching similar to echo-planar imaging (Fig. 1.3.5, top), and in the second case multiple dimensions can be encoded at the same time by spiraling through a 2D or 3D k-space (Fig. 1.3.5, bottom). Both

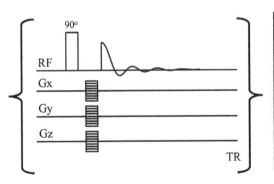
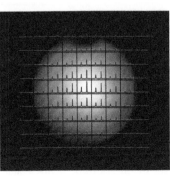

FIGURE 1.3.3 Pulse acquire sequence (right) with phase-encoding steps in two directions to encode a 2D data set. The resulting dataset consists of a 2D array of spectra (left). This figure is reproduced in color in the color plate section.

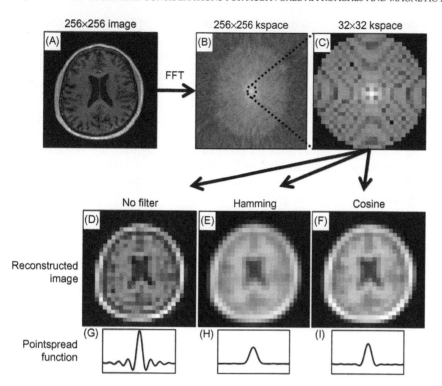

FIGURE 1.3.4 Effects of the limited resolution generally used in MRSI. A high-resolution image (A) after Fourier transform (B, log scale) shows a lot of high spatial frequency information. If only the central part of k-space is sampled (C, log scale), this results in a low-resolution image (D), where the voxel definition suffers from severe rippling (G). Using a either a Hamming (E) or cosine (F) filter results in reduced rippling and thus improved voxel localization, at the cost of increased voxel size as seen from the width of the point spread function (H, I) and blurring of the corresponding images.

types of readouts can be combined with traditional phase encoding to allow for 3D encoding.

To maximize the signal-to-noise ratio (SNR), the receive sensitivity should also be maximized. This is generally performed with a close fitting receiver array to the tissue of interest. Signal from the different receiver coils is to be phased and weighted in an optimal way for every voxel to generate the highest SNR (Wald et al., 1995). If such a receive array is used, parallel imaging strategies also can be employed to speed up the MRSI acquisition. As with imaging, the coil sensitivity patterns in a multi-element receiver coil can be used for spatial encoding and therefore can be used to perform acceleration. For example, the SENSE algorithm has been extended for use with spectroscopic imaging (Dydak et al., 2003). However, with SENSE acceleration, the point spread function shows a more complex shape, and possible contamination from other regions can be a complicating factor. Along the same lines, strategic undersampling of k-space, combined with iterative reconstruction algorithms (compressed sensing), has shown great potential for further acceleration in MRSI (Askin et al., 2012).

ENCODING BASED ON PRIOR KNOWLEDGE

To reduce the required amount of phase-encoding steps prior knowledge can be included into the encoding and reconstruction algorithm (Hu et al., 1988).

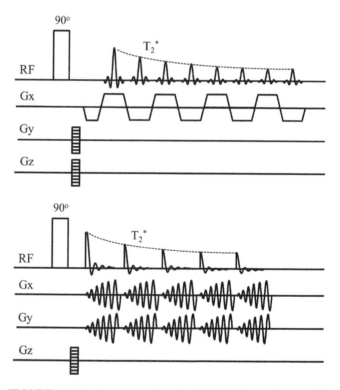

FIGURE 1.3.5 Two examples of a fast MRSI sampling. A 1D echo-planar imaging-based readout (top) allows for spectral and spatial mapping in the x-direction in every shot. It is here combined with 2D phase encoding to allow for 3D spatial mapping of metabolites. The second example (bottom) shows a spiral that collects a 2D MRSI dataset in one shot.

Instead of acquiring a large k-space span to reconstruct a large matrix with spectra, the area of interest could be subdivided into several compartments from which similar spectral information is acquired. If a region can, for example, be subdivided into three well-separated compartments, in principle only three phase-encoding steps are required to allow for separation of the three signals. Instead of Fourier reconstruction, a signal model is used to reconstruct the data. For this, the spatial distribution of the signal has to be known from a segmented image, and this information is used to generate a signal model. In addition, prior information such as B_0 or B_1 variation or spin density can be incorporated. With such a method, tremendous time gains can be achieved since less than the full matrix has to be encoded, but only if prior to the scan it is clear that only a limited number of areas will have different metabolite signals. Note that this method would fail if artifacts or unexpected sources of signal are present in the data.

WATER SUPPRESSION

Similarly to ^{1}H single-voxel MRS, it is of the utmost importance to have a good water suppression in ^{1}H MRSI. Any sidebands of the water signal might obscure the metabolites of interest (Nixon et al., 2008). Even more so with MRSI, the water from other regions might show up in a region of interest due to the point spread function or due to instabilities in the spatial-encoding scheme. Therefore, with MRSI, the water suppression has to be optimized for the whole area included in the preselected volume. As a consequence, a water-suppression technique has to be used that is robust enough to perform a good suppression taking the off-resonance effects (B_0) and B_1 variations in this large region into account.

To counter any off-resonance effects it is important to perform shimming over the whole volume to prevent any region falling out of the bandwidth of the suppression pulse. Also careful placement of the excitation volume will help in this respect, particularly if areas with a large off-resonance can be excluded in the preselected volume.

A whole family of water-suppression techniques has been described in literature. Most techniques use chemical shift-selective RF pulses to either saturate the water signal before the volume excitation, or selectively refocus the metabolites of interest while excluding the water resonance. In combination with crusher gradients the water signal is dephased where the metabolites are either not affected (presaturation) or rephased (selective refocusing).

To date, various flavors of preselection water signal saturation still exist using one or multiple pulses with varying flip angles and varying delays between the pulses. In this way, a train of suppression pulses can be numerically optimized to perform well for a range of B_1 values and different T_1 relaxation times of the water signal in different tissue types. The most simple sequence consists of a single frequency-selective pulse combined with a CHEmical Shift Selective (CHESS) crusher gradient (Haase et al., 1985), whereas a more complicated implementation is the VAriable Pulse power and Optimized Relaxation (VAPOR; Tkac et al., 1999) suppression technique with several RF pulses with various interpulse timings to allow for superb suppression within a range of B_1 and T_1 values. Disadvantages include the long duration of the suppression train (>500 ms) and the fact that full relaxation is required for optimal suppression. This principle has been extended to a shorter version (~ 250 ms) (Starcuk et al., 2011), and a version that performs well in steady state (~ 300 ms) (Boer et al., 2012).

The second, very effective suppression technique is chemical shift-selective refocusing, where a selective RF pulse in combination with crusher gradients is incorporated in the echo time such as the BASING (Star-Lack et al., 1997) or MEscher–GArwood (MEGA; Mescher et al., 1996) approach. This is, however, not possible for short TE sequences, but can be incorporated into most longer TE acquisitions.

LIPID SUPPRESSION

With MRSI of the brain it is important to prevent the occurrence of lipid signals in the selected volume since these very high signals generally tend to show ghosting and point spread effects over the whole encoded volume, potentially distorting the spectra throughout the 2D/3D dataset (Fig. 1.3.7). For this reason, generally volume preselection with a STimulated Echo Acquisition Mode (STEAM), Point RESolved Spectroscopy (PRESS), or Localization by Adiabatic SElective Refocusing (LASER) or a similar sequence is performed to exclude lipid tissue in the excited volume. These sequences use slice-selective RF pulses, where the location of the volume depends on the difference in carrier frequency of the RF pulse and the Larmor frequency of the spins. However, as the metabolites have different chemical shifts, the location of the selected volume will shift accordingly, which is called chemical shift displacement artifact (CSDA; Fig. 1.3.6). For instance, the selected volume for lipids will be shifted from the selection of choline, which needs to be considered when preventing inclusion of lipids in the selected volume. In fact, when using a PRESS sequence at 3 T, this shift can be more than 36% (Scheenen et al., 2008). The CSDA can be minimized using high bandwidth RF pulses, which can be realized using high B_1 fields with

efficient transmit coils, or by using adiabatic RF pulses as used in (semi)LASER sequences at high field (Boer et al., 2011b).

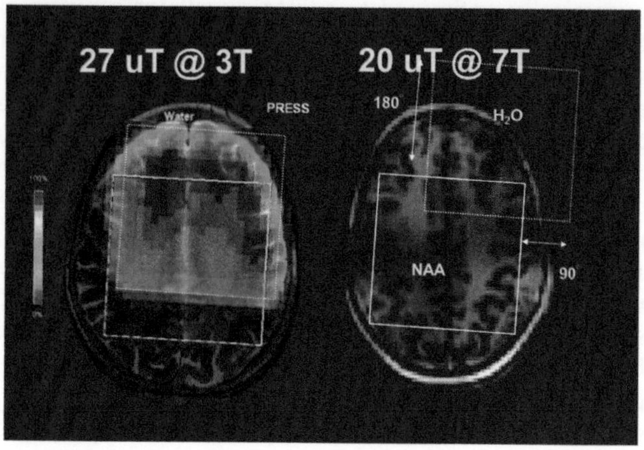

In most cases the volume preselection is combined with outer volume suppression pulses to further suppress the potential signal coming from lipid tissue (Fig. 1.3.7). Unfortunately, due to specific absorption rate limitations, the combination of a train of outer volume suppression pulses and volume preselection put a restraint on the minimum TR that can be used. Therefore less power-demanding lipid-suppression schemes have been developed; for example, by frequency-selective lipid suppression, in combination with proper B_0 shimming (Boer et al., 2011a). Particularly when excluding the volume preselection scheme, this requires fewer RF pulses and less CSDA, but on the downside this also suppresses metabolites around the 1.3 ppm resonance such as lactate. Other types of spatial lipid saturation include local excitation of the skull by an RF-shimmed B_1 distribution (Hetherington et al., 2010), however, this requires the use of multiple transmit coil elements and a multi-transmit MR system.

FIGURE 1.3.6 Demonstration of CSDA when using a volume preselection box to exclude signals from the skull while obtaining signals from the brain. Examples are shown for 3 T (left; Scheenen, et al., 2008) and extrapolated to 7 T (right) demonstrating that the PRESS box fails its task. This figure is reproduced in color in the color plate section.

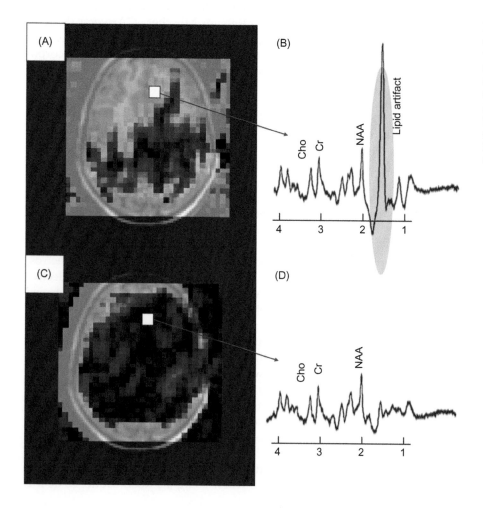

FIGURE 1.3.7 Lipids from the skull and skin can lead to large artifacts over the whole brain as seen in the lipid integration map (A). Voxels located fully in the brain still show a large lipid artifact due to point spread and ghosting effects (B). After lipid suppression the residual lipid signal over the whole slice is suppressed (C) and voxels in the brain do not suffer from large lipid artifacts (D). This figure is reproduced in color in the color plate section.

B₀ SHIMMING

Linewidth in the MR spectra, and therefore the SNR, is affected by B_0 inhomogeneities. Hence it is crucial to compensate for distortions in the B_0 field to ensure uniform spectral quality over the MRSI volume. Apart from very local susceptibility transitions, such as close to the nasal cavity, it is possible to compensate for B_0 field distortions by shimming.

Compensation is generally performed with external shim coils with spherical harmonic spatial distributions. All MR systems are capable of linear shimming. On top of that, in high-field MR systems, second- or third-order shims are available, and higher than third-order shimming has been shown with a brain insert shim setup at 7 T (Pan et al., 2012) where the magnetic field homogeneity increases with the amount of shim coils, and decreases with the size of the area under investigation. Since large frequency offsets can be generated outside the shimmed region due to high-order shimming, it can be advantageous also to take these into account during shimming (Fig. 1.3.8). For example, a cost function can be defined where both the homogeneity in a region of interest is optimized, and large offsets in neighboring regions are minimized (Boer et al., 2011a).

Another further gain can be found in dynamic shimming. Since the shim will be compromised for a large heterogeneous region of interest, the volume of interest can be divided into multiple acquisition stacks or slices, so that the magnetic field can be optimized for every stack individually (Fig. 1.3.9). For example, multiple voxels can be interleaved in a scan (Koch et al., 2007). Since the B_0 shim demands can even be different during different sequence elements (e.g.,

water suppression and signal excitation or acquisition), the B_0 field can be optimized for every sequence element individually (Boer et al., 2012).

Apart from static field distortions, dynamic B_0 field variation also plays an important role in MRSI, since a changing B_0 field over time can lead to errors in spatial encoding. Furthermore, a fluctuating field over time can cause line broadening. Whilst in single-voxel MRS it is generally possible to perform alignment of the spectra in postprocessing to remove such fluctuations, in MRSI this is not possible. For this end a separate frequency reference can be required. This can be collected by measuring the localized water frequency by a fast scan, interleaved with the MRSI acquisition (Hess et al., 2012). Alternatively, a fast coil-localized reference signal on specific points in space close to the object of interest can be obtained with field probes to monitor and correct for field changes over time (De Zanche et al., 2008).

The processing of MRSI data is similar to any single-voxel reconstruction; however, in general more data is processed. This raises questions as to the optimal processing and display methods for 3D or even 4D data. Spectral fitting or integration can be performed for all voxels, and the signal has to be normalized to a certain reference (e.g., water) to remove the effects of coil sensitivity profiles. The resulting normalized signal is generally displayed per metabolite as a color map over an MR image (Fig. 1.3.10). To minimize the chance of bias in the spectral processing, however, strict quality checks on the SNR, linewidth, and water/lipid artifact levels have to be performed on every spectrum in a dataset to ensure consistent data over the volume of interest (Wright et al., 2013).

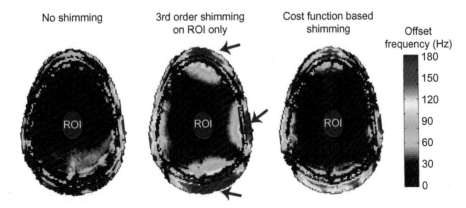

FIGURE 1.3.8   Shimming in a slice through the human brain for MRSI. Without shimming (left) the magnetic field homogeneity in the region of interest (ROI; black) is poor with 10 Hz standard deviation. After third-order shimming the magnetic field homogeneity improves to 3 Hz; however, large frequency offsets are generated outside the ROI, which compromise water and lipid suppression (middle). By taking two regions into account, the homogeneity in the ROI is not affected, and the homogeneity over the slice is good enough to perform adequate water and lipid suppression (right). This figure is reproduced in color in the color plate section.

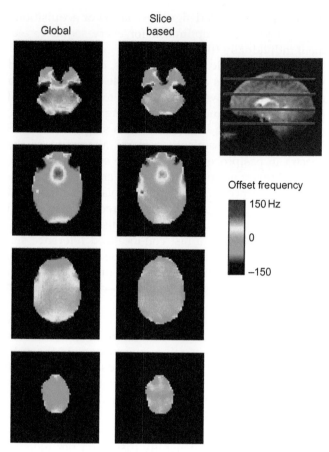

FIGURE 1.3.9   If the acquisition can be separated into multiple slices, the B_0 shim can be optimized for every slice individually. A clear gain in B_0 field homogeneity for the brain at 7 T can be seen between global third-order shimming on the whole brain (left) and a third-order slice-based optimization (right), resulting in improved linewidth. This figure is reproduced in color in the color plate section.

CONCLUSIONS

Metabolic images of the human brain can be obtained with MRSI. When excluding the edges of the brain and areas of strong susceptibility differences, standard MR systems can be used to generate metabolic maps. Using the latest state-of-the-art technology, which enables dynamic steering of B_1 and B_0, MRSI becomes feasible for the entire brain at improved spectral quality. Particularly in combination with acceleration techniques, metabolic imaging may find its way into clinical practice.

References

Adalsteinsson, E., Irarrazabal, P., Topp, S., Meyer, C., Macovski, A., & Spielman, D. M. (1998). Volumetric spectroscopic imaging with spiral-based k-space trajectories. *Magnetic Resonance in Medicine, 39*(6), 889–898.

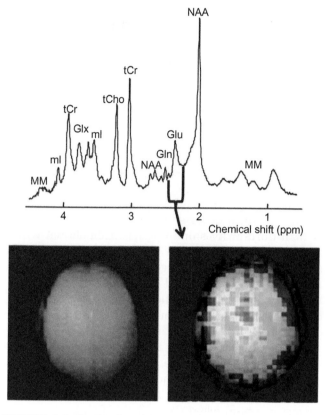

FIGURE 1.3.10   Display of the glutamate signal from a 2D MRSI dataset. A specific part of the spectrum is integrated, or fitted, normalized to a general reference signal (e.g., water) and displayed as a color map over an image. This figure is reproduced in color in the color plate section.

Askin, N. C., Atis, B. & Ozturk-Isik, E. (2012). Accelerated phosphorus magnetic resonance spectroscopic imaging using compressed sensing. *Conference Proceedings of the IEEE, Engineering in Medicine and Biology Society, 2012*, 1106–1109.

Boer, V. O., Klomp, D. W., Juchem, C., Luijten, P. R., & de Graaf, R. A. (2012). Multislice (1)H MRSI of the human brain at 7 T using dynamic B(0) and B(1) shimming. *Magnetic Resonance in Medicine, 68*(3), 662–670.

Boer, V. O., Siero, J. C., Hoogduin, H., van Gorp, J. S., Luijten, P. R., & Klomp, D. W. (2011a). High-field MRS of the human brain at short TE and TR. *NMR in Biomedicine, 24*(9), 1081–1088.

Boer, V. O., van Lier, A. L., Hoogduin, J. M., Wijnen, J. P., Luijten, P. R., & Klomp, D. W. (2011b). 7-T (1)H MRS with adiabatic refocusing at short TE using radiofrequency focusing with a dual-channel volume transmit coil. *NMR in Biomedicine, 24*(9), 1038–1046.

Bolinger, L., & Leigh, J. S. (1988). Hadamard spectroscopic imaging (HSI) for multivolume localization. [Note]. *Journal of Magnetic Resonance, 80*(1), 162–167.

Brown, T. R., Kincaid, B. M., & Ugurbil, K. (1982). NMR chemical shift imaging in three dimensions. *Proceedings of the National Academy of Sciences USA, 79*(11), 3523–3526.

de Graaf, R. A. (2008). *In Vivo Nmr Spectroscopy: Principles and Techniques.* New York: John Wiley & Sons.

De Zanche, N., Barmet, C., Nordmeyer-Massner, J. A., & Pruessmann, K. P. (2008). NMR probes for measuring magnetic fields and field dynamics in MR systems. *Magnetic Resonance in Medicine, 60*(1), 176–186.

Duyn, J. H., & Moonen, C. T. (1993). Fast proton spectroscopic imaging of human brain using multiple spin-echoes. *Magnetic Resonance in Medicine, 30*(4), 409–414.

Dydak, U., Pruessmann, K. P., Weiger, M., Tsao, J., Meier, D., & Boesiger, P. (2003). Parallel spectroscopic imaging with spin-echo trains. *Magnetic Resonance in Medicine, 50*(1), 196–200.

Ernst, T., & Hennig, J. (1991). Double-volume 1H spectroscopy with interleaved acquisitions using tilted gradients. *Magnetic Resonance in Medicine, 20*(1), 27–35.

Haase, A., Frahm, J., Hanicke, W., & Matthaei, D. (1985). 1H NMR chemical shift selective (CHESS) imaging. *Physics in Medicine and Biology, 30*(4), 341–344.

Hess, A. T., Andronesi, O. C., Tisdall, M. D., Sorensen, A. G., van der Kouwe, A. J., & Meintjes, E. M. (2012). Real-time motion and B0 correction for localized adiabatic selective refocusing (LASER) MRSI using echo planar imaging volumetric navigators. *NMR in Biomedicine, 25*(2), 347–358.

Hetherington, H. P., Avdievich, N. I., Kuznetsov, A. M., & Pan, J. W. (2010). RF shimming for spectroscopic localization in the human brain at 7 T. *Magnetic Resonance in Medicine, 63*(1), 9–19.

Hu, X., Levin, D. N., Lauterbur, P. C., & Spraggins, T. (1988). SLIM: spectral localization by imaging. *Magnetic Resonance in Medicine, 8*(3), 314–322.

Koch, K. M., Sacolick, L. I., Nixon, T. W., McIntyre, S., Rothman, D. L., & de Graaf, R. A. (2007). Dynamically shimmed multivoxel 1H magnetic resonance spectroscopy and multislice magnetic resonance spectroscopic imaging of the human brain. *Magnetic Resonance in Medicine, 57*(3), 587–591.

Mansfield, P. (1984). Spatial mapping of the chemical shift in NMR. *Magnetic Resonance in Medicine, 1*(3), 370–386.

Mescher, M. , A. , T., Johnson, M. O., & Garwood, M. (1996). Solvent suppression using selective echo dephasing. *Journal of Magnetic Resonance, Series A, 123*(2), 226–229.

Nixon, T. W., McIntyre, S., Rothman, D. L., & de Graaf, R. A. (2008). Compensation of gradient-induced magnetic field perturbations. *Journal of Magnetic Resonance, 192*(2), 209–217.

Pan, J. W., Lo, K. M., & Hetherington, H. P. (2012). Role of very high order and degree B0 shimming for spectroscopic imaging of the human brain at 7 tesla. *Magnetic Resonance in Medicine, 68*(4), 1007–1017.

Pohmann, R., & von Kienlin, M. (2001). Accurate phosphorus metabolite images of the human heart by 3D acquisition-weighted CSI. *Magnetic Resonance in Medicine, 45*(5), 817–826.

Scheenen, T. W., Klomp, D. W., Wijnen, J. P., & Heerschap, A. (2008). Short echo time 1H-MRSI of the human brain at 3T with minimal chemical shift displacement errors using adiabatic refocusing pulses. *Magnetic Resonance Medicine, 59*(1), 1–6.

Star-Lack, J., Nelson, S. J., Kurhanewicz, J., Huang, L. R., & Vigneron, D. B. (1997). Improved water and lipid suppression for 3D PRESS CSI using RF band selective inversion with gradient dephasing (BASING). *Magnetic Resonance in Medicine, 38*(2), 311–321.

Starcuk Jr., Z., Starcukova, J., & Starcuk, Z. (2011). Short dual-band VAPOR-like pulse sequence for simultaneous water and lipid suppression for in vivo MR spectroscopy and spectroscopic imaging. Paper presented at the ISMRM, Montreal, Canada.

Tkac, I., Starcuk, Z., Choi, I. Y., & Gruetter, R. (1999). In vivo ^{1}H NMR spectroscopy of rat brain at 1 ms echo time. *Magnetic Resonance in Medicine, 41*(4), 649–656.

Wald, L. L., Moyher, S. E., Day, M. R., Nelson, S. J., & Vigneron, D. B. (1995). Proton spectroscopic imaging of the human brain using phased array detectors. *Magnetic Resonance in Medicine, 34*(3), 440–445.

Wright, A. J., Kobus, T., Selnaes, K. M., Gribbestad, I. S., Weiland, E., Scheenen, T. W., et al. (2013). Quality control of prostate (1)H MRSI data. *NMR in Biomedicine, 26*(2), 193–203.

Spectral Editing and 2D NMR

Robin A. de Graaf

Magnetic Resonance Research Center, Yale University, School of Medicine, New Haven, Connecticut, USA

INTRODUCTION

[1]H nuclear magnetic resonance (NMR) spectroscopy is a powerful method to study the metabolic content of living tissues *in vivo*. ^{1}H NMR, often referred to as magnetic resonance spectroscopy (MRS), provides information about energy metabolism in the form of creatine, phosphocreatine, glucose, and lactate; about neurotransmission through the detection of glutamate, γ-amino butyric acid (GABA), aspartate, and glycine; and about membrane metabolism and integrity via choline detection. The detection of *N*-acetylaspartate (NAA) and myo-inositol has frequently been used as neuronal and astroglial markers, respectively. The combined detection of ascorbic acid and glutathione provides the *in vivo* antioxidant profile.

Fig. 1.4.1 shows a typical ^{1}H NMR spectrum from human brain at 7 T. The high magnetic field strength in combination with an optimized magnetic field homogeneity allows the detection of up to 15 metabolites. The singlet resonances from NAA (2.01 parts per million, ppm), total creatine (=sum of creatine and phosphocreatine, tCr, 3.02 ppm) and total choline (=sum of choline, phosphorylcholine, and glycerophosphorylcholine, tCho, 3.21 ppm) dominate the spectrum. These singlet resonances can be readily measured at any magnetic field strength. However, at lower magnetic fields many resonances from other metabolites, like glutamate, glutamine, and GABA, cannot easily be detected and quantified due to spectral overlap. The improved spectral resolution that can be achieved at 7 T allows, for example, the separation of glutamate from glutamine. However, despite the improved spectral resolving power, spectral overlap between resonances from other compounds is still abundant. Examples include the overlap between GABA and total creatine, between lactate and macromolecules/lipids, and between glutathione and a

variety of compounds. Whereas some examples of spectral overlap can be accommodated during spectral fitting, the majority of examples require some form of spectral manipulation or editing for a reliable separation.

Spectral editing can, in the broadest sense, be described as any technique that separates overlapping NMR resonances by utilizing differences in NMR or other physical properties. Under this definition spectral editing includes techniques that utilize differences in T_1 or T_2 relaxation, diffusion, or chemical exchange to achieve separation. While all of these techniques have been applied *in vivo*, their success is in most cases limited due to the fact that differences between metabolites in the aforementioned parameters are generally small. As a result the separation is either incomplete or comes at the cost of a greatly reduced signal-to-noise ratio. A noticeable exception is the excellent separation between metabolites and macromolecules due to the large difference in T_1 and T_2 relaxation, as well as diffusion.

Spectral editing is therefore typically defined as a technique that utilizes scalar coupling to achieve spectral simplification. Since chemical groups within a metabolite either have scalar coupling (e.g., glutamate, GABA) or not (e.g., creatine, water), the spectral separation can be expected to be absolute.

SCALAR COUPLING

A rigorous description of NMR for scalar-coupled spin systems requires the involvement of quantum mechanics, which is outside the scope of this chapter. Therefore, the interested reader is referred to excellent textbooks dealing with the quantum mechanics of NMR (Ernst et al., 1987; Levitt, 2005). Here we will proceed with more intuitive and qualitative arguments to explain scalar coupling and formulate a number of practical rules that will allow one to understand the principle of the experiments described in the next section.

At first sight an NMR spectrum is completely characterized by the resonance frequencies and relative amplitudes originating from the nuclei under investigation. However, closer inspection reveals that some

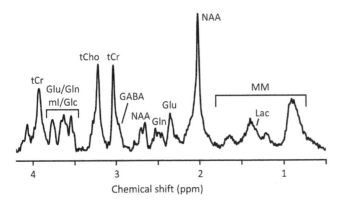

FIGURE 1.4.1 ^{1}H NMR spectrum extracted from an ultrashort TE MRSI dataset (TE = 2.75 ms, actual voxel size = 875 μL) acquired from the human brain at 7T. Macromolecular resonances, present under the entire spectrum but directly visible only between 0 and 2 ppm, are enhanced due to the short echo time. GABA, γ-aminobutyric acid; Glc, glucose; Glu, glutamate; Gln, glutamine; MM, macromolecules; mI, myo-inositol; NAA, N-acetyl aspartate; Lac, lactate; tCho, total choline; tCr, total creatine.

resonances are split into several smaller lines. This phenomenon of spin—spin or scalar coupling originates from the fact that nuclei with magnetic moments can influence each other, both directly through space (dipolar coupling) and also through electrons in chemical bonds (scalar coupling). Even though dipolar interactions are the main mechanism for relaxation in a liquid, there is no net interaction between nuclei since rapid molecular tumbling averages the dipolar interactions to zero. However, interactions through chemical bonds do not average to zero and give rise to the phenomenon of scalar (or J) coupling.

In order to understand scalar coupling, consider the interaction between two spin-1/2 nuclei, a proton and a ^{13}C nucleus (e.g., in [1-^{13}C]-glucose). For the proton there are two distinct states in which the magnetic moment of the scalar-coupled ^{13}C nucleus is either parallel or antiparallel to the external magnetic field. The proton "senses" these different states, which are conveyed through the electron spin in the covalent ^{1}H—^{13}C chemical bond. As a result the energy levels of the proton will degenerate, leading to two frequencies separated by the scalar coupling constant J (Fig. 1.4.2A). The scalar coupling is dependent on the nuclei involved, but is independent of the magnetic field strength. The same situation arises for the ^{13}C nucleus that senses two different orientations for the proton and also splits into two resonances at slightly different frequencies (Fig. 1.4.2A). When there are

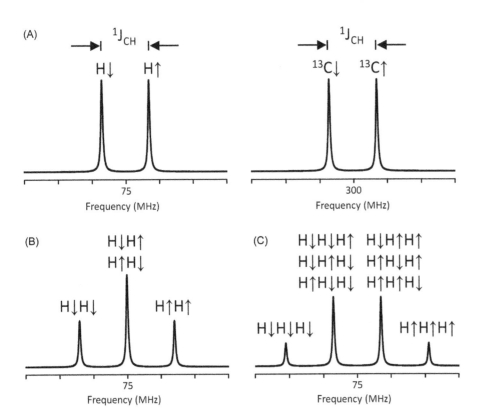

FIGURE 1.4.2 Effect of scalar coupling on the spectral appearance of resonances. For a heteronuclear ^{1}H/^{13}C two-spin system, scalar coupling leads to the formation of two doublet signals, one in the ^{1}H NMR spectrum and one in the ^{13}C NMR spectrum. For illustration purposes the spectra are drawn at 7 T. The ^{13}C resonances with the lower/higher frequencies originate from ^{13}C nuclei, which are coupled to protons with their spins antiparallel/parallel to the external magnetic field. Similar arguments hold for the splitting in the ^{1}H NMR spectrum. (B, C) Splitting patterns in the ^{13}C NMR spectrum for heteronuclear (B) three-spin H$_2^{13}$C and (C) four-spin H$_3^{13}$C systems. The spin states of the protons are indicated above each resonance line. In general, the higher frequencies originate from ^{13}C nuclei that are scalar coupled to protons in a parallel state.

more than two nuclei involved [as in $H_2{}^{13}C$ methylene (Fig. 1.4.2B) or $H_3{}^{13}C$ methyl (Fig. 1.4.2C) groups] the resonances split in a binomial pattern. For example, signal from the ^{13}C nucleus splits into two resonances by the first proton. Each resonance splits again due to the second proton and again due to the third proton, finally appearing as four resonances, each separated by the scalar coupling constant at relative intensities of 1:3:3:1 (a so-called quartet; Fig. 1.4.2C). The protons only experience a single ^{13}C nucleus and therefore only split once into a doublet of relative intensity 1:1. Note that magnetically equivalent protons, like protons in a methyl group, do not split among themselves due to magnetic equivalence rules. Further note that these splitting rules are only valid in the weak coupling approximation when the frequency difference between the resonances (e.g., ^{1}H and ^{13}C) is much larger than the scalar coupling constant. All heteronuclear scalar couplings are weak couplings, while most of the homonuclear scalar couplings (especially in proton NMR) are in the strong coupling limit. A noticeable exception is lactic acid, which is represented by a doublet resonance at 1.32 ppm and a quartet resonance at 4.10 ppm, even at low magnetic field strengths. The scalar couplings in proton NMR operate over multiple chemical bonds. In general, the strength of the scalar coupling (and thus the magnitude of the scalar coupling constant) diminishes with the increasing number of chemical bonds, typically becoming negligible for four or more bonds. As a final observational rule, the scalar coupling with exchangeable protons (in NH or OH groups) is typically not observed due to fast exchange of those protons with water.

Scalar Coupling Evolution

Scalar coupling between spins provides a large amount of information on the spin system under investigation. For instance, observing a quartet resonance in a ^{1}H NMR spectrum implies the presence of an $RR'CH-CH_3$ moiety in the molecule of interest. If the spectrum also contains a triplet with an equal scalar coupling constant and 50% more intensity than the quartet resonance, then it can be inferred that $R' = H$ and R does not contain any other protons within three chemical bonds. Depending on the molecule of interest, analysis of the scalar coupling patterns and chemical shifts in a ^{1}H NMR spectrum can often provide a partial or even complete structure elucidation. In some cases additional information from 2D NMR or heteronuclear studies are necessary. However, despite this powerful feature, scalar coupling does not provide a means to separate overlapping resonances *per se*. In order to fully utilize the power of scalar coupling in

separating overlapping resonances, it is necessary to let the spins evolve in the transverse plane during a Hahn spin-echo sequence. Fig. 1.4.3A shows a Hahn spin-echo sequence, which is characterized by six distinct periods/operations. Following a recovery delay (TR) in which the longitudinal magnetization is restored after any previous perturbations, the magnetization is excited onto the transverse plane by a 90° excitation pulse. During a time period TE/2, the transverse magnetization evolves under the influence of chemical shift, magnetic field inhomogeneity, T_2 relaxation, and scalar coupling. The 180° refocusing pulse inverts the acquired phase evolution due to chemical shift and magnetic field inhomogeneity, which will be perfectly refocused after the second TE/2 delay at the start of the signal detection period (Fig. 1.4.3B). However, the effects of T_2 relaxation and scalar coupling are not refocused by the 180° pulse and lead to echo-time (TE)-dependent signal loss and phase evolution, respectively (Fig. 1.4.3C). A complete description

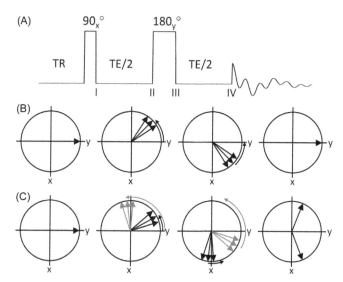

FIGURE 1.4.3 (A) Hahn spin-echo sequence with a repetition time TR and an echo time TE. (B) Evolution of transverse magnetization for uncoupled spins drawn at time points (I) following excitation, (II) prior to refocusing, (III) following refocusing, and (IV) prior to signal acquisition. The phase acquired between (I) and (II) due to chemical shift and magnetic field inhomogeneity is inverted by the 180° refocusing pulse. As the magnetization accrues an equal amount of phase between (III) and (IV), the magnetization has a zero net phase at the start of acquisition. (C) Evolution of transverse magnetization for a scalar-coupled two-spin system shown at the same time points as in (B). Half of the spins in a doublet have a higher chemical shift, such that they rotate faster in the transverse plane. The 180° refocusing pulse inverts the accumulated phase. As the 180° pulse is nonselective it also inverts the spin states of the scalar-coupled spins. This means that spins that rotated faster prior to the 180° pulse will rotate slower following the 180° pulse. As a result, chemical shift and magnetic field inhomogeneity will still be refocused, but scalar coupling is not, leading to an echo-time-dependent phase as shown in Fig. 1.4.4 in more detail.

of the phase evolution due to scalar coupling ("J-evolution") is beyond the scope of this chapter, but Fig. 1.4.4 summarizes the evolution of three important spin systems *in vivo*, namely creatine, lactic acid, and GABA. It follows that the integrated transverse magnetization for the creatine protons does not, besides T_2 relaxation, modulate as a function of the TE. The lactate protons modulation is cosinusoidal. At TE = 1/J ($\sim$144 ms) the lactate doublet (1.32 ppm) will be inverted relative to uncoupled spins (like creatine), while at TE = 1/(2J) ($\sim$72 ms) the resonance appears as an antiphase doublet, with zero integrated intensity. GABA-H4, which is scalar coupled to two protons of GABA-H3, appears as a triplet at 3.01 ppm and will therefore have a more complicated J-coupling modulation. The inner resonance of GABA-4 does not modulate as a function of TE and essentially behaves as an uncoupled spin. The outer resonances have a cosinusoidal modulation and are completed inverted at TE = 1/(2J) ($\sim$68 ms). Uncoupled spin systems do not have scalar coupling modulation and decrease exponentially with increasing echo time. This difference is utilized in spectral editing to differentiate between scalar-coupled and uncoupled spin systems.

One additional tool is required to achieve homonuclear spectral editing, namely frequency-selective radiofrequency (RF) pulses. An RF pulse that selectively refocuses one spin in a scalar-coupled multispin system effectively inhibits J-evolution, such that only T_2 relaxation affects the signal intensity as a function of the TE (Fig. 1.4.5). The results in Fig. 1.4.5 indicate that the simplest form of homonuclear spectral editing, namely J-difference editing (Rothman et al., 1984), comes down to the acquisition of two experiments. In the first experiment a nonselective spin-echo is employed, leading to J-evolution of the spin system of interest. At a total TE of 1/(2J), the outer resonances of GABA-H2 and GABA-H4 are inverted (Fig. 1.4.5A). In the second experiment a frequency-selective spin-echo is executed, with a refocusing pulse that is selective for GABA-H3. As a result, the J-evolution of GABA is inhibited leading to positive resonances for GABA-H2 and GABA-H4 (Fig. 1.4.5B). Spectral editing is achieved by subtracting the two datasets from each other. The resonances from uncoupled metabolites appear identical in both experiments, such that subtraction of the two datasets will lead to a cancellation of the unwanted resonances (Fig. 1.4.5C). The outer resonances of GABA-H2 and GABA-H4 modulate between the two experiments and will therefore survive the subtraction, forming the edited signal. The inner resonance of GABA-H2 and GABA-H4 behaves as an uncoupled spin system and is lost in the subtraction process. By changing the echo time and frequency offset of the selective refocusing pulse, any scalar-coupled

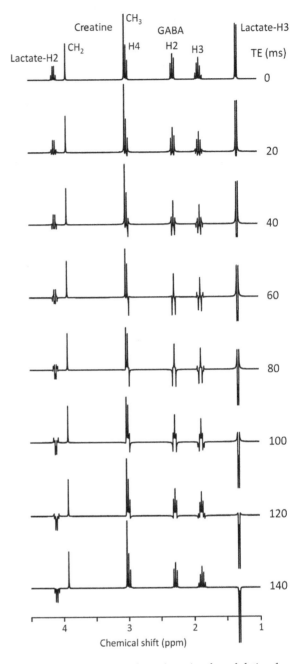

FIGURE 1.4.4 Echo-time dependent signal modulation for creatine, GABA, and lactate. The creatine signals originate from isolate methylene and methyl groups without scalar coupling. As a result, the creatine signals do not modulate as a function of TE. The GABA signals originate from three methylene groups, forming (to a first approximation) triplets for GABA-H2 and GABA-H4 and a quintet for GABA-H3. The lactate signals are split into a doublet at 1.32 ppm and a quartet at 4.11 ppm. The lactate resonances are inverted relative to creatine at an echo time of 140 ms, which equals J^{-1}. At an echo time of $(2J)^{-1}$ the lactate signals are in an antiphase state, with a net integrated intensity of zero. For GABA-H2 and H4 only the outer resonances modulate with the echo time, reaching complete inversion at TE = 68 ms = $(2J)^{-1}$.

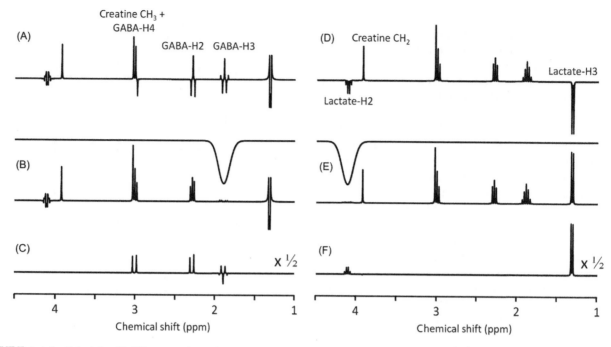

FIGURE 1.4.5   Principle of J-difference editing illustrated for (A–C) GABA and (D–F) lactate. (A, D) ^{1}H NMR spectrum acquired without selective refocusing at TE = $(2J)^{-1}$ and J^{-1} for (A) GABA and (D) lactate. (B, E) ^{1}H NMR spectrum acquired with selective refocusing at TE = $(2J)^{-1}$ and J^{-1} for (B) GABA and (E) lactate. The selective refocusing pulses were applied to (B) GABA-H3 and (E) lactate-H2. The J-difference editing difference spectrum for (C) = (B) − (A) GABA and (F) = (E) − (D) lactate. Note that all other resonances are identical between the two scans, such that they are subtracted out.

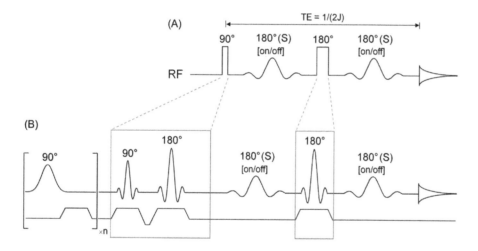

FIGURE 1.4.6   Required modifications to convert (A) the basic J-difference editing sequence into (B) a 3D localized, water-suppressed MEGA-PRESS editing method. CHESS water suppression (ref) is depicted, but can easily be changed to VAPOR (ref) or MEGA (ref). When using MEGA water suppression, the frequency-selective refocusing pulses are made double banded, with one frequency band selectively refocusing (and thus dephasing) the water resonance, while the other frequency band is used for spectral editing.

compound can, in principle, be editing as is shown for lactate in Fig. 1.4.5D–F.

The pulse sequence for homonuclear J-difference editing as depicted in Fig. 1.4.3A is purely theoretical and needs to be augmented with spatial localization and water-suppression techniques for applications *in vivo*. Fig. 1.4.6 shows a popular implementation of J-difference editing, commonly referred to as MEscher–GArwood-Point RESolved Spectrometry (MEGA-PRESS; Mescher et al., 1998). It utilizes PRESS for spatial localization and can accommodate a range of water-suppression techniques, of which VAriable Pulse

power and Optimized Relaxation (VAPOR) and MEGA are most commonly used. The combination of two frequency-selective refocusing pulses ensures the absence of any editing pulse-related phase effects.

IN VIVO GABA EDITING

When the described spectral editing methods are applied *in vivo*, the results are typically complicated by a number of effects, some of which will be described for *in vivo* GABA editing in the human brain at 7 T.

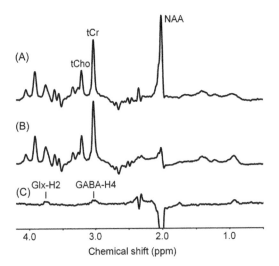

FIGURE 1.4.7   *In vivo* GABA editing on the human brain at 7 T (2 × 2 × 2 cm volume, repetition time TR = 3000 ms, TE = 68 ms, number of averages = 2 × 64). The frequency-selective spectral editing pulse is applied at (A) 4.13 ppm and (B) 1.89 ppm in order to manipulate the J-evolution of GABA. The difference between (A) and (B) gives the edited GABA-H4 signal. Note the co-edited signals from glutamate/glutamine (Glx) H2 at 3.75 ppm, *N*-acetyl aspartate (NAA) at 2.01 ppm and macromolecules at circa 0.9 ppm. Data are courtesy of Christoph Juchem.

Under ideal conditions, the magnetic environment of the location from which the signal is acquired is completely stable. However, the magnetic field in the human brain can vary over time due to respiration, cardiac-related pulsations, head or limb movement, magnet drift, or heating of the gradient/shim coils. These temporal magnetic field variations can lead to phase, frequency, and linewidth variations in the acquired NMR spectra, which in turn can lead to subtraction artifacts in the edited NMR spectrum. Several strategies can be employed to minimize these variations, including respiratory and cardiac triggering and real-time magnetic field monitoring and correction (Henry et al., 1999). One of the simplest strategies to minimize the effects of magnetic field variation is to acquire the editing data in an interleaved manner and store each free induction decay separately (de Graaf, 2007). Phase and frequency variations can then be corrected post acquisition. This strategy can be completely automated and user transparent on both the acquisition and processing sides and should be the default mode for any difference (editing) experiment.

Fig. 1.4.7 shows the detection of GABA in the human brain at 7 T by MEGA-PRESS spectral editing. In Fig. 1.4.7A the frequency-selective refocusing pulses are applied at 4.13 ppm, such that scalar coupling evolution is not inhibited thereby leading to an inversion of the outer resonance lines of GABA-H4 at 3.01 ppm relative to creatine. In Fig. 1.4.7B the editing pulses are applied to the GABA-H3 resonance at 1.89 ppm, thereby inhibiting the scalar coupling evolution and thus making all GABA-H4 resonance lines positive. The difference between the two spectra, as shown in Fig. 1.4.7C, gives the edited spectrum in which the GABA-H4 resonance is clearly visible without spectral overlap of creatine. Besides the GABA-H4 signal at 3.01 ppm, the difference spectrum also holds other signals, most noticeably an inverted signal from NAA. This is a so-called co-edited signal and is due to the finite bandwidth of the frequency-selective refocusing pulses. Ideally, the selective refocusing only affects the GABA-H3 resonance at 1.89 ppm. However, the echo time of $1/(2J)$ ~68 ms limits the length of the frequency-selective refocusing pulses to a maximum of about 20 ms. A 20 ms Gaussian refocusing pulse (truncated at 10%) has a bandwidth at half maximum of about 60 Hz = 0.2 ppm at 7 T, such that the NAA resonance at 2.01 ppm is also partially affected. The co-editing of NAA is inconsequential for GABA-H4 detection, as the NAA and GABA-H4 resonances are not overlapping. However, there are examples in which the unwanted co-edited signal is overlapping with the edited signal of interest. For GABA-H4 detection this situation arises with the co-editing of macromolecular (MM) signals. Macromolecules represent a large collection of proteins that gives broad, but detectable signals in ^1H NMR spectra. In Fig. 1.4.1 a number of MM resonances are visible between 1 and 2 ppm, with many other signals residing between 2 and 4 ppm underneath the metabolites signals. ^1H NMR spectra from rat (Behar & Ogino, 1991, 1993) and human (Hwang et al., 1996) brain contain MM resonances at 3.00 and 1.72 ppm that are scalar coupled to each other (J ~ 7 Hz). It follows that if the MM signal at 1.72 ppm is (partially) refocused when the editing pulses are applied at the GABA-H3 frequency at 1.89 ppm, the MM signal at 3.00 ppm is co-edited with GABA-H4. At lower magnetic field strengths the total edited signal at 3.0 ppm can contain as much as 50% MM contamination. A useful strategy to minimize the co-editing of MM signal is the symmetrical editing method proposed by Henry et al. (2001). Here the editing pulses are applied at 1.89 ppm in one experiment and symmetrical around the MM signal at $1.72 − (1.89 − 1.72) = 1.55$ ppm in the second experiment. Under the assumption that the MM signal at 1.72 ppm is symmetrical, the MM contribution is the same in both experiments and will thus be subtracted out in the difference spectrum. Fortunately, the frequency difference between GABA-H3 and MM at 7 T becomes large enough that the selectivity of the editing pulses is sufficient to avoid perturbation of the MM signal. However, co-editing of signals is the rule rather than the exception and the exact composition of the edited signal should always be established before conclusions are drawn.

2D NMR SPECTROSCOPY

The concept of 2D NMR was first described by Jeener in 1971 and was theoretically and experimentally formalized by Ernst and coworkers in 1976 (Aue et al., 1976a,b). To stay in line with the rest of this chapter 2D NMR spectroscopy can be seen as a generalization of spectral editing in which no assumptions are made about the spin systems or their spectral overlap. The number of different 2D NMR methods currently reaches into the hundreds as researchers are pushing the boundaries on manipulation and detection opportunities, especially in large spin systems like proteins and DNA. However, the number of 2D NMR methods that have been used, and are suitable for, *in vivo* applications is limited, largely due to time and sensitivity restrictions. The very first method described by Jeener in 1971, which is now known as correlation spectroscopy (COSY), is still one of the most commonly used sequences for *in vivo* 2D NMR. In its most basic form, COSY is a two-pulse sequence consisting of two 90° pulses separated by a variable delay t_1 and signal acquisition immediately following the second 90° pulse. Following excitation, uncoupled spins evolve in the transverse plane under the influence of chemical shift, T_2 relaxation, and magnetic field inhomogeneity. Following a delay t_1, the second 90° pulse transfers part of the magnetization to the longitudinal axis and leaves the rest in the transverse plane. During the acquisition time t_2, the chemical shift is identical to that during the evolution time t_1. Acquiring a full 2D dataset $S(t_1, t_2)$ by linearly incrementing t_1 in subsequent scans will thus give a spectrum $F(\nu_1, \nu_2)$ in which all resonances are on the diagonal where $\nu_1 = \nu_2$. For uncoupled spins the acquisition of a 2D dataset thus provides no additional information relative to a conventional 1D NMR spectrum. However, the situation for scalar-coupled spins is distinctly different. Consider a scalar-coupled two-spin system AX with resonance frequencies ν_A and ν_X and scalar coupling J_{AX}. Following excitation, spin A will evolve under the influence of chemical shift, T_2 relaxation, magnetic field inhomogeneity, and scalar coupling. During the evolution time t_1 spin A will precess at resonance frequency ν_A. The second 90° pulse again transfers part of the magnetization to the longitudinal axis, leaves part in the transverse plane evolving at frequency ν_A, and now also converts part of the spin A magnetization to spin X magnetization. This process is referred to as polarization transfer and has the effect that the precession of magnetization during the t_1 and t_2 evolution periods is no longer equal. Acquiring a full 2D dataset $S(t_1, t_2)$ now gives a spectrum $F(\nu_1, \nu_2)$, which contains, along with the diagonal signal

(ν_A, ν_A), also a cross-peak at (ν_A, ν_X). Using similar arguments, it can be readily be shown that the X spins have signals at (ν_X, ν_X) and (ν_X, ν_A). By observing cross-peaks between spins A and X, it is immediately revealed that spins A and X are scalar coupled. This information is invaluable for the determination of the chemical structure of unknown compounds. For purposes of spectral editing, uncoupled spins do not generate cross-peaks, such that cross-peaks are typically not hampered by spectral overlap. Fig. 1.4.8A shows a theoretical 2D COSY spectrum for a mixture of creatine, GABA, and lactate. It can be seen that creatine only has diagonal signals. GABA-H3 has cross-peaks with GABA-H2 and GABA-H4, but there is no cross-peak between GABA-H2 and GABA-H4 since they are not (directly) scalar coupled. Even though the GABA-H4 resonance is overlapping with creatine in a regular 1D NMR spectrum, the cross-peaks between GABA-H4 and GABA-H3 are free from spectral overlap, allowing the unambiguous detection of GABA.

The basic two-pulse implementation of COSY has a number of limitations. First, the polarization transfer between two spins is dependent on the scalar coupling constant and can thus not be optimal for all metabolites simultaneously. Second, all 2D NMR peaks have a fine structure in which multiple resonance lines contribute to a diagonal or cross-peak. For cross-peaks this fine structure contains both positive and negative signals, such that the total peak intensity depends on the magnetic field homogeneity, as positive and negative peaks cancel each other more for wider lines. Third, small cross-peaks close to larger diagonal peaks often get obscured by the "tails" of the diagonal signals. Fourth, as the sequence only has two pulses, COSY cannot achieve 3D spatial localization. For these and other reasons, the basic two-pulse COSY sequence is rarely used *in vivo*. There are many variants of COSY to enhance cross-peaks, remove diagonal peaks, or allow spatial localization. TOCSY (Braunschweiler & Ernst, 1983) can be seen as an ultimate extension of COSY in that a TOCSY spectrum shows all possible correlations even between spins that are not directly coupled. Fig. 1.4.8B shows the general layout for a 2D TOCSY spectrum for a mixture of creatine, GABA, and lactate. The main difference is that the spectrum now also shows a 2D cross-peak between GABA-H2 and GABA-H4, even though they are not directly coupled. Another difference is that TOCSY signals tend to be all positive and in-phase.

A final 2D NMR method that has acquired some popularity for *in vivo* use is the 2D J-resolved (JRES) experiment. The primary purpose of a 2D JRES experiment is to separate chemical shifts and scalar couplings along two orthogonal axes. The basic pulse

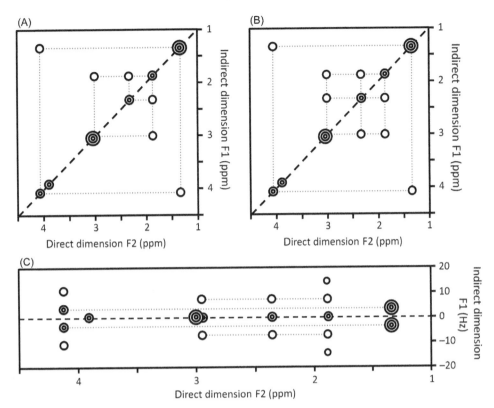

FIGURE 1.4.8 Theoretical (A) COSY, (B) TOCSY, and (C) J-resolved 2D NMR spectra for a mixture of creatine, GABA, and lactate. Traditionally 2D NMR spectra are plotted as contour plots in which closed loops drawn at fixed heights indicate equal intensity. Intense and weak signals can then be distinguished by the number of contour lines. Note that in reality all 2D NMR signals have a fine structure, often with both positive and negative resonances within a single cross or diagonal peak.

sequence for 2D JRES is shown in Fig. 1.4.3A and is essentially a Hahn spin echo with $t_1 = TE$. For every t_1 increment the chemical shifts are refocused, such that the t_1 dimension only holds information on scalar couplings. The direct t_2 dimension holds the regular spectrum with both chemical shift and scalar coupling information. Following Fourier transformation of a dataset $S(t_1, t_2)$ the 2D NMR spectrum $F(\nu_1, \nu_2)$ holds signals that appear to stand along a 45° rotated axis. After the 2D NMR spectrum is rotated by 45°, a final 2D JRES spectrum as shown in Fig. 1.4.8C is obtained. Along the F1 dimension all signals are centered on zero, as the chemical shifts are refocused, and only show the scalar coupling splitting pattern (e.g., a doublet for lactate at 1.32 ppm and a quintet for GABA-H3 at 1.89 ppm). Along the F2 dimension the regular ^{1}H NMR spectrum is visible, with the exception that the scalar coupling appears to have been removed. Summing the 2D NMR spectrum over the F1 dimension will therefore provide a homonuclear decoupling NMR spectrum. In addition to the aforementioned methods (COSY, TOCSY, JRES), there have been a limited number of papers of more "exotic" 2D NMR methods. These include heteronuclear methods (van

Zijl et al., 1993; Watanabe et al., 2000) and multiple quantum-based methods (de Graaf et al., 2007).

In conclusion, at the currently available magnetic field strengths, spectral overlap of resonances from different compounds is routinely observed. Primary examples are the overlap of GABA and creatine, glutamate, and glutamine and lactate and lipids. In the case of partial spectral overlap, the compounds may be separated through a spectral fitting routine and going to a higher magnetic field strength. However, in the case of complete spectral overlap, the use of spectral editing or 2D NMR is mandatory. On relatively stable organs like the brain or muscle, the use of J-difference editing is most straightforward and can provide consistent and reliable results.

References

Aue, W. P., Bartholdi, E., & Ernst, R. R. (1976a). Two-dimensional spectroscopy. Application to nuclear magnetic resonance. *Journal of Chemical Physics, 64*, 2229–2246.

Aue, W. P., Karhan, J., & Ernst, R. R. (1976b). Homonuclear broadband decoupling in two-dimensional J-resolved NMR spectroscopy. *Journal of Chemical Physics, 64*, 4226–4227.

Behar, K. L., & Ogino, T. (1991). Assignment of resonance in the ^{1}H spectrum of rat brain by two-dimensional shift correlated and J-resolved NMR spectroscopy. *Magnetic Resonance in Medicine, 17,* 285–303.

Behar, K. L., & Ogino, T. (1993). Characterization of macromolecule resonances in the ^{1}H NMR spectrum of rat brain. *Magnetic Resonance in Medicine, 30,* 38–44.

Braunschweiler, L., & Ernst, R. R. (1983). Coherence transfer by isotropic mixing: application to proton correlation spectroscopy. *Journal of Magnetic Resonance, 53,* 521–528.

de Graaf, R. A. (2007). *In vivo NMR spectroscopy. Principles and Techniques.* Chichester, UK: John Wiley.

de Graaf, R. A., Rothman, D. L., & Behar, K. L. (2007). High resolution NMR spectroscopy of rat brain *in vivo* through indirect zero-quantum-coherence detection. *Journal of Magnetic Resonance, 187,* 320–326.

Ernst, R. R., Bodenhausen, G., & Wokaun, A. (1987). *Principles of Nuclear Magnetic Resonance in One and Two Dimensions.* Oxford, UK: Clarendon Press.

Henry, P. G., Dautry, C., Hantraye, P., & Bloch, G. (2001). Brain GABA editing without macromolecule contamination. *Magnetic Resonance in Medicine, 45,* 517–520.

Henry, P. G., van de Moortele, P. F., Giacomini, E., Nauerth, A., & Bloch, G. (1999). Field-frequency locked *in vivo* proton MRS on a whole-body spectrometer. *Magnetic Resonance in Medicine, 42,* 636–642.

Hwang, J. H., Graham, G. D., Behar, K. L., Alger, J. R., Prichard, J. W., & Rothman, D. L. (1996). Short echo time proton magnetic resonance spectroscopic imaging of macromolecule and metabolite signal intensities in the human brain. *Magnetic Resonance in Medicine, 35,* 633–639.

Levitt, M. H. (2005). *Spin dynamics. Basics of Nuclear Magnetic Resonance.* New York: Wiley.

Mescher, M., Merkle, H., Kirsch, J., Garwood, M., & Gruetter, R. (1998). Simultaneous *in vivo* spectral editing and water suppression. *NMR in Biomedicine, 11,* 266–272.

Rothman, D. L., Behar, K. L., Hetherington, H. P., & Shulman, R. G. (1984). Homonuclear ^{1}H double-resonance difference spectroscopy of the rat brain *in vivo*. *Proceedings of the National Academy of Sciences USA, 81,* 6330–6334.

van Zijl, P. C., Chesnick, A. S., DesPres, D., Moonen, C. T., Ruiz-Cabello, J., & van Gelderen, P. (1993). *In vivo* proton spectroscopy and spectroscopic imaging of [1-^{13}C]-glucose and its metabolic products. *Magnetic Resonance in Medicine, 30,* 544–551.

Watanabe, H., Umeda, M., Ishihara, Y., Okamoto, K., Oshio, K., Kanamatsu, T., et al. (2000). Human brain glucose metabolism mapping using multislice 2D ^{1}H-^{13}C correlation HSQC spectroscopy. *Magnetic Resonance in Medicine, 43,* 525–533.

Spectral Quantification and Pitfalls in Interpreting Magnetic Resonance Spectroscopic Data: What To Look Out For

Jamie Near

Department of Psychiatry, McGill University, and the Centre d'Imagerie du Cerveau, Douglas Mental Health
University Institute, Montreal, QC, Canada

INTRODUCTION: A SIMPLE EXAMPLE OF SPECTRAL QUANTITATION

Spectral quantification generally involves measuring the intensity of a spectral peak or a group of peaks, and then converting the measured peak intensity into a metabolite concentration estimate. On its own, peak intensity is a meaningless quantity, usually in arbitrary units, whose value is influenced by numerous factors such as voxel size, voxel placement, radiofrequency (RF) coil sensitivity, receiver gain, and other experimental factors. The conversion of a peak intensity into a meaningful quantitative metabolite concentration is a critical step that requires the use of a reference peak: a spectral peak from a compound whose concentration is known. A metabolite concentration estimate, then, is obtained by comparing the intensity of the desired metabolite peak with the intensity of a reference peak.

To illustrate the process of spectral quantification, consider the following simple example. Imagine a sample containing two magnetic resonance (MR)-visible compounds, compound A and compound B. Suppose that the concentration of compound A is well known to be 10 mM, and that the concentration of compound B is unknown. Finally, we know that compound A contains two MR-visible protons, which give rise to a singlet peak at 3 parts per million (ppm), and that compound B contains three MR-visible protons, which give rise to a singlet peak at 2 ppm. Assume for simplicity that the two compounds have identical relaxation properties. Fig. 1.5.1

shows an example of a processed spectrum that might be obtained from this hypothetical sample.

Before we go on to perform spectral quantification on this example spectrum, we note that the peak intensity, I_j, for a given compound, j, is proportional to the concentration of that compound, $[j]$, as well as the number of MR-visible protons per molecule, N_j. Therefore in the following equation:

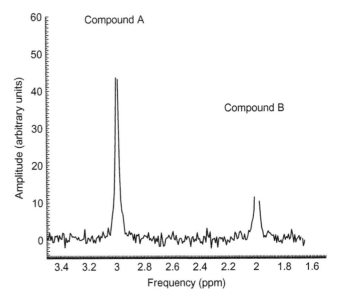

FIGURE 1.5.1 Example of processed spectrum that might be obtained by a hypothetical sample containing only two MR-visible compounds.

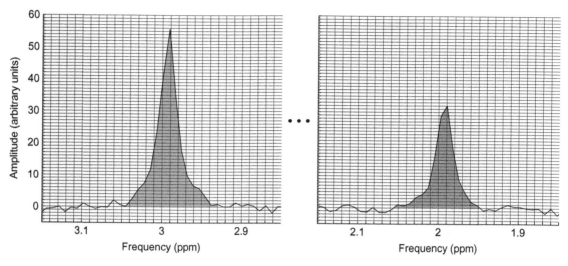

FIGURE 1.5.2　Calculation of peak intensities by overlaying the spectrum with a grid and shading the area under the peaks of interest.

$$I_A = [A] \cdot N_A \cdot e^{-TE/T2_A} \cdot \left(1 - e^{-TR/T1_A}\right) \cdot K \qquad (1)$$

$$I_B = [B] \cdot N_B \cdot e^{-TE/T2_B} \cdot \left(1 - e^{-TR/T1_B}\right) \cdot K \qquad (2)$$

$T1_j$ and $T2_j$ are the longitudinal and transverse relaxation rates, respectively, of compound j, TR is the repetition time, TE is the echo time, and the proportionality constant, K, accounts for effects such as coil sensitivity, voxel volume, receiver gain, and field strength.

Now, in order to determine the unknown concentration of compound B, we must measure its peak intensity. A number of methods exist for the measurement of peak intensities, but for this example let us use the simple method of peak integration, which involves calculating the area under (or integrating) each peak. While peak integration is most often done using software, it can also be done manually, simply by overlaying the spectrum with a grid and shading the area under the peaks of interest, as shown in Fig. 1.5.2. (In fact, this is likely how most of us learned how to calculate the areas of 2D shapes back in elementary school.)

By counting the shaded boxes and fractions thereof, we can obtain an estimate of the area under each peak. Importantly, measuring peak intensities in this manner gives us a value in units of "boxes," which is a completely arbitrary unit that depends on the size of the grid that we choose. Furthermore, we cannot directly use Equation 2 to calculate the concentration of B, because the factor K is unknown. However, by rearranging Equations 1 and 2 we can obtain the following expression for the relative concentrations of compounds A and B:

$$\frac{[B]}{[A]} = \frac{I_B}{I_A} \cdot \frac{N_A}{N_B} \qquad (3)$$

Note that the factor K has vanished. Note also that if compounds A and B have the same relaxation rates (as we assume in this example), the exponential relaxation terms also vanish. Given this estimated concentration ratio, and given that the concentration of the reference compound is known, we can finally calculate the concentration of compound B. In the previous example, the intensity of peak B was approximately 98 boxes, while the intensity of the reference peak, A, was approximately 176 boxes. Recall that each molecule of compound B contained three MR-visible protons ($N_B = 3$), while the reference compound, A, contained two MR-visible protons ($N_A = 2$). Then, from Equation 3, the concentration ratio [B]/[A] is 0.37. Since we know that the concentration of the reference metabolite is 10 mM, it follows that the concentration of compound B is 3.7 mM. If the concentration of the reference metabolite was unknown, then we would not have been able to calculate the concentration of metabolite B in absolute units. We would still, however, have been able to calculate the concentration ratio, which may be a useful quantity. Furthermore, it is important to note that our measurement of [B] has some uncertainty associated with it, and that the magnitude of that uncertainty depends on the uncertainty of the peak intensity measurements.

The previous example was intended to demonstrate the process of spectral quantification, and to show that spectral quantification is, at least in principle, fairly straightforward. Under more realistic circumstances, spectral quantification can be significantly more complicated due to the presence of more complex spectral lineshapes, overlapping peaks, macromolecule signal contamination, and T_1 and T_2 relaxation.

In this chapter, we will discuss some of the more commonly used spectral quantification approaches, and ways of dealing with the issues mentioned earlier. We will introduce some of the most commonly used spectral quantification software packages, and their various applications. We will discuss some of the most commonly used reference compounds *in vivo*, and the advantages and disadvantages of each. Finally, we will outline some of the most commonly used methods for ensuring the accuracy and reliability of MR spectroscopic (MRS) methods.

MEASURING PEAK INTENSITY

As mentioned previously, there are a number of methods of measuring peak intensity in MR spectra. Among the methods that exist, the three most common are peak integration, peak fitting, and basis spectrum fitting.

Peak Integration

Peak integration is the simplest and most antiquated method of determining peak intensities. The strength of peak integration is its simplicity and ease of implementation: as demonstrated in the introduction to this chapter, it is easily done even without the aid of a computer. However, there are a number of major drawbacks of peak integration that limit its applicability in real-world situations. Namely, peak integration cannot effectively separate the contributions from overlapping, or even partially overlapping peaks. This is a severely limiting factor in the case of *in vivo* MRS, where spectra may consist of overlapping peaks from more than 15 metabolites as well as broad signals from macromolecules. Furthermore, peak integration measurements are influenced by errors in the phase of the spectrum, as well as the choice of the frequency range over which the peaks are integrated.

Despite its drawbacks, peak integration warrants some discussion in any text on spectral quantification. It was, after all, the method of choice for most early papers on *in vivo* MRS (Arus et al., 1985; Cady & Azzopardi, 1989; Matson et al., 1993). Peak integration is normally performed in the frequency domain (the domain in which the spectral peaks are observed). However, an important property of the Fourier transform results in the area of a signal in the frequency domain being exactly equal to the amplitude of the first point of the same signal in the time domain. Therefore, if a spectrum consists of only a single spectral peak (such as is approximately the case in a water-unsuppressed spectrum, for example), the peak "integration" can be performed simply by reading the amplitude of the first point in the free induction decay

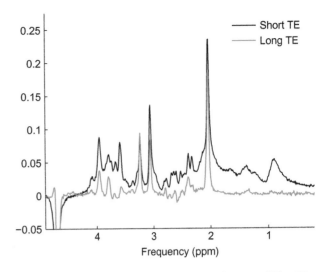

FIGURE 1.5.3 A comparison of short echo time (TE = 8.5 ms, blue curve) and long echo time (270 ms, green curve) spectra in the same subject (different voxel locations). The metabolite signals in the short echo-time spectrum are superimposed on a background of broad baseline resonances. At long echo times, the short-T_2 baseline resonances have decayed away, and the metabolites are observed with a flat baseline.

(FID). In the case of a spectrum containing multiple peaks, however, the amplitude of the first point in the FID is equal to the sum of the peak areas in the spectrum, and can therefore no longer be used to estimate the area under any individual peaks.

Although the requirement of nonoverlapping peaks is a major limiting factor for the applicability of peak integration, this requirement can be satisfied in some real-life situations. For example, at long echo times, the signals from macromolecules and coupled metabolites are relatively small due to T_2 decay and scalar evolution, and spectra are dominated by large singlet resonances from *N*-acetylaspartate (NAA), choline, and creatine (Fig. 1.5.3). In such spectra, the peak amplitudes of the large singlet resonances can be estimated using peak integration. A second example where peak integration is sometimes feasible is phosphorus 31 (^{31}P) or carbon 13 (^{13}C) MRS. For both of these nuclei, the resonances observed *in vivo* span a very large range of chemical shift values, resulting in fewer overlapping peaks than typical proton spectra.

There are several ways to perform peak integration in practice. Here is a brief step-by-step example of one possible method:

1. Ensure that the spectrum is properly phased by adjusting the zero-order and (if necessary) first-order phase of the spectrum until all of the singlet peaks are perfectly upright (Fig. 1.5.4A). If the phase is not properly adjusted, then the peak amplitude will be underestimated.

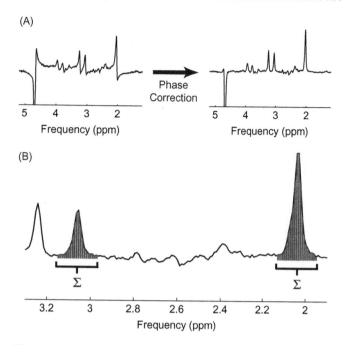

FIGURE 1.5.4 The method of peak integration. (A) First the phase of the spectrum is adjusted such that the metabolite peaks are upright. (B) Peaks of interest are then integrated numerically by summing the discrete spectral points under within a specified range.

2. Choose a frequency range over which to perform the peak integration. If multiple peaks are to be integrated, the chosen range should be a constant fraction of the peak width, or at least twice the width of the broadest peak.

3. Calculate the peak area (Fig. 1.5.4B) by taking the real part of the sum of the discrete spectral points within the integration range, and multiplying by the spectral resolution (the frequency difference between adjacent spectral points). Such numerical integration can be done using any software that allows you to view the spectrum as a vector of intensity values, such as MATLAB, IDL, or even Microsoft Excel.

As mentioned earlier, the method of peak integration is severely limited in the presence of overlapping peaks. One way to improve the handling of overlapping signals is to fit peaks to a model function, a method known as peak fitting.

Peak Fitting

Peak fitting involves choosing a model function that best describes the shape of the peak of interest, and then fitting that function to the data. The fit can sometimes be improved by imposing some restrictions, known as prior knowledge, on some of the model parameters. The quality of the fit is assessed by the difference between the data and the fitted curve, or the residual, with small residuals indicative of a good fit. Once the model function has been fit to the data, the estimated peak intensity is given by the intensity of the fitted model function. Fig. 1.5.5 shows an example of the peak fitting method.

The three most commonly used model functions are Lorentzian, Gaussian, and Voigt lineshapes. Each model is described briefly in the following paragraph.

MRS FIDs are often roughly approximated as decaying monoexponential signals in the time domain. A Lorentzian lineshape is simply the frequency domain representation of such a decaying monoexponential. In other words, if we were to measure the MR signal from an ensemble of spins undergoing perfect monoexponential T_2 decay, the complex Fourier transform of this signal would be a Lorentzian function. For this reason, the Lorentzian function seems a natural choice of modeling function for fitting MRS peaks; indeed they are probably the most commonly used fitting model functions in MR spectral quantification. In the MRS literature, the term "Lorentzian fitting" generally refers to the process of fitting the data to a Lorentzian curve in the frequency domain, *or* to a decaying exponential in the time domain. Mathematically, the Lorentzian function is most intuitively represented in the time domain, as a decaying complex exponential as seen Equation 4:

$$s(t) = A \cdot e^{-i(\omega_0(t+t_0)+\phi)} \cdot e^{-(t+t_0)/T2} \qquad (4)$$

where A is the signal amplitude, $T2$ is the transverse relaxation rate, ω_0 is the frequency offset in radians per second, t_0 is the temporal shift between $t = 0$ and the top of the echo, and ϕ is the global phase offset in radians.

The assumption of a monoexponential decay of a single frequency (on which the Lorentzian model is based) is somewhat simplistic. In real-world situations, the NMR signal consists of a distribution of frequencies due to spatial variations in the static magnetic field. This spread of frequencies can be approximated as a Gaussian distribution. Therefore, the use of Gaussian fitting functions has also been proposed (Vanhamme et al., 2001). Because the Fourier transform of a Gaussian is, itself, Gaussian, the corresponding time domain and frequency domain model functions are of the same form, and the relationship between the time and frequency domains is such that a quickly decaying Gaussian-shaped signal in the time domain leads to a broad Gaussian-shaped peak in the frequency domain. Conversely, a slowly decaying Gaussian-shaped signal in the time domain leads to a sharp Gaussian-shaped peak in the frequency domain.

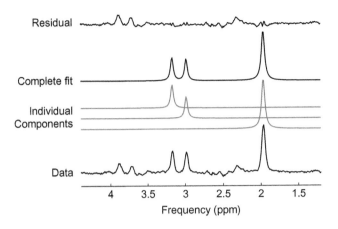

FIGURE 1.5.5 The method of peak fitting. Peaks of interest are each fit to a Lorentzian lineshape model to estimate their intensities. The quality of the fit is assessed by looking at the flatness of the residual.

The time domain representation of a Gaussian MRS signal is expressed in the following way:

$$s(t) = A \cdot e^{-i(\omega_0(t+t_0)+\phi)} \cdot e^{-(\pi\beta(t+t_0))^2/4 \cdot \log 2} \qquad (5)$$

where β is the Gaussian damping factor.

Like the Lorentzian model, the Gaussian model is also somewhat oversimplified. It assumes purely Gaussian broadening, but ignores any monoexponential decay component. A third model, called the Voigt model, addresses the shortcomings of both the Lorentzian and Gaussian lineshape models simply by combining them. The Voigt model consists of a monoexponential decay (Lorentzian) component to account for T_2 relaxation, as well as a Gaussian broadening component to account for magnetic field inhomogeneity. The Voigt model has been shown to provide improved fitting performance in comparison with both Lorentzian and Gaussian models (Marshall et al., 1997; Bartha et al., 1999). An expression for the Voigt model in the time domain is shown in Equation 6:

$$s(t) = A \cdot e^{-i(\omega_0(t+t_0)+\phi)} \cdot e^{-(t+t_0)/T2} \cdot e^{-(\pi\beta(t+t_0))^2/4\log 2} \qquad (6)$$

One potential drawback of the Voigt method is that inclusion of both Gaussian and Lorentzian damping factors introduces an extra parameter into the model, which may be a source of error (Jansen et al., 2006).

MRS data can be fit to any of the previous models in the time domain using Equations 4, 5, or 6. These models can also be adapted to some extent to allow for fitting in the frequency domain; however, time domain models are often more convenient because subtle yet important effects such as time shifting or FID truncation are not easily modeled in the frequency domain (Joliot et al., 1991; Marshall et al., 1997; Bartha et al., 1999). However, provided that the fitting is done correctly, time domain and frequency domain fitting

methods should produce similar results (Joliot et al., 1991; van den Boogaart et al., 1994).

Fitting the earlier models to the data is achieved by adjusting the parameters (A, T_2, and/or β, ω_0, t_0, and ϕ) until the model function matches the data as closely as possible, or more accurately, until the square of the absolute value of the residual is minimized as follows:

$$minimize |\mathscr{S} - s|^2 \qquad (7)$$

where $\mathscr{S}$ is the data and s is the model function.

Efficient and accurate methods of performing this minimization are numerous and varied; however, such methods involve advanced mathematics, and are beyond the scope of this text. Fortunately, there are a number of user-friendly software programs available that provide state-of-the-art spectral fitting algorithms in an easy-to-use graphical user interface, meaning that you do not have to be an expert in mathematics to perform spectral fitting. Some of the available software packages will be discussed later in this chapter.

As mentioned previously, the quality of the fit can sometimes be improved by placing restrictions on one or more of the model parameters based on prior knowledge of the spectral appearance. While some fitting routines require very little prior knowledge in order to perform effectively, others benefit from a very large amount of prior knowledge. For example, since metabolite concentrations are necessarily positive values, it would make sense to ensure that the signal amplitudes, A, must also be positive. By enforcing this type of prior knowledge, we can prevent the fitting algorithm from finding "nonphysical" solutions, as well as improve the speed and efficiency of the algorithm. Another example of commonly used prior knowledge is the frequency of the spectral peaks. Because the frequencies of metabolite peaks are highly reproducible, and are generally well known a priori, it is often helpful to include this information in the model to reduce the computational workload and improve accuracy.

Not only can we specify the absolute frequency of individual peaks, but we can also place prior knowledge restrictions on the relative frequency offsets and the relative amplitudes between different spectral peaks. This is particularly helpful in the case of metabolites that have complex spectral patterns. For example, the spectral signature of NAA consists of at least five individual peaks whose relative frequencies and intensities are fixed, and can be determined a priori (Bartha et al., 1999). If the concentration of NAA changes, the signal intensity of each of these five peaks changes proportionally, but their relative frequencies and intensities remain unchanged. Indeed, the vast majority of metabolites found *in vivo* consist of a series of peaks whose relative frequencies and intensities are fixed. Therefore, the inclusion of this type of prior knowledge can be extremely valuable in improving the quality and efficiency of spectral fitting.

Basis Spectrum Fitting

The earlier discussion suggests that it may be beneficial to include "within metabolite" prior knowledge by fixing the relative peak intensities and frequencies for each fitted peak. However, given that there are upward of 15 different metabolite signals in a typical MR spectrum, some of which consist of over 10 individual peaks, the total number of modeled peaks (and the amount of prior knowledge required to specify their relative frequencies and intensities) would become very large. One way of simplifying this situation is to model each metabolite spectrum not as the sum of individual peaks, or model functions, but as a single "basis spectrum." A basis spectrum is a complete representation of an individual metabolite's spectral shape, or signature, and it is usually defined numerically; it is not expressed using a mathematical formula. The method of basis spectrum fitting is highly intuitive, and is based on the logical principle that if the shape (or basis spectrum) of each individual metabolite signal is known, then an MRS spectrum can be modeled as a linear combination of the individual metabolite basis spectra. In current MRS literature, the method of basis spectrum fitting is probably the most commonly used method of spectral quantification. As the name suggests, basis spectrum fitting differs from peak fitting in that spectral fitting generally involves fitting the entire spectrum to a series of basis functions, whereas peak fitting may involve fitting as little as one single peak of interest. Basis spectrum fitting has been shown to outperform peak fitting in terms of quantification accuracy for the analysis of *in vivo* short echo-time MRS data (Kanowski et al., 2004). Fig. 1.5.6 shows an example spectrum that was fit using the method of basis spectrum fitting, we well as the individual basis spectrum components of the fit.

There are two methods of determining the basis spectrum for an individual metabolite. The first, and probably more outdated method is to determine the basis spectrum simply by measuring it experimentally. This is achieved by preparing an aqueous solution of the metabolite of interest, and acquiring a MR spectrum directly from this solution. Experimentally acquiring the basis spectra has the advantage that experimental imperfections present in the *in vivo* data will be accounted for by the basis spectra, provided

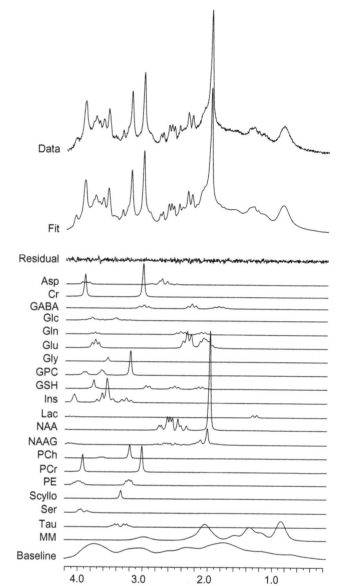

FIGURE 1.5.6 The method of basis spectrum fitting. The entire spectrum is fit to a linear combination of model spectra, or basis spectra. Each basis spectrum corresponds to an individual metabolite, and the amplitude of the basis spectra corresponds to the metabolite concentrations. Once again, the residual is an indicator of the goodness of fit.

that the experimental basis spectra are acquired on the same scanner and with the same pulse sequence that will be used to acquire the *in vivo* MRS data. On the other hand, the biggest drawback to measuring the basis spectra experimentally is that, given the large number of metabolites of interest, it is very expensive and time-consuming to purchase the necessary chemicals, to carefully prepare the phantoms, and to physically acquire the MRS data and to process the results for each of the metabolites of interest.

The second method of determining the basis spectra is to use quantum mechanical simulations. This involves predicting the signal that would be observed from an individual metabolite based on the known properties of the spin system, and the specific sequence of pulses used in the acquisition. The most relevant spin-system properties are the number of MR-visible protons, their chemical shifts, and the couplings between them. For most metabolites observed *in vivo*, the chemical shifts and coupling constants have been estimated using high-resolution NMR, and are available in literature (Govindaraju et al., 2000; de Graaf, 2007; Near et al., 2012). The minimum required information about the acquisition is the field strength, number of RF pulses in the pulse sequence, the flip angle of each of the pulses, and their exact timings, although it is often beneficial to include additional information, such as the exact shape of the RF pulses and the slice-selective gradient strengths. Given all of the information regarding both the spin system and the acquisition, it is possible to simulate the experiment to predict the resulting signal. This is done using a quantum mechanical approach called the density matrix formalism, the details of which are beyond the scope of this text. For the interested reader, a number of resources are available on the topic of the density matrix formalism (Slichter, 1992; Mulkern & Bowers, 1994). One of the major drawbacks of the use of the density matrix formalism is that basis spectra produced using this method do not necessarily take into account system imperfections that are observed in real-world experimental data. Specifically, simulations do not generally account for gradient-induced eddy currents, receiver digitization errors, and chemical shift displacement errors induced by slice-selective refocusing pulses (although it is possible to account for the latter using spatially resolved simulations; Maudsley et al., 2005). A second drawback of the density matrix approach is its relative mathematical complexity, and the computational workload required to perform simulations for large spin systems (especially when the effects of shaped RF pulses and gradients are taken into account). Despite this limitation, a number of user-friendly software packages have been developed for the express purpose of generating simulated metabolite basis spectra for *in vivo* MR spectroscopy. Available packages include the GAMMA software library (Smith et al., 1994), GAVA (Soher et al., 2007), NMR-SCOPE (Stefan et al., 2009), and Vespa (http://scion.duhs.duke.edu/vespa/).

Whether the basis set is generated experimentally or using simulations, it is important to note that the basis set is specific to the pulse sequence and timing parameters. For example, analyzing data from two separate Point RESolved Spectroscopy (PRESS) acquisitions with different echo times would require the use of two separate basis sets. Likewise, separate basis sets would also be required to analyze separate datasets acquired using a PRESS acquisition and a STimulated Echo Acquisition Mode (STEAM) acquisition, regardless of whether or not the echo times of the two acquisitions were the same.

Finally, once the basis sets have been properly generated, the processed data can be analyzed by fitting the data to a linear combination of the basis spectra. As with peak fitting, this can either be performed in the time domain (Vanhamme et al., 2001) or the frequency domain (Slotboom et al., 1998; Mierisova & Ala-Korpela, 2001). These data are fit to a linear combination of the metabolite basis spectra, and the relative metabolite concentrations are estimated based on the amplitude weightings in the linear combination that produces the best fit. In addition to the amplitude of the basis spectra, a number of other parameters may be adjusted to achieve the best fit to the data, including the zero-order phase, time shift (first-order phase), frequency (the allowed frequency shift of each basis spectrum is usually very small, on the order of a few Hertz), and the lineshape and broadening (Gaussian, Lorentzian, or Voigt). The quality of fitting, particularly for peaks with low signal-to-noise ratio (SNR), is greatly improved by accurately modeling the *in vivo* lineshape, including lineshape distortions due to eddy currents. Fortunately, these factors can be accurately estimated based on the shape of higher SNR peaks (such as unsuppressed water or NAA).

Another advantage of the method of basis spectrum fitting is its relative insensitivity to overlapping peaks. It is often possible to separate the contributions of two metabolites whose basis spectra have substantial peak overlap, provided that they contain at least a small amount of nonoverlapping peak information, or independence. For example, the proton NMR spectra of glutamate (Glu) and glutamine (Gln) contain substantial spectral overlap, and yet at field strengths of 3 T and above, their signals can be separated from one another using spectral fitting at short echo times (Wijtenburg & Knight-Scott, 2011). The ability to separate these two signals is made possible based on only a small spectral region (~2.3 ppm) where their basis spectra differ. In contrast, some other metabolites have very strongly overlapping spectral patterns, and cannot be separated by basis spectrum fitting (or any other analysis method). The pair of creatine (Cr) and phosphocreatine (PCr) is one example of two metabolites whose contributions cannot be separated due to spectral overlap. The separable signals of Glu and Gln, as well as the inseparable signals of Cr and PCr are shown in Fig. 1.5.7.

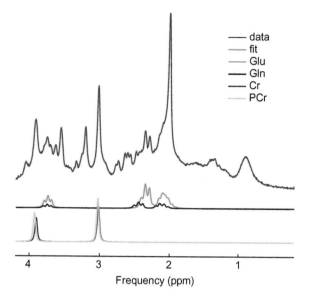

FIGURE 1.5.7 Separation of similar basis spectra. The basis spectra of glutamate (Glu, green curve) and glutamine (Gln, blue curve), are similar in shape, but their contributions can be separated using the method of basis spectrum fitting. The basis spectra of creatine (Cr, cyan curve) and phosphocreatine (PCr, yellow curve), on the other hand, are nearly identical, and cannot generally be separated *in vivo*.

In most cases, a simple linear combination of metabolite basis spectra is not enough to produce a good fit to the data. This is because a number of additional signals are present in *in vivo* MR spectra from sources other than metabolites. These sources include lipids, macromolecules, unsuppressed water, and other unknown resonances. In order to produce a good fit to the data, all of these additional so-called "nuisance signals" must be taken into account. Methods for handling such signals are discussed in the following section.

NUISANCE SIGNALS

Most MR spectra contain a significant amount of signal from unwanted sources, including macromolecules (MM), lipids, unsuppressed water, and other unknown sources. These signals cannot be completely removed by preprocessing, and therefore must be considered when performing spectral quantification. Regardless of the chosen method of measuring peak intensity, it is important for the user to be aware of these so-called nuisance signals, and to try to minimize their impact on the accuracy of metabolite peak intensity measurements. This section deals with the most common nuisance signals observed in *in vivo* MRS.

Macromolecules

MM are relatively immobile, high molecular weight (>3500 DA) compounds that give rise to broad (short T_2) resonances in proton MR spectra of the brain. Failure to account for these macromolecular resonances will generally lead to an overestimation of the metabolite concentrations whose signals overlie the MM signals. Due to their short T_2 and broad spectral signatures, the molecular compounds that give rise to MM signals in the brain are not as well characterized as the low molecular weight metabolite signals. Some authors, however (Behar & Ogino, 1993; Behar et al., 1994), have speculated on the origins of the MM signals based on the chemical shifts and couplings of the peaks observed *in vivo* and *in vitro*. Specifically, the MM signals between 0.9 and 2.4 ppm are believed to arise from the methyl (CH_3) and methylene (CH_2) resonances of amino acids such as leucine, isoleucine, valine, threonine and alanine, lysine and arginine, and glutamate and glutamine. Other MM resonances between 3.5 and 4.5 ppm have been attributed to α-methine (CH) protons, and the macromolecule resonance at 3.0 ppm is attributed to the εCH_2 resonance of Lysine, with possible contributions as well from cysteine.

Despite being less well characterized than the low molecular weight metabolite signals, it has been shown that the MM signals appear reproducibly (in short-TE MRS) at certain frequencies and that these resonances can be modeled using a series of broad Gaussian functions (Seeger et al., 2003), as shown in Fig. 1.5.8. Therefore, in the case of basis spectrum fitting, the MM signals can be accounted for by including basis spectra for the macromolecule signals that typically arise in the spectrum, and omission of these MM basis spectra may result in failure of the fitting algorithm (Auer et al., 2001; Seeger et al., 2003). It should be

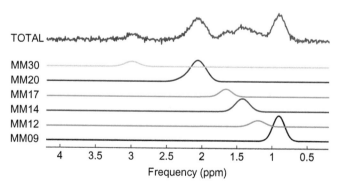

FIGURE 1.5.8 MM resonances in the brain can be modeled as a series of Gaussian peaks at specific frequencies. At 3 T, the most commonly observed MM resonances occur at 0.9 ppm (MM09, blue curve), 1.2 ppm (MM12, green curve), 1.4 ppm (MM14 red curve), 1.7 ppm (MM17, cyan curve), 2.0 ppm (MM20, purple curve), and 3.0 ppm (MM30, yellow curve).

noted, though, that rather than assigning specific basis spectra to each individual compound (as is the case with the metabolite signals) this method models the MM peaks in more of an empirical fashion, with the individual peaks labeled simply MM09, MM12, MM14, etc. As a result, the modeling of MM peaks in basis spectrum fitting provides a useful means of accounting for the MM signals in the spectrum, but does not enable the quantification of specific macromolecular compounds.

It is possible to separate the MM resonances from the metabolite resonances based on the fact that they have very different T_1 relaxation rates. Specifically, the metabolite signals have a relatively long T_1 (~ 1500 ms), whereas MM have relatively short T_1 (~ 250 ms) (Behar et al., 1994; Seeger et al., 2001; Kassem & Bartha, 2003). Therefore, it is possible to measure the MM baseline directly by acquiring a "metabolite-nulled" spectrum in which an inversion pulse is applied prior to the acquisition, and the inversion recovery time is chosen such that the metabolite signals are approximately nulled at the time of excitation. Once the MM signals have been measured directly, it is possible to remove the MM contribution from the original spectrum (thereby producing a "metabolite only" spectrum) simply by subtracting the measured MM component. Spectral analysis can then be performed on the "metabolite only" spectrum without the need for modeling of the MM signals (Kassem & Bartha, 2003; Penner et al., 2010). Alternatively, the measured MM component can be included as a basis spectrum in spectral analysis.

Due to the short T_2 of the MM signals, the macromolecular resonances can be almost completely eliminated simply by using acquisitions with long echo times (Fig. 1.5.3), thus simplifying the detection of metabolite signals. However, the utility of long echo-time MRS is limited, since many metabolite signals also become undetectable at long echo times.

There are some instances when the MM signal cannot be accounted for or removed, and metabolite measurements include an acknowledged component of MM contamination as a result. One such example is in the edited detection of GABA using the MEscher–GArwood (MEGA)-PRESS pulse sequence. Because the observed edited GABA resonance overlaps directly with a co-edited MM resonance at 3 ppm, the two signals are not separable. Therefore, the total peak intensity at 3 ppm is generally measured using a peak fitting method, and GABA concentrations are often reported as GABA + MM (Bogner et al., 2010; Near et al., 2011). However, at higher field strengths, MM contamination can be minimized in MEGA-PRESS-edited GABA spectra by employing more advanced acquisition strategies (Henry et al., 2001).

Lipids

Lipids in the human brain are normally very immobile, held tightly in bilayer membranes. As a result, lipids in the healthy human brain are generally MR invisible. However, lipid signals may be present in MR spectra of the human brain if either (1) the volume of interest is placed too close to the skull (Fig. 1.5.9, top), allowing extracranial lipid signals to contaminate the spectrum or (2) mobile lipids are present in the brain tissue itself due to pathologies such as brain tumors or multiple sclerosis (Fig. 1.5.9, bottom). Like macromolecules, lipids produce broad (short T_2) resonances that appear in the spectrum between 0.9 and 2.8 ppm. Failure to account for lipid signals may result in failure of the spectral quantification, or overestimation of the metabolite resonances. In some cases, the lipid signals

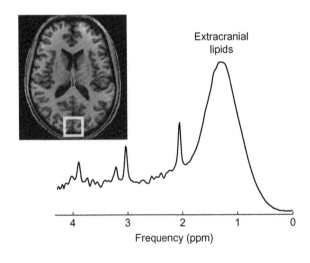

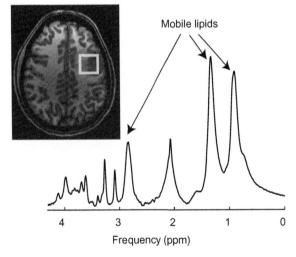

FIGURE 1.5.9 Lipid resonances in the human brain. Top, extracranial lipids are observed if the volume of interest (yellow box) is placed too close to the scalp. Bottom, prominent resonance from mobile lipid are often observed in malignant brain tumors, as shown in this example.

themselves are of clinical interest (Poptani et al., 1995; Calvar et al., 2005), and in such cases are targets for quantification. The most common way of accounting for lipid signals is to include parameterized models of their resonances in a spectral fitting approach, as described previously (Auer et al., 2001; Seeger et al., 2003). In the case of extracranial lipids, their contribution can be minimized using outer volume presaturation pulses.

Unsuppressed Water

Water is by far the most abundant MR-visible substance in the human brain, and the most prominent resonance in any *in vivo* MR spectrum. Even though most MRS acquisitions make use of water-suppression techniques to minimize its contribution to the spectrum, a significant residual water signal can often still remain. In some cases, the residual water signal can perturb the entire baseline of the spectrum, even at frequencies far from the water resonance, resulting in over or under estimation of the metabolite signals of interest. Therefore, handling of the residual water resonance is critical to proper spectral quantification.

One commonly used approach is to simply remove the water resonance in processing prior to analysis. In theory, one could fit the water peak to a model function (Gaussian, Lorentzian, or Voigt) as described earlier, and then subtract the fitted curve from the spectrum. In practice, however, the water signal can be difficult to parameterize due to multi-exponential decay. To account for this, the residual water peak can be modeled as the sum of multiple Lorentzian peaks. A method called the Hankel–Lanczos singular value decomposition (HLSVD; Pijnappel et al., 1992) is commonly used, in which the user needs only to estimate the number of components and to specify the frequency range of the water peak. The water peak is then fit and subtracted from the spectrum.

Spectral Baseline

All of the MRS signals that we have identified so far (metabolites, macromolecules, lipids, and water) are superimposed on a background of resonances whose origins are not well characterized. These signals generally have very short T_2, and therefore have very broad spectral peaks and are not observed at long echo times. This background of unidentified resonances is often referred to as the spectral baseline. Regardless of the method used for spectral quantification, the baseline must be accounted for to avoid overestimation of the resonances of interest. An example of the spectral baseline can be seen in Fig. 1.5.6.

Methods of handling the baseline signal can be divided into time domain and frequency domain methods. In the time domain, the baseline signal is generally removed by truncating or downweighting the initial part of the FID (Ratiney et al., 2004). Since the baseline signals have an extremely short T_2, this approach is generally effective at removing the spectral baseline. In the frequency domain the baseline is most commonly estimated using a spline model (Provencher, 1993; Poullet et al., 2007), which essentially acts as an efficient high-pass filter.

Since, almost by definition, very little is known about the origins of the baseline signal, the methods of accounting for the baseline are relatively "model-free." In other words, we do not have a great deal of prior knowledge about the shape of the baseline, and the existing methods of dealing with the spectral baseline have very few restrictions on their shape. Furthermore, because it is very difficult to isolate the baseline signal, it is equally difficult to properly validate the various methods of baseline accommodation. As a result, even the most commonly used methods of handling the baseline signal are often viewed with caution, or even suspicion. In general, the fitted baseline signal should contain fairly low-order fluctuations (i.e., it should be smoothly varying), particularly if the MMs are included in the basis set. The presence of a more "wobbly" baseline suggests either incomplete characterization of metabolite peaks or breakthrough of susceptibility-shifted nuisance signals such as water or lipids due to poor spatial localization.

SOFTWARE PACKAGES FOR SPECTRAL QUANTIFICATION

A number of different software packages are available for the analysis of MRS data. Listed in the following sections, in alphabetical order, are just a few of the most commonly used packages, and some details about them.

AQSES

AQSES (Automated Quantitation of Short Echo-time MRS Spectra) (Poullet et al., 2007) is a freely available software package that was developed in JAVA, and is platform independent (Windows, Linux, OSX, and Solaris). AQSES includes a graphical user interface as well as a selection of spectral preprocessing tools. It supports most clinical MRS data formats, and it can be obtained from http://homes.esat.kuleuven.be/~biomed/software.php. In AQSES, MRS data are fit in the time domain using the basis spectrum fitting method, with a set of user-defined (either experimental or simulated) basis spectra. The basis spectrum weights are estimated using an algorithm called variable projection (VARPRO) (van der Veen et al., 1988). Residual water signals are removed automatically prior to analysis using a maximum-phase, finite impulse response filter. The MM signal and the spectral baseline are not considered separately, but rather, they are modeled together as a single entity. This "macromolecular baseline" is accounted for during spectral fitting, and is modeled in the time domain using a nonparametric penalized spline. The lack of any prior knowledge of the MM signals may be viewed as a shortcoming of this software package.

jMRUI

jMRUI is a widely used, JAVA-based user interface for the processing and analysis of both high-resolution NMR data and *in vivo* MR spectroscopy data (Naressi et al., 2001a,b; Stefan et al., 2009). This software package is freely available, and is used by more than 1400 research labs worldwide. jMRUI is a highly versatile software package that includes a full complement of preprocessing and analysis tools including both peak fitting and basis spectrum fitting, spectral simulation, as well as batch processing tools, and support for both single-voxel MRS and MRS imaging data analysis. It supports most clinical MRS data formats. Because of the difficulties of modeling certain data imperfections (signal truncation, echo timing errors, and spectral baseline) in the frequency domain, jMRUI performs all of its fitting procedures in the time domain, which enables handling of these issues with fewer assumptions and approximations. Peak fitting in jMRUI is performed using an algorithm called the advanced method for accurate, robust, and efficient spectral fitting (AMARES) (Vanhamme et al., 1997), which is similar to the VARPRO method, except that it can incorporate a greater range of prior knowledge constraints. Fig. 1.5.10 shows an example of peak fitting using the AMARES package in jMRUI. The AMARES algorithm provided within jMRUI is highly cited in literature (Torriani et al., 2005; Stagg et al., 2009; Near et al., 2011), and certainly one of the most commonly used peak fitting software packages for *in vivo* MRS. Basis spectrum fitting in jMRUI is performed using an algorithm called QUantitation based on QUantum ESTimation (QUEST) (Ratiney et al., 2004, 2005), which fits the data to a basis set in the time domain, and the simulation of the basis spectra is also possible within jMRUI using the NMR-SCOPE tool. Both AMARES and QUEST enable the handling of MM signals and spectral baseline in a number of ways, including truncation or downweighting of the initial points in FID. MM signals can also be modeled in QUEST using MM basis spectra (Ratiney et al., 2004). Finally, jMRUI also includes a set of state-space, or "black-box" fitting methods (HSVD, HSLVD, etc.), which can be used to remove residual water signals prior to analysis, or to perform an entire spectral fit using little or no prior knowledge.

LCModel

This software is so-called because it analyzes *in vivo* MRS data as a linear combination of model (LCModel) spectra, or basis spectra (Provencher, 1993, 2001). LCModel was initially developed in the early 1990s and is almost certainly the most commonly used basis spectrum fitting tool for *in vivo* MRS. This software is not freely available, and requires a license to run. The software package comes with a graphical user interface, but one of its major strengths is the ability to also run analyses from the command line, making the program easily scriptable and very useful for high throughput MRS studies. LCModel is different in several respects to other MRS fitting software packages: First, while the majority of other fitting tools perform fitting in the time domain, LCModel performs fitting in the frequency domain. Second, LCModel presumes neither a Lorentzian nor a Gaussian lineshape model to account for shim-related line broadening. Rather, it uses a nearly model-free lineshape function, the shape of which is estimated using the data itself. This feature is meant to account for the fact that the lineshape may differ depending on experimental conditions. Finally, to avoid either underfitting or overfitting the baseline, LCModel uses a nearly model-free baseline, which attempts to find the smoothest function that is still consistent with the data. Removal of the residual water signal is not necessary prior to analysis; the tail of the water signal is accounted for as part of the model-free baseline, and large residual water signals can be handled. An example of an LCModel fit output is shown in Fig. 1.5.11. LCModel is highly automated, and requires little or no user input, which is advantageous when performing large MRS studies or studies across centers. Metabolite basis sets for commonly used MRS pulse sequences are available from the software vendor, but custom basis sets can also be generated by the user. The software has built-in corrections for eddy current artifacts, global frequency and phase offsets of the input data, and small frequency offsets of individual basis spectra. LCModel is compatible with most clinical MRS data formats. In general, the best results are obtained with LCModel if an MM basis set is included in the fitting (for low field strength data, this

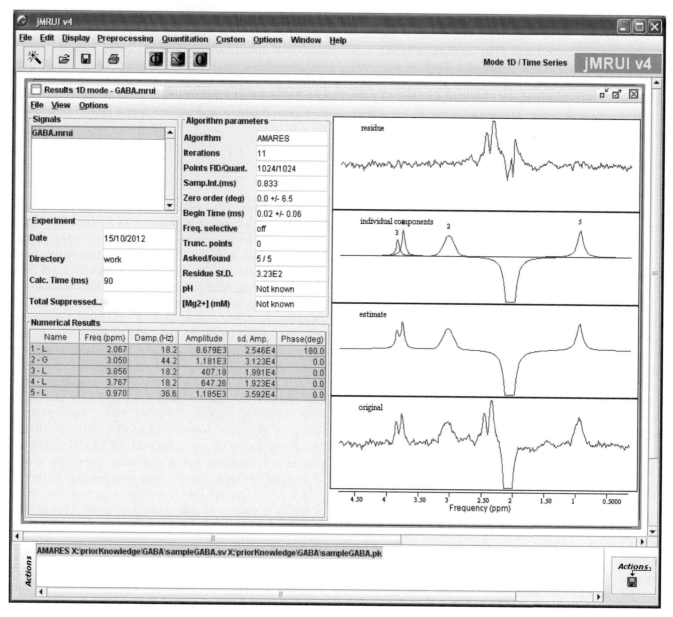

FIGURE 1.5.10   Example output from the AMARES fitting package within the jMRUI software.

is provided with the software), and if there is a high SNR reference signal such as unsuppressed water or NAA from which to estimate the lineshape.

PROFit

PROFit (PRiOr knowledge Fitting) is a basis spectrum fitting software package that is specifically designed for the analysis of 2D MRS data (Schulte & Boesiger, 2006). 2D MRS is a method that involves acquiring multiple conventional (1D) spectra from a sample using different timing parameters (i.e., echo time), and then combining them to make a 2D dataset.

Although not used as commonly as conventional spectroscopy, 2D MRS is advantageous because it enables the separation of peaks that would normally be overlapping and inseparable in 1D spectra. Basis spectrum fitting of 2D MRS data is analogous to basis spectrum fitting of 1D data: each individual metabolite gives rise to a unique 2D spectral signature, or basis spectrum that is know a priori, and the experimental 2D MRS data is fit to a linear combination of the 2D basis spectra. As with conventional MRS, the 2D basis spectra can be obtained either through phantom experiments or through simulations. PROFit makes use of the VARPRO algorithm for the estimation of the amplitudes of the 2D basis spectra.

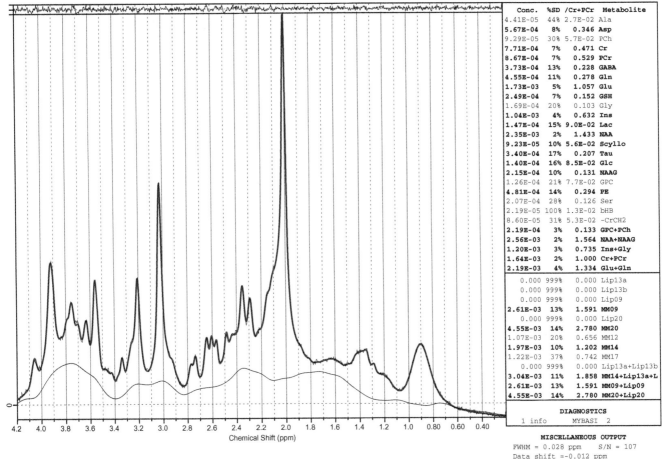

Pulse Sequence Name
Data of: MRS Laboratory Name

LCModel (Version 6.2-2B) Copyright: S.W. Provencher.   *Ref.: Magn. Reson. Med. 30:672-679 (1993).*   *dd-mm-yyyy hh:mm*

Conc.	%SD	/Cr+PCr	Metabolite
4.41E-05	44%	2.7E-02	Ala
5.67E-04	8%	0.346	Asp
9.29E-05	30%	5.7E-02	PCh
7.71E-04	7%	0.471	Cr
8.67E-04	7%	0.529	PCr
3.73E-04	13%	0.228	GABA
4.55E-04	11%	0.278	Gln
1.73E-03	5%	1.057	Glu
2.49E-04	7%	0.152	GSH
1.69E-04	20%	0.103	Gly
1.04E-03	4%	0.632	Ins
1.47E-04	15%	9.0E-02	Lac
2.35E-03	2%	1.433	NAA
9.23E-05	10%	5.6E-02	Scyllo
3.40E-04	17%	0.207	Tau
1.40E-04	16%	8.5E-02	Glc
2.15E-04	10%	0.131	NAAG
1.26E-04	21%	7.7E-02	GPC
4.81E-04	14%	0.294	PE
2.07E-04	28%	0.126	Ser
2.19E-05	100%	1.3E-02	bHB
8.60E-05	31%	5.3E-02	-CrCH2
2.19E-04	3%	0.133	GPC+PCh
2.56E-03	2%	1.564	NAA+NAAG
1.20E-03	3%	0.735	Ins+Gly
1.64E-03	2%	1.000	Cr+PCr
2.19E-03	4%	1.334	Glu+Gln
0.000	999%	0.000	Lip13a
0.000	999%	0.000	Lip13b
0.000	999%	0.000	Lip09
2.61E-03	13%	1.591	MM09
0.000	999%	0.000	Lip20
4.55E-03	14%	2.780	MM20
1.07E-03	20%	0.656	MM12
1.97E-03	10%	1.202	MM14
1.22E-03	37%	0.742	MM17
0.000	999%	0.000	Lip13a+Lip13b
3.04E-03	11%	1.858	MM14+Lip13a+L
2.61E-03	13%	1.591	MM09+Lip09
4.55E-03	14%	2.780	MM20+Lip20

DIAGNOSTICS
1 info   MYBASI 2

MISCELLANEOUS OUTPUT
FWHM = 0.028 ppm   S/N = 107
Data shift =-0.012 ppm

Chemical Shift (ppm)

FIGURE 1.5.11   Example output from the LCModel software.

TARQUIN

TARQUIN (Totally Automatic Robust QUantitation In NMR) is a freely available software package for basis spectrum fitting of MRS data. Initially published as a method for the analysis of *ex vivo* or *in vitro* MRS and NMR studies (Reynolds et al., 2006), the method has since been adapted for the analysis of *in vivo* MRS data (http://tarquin.sourceforge.net/paper/tarquin_paper.pdf). This method models the metabolite, lipid, and MM signals using basis spectra in the time domain with Voigt lineshape models, and the spectral baseline is accounted for by signal truncation in the time domain. One unique feature of TARQUIN is that it enforces soft constraints on the relative amplitudes of the various basis spectra based on prior knowledge of the approximate relative concentrations of metabolites, MM, and lipids *in vivo*. In addition, for conventional pulse sequences (PRESS, STEAM), the basis spectra can be calculated automatically within

the software using simulations based on the pulse sequence parameters specified in the header of the input data file. Most clinical MRS data formats are accepted.

SIGNAL REFERENCING AND ABSOLUTE QUANTIFICATION

As mentioned in the introduction, metabolite quantification is performed by comparing the metabolite signal intensity with a reference compound signal. If the concentration of the reference compound is well known, then the absolute concentration of the metabolite of interest can be calculated based on the relative peak intensities, as in Equation 3. Metabolite concentrations can either be determined in molar units (moles per unit volume) or molal units (moles per unit mass of tissue). The two units are related and are interchangeable if the density of brain tissue is known. A number of referencing methods are available to the experimenter, including internal (metabolite or water) referencing, external referencing, the phantom replacement method, and the electrical reference methods. Each of these has its own advantages and disadvantages, and the choice of reference compound is generally a trade-off between quantification accuracy, and ease of implementation.

Internal Metabolite Referencing

Internal metabolite referencing involves choosing a metabolite to serve as the reference compound. All other metabolite concentrations are then expressed as a ratio, with the signal intensity of the metabolite of interest in the numerator, and the signal intensity of the reference metabolite in the denominator. For this reason, the method of internal referencing is considered a relative (not absolute) quantification technique. An obvious drawback of this approach is that metabolite ratios are influenced by changes in both the metabolite of interest and the reference compound, making it difficult or impossible to determine which signal is changing. The most commonly used reference signal is that of total creatine (creatine + phosphocreatine), which displays a prominent singlet resonance at 3.02 ppm, and whose concentration is relatively stable at around 8 mM. It has been shown, however, that creatine levels are unstable in many pathologies, and therefore the use of creatine as an internal reference is not always appropriate. Other commonly used internal references include NAA and total choline (free choline + phosphorylcholine + glycerophosphorylcholine), although the stability of these compounds is also reduced in certain pathologies. Despite all of its drawbacks, internal metabolite referencing still enjoys widespread use due to its convenience and ease of implementation. The method does not require any additional scans, since the reference peak and metabolite peaks of interest are present in the same acquired spectrum, thus saving valuable scan time. Furthermore, because the reference signal and the metabolite of interest are acquired from the same region of interest, no RF field corrections are necessary.

Internal Water Referencing

Internal water referencing requires a measurement of the water signal intensity from the same volume of interest as the metabolite signal measurement. This is achieved by using the identical localized MRS sequence that was used to acquire the metabolite

spectrum, only with the water-suppression pulses turned off. Due to the high SNR of the water peak, only a few signal averages are required, meaning that the added scan time for the acquisition of the unsuppressed water signal is usually less than one minute. If water is to serve as the reference compound, its concentration in the volume of interest must be well known. However, the water concentration in any volume of interest in the brain depends on the tissue composition within that volume. Methods to determine the tissue composition involve either tissue segmentation of a structural image with appropriate contrast (Barker et al., 1993), or measurement of the multicomponent T_2 decay curve of the water signal to estimate chemical shift imaging versus tissue signal fraction (Ernst et al., 1993; Kreis et al., 1993; Knight-Scott et al., 2003). Once the tissue composition within the volume of interest is known, the water concentration can be estimated using literature values for the water content of various tissue types. In some pathologies, however, the water content of brain tissue may be significantly altered, making internal water referencing an inappropriate choice of quantification method.

External Reference Method

The external reference method involves preparing a small vial with a known concentration of reference material and placing it in the scanner (close to the subject's head) during the examination (Roth et al., 1989), as shown in Fig. 1.5.12A. Either before or after the *in vivo* MRS acquisition, a second, identical acquisition is performed with the region of interest (ROI) placed

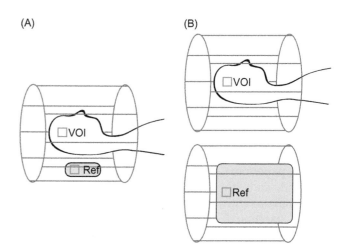

FIGURE 1.5.12 *Absolute quantification methods. (A) The external reference method is performed by preparing a vial with a known (MR-visible) concentration reference, and placing it in the RF coil next to the subject's head. (B) The phantom replacement method is performed by replacing the subject with a large phantom containing a known concentration reference. VOI, volume of interest.*

inside the reference material. This method has the advantage because it enables the detection of a reference signal whose concentration is very accurately known, and the signal can be detected within the same session as the *in vivo* exam. However, because the reference signal comes from a different spatial region from the *in vivo* ROI, the reference signal intensity will be affected by inhomogeneities in the RF field. This must be accounted for by either RF field simulations, or by additional scans to map the RF field inhomogeneity.

Phantom Replacement Method

The phantom replacement method involves preparing a large phantom, similar in size to a human head, with a known concentration of reference material (Duc et al., 1998). Following the *in vivo* scan, the subject is removed from the scanner and replaced with the reference phantom. The electrical properties of the phantom and the positioning of the phantom are carefully optimized such that the coil loading is identical between the *in vivo* and the phantom scans. The reference signal is then measured using the same acquisition as the *in vivo* scan, and the same volume of interest, as shown in Fig. 1.5.12B. The assumption is that since the electrical properties of the two samples are similar, and the volume of interest is identical, RF scaling effects will not need to be considered. However, this assumption is somewhat flawed, since a phantom is unlikely to perfectly mimic the electrical properties of a human head. Therefore, corrections are generally required to account for differences in flip angle and receiver sensitivity between the *in vivo* scan and the replacement phantom scan (Shulman et al., 1990; Jost et al., 2005).

Electrical Referencing

A recently developed method for absolute *in vivo* quantification involves the use of a synthetic reference signal that is introduced into the MR spectrum through magnetic induction. This method is called the ERETIC (Electric REference to access *In vivo* Concentrations) method. In this approach, an inductive coupling loop is placed close to the RF receive coil and driven with a mono-exponentially decaying sinusoid with a precisely known amplitude, as shown in Fig. 1.5.13. To eliminate electrical interference from spurious signals the inductive loop can be driven using a fiber optic cable. This synthetic signal produces a reference peak in the acquired spectrum whose amplitude and frequency can be controlled by the user. The synthetic peak can be used as a concentration reference, provided that it has been calibrated in a separate experiment by comparing

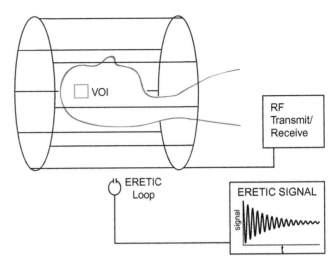

FIGURE 1.5.13 In the ERETIC method, a synthetic reference signal is introduced into the *in vivo* MRS scan using an inductive coupling loop next to the RF coil. The synthetic ERETIC signal is calibrated to produce a resonance that corresponds to a known concentration level. VOI, volume of interest.

its intensity to a phantom reference signal. By carefully designing the inductive coupling loop, the ERETIC signal can be made relatively insensitive to changes in coil loading. The primary advantage of this method is that it enables the observation of a reliable reference signal in the same scan as the metabolite data acquisition, without the need for extra scans, and calibration scans need not be repeated for each subject. Furthermore, the stable frequency of the ERETIC signal can be used to correct scanner frequency drift (Heinzer-Schweizer et al., 2010).

Regardless of what referencing method is used, it is important to take into account the relaxation of both the metabolites of interest and the reference signal. T_1 and T_2 values of metabolites and brain water can be found in literature, and in the case of an external reference compound, the T_1 and T_2 relaxation rates should be determined experimentally.

QUALITY CONTROL

This section discusses some basic tools and metrics that can be used to evaluate the accuracy and reproducibility of MRS data. These include the Cramér-Rao lower bounds (CRLB), data quality, fit residuals, metabolite correlation coefficients, and Monte Carlo simulations.

CRLB of Variance

The spectral fitting methods described earlier in this chapter enable the estimation of metabolite peak amplitudes, but it is not possible to directly access the uncertainty on these peak amplitudes without performing repeated measurements. Since we do not generally have time to perform repeated MRS measurements to assess reproducibility, the uncertainty on a metabolite measurement is usually estimated using the CRLB of variance (Cavassila et al., 2001). The CRLB is a measure of the minimum possible variance on a fit parameter, assuming that the model used is an accurate representation of the data. As a rule of thumb, metabolite concentration estimates are only considered reliable if the corresponding CRLB variance is <20% of the estimated value. Metabolites with CRLB values ≥20% should therefore be discarded. Most spectral fitting software packages provide CRLB estimates for all peak intensity measurements. While the CRLB is a useful quality control tool, it should be noted that a low CRLB value does not guarantee an accurate or reproducible concentration estimate, and can sometimes be misleading (Kreis & Boesch, 2003). This is especially true since the models that are used to fit MRS data (especially the baseline models) are known to be flawed. Therefore the use of other quality control metrics, in addition to the CRLB, is recommended (Kreis, 2004).

Although it is time-consuming, one should not discount the idea of determining the measurement uncertainty directly using repeated measurements (Bogner et al., 2010). Repeated measurements are a good way to validate the reproducibility of a given pulse sequence, with a specific set of acquisition parameters. Repeated measurements can either be done within session, or between sessions. While the within-session reproducibility reflects on the reproducibility of the pulse sequence and analysis method, the between-session reproducibility is affected by more operator-dependent factors such as the reproducibility of voxel positioning and prescan procedures such as shimming and pulse calibrations.

Data Quality

One of the easiest and most effective ways of controlling the quality of MRS data is to enforce strict limits on the SNR and the linewidth of the data. This is a good idea for several reasons. First, it is possible for the CRLB values to be low, even if the data quality is poor and the concentration estimates are unreliable (Kreis & Boesch, 2003). Second, changing the SNR and linewidth significantly can introduce biases in the metabolite concentration estimates. In addition to the monitoring of linewidth and SNR, spectra should always be checked for the presence of unwanted signals (residual water, lipid contamination, and spurious

echoes), and postprocessing techniques should be employed to remove artifacts such as subject motion and scanner drift. Any spectra that do not conform to a predefined standard of data quality should be discarded from further analysis.

Fit Residuals

The difference between the data and the model fit is called the fit residual, and it can be a good indicator of whether or not the fitting procedure was a success. Examples of fit residuals can be seen in Figs. 5.5, 5.6, 5.10, and 5.11. Ideally, the fit residual should be flat, and as close to zero as possible (although it should still include noise). Problems with the fit are identified by peaks (positive or negative) in the fit residual, which indicate either that one or more peaks have been over or under estimated, or that an inappropriate model function (Gaussian, Lorentzian, etc.) was chosen. It is important to note that, while peaks in the residual always indicate a poor fit, a flat residual is not always indicative of a good fit. For example, in spectral fitting, if two or more metabolite signals are highly correlated (having many overlapping peaks), it is possible to produce a good fit to the data using the incorrect combination of basis spectra. For this reason, the fit residuals are useful for spotting problems, but are not useful on their own for validating the success of the quantification.

Metabolite Correlation Coefficients

As alluded to in the previous paragraph, metabolites whose basis spectra contain significant overlap are said to be correlated. The correlation between two metabolites can be quantified using a correlation coefficient, C. If the absolute value of the correlation coefficient between two metabolites, $|C|$, is >0.5, then the two metabolites are considered highly correlated and cannot be separated. In this case, the sum of the two metabolite concentrations may be reported (as is commonly done with Cr + PCr, or Glu + Gln), but the individual metabolite concentrations should not, even if their individual CRLB values are <20%. Several of the basis spectrum fitting software packages described above will automatically calculate a matrix of correlation coefficient values between all of the metabolite basis spectra (Ratiney et al., 2005), as shown in Fig. 1.5.14.

Monte Carlo Simulations

Monte Carlo simulations are a useful way of evaluating both the accuracy and reproducibility of a

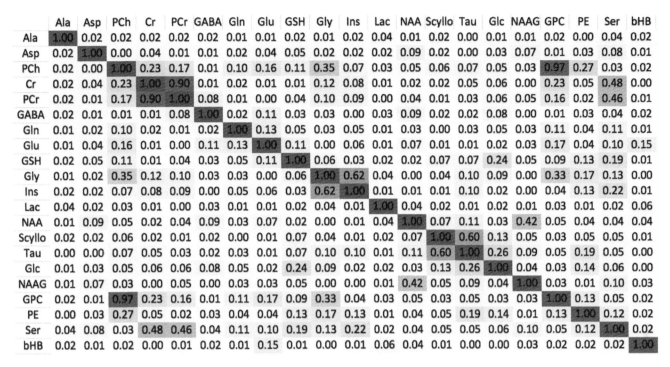

	Ala	Asp	PCh	Cr	PCr	GABA	Gln	Glu	GSH	Gly	Ins	Lac	NAA	Scyllo	Tau	Glc	NAAG	GPC	PE	Ser	bHB
Ala	1.00	0.02	0.02	0.02	0.02	0.02	0.01	0.01	0.02	0.01	0.02	0.04	0.01	0.02	0.00	0.01	0.01	0.02	0.00	0.04	0.02
Asp	0.02	1.00	0.00	0.04	0.01	0.01	0.02	0.04	0.05	0.02	0.02	0.02	0.09	0.02	0.00	0.03	0.07	0.01	0.03	0.08	0.01
PCh	0.02	0.00	1.00	0.23	0.17	0.01	0.10	0.16	0.11	0.35	0.07	0.03	0.05	0.06	0.07	0.05	0.03	0.97	0.27	0.03	0.02
Cr	0.02	0.04	0.23	1.00	0.90	0.01	0.02	0.01	0.01	0.12	0.08	0.01	0.02	0.02	0.05	0.06	0.00	0.23	0.05	0.48	0.00
PCr	0.02	0.01	0.17	0.90	1.00	0.08	0.01	0.00	0.04	0.10	0.09	0.00	0.04	0.01	0.03	0.06	0.05	0.16	0.02	0.46	0.01
GABA	0.02	0.01	0.01	0.01	0.08	1.00	0.02	0.11	0.03	0.03	0.00	0.03	0.09	0.02	0.02	0.08	0.00	0.01	0.03	0.04	0.02
Gln	0.01	0.02	0.10	0.02	0.01	0.02	1.00	0.13	0.05	0.03	0.05	0.01	0.03	0.00	0.03	0.05	0.03	0.11	0.04	0.11	0.01
Glu	0.01	0.04	0.16	0.01	0.00	0.11	0.13	1.00	0.11	0.00	0.06	0.01	0.07	0.01	0.01	0.02	0.03	0.17	0.04	0.10	0.15
GSH	0.02	0.05	0.11	0.01	0.04	0.03	0.05	0.11	1.00	0.06	0.03	0.02	0.02	0.07	0.07	0.24	0.05	0.09	0.13	0.19	0.01
Gly	0.01	0.02	0.35	0.12	0.10	0.03	0.03	0.00	0.06	1.00	0.62	0.04	0.00	0.04	0.10	0.09	0.00	0.33	0.17	0.13	0.00
Ins	0.02	0.02	0.07	0.08	0.09	0.00	0.05	0.06	0.03	0.62	1.00	0.01	0.01	0.01	0.10	0.02	0.00	0.04	0.13	0.22	0.01
Lac	0.04	0.02	0.03	0.01	0.00	0.03	0.01	0.01	0.02	0.04	0.01	1.00	0.04	0.02	0.01	0.02	0.01	0.03	0.01	0.02	0.06
NAA	0.01	0.09	0.05	0.02	0.04	0.09	0.03	0.07	0.02	0.00	0.01	0.04	1.00	0.07	0.11	0.03	0.42	0.05	0.04	0.04	0.04
Scyllo	0.02	0.02	0.06	0.02	0.01	0.02	0.00	0.01	0.07	0.04	0.01	0.02	0.07	1.00	0.60	0.13	0.05	0.03	0.05	0.05	0.01
Tau	0.00	0.00	0.07	0.05	0.03	0.02	0.03	0.01	0.07	0.10	0.10	0.01	0.11	0.60	1.00	0.26	0.09	0.05	0.19	0.05	0.00
Glc	0.01	0.03	0.05	0.06	0.06	0.08	0.05	0.02	0.24	0.09	0.02	0.02	0.03	0.13	0.26	1.00	0.04	0.03	0.14	0.06	0.00
NAAG	0.01	0.07	0.03	0.00	0.05	0.00	0.03	0.03	0.05	0.00	0.00	0.01	0.42	0.05	0.09	0.04	1.00	0.03	0.01	0.10	0.03
GPC	0.02	0.01	0.97	0.23	0.16	0.01	0.11	0.17	0.09	0.33	0.04	0.03	0.05	0.03	0.05	0.03	0.03	1.00	0.13	0.05	0.02
PE	0.00	0.03	0.27	0.05	0.02	0.03	0.04	0.04	0.13	0.17	0.13	0.01	0.04	0.05	0.19	0.14	0.01	0.13	1.00	0.12	0.02
Ser	0.04	0.08	0.03	0.48	0.46	0.04	0.11	0.10	0.19	0.13	0.22	0.02	0.04	0.05	0.05	0.06	0.10	0.05	0.12	1.00	0.02
bHB	0.02	0.01	0.02	0.00	0.01	0.02	0.01	0.15	0.01	0.00	0.01	0.06	0.04	0.01	0.00	0.00	0.03	0.02	0.02	0.02	1.00

FIGURE 1.5.14 Table of metabolite correlation coefficients (absolute values shown). Any two metabolites whose correlation coefficient is >0.5 are said to be highly correlated, meaning that their individual concentration values cannot be separated.

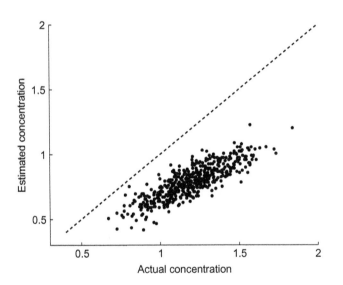

FIGURE 1.5.15 Monte Carlo simulations. This plot shows the estimated versus actual metabolite concentrations following the analysis of 500 simulated spectra with known metabolite concentrations. Monte Carlo simulations like this can be used to evaluate the accuracy and reproducibility of MRS techniques.

broadened to simulate various shimming conditions. Finally, the simulated spectra are analyzed using the fitting method of choice, and the resulting estimated metabolite concentrations are compared with the known input concentrations (Hancu, 2009; Hancu & Port, 2011). By repeating this procedure many times, using different noise seeds, it is possible to generate an estimate of both the accuracy and the reproducibility of the analysis method. Fig. 1.5.15 shows an example plot of the estimated versus actual metabolite concentration that can be generated using Monte Carlo simulations to assess both accuracy and reproducibility. One criticism of Monte Carlo simulations is that the simulated spectra often do not include any of the experimental imperfections that are observed in real data, and so the accuracy and reproducibility may be overestimated.

CONCLUSIONS

In conclusion, MRS is a very powerful tool that can provide *in vivo* measurements of metabolite concentrations. There are a variety of methods available for quantitative analysis of MRS data, and all of these methods should be used with extreme care to ensure that metabolite measurements are as reliable and as accurate as possible.

particular pulse sequence and analysis method. They involve generating a simulated spectrum by combining simulated or experimental basis spectra together in approximately physiological concentrations and then adding noise to achieve SNR that is experimentally realistic. The simulated spectra can also be line

References

Arus, C., Chang, Y. C., & Barany, M. (1985). The separation of phosphocreatine from creatine, and pH determination in frog muscle by natural abundance 13C-NMR. *Biochim Biophys Acta*, *844*(1), 91–93.

Auer, D. P., Gossl, C., Schirmer, T., & Czisch, M. (2001). Improved analysis of 1H-MR spectra in the presence of mobile lipids. *Magnetic Resonance in Medicine*, *46*(3), 615–618.

Barker, P. B., Soher, B. J., Blackband, S. J., Chatham, J. C., Mathews, V. P., & Bryan, R. N. (1993). Quantitation of proton NMR spectra of the human brain using tissue water as an internal concentration reference. *NMR in Biomedicine*, *6*(1), 89–94.

Bartha, R., Drost, D. J., & Williamson, P. C. (1999). Factors affecting the quantification of short echo in-vivo 1H MR spectra: prior knowledge, peak elimination, and filtering. *NMR in Biomedicine*, *12*(4), 205–216.

Behar, K. L., & Ogino, T. (1993). Characterization of macromolecule resonances in the 1H NMR spectrum of rat brain. *Magnetic Resonance in Medicine*, *30*(1), 38–44.

Behar, K. L., Rothman, D. L., Spencer, D. D., & Petroff, O. A. (1994). Analysis of macromolecule resonances in 1H NMR spectra of human brain. *Magnetic Resonance in Medicine*, *32*(3), 294–302.

Bogner, W., Gruber, S., Doelken, M., Stadlbauer, A., Gansland, O., Boettcher, U., et al. (2010). In vivo quantification of intracerebral GABA by single-voxel (1)H-MRS-How reproducible are the results?. *European Journal of Radiology*, *73*(3), 526–531.

Cady, E. B., & Azzopardi, D. (1989). Absolute quantitation of neonatal brain spectra acquired with surface coil localization. *NMR in Biomedicine*, *2*(5-6), 305–311.

Calvar, J. A., Meli, F. J., Romero, C., Calcagno, M. L., Yanez, P., Martinez, A. R., et al. (2005). Characterization of brain tumors by MRS, DWI and Ki-67 labeling index. *Journal of Neurooncology*, *72* (3), 273–280.

Cavassila, S., Deval, S., Huegen, C., van Ormondt, D., & Graveron-Demilly, D. (2001). Cramer-Rao bounds: an evaluation tool for quantitation. *NMR in Biomedicine*, *14*(4), 278–283.

de Graaf, R. A. (2007). *In vivo NMR spectroscopy* (2nd ed.). Chichester, UK: John Wiley & Sons Ltd.

Duc, C. O., Weber, O. M., Trabesinger, A. H., Meier, D., & Boesiger, P. (1998). Quantitative 1H MRS of the human brain in vivo based on the stimulation phantom calibration strategy. *Magnetic Resonance in Medicine*, *39*(3), 491–496.

Ernst, T., Kreis, R., & Ross, B. D. (1993). Absolute Quantitation of Water and Metabolites in the Human Brain. I. Compartments of Water. *Journal of Magnetic Resonance B*, *102*, 1–8.

Govindaraju, V., Young, K., & Maudsley, A. A. (2000). Proton NMR chemical shifts and coupling constants for brain metabolites. *NMR in Biomedicine*, *13*(3), 129–153.

Hancu, I. (2009). Which pulse sequence is optimal for myo-inositol detection at 3T?. *NMR in Biomedicine*, *22*(4), 426–435.

Hancu, I., & Port, J. (2011). The case of the missing glutamine. *NMR in Biomedicine*, *24*(5), 529–535.

Heinzer-Schweizer, S., De Zanche, N., Pavan, M., Mens, G., Sturzenegger, U., Henning, A., et al. (2010). In-vivo assessment of tissue metabolite levels using 1H MRS and the Electric REference To access In vivo Concentrations (ERETIC) method. *NMR in Biomedicine*, *23*(4), 406–413.

Henry, P. G., Dautry, C., Hantraye, P., & Bloch, G. (2001). Brain GABA editing without macromolecule contamination. *Magnetic Resonance Medicine*, *45*(3), 517–520.

Jansen, J. F., Backes, W. H., Nicolay, K., & Kooi, M. E. (2006). 1H MR spectroscopy of the brain: absolute quantification of metabolites. *Radiology*, *240*(2), 318–332.

Joliot, M., Mazoyer, B. M., & Huesman, R. H. (1991). In vivo NMR spectral parameter estimation: a comparison between time and frequency domain methods. *Magnetic Resonance in Medicine*, *18*(2), 358–370.

Jost, G., Harting, I., & Heiland, S. (2005). Quantitative single-voxel spectroscopy: the reciprocity principle for receive-only head coils. *Journal of Magnetic Resonance Imaging*, *21*(1), 66–71.

Kanowski, M., Kaufmann, J., Braun, J., Bernarding, J., & Tempelmann, C. (2004). Quantitation of simulated short echo time 1H human brain spectra by LCModel and AMARES. *Magnetic Resonance in Medicine*, *51*(5), 904–912.

Kassem, M. N., & Bartha, R. (2003). Quantitative proton short-echo-time LASER spectroscopy of normal human white matter and hippocampus at 4 Tesla incorporating macromolecule subtraction. *Magnetic Resonance in Medicine*, *49*(5), 918–927.

Knight-Scott, J., Haley, A. P., Rossmiller, S. R., Farace, E., Mai, V. M., Christopher, J. M., et al. (2003). Molality as a unit of measure for expressing 1H MRS brain metabolite concentrations in vivo. *Magnetic Resonance Imaging*, *21*(7), 787–797.

Kreis, R. (2004). Issues of spectral quality in clinical 1H-magnetic resonance spectroscopy and a gallery of artifacts. *NMR in Biomedicine*, *17*(6), 361–381.

Kreis, R., Boesch, C. (2003). Bad spectra can be better than good spectra. Paper presented at the International Society for Magnetic Resonance in Medicine, Toronto, Canada.

Kreis, R., Ernst, T., & Ross, B. D. (1993). Absolute quantitation of water and metabolites in the human brain. II. Metabolite concentrations. *Journal of Magnetic Resonance B*, *102*, 9–19.

Marshall, I., Higinbotham, J., Bruce, S., & Freise, A. (1997). Use of Voigt lineshape for quantification of in vivo 1H spectra. *Magnetic Resonance in Medicine*, *37*(5), 651–657.

Matson, G. B., Meyerhoff, D. J., Lawry, T. J., Lara, R. S., Duijn, J., Deicken, R. F., et al. (1993). Use of computer simulations for quantitation of 31P ISIS MRS results. *NMR in Biomedicine*, *6*(3), 215–224.

Maudsley, A. A., Govindaraju, V., Young, K., Aygula, Z. K., Pattany, P. M., Soher, B. J., et al. (2005). Numerical simulation of PRESS localized MR spectroscopy. *Journal of Magnetic Resonance*, *173*(1), 54–63.

Mierisova, S., & Ala-Korpela, M. (2001). MR spectroscopy quantitation: a review of frequency domain methods. *NMR in Biomedicine*, *14*(4), 247–259.

Mulkern, R., & Bowers, J. (1994). Density matrix calculations of AB spectra from multipulse sequences: quantum mechanics meets in vivo spectroscopy. *Concepts of Magnetic Resonance*, *6*, 1–23.

Naressi, A., Couturier, C., Castang, I., de Beer, R., & Graveron-Demilly, D. (2001a). Java-based graphical user interface for MRUI, a software package for quantitation of in vivo/medical magnetic resonance spectroscopy signals. *Computers in Biology and Medicine*, *31*(4), 269–286.

Naressi, A., Couturier, C., Devos, J. M., Janssen, M., Mangeat, C., de Beer, R., et al. (2001b). Java-based graphical user interface for the MRUI quantitation package. *Magnetic Resonance Materials in Physics, Biology and Medicine (MAGMA)*, *12*(2-3), 141–152.

Near, J., Leung, I., Claridge, T., Cowen, P., Jezzard, P. (2012). Chemical shifts and coupling constants of the GABA spin system. Paper presented at the International Society for Magnetic Resonance in Medicine, Melbourne, Australia.

Near, J., Simpson, R., Cowen, P., & Jezzard, P (2011). Efficient gamma-aminobutyric acid editing at 3T without macromolecule contamination: MEGA-SPECIAL. *NMR in Biomedicine*, *24*(10), 1277–1285.

Penner, J., Rupsingh, R., Smith, M., Wells, J. L., Borrie, M. J., & Bartha, R. (2010). Increased glutamate in the hippocampus after galantamine treatment for Alzheimer disease. *Progress in Neuro-Psychopharmacoly & Biological Psychiatry*, *34*(1), 104–110.

Pijnappel, W. W. F., van den Boogaart, A., de Beer, R., & van Ormondt, D. (1992). SVD-Based Quantification of Magnetic Resonance Signals. *Journal of Magnetic Resonance, 97*, 122–134.

Poptani, H., Gupta, R. K., Jain, V. K., Roy, R., & Pandey, R. (1995). Cystic intracranial mass lesions: possible role of in vivo MR spectroscopy in its differential diagnosis. *Magnetic Resonance Imaging, 13*(7), 1019–1029.

Poullet, J. B., Sima, D. M., Simonetti, A. W., De Neuter, B., Vanhamme, L., Lemmerling, P., et al. (2007). An automated quantitation of short echo time MRS spectra in an open source software environment: AQSES. *NMR in Biomedicine, 20*(5), 493–504.

Provencher, S. W. (1993). Estimation of metabolite concentrations from localized in vivo proton NMR spectra. *Magnetic Resonance in Medicine, 30*(6), 672–679.

Provencher, S. W. (2001). Automatic quantitation of localized in vivo 1H spectra with LCModel. *NMR in Biomedicine, 14*(4), 260–264.

Ratiney, H., Coenradie, Y., Cavassila, S., van Ormondt, D., & Graveron-Demilly, D. (2004). Time-domain quantitation of 1H short echo-time signals: background accommodation. *Magnetic Resonance Materials in Physics, Biology and Medicine (MAGMA), 16*(6), 284–296.

Ratiney, H., Sdika, M., Coenradie, Y., Cavassila, S., van Ormondt, D., & Graveron-Demilly, D. (2005). Time-domain semi-parametric estimation based on a metabolite basis set. *NMR in Biomedicine, 18*(1), 1–13.

Reynolds, G., Wilson, M., Peet, A., & Arvanitis, T. N. (2006). An algorithm for the automated quantitation of metabolites in in vitro NMR signals. *Magnetic Resonance in Medicine, 56*(6), 1211–1219.

Roth, K., Hubesch, B., Meyerhoff, D. J., Naruse, S., Gober, J. R., Lawry, T. J., et al. (1989). Noninvasive quantitation of phosphorus metabolites in human tissue by NMR spectroscopy. *Journal of Magnetic Resonance, 81*, 299–311.

Schulte, R. F., & Boesiger, P. (2006). ProFit: two-dimensional prior-knowledge fitting of J-resolved spectra. *NMR in Biomedicine, 19*, 255–263.

Seeger, U., Klose, U., Mader, I., Grodd, W., & Nagele, T. (2003). Parameterized evaluation of macromolecules and lipids in proton MR spectroscopy of brain diseases. *Magnetic Resonance in Medicine, 49*(1), 19–28.

Seeger, U., Mader, I., Nagele, T., Grodd, W., Lutz, O., & Klose, U. (2001). Reliable detection of macromolecules in single-volume 1H NMR spectra of the human brain. *Magnetic Resonance in Medicine, 45*(6), 948–954.

Shulman, G. I., Rothman, D. L., Jue, T., Stein, P., DeFronzo, R. A., & Shulman, R. G. (1990). Quantitation of muscle glycogen synthesis in normal subjects and subjects with non-insulin-dependent diabetes by 13C nuclear magnetic resonance spectroscopy. *New England Journal of Medicine, 322*(4), 223–228.

Slichter, C. P. (1992). *Principles of Magnetic Resonance* (3rd ed.). Berlin: Springer-Verlag.

Slotboom, J., Boesch, C., & Kreis, R. (1998). Versatile frequency domain fitting using time domain models and prior knowledge. *Magnetic Resonance in Medicine, 39*, 899–911.

Smith, S. A., Levante, T. O., Meier, B. H., & Ernst, R. R. (1994). Computer simulations in magnetic resonance. An object-oriented programming approach. *Journal of Magnetic Resonance A, 106*, 75–105.

Soher, B. J., Young, K., Bernstein, A., Aygula, Z., & Maudsley, A. A. (2007). GAVA: spectral simulation for in vivo MRS applications. *Journal of Magnetic Resonance, 185*(2), 291–299.

Stagg, C. J., Wylezinska, M., Matthews, P. M., Johansen-Berg, H., Jezzard, P., Rothwell, J. C., et al. (2009). Neurochemical effects of theta burst stimulation as assessed by magnetic resonance spectroscopy. *Journal of Neurophysiology, 101*(6), 2872–2877.

Stefan, D., Di Cesare, F., Andreasescu, A., Popa, E., Lazariev, A., Vescovo, E., et al. (2009). Quantitation of magnetic resonance spectroscopy signals: the jMRUI software package. *Measurement of Science and Technology, 20*, 104035–104044.

Torriani, M., Thomas, B. J., Halpern, E. F., Jensen, M. E., Rosenthal, D. I., & Palmer, W. E. (2005). Intramyocellular lipid quantification: repeatability with 1H MR spectroscopy. *Radiology, 236*(2), 609–614.

van den Boogaart, A., Ala-Korpela, M., Jokisaari, J., & Griffiths, J. R. (1994). Time and frequency domain analysis of NMR data compared: an application to 1D 1H spectra of lipoproteins. *Magnetic Resonance in Medicine, 31*(4), 347–358.

van der Veen, J. W., de Beer, R., Luyten, P. R., & van Ormondt, D. (1988). Accurate quantification of in vivo 31P NMR signals using the variable projection method and prior knowledge. *Magnetic Resonance in Medicine, 6*(1), 92–98.

Vanhamme, L., Sundin, T., Hecke, P. V., & Huffel, S. V. (2001). MR spectroscopy quantitation: a review of time-domain methods. *NMR in Biomedicine, 14*(4), 233–246.

Vanhamme, L., van den Boogaart, A., & Van Huffel, S. (1997). Improved method for accurate and efficient quantification of MRS data with use of prior knowledge. *Journal of Magnetic Resonance, 129*(1), 35–43.

Wijtenburg, S. A., & Knight-Scott, J. (2011). Very short echo time improves the precision of glutamate detection at 3T in 1H magnetic resonance spectroscopy. *Journal of Magnetic Resonance Imaging, 34*(3), 645–652.

BIOCHEMISTRY—WHAT UNDERLIES THE SIGNAL?

N-Acetylaspartate and N-Acetylaspartylglutamate in Central Nervous System Health and Disease

John R. Moffett, Prasanth Ariyannur, Peethambaran Arun and Aryan M.A. Namboodiri

Department of Anatomy, Physiology and Genetics, and Neuroscience Program, Uniformed Services University of the Health Sciences, Bethesda, Maryland, USA

INTRODUCTION

Brain metabolites are most often defined by their functions, but one brain metabolite stands out as being defined by its utility to magnetic resonance spectroscopists; namely *N*-acetylaspartate (NAA). The utility afforded by NAA is that it represents the most reliable marker for neuronal health and integrity using water-suppressed proton magnetic resonance spectroscopy (MRS). Its utility as a marker for neuronal health is not based on a mature understanding of the functions served by NAA, but primarily through empirical evidence derived from MRS studies of brain injury, disease, mental disorders, and drug abuse, where NAA levels in the brain are typically reduced.

Also known as *N*-acetyl-L-aspartic acid, NAA is the acetylated form of the amino acid aspartate, and is present at very high concentrations in the brain. In rat brain the concentration is between 9.2 and 9.3 mM (Mlynarik et al., 2008). In humans it has been measured at approximately 12 mM (Rigotti et al., 2007, 2011b), making NAA one of the most concentrated metabolites in the human brain. The concentration of NAA in other tissues and serum is low, typically <40−50 μM (Miyake et al., 1981). One documented function of NAA in the nervous system is that it serves as a precursor for the biosynthesis of the neuronal peptide *N*-acetylaspartylglutamate or NAAG. NAAG has been described as the most concentrated neuroactive peptide in the human brain (Tsai & Coyle, 1995; Neale et al., 2000). NAAG can also be measured by MRS, but

because the NAAG peak is smaller and appears as a shoulder on the NAA peak, its quantification is more difficult (Edden et al., 2007). Research into the functions of NAA and NAAG have begun to reveal roles in central nervous system (CNS) function, but controversies still surround many of the proposed functions.

Recently the genes for the biosynthetic enzymes for NAA (Wiame et al., 2010; Ariyannur et al., 2010b) and NAAG (Becker et al., 2010; Collard et al., 2010) have been identified providing much needed data on protein structure, mechanisms of synthesis, and tissue distribution, as well as providing new tools for identifying key functional roles. These recent discoveries raise hopes that definitive roles for both of these related metabolites will be determined in the relatively near future. Several earlier reviews of NAA and NAAG have been published (Neale et al., 2000; Demougeot et al., 2004; Moffett et al., 2006, 2007; Benarroch, 2008), so this review will focus somewhat more on recent developments and controversies.

NAA

NAA in MRS

NAA is a relatively small molecule, only 174 Da in its ionized form, and it has a methyl (CH_3) group associated with the acetate group. The three hydrogen atoms on the methyl group all resonate with a single frequency in water-suppressed proton MRS at a value of 2.0 parts per million. Because the methyl hydrogen atoms all resonate with the same frequency, and because NAA is one of the most concentrated molecules in the brain, NAA provides the largest peak on proton MR spectrograms of healthy human brain tissue. For this reason most investigations have focused on determining the utility of NAA measurements in various brain diseases and disorders. NAA is reduced, often in specific brain areas, in a wide array of brain diseases, disorders, and neuropsychiatric conditions. Schizophrenia is one neuropsychiatric disorder in particular that has been relatively well studied with regard to reduced NAA levels in specific brain areas (Brugger et al., 2011). Reductions were consistently observed in frontal lobes, temporal lobes, and thalamus in both first episode and chronic patients. The observed reductions are generally modest, often around 5% relative to controls. In contrast, NAA is substantially reduced after severe brain injury or stroke, and levels may recover after several weeks, depending on the severity of the injury (Wardlaw et al., 1998; Signoretti et al., 2010, 2011; Vagnozzi et al., 2010). Recovery of NAA to normal levels is seen after milder brain injuries, but not in the case of severe injuries, or in the case of multiple milder injuries spaced closely in time as often occurs in contact sports. NAA decreases are also observed in a wide array of brain disorders including epilepsy (Savic et al., 2000, 2004; Riederer et al., 2006), multiple sclerosis (Gonzalez-Toledo et al., 2006; Rigotti et al., 2011a), Alzheimer's disease (Passani et al., 1997a; Kantarci & Jack, 2003; Watanabe et al., 2010), and human immunodeficiency virus (Suwanwelaa et al., 2000; Edden et al., 2007). NAA levels in the brain are increased in Canavan's disease (CD) due to genetic defects in the enzyme that degrades NAA (Wittsack et al., 1996), as will be discussed in detail below.

NAA Synthesis

NAA was first identified in brain extracts in 1956 (Tallan et al., 1956) and biosynthesis was tentatively observed in 1959 (Goldstein, 1959) and subsequently confirmed in 1969 (Goldstein, 1969). NAA is synthesized from L-aspartate and acetyl coenzyme A (acetyl CoA) by the enzyme aspartate N-acetyltransferase (Asp-NAT; Truckenmiller et al., 1985). In the adult brain, NAA synthesis occurs mostly in neurons (Urenjak et al., 1992). The corresponding gene for Asp-NAT is Nat8l, and is expressed predominantly in the brain (Wiame et al., 2010; Ariyannur et al., 2010b). It is not known if other cell types can synthesize NAA, but mRNA for Asp-NAT is expressed at low levels in the spleen and thymus (Wiame et al., 2010) suggesting

that some immune cells may also synthesize NAA under some conditions. In fact, NAA levels have been reported to be relatively high in histamine-containing rat peritoneal mast cells, and it was found that compounds, which result in histamine depletion in these cells, also caused a reduction in NAA levels (Burlina et al., 1997).

Asp-NAT has not been extensively studied because of the difficulties in purifying and characterizing the enzyme activity from brain. An early examination of the tissue distribution of enzyme activity found it present only in the brain, spinal cord, and retina, but in this early study the spleen and thymus were not among the peripheral organs tested (Truckenmiller et al., 1985). It was found that caudal CNS structures such as the spinal cord and brainstem had the highest Asp-NAT activity levels, whereas retina had the lowest level. Now that the gene for Asp-NAT has been identified as Nat8l, it will be possible to study the enzyme in much greater detail. For example, recent studies have shown that the Asp-NAT protein sequence can be subdivided into five functional domains (regions 1–5) including a putative membrane associated domain (region 4), which is closely associated with the catalytic domains. This close association between membrane and catalytic domains may explain the lability of Asp-NAT activity in detergent-solubilized brain homogenates (Tahay et al., 2012). Enzyme purification studies using mild detergent homogenization, native gel electrophoresis, and size-exclusion chromatography indicated that the functional enzyme existed as a large, multiprotein complex with an apparent molecular weight exceeding 600 kDa (Madhavarao et al., 2003; Ariyannur et al., 2008). These findings suggest that in the mammalian brain Asp-NAT is part of a membrane-associated protein complex, and that dissociation from the complex or the membrane disrupts the catalytic site and abolishes enzyme activity.

The fact that NAA levels are decreased in many neurological disorders and disease states raises the question of whether the loss of NAA results from reduced NAA synthesis or increased NAA catabolism. The synthesis of NAA can be monitored noninvasively using ^{13}C MRS using 1-^{13}C-labeled glucose administration. NAA synthesis rates measured by this method indicate a reduction by approximately 60% in CD patients, whereas synthesis rates appear to be modestly increased in Alzheimer's disease and schizophrenia patients (Moreno et al., 2001; Harris et al., 2006). This provides in vivo evidence for the regulation of NAA synthesis under different pathological conditions. Based on the observations that brain NAA levels are reduced in Alzheimer's disease (Passani et al., 1997a; Watanabe et al., 2010) and schizophrenia (Brugger et al., 2011), the finding that synthesis rates are modestly increased under these conditions could suggest that increased catabolism is responsible for the observed decreases. However, in conditions where significant neuronal loss is involved, such as late stage Alzheimer's disease, it is also possible that the observed reductions in NAA levels are associated directly with the loss of biosynthetic capacity, with a concomitant increase in the rate of synthesis in the remaining neurons.

Using ^{13}C MRS and 1-^{13}C-labeled glucose administration in rats, Choi and Gruetter (2004) studied NAA synthesis *in vivo* and found that incorporation was detected in the acetyl group of NAA about 1.5 h earlier than in the aspartate group, indicating a delay in labeling of aspartate as compared to acetyl CoA. This finding would be expected based on the rapid conversion of glucose to pyruvate and subsequently acetyl CoA, which then could be used for the synthesis of NAA. The incorporation of label from glucose into aspartate would follow later after acetyl CoA entered the citric acid cycle, eventually forming oxaloacetate and then aspartate. Based on their findings, Choi and Gruetter (2004) concluded that NAA synthesis occurs in a single metabolic compartment (neurons), that it exhibits a relatively low turnover rate (up to 72 h for complete turnover), and that it is not likely to be involved as a major source of energy when the brain is in a resting state. These findings are in agreement with earlier studies that showed NAA is a substantial source of acetyl groups for lipid synthesis (Burri et al., 1991), which is a metabolic process that is relatively slow compared with energy derivation. In the same study, Burri and coworkers (1991) found that between 7 and 9% of the acetate moiety of NAA ended up in the protein fraction after 4 h incubation. Although this finding was not discussed by these investigators, their finding of rapid protein labeling from NAA-derived acetate suggests that some portion of this acetate may be employed in protein acetylation reactions because this is the most rapid route by which acetate could be incorporated into the protein fraction. This will be discussed in more detail in the following sections.

NAA and Asp-NAT Cellular Localization

Early studies of the levels of NAA in different dissected brain regions suggested that NAA might be localized predominantly in neurons (Tallan, 1957). An examination of human nervous system tumors and peripheral neural tissues from cows strongly suggested that NAA was predominantly localized in neurons (Nadler & Cooper, 1972b). Gas chromatography of various tissue extracts indicated that NAA was present in the brain at concentrations over 100 times greater than found in non-neural tissues suggesting that neurons were a major source of NAA (Miyake et al., 1981). A later *in vitro* study on purified brain cell types using MRS and high-performance liquid chromatography (HPLC) indicated that neurons such as cerebellar granule cells contained high levels of NAA, whereas astrocytes and mature oligodendrocytes contained undetectable levels (Urenjak et al., 1992). They also found high levels of NAA in oligodendrocyte-type-2 astrocyte progenitor cells and immature oligodendrocytes.

Antibodies to protein-coupled NAA used in conjunction with specialized tissue fixation methods for coupling NAA to tissue proteins provided a method of looking at NAA localization directly in brain tissue via immunohistochemistry (Moffett et al., 1991; Simmons et al., 1991). NAA was found to be present predominantly in neurons throughout the CNS. The methods were refined by the use of highly purified antibodies to protein-coupled NAA and enhanced NAA-fixation techniques allowing for the visualization of NAA in neurons and their processes (Moffett et al., 1993; Moffett & Namboodiri, 1995, 2006). NAA in the rat brain was present in most neurons, some dendritic processes, and in the axons of most fiber pathways throughout the CNS. In the rat, NAA was found to be present at different levels in different neuronal populations, with pyramidal neurons having higher levels than smaller interneurons (Fig. 2.1.1). This suggests that NAA may be more important in larger projection neurons with longer axons and more extensive myelination.

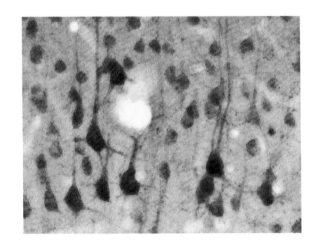

FIGURE 2.1.1 NAA immunoreactivity in motor cortex of the rat. Highly purified antibodies to protein-coupled NAA were used to visualize NAA in carbodiimide-fixed brain tissue. NAA was observed predominantly in neurons, with staining in cell bodies, dendrites, and axons. Much lighter staining was observed in oligodendrocytes, ependymal cells, and some blood vessels (40× objective with enhanced depth of field). This figure is reproduced in color in the color plate section.

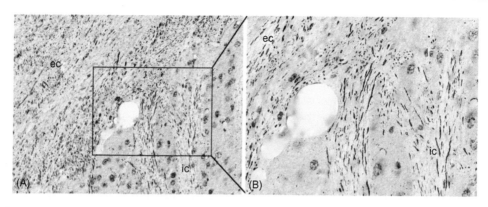

FIGURE 2.1.2   Immunostaining for the NAA biosynthetic enzyme Asp-NAT in the corpus callosum and internal capsule of the rat. Affinity-purified polyclonal antibodies to a 19 amino acid sequence unique to Asp-NAT were used to demonstrate cellular expression levels. Asp-NAT immunoreactivity was present at low levels in neuronal cell bodies, and at substantially higher levels in axons throughout the brain. Staining was present in discontinuous patches along the length of axons. Image in (A) is shown at higher magnification in (B) (20 × objective, A; 40 × , B). ec, external capsule; ic, internal capsule. This figure is reproduced in color in the color plate section.

Detailed studies of Asp-NAT cellular localization in brain have not been done to date. Using uncharacterized and unpurified antibodies, Niwa and coworkers (2007) showed that neurons of the nucleus accumbens expressed *Nat8l*, but at the time it had not been determined that the corresponding gene encoded Asp-NAT. Our laboratory has affinity purified the same antibody obtained from the Niwa group (2007) and applied it to rat brain slices, and have found the expression to be generally light in neuronal somata, and stronger in neuronal axons. Interestingly the expression in axons was not homogeneous, but appeared to be present in discontinuous patches (Fig.2.1.2).

Asp-NAT Subcellular Localization

Pioneering studies on NAA production in the brain provided strong evidence for mitochondria being one major site of NAA synthesis. Using purified mitochondrial preparations Patel and Clark (1979) found that brain mitochondria oxidizing pyruvate or 3-hydroxybutyrate to acetyl CoA produced and exported NAA in an inverse relationship to aspartate. As more pyruvate or 3-hydroxybutyrate was added to the incubation medium, they observed increasing NAA export and decreasing aspartate export. They concluded that NAA synthesis depended on and was regulated by aspartate synthesis in mitochondria. They noted that intramitochondrial aspartate synthesis depended on the supply of cytoplasmic glutamate, which is transported into the mitochondrial matrix in brain by the aspartate-glutamate exchanger now known as aralar1.

This conclusion brings up an interesting connection between mitochondrial function and NAA synthesis that was discovered during studies of aralar1 knockout mice. Aralar1 is the main mitochondrial aspartate-glutamate carrier expressed in the brain and skeletal muscle, and it is part of a larger complex that comprises the so-called mitochondrial malate-aspartate shuttle. This key metabolite exchanger system acts in bulk to move reducing equivalents into the mitochondrial matrix in the form of malate. Aralar1, as a component of this complex, acts to move cytoplasmic glutamate into mitochondria, while also moving mitochondrially synthesized aspartate out. Without aralar1, mitochondrial glutamate import and aspartate export are crippled. Studies with aralar1 knockout mice showed a dramatic drop in aspartate levels, and in turn dramatic reductions in NAA synthesis in the brain (Satrustegui et al., 2007). The finding that lack of aralar1 dramatically reduces NAA synthesis has at least two possible explanations. First, it could be due to the lack of aspartate output from mitochondria, which would limit the ability of microsomal Asp-NAT to synthesize NAA due to a lack of substrate. Second, it could be that the lack of glutamate uptake into mitochondria prevents intramitochondrial aspartate synthesis due to the lack of substrate for the mitochondrial aspartate aminotransferase reaction, which interconverts glutamate and oxaloacetate with aspartate and α-ketoglutarate. In this case the lack of intramitochondrial aspartate synthesis limits NAA production. It is possible that both of these mechanisms are involved in the drop in brain NAA levels in aralar1-deficient mice. The earlier work by Patel and Clark (1979) would suggest that the second alternative was more likely; however, more recent work with *Nat8l* transfection and bioinformatics studies call this conclusion into question, as discussed later.

One of the more interesting outcomes of aralar1 deficiency in addition to the large decrease in brain NAA levels is hypomyelination (Jalil et al., 2005; Wibom et al., 2009). The hypomyelination is hypothesized to result from the lack of availability of NAA, and this conclusion is supported by the fact that galactocerebrosides were reduced in aralar1 knockout mice, one of the myelin lipid classes that are reduced in CD (Madhavarao et al., 2005; Arun et al., 2010). CD will be discussed in more detail in the next section.

The majority of studies on NAA synthesis have suggested that NAA is synthesized in both mitochondria and in the microsomal fraction, which probably represents endoplasmic reticulum synthesis (Patel & Clark, 1979; Clark, 1998; Wang et al., 2007; Ariyannur et al., 2008; Arun et al., 2009). However, recent bioinformatics and *Nat8l* transfection studies have suggested that based on the protein sequence Asp-NAT is always retained in the endoplasmic reticulum (ER), and is not targeted to mitochondria (Wiame et al., 2010). These investigations included *Myc*-tagged *Nat8l* construct transfection experiments *in vitro*, which showed Asp-NAT to have predominantly perinuclear and ER localization, without any detectable mitochondrial localization (Tahay et al., 2012). The investigators concluded that Asp-NAT is localized almost exclusively in the ER when expressed under *in vitro* conditions. Verifying that Asp-NAT is also present in neuronal mitochondria *in vivo* awaits future studies. Nonetheless, dual targeting of proteins to both the ER and mitochondria is a common expression pattern for many proteins. Unlike proteins with N-terminal mitochondrial targeting sequences, a number of proteins with dual localization expression patterns have subcellular targeting sequences that are internal to the protein, and these are known as cryptic targeting sequences (Anandatheerthavarada et al., 2008; Sangar et al., 2010; Avadhani et al., 2011). Also there are instances in which proteins lacking any targeting sequence are associated with other proteins that have mitochondrial targeting sequences. Because Asp-NAT appears to exist as a part of a multiprotein complex, this may be how Asp-NAT could also be targeted to mitochondria (Madhavarao et al., 2003).

NAA and CD

Prior to identifying the connection between NAA and CD, NAA was considered metabolically inert, and therefore attracted little attention from neuroscientists or clinicians (Nadler & Cooper, 1972a). CD was first described in the 1930s (Canavan, 1931) and was recognized as a unique infantile disorder in the 1940s, but the cause remained unknown (van Bogaert & Bertrand, 1949). It was not until the 1980s that the connection to NAA catabolism was made (Hagenfeldt et al., 1987; Matalon et al., 1988). The enzyme that catabolizes NAA is designated aspartoacylase (ASPA), and

is also known as amidohydrolase II. Amidohydrolases including ASPA act to remove acetate from acetylated amino acids in order to allow for metabolism and recycling of the deacetylated amino acids, and reclamation of the released acetate (Lindner et al., 2000; Perrier et al., 2005). In CD mutations in the ASPA gene result in greatly reduced enzyme activity, and therefore NAA catabolism is substantially blocked because there are no alternative enzyme pathways. As such, NAA levels build up in the brain and greatly increased levels of NAA appear in the urine. Despite the understanding that CD is associated with ASPA deficiency, resulting in increased NAA levels in the brain, the pathophysiology of CD remains uncertain because the functions of NAA in the nervous system are far from completely understood.

CD is classified as an autosomal recessive spongiform leukodystrophy, and a number of previous reviews have detailed the clinical symptoms, and possible biochemical mechanisms, involved in this fatal genetic disorder (Kaul et al., 1994b; Matalon & Michals-Matalon, 1998; Traeger & Rapin, 1998; Kumar et al., 2006a; Moffett et al., 2007). CD infants appear normal at birth, and symptoms typically occur by 4–6 months of age. The clinical symptoms of CD include poor head control, macrocephaly, marked developmental delay, optic atrophy, seizures, hypotonia, and for most of those afflicted, death in childhood. Postmortem analyses of the brains of CD patients indicate severe vacuolation in both white and gray matter and enlargement of the ventricles. Cloning of the human ASPA gene has enabled molecular genetic studies of CD (Kaul et al., 1993; Namboodiri et al., 2000). Two mutations were found to be prevalent among Ashkenazi Jewish patients with CD (Kaul et al., 1994b). A missense mutation in codon 285 causing substitution of glutamic acid to alanine accounts for 83.6 % mutations identified in 104 alleles from 52 unrelated Ashkenazi Jewish patients. A nonsense mutation on codon 231, which converts tyrosine to a stop codon, was found in 13.4% of the alleles from the Jewish patients. Among non-Jewish patients, the mutations are different and more diverse (Kaul et al., 1996; Sistermans et al., 2000). The most common is in codon 305, a missense mutation substituting alanine for glutamic acid. This mutation was observed in 35.7% of the 70 alleles from 35 unrelated non-Jewish patients (Kaul et al., 1994a). Fifteen other mutations were detected in 24 other CD patients. Additional mutations, some with the children dying immediately after birth, have also been reported (Zeng et al., 2002). The diverse mutations limit the use of prenatal diagnosis to couples who are both carriers with known mutations. Very recently a study has looked at the correlation between enzyme activity levels associated with various ASPA mutations and the severity of CD phenotype, and observed that a good correlation existed between reduction in enzyme activity and disease severity (Zano et al., 2012). However, there were exceptions to this rule where two mutations in which enzyme activity was very low but the disease progression was relatively mild. It was found that enzyme stability may be a more significant factor in disease progression than catalytic activity wherein milder forms of CD are associated with ASPA enzyme that is conformationally stable despite the mutations.

Mechanisms of CD Pathogenesis

There are two primary hypotheses on the pathogenic mechanisms of CD that are not mutually exclusive. One hypothesis posits that the accumulation of excess NAA in the brain impairs osmotic regulation in neurons (Baslow, 1999, 2003), or causes neuronal overexcitation (Kitada et al., 2000). This hypothesis suggested that ASPA gene therapy with a neurotrophic viral vector could overcome the problem and serve as a cure for the disease by reducing brain NAA levels. Similarly, efforts toward decreasing the synthesis of NAA by selective inhibitors of the NAA synthesizing enzyme have been attempted. In the other hypothesis it is proposed that NAA-derived acetate is a significant source of acetyl CoA during brain development, which is synthesized in neurons and transferred to oligodendrocytes as a trophic support mechanism. The transferred NAA is then used in the synthesis of fatty acids and myelin lipids in the brain, as well as in protein acetylation reactions including histone acetylation. Under this hypothesis, a lack of ASPA activity in the brain impairs oligodendrocyte development and maturation through an acetyl CoA deficit leading to oligodendrocyte death and defective myelin synthesis during the period of postnatal myelination.

Our laboratory has directly tested the acetate deficiency hypothesis in ASPA − / − mice providing data showing significant decreases in both brain acetate levels, and the synthesis of myelin lipids, during the peak period of postnatal myelination (Madhavarao et al., 2005). More recently we have shown that dietary acetate supplementation using a potent, hydrophobic acetate source, glyceryl triacetate (GTA), significantly improves the phenotype in the tremor rat model of CD (Arun et al., 2010). Tremor rats are a naturally occurring mutant strain that lacks the entire genetic sequence for ASPA (Kitada et al., 2000). Motor performance of the GTA-treated tremor rats was significantly improved, and brain vacuolation was modestly reduced. Further, galactocerebroside levels in myelin were also improved with GTA treatment. Nonetheless, the pathogenic mechanisms of CD remain a controversial issue. This is primarily due to our lack of understanding the

role of NAA in the nervous system. Our laboratory has proposed that NAA acts as a storage form of acetyl CoA that can be transported from the site of synthesis in neurons, to the site of utilization in oligodendrocytes, representing a trophic interaction between the two cell types (Ariyannur et al., 2010b). Therefore, CD results in a lack of acetyl CoA in oligodendrocytes, especially during the period of postnatal myelination, impairing oligodendrocyte maturation, possibly by disrupting histone acetylation and epigenetic gene regulation (Kumar et al., 2006b, 2009; Mattan et al., 2010). It is also likely that the excess levels of NAA in the brain are responsible for some of the pathological consequences of ASPA deficiency, for example epileptic seizures (Klugmann et al., 2005).

Increased NAA and CD Pathogenesis

An unresolved issue concerning NAA surrounds its potential toxicity to neurons or oligodendrocytes when the concentration is elevated in the brain, as is the case with CD patients (Matalon & Michals-Matalon, 1998). Based on the assumption that the primary etiology of CD involves toxic NAA buildup in the brain, adenoviral transfer of the ASPA gene to the brains of humans has been performed in an attempt to reverse brain edema and vacuolation (Janson et al., 2002). The only available viral vectors for gene introduction into the CNS are neurotrophic in nature, and will primarily target genes to neurons rather than oligodendrocytes. Adenoviral gene transfer studies using the tremor rat ASPA-null mutant strain have yielded generally negative results on the efficacy of this approach using current technology. In one study, NAA levels were reduced, and seizure activity was diminished, but brain vacuolation, motor performance, and dysmyelination were unaffected, suggesting that some of the pathological features of the disease are not mediated only by excessive NAA concentrations (Klugmann et al., 2005). A very recent follow-up study of the children who underwent ASPA gene therapy has indicated that NAA levels in the brain were modestly reduced, and that this was accompanied by reduced seizure activity and a stabilization of the children's condition (Leone et al., 2012). These results strongly suggest that excess NAA is in part responsible for the pathogenesis of CD, especially with regard to seizure activity.

NAA and Osmoregulation

NAA synthesis and breakdown have been proposed as an osmoregulatory mechanism for removing metabolic water from neurons (Baslow, 1997, 1999, 2002; Baslow et al., 2007). The existing empirical data on an osmoregulatory role for NAA are sparse and suggest that NAA is not one of the major osmolytes that move in response to changes in extracellular tonicity (reviewed in Moffett et al., 2007). It is well documented that many inorganic ions and organic metabolites, including a number of amino acids, move in response to osmotic stress (Gullans & Verbalis, 1993), so NAA represents a viable candidate for this role. However, studies of the organic compounds that respond to hyponatremia often do not include NAA in the list of responsive metabolites (Soupart et al., 2007). Studies that looked directly at NAA responsiveness to osmotic stress indicate that it is a minor contributor to osmoregulatory responses in the brain when compared with other osmolytes such as taurine (Taylor et al., 1994, 1995; Verbalis, 2006).

The NAA osmolyte hypothesis is distinct from standard models of water homeostasis in the brain in that it does not view NAA as responsive to osmotic stress, but rather that it acts as a water cotransporter that removes metabolically produced water from neurons (Baslow et al., 2012). This is hypothesized to be a continuous process linked only to neuronal depolarization, which is said to move NAA-bound water to the extracellular space by way of an uncharacterized transporter. So technically NAA would not be considered a standard osmolyte under this hypothesis, but rather that in conjunction with an uncharacterized transporter protein would be classified specifically as a "molecular water pump" found only in nerve cells. Catabolism by ASPA is thought to dewater the NAA, and allow the water to exit the extracellular fluid more rapidly than bound water. Therefore, under this hypothesis CD is an osmotic disorder of the nervous system associated with the inability to move metabolic water generated in neurons to the vasculature in a timely manner. Currently there is no data on depolarization-induced NAA release from neurons or any potential NAA transporter protein that moves both NAA and its bound water out of neurons during neuronal depolarization. Until such a transport protein is identified and characterized the molecular water pump hypothesis remains both intriguing and hypothetical.

NAA, Acetyl CoA, and Lipid Synthesis

Neurons are known to provide metabolites, which include choline, palmitate, acetate, phosphate and ethanolamine (Ledeen, 1984), as well as NAA (Chakraborty et al., 2001) their ensheathing oligodendrocytes for the purpose of myelination. It has also been known for some time that NAA supplies acetate groups for the synthesis of acetyl CoA (D'Adamo & Yatsu, 1966; Burri et al., 1991; Mehta & Namboodiri, 1995), but the quantitative contribution to total acetyl CoA synthesis under different physiological conditions is uncertain. The synthesis of NAA requires the utilization of existing acetyl CoA and therefore NAA is not a primary source of acetyl CoA as is the case with pyruvate. Because NAA concentrations in the brain are exceptionally high, NAA synthesis probably consumes a substantial proportion of the acetyl CoA pool in brain. It seems likely that NAA may be acting in part as a storage and transport form of acetate in the CNS that can be used for subsequent *de novo* synthesis of acetyl CoA (Ariyannur et al., 2010b). This arrangement makes sense when viewed in light of the localization of the biosynthetic and degradatory enzymes for NAA wherein Asp-NAT is present primarily in neurons (Truckenmiller et al., 1985; Madhavarao et al., 2003; Wiame et al., 2010), and ASPA is present primarily in oligodendrocytes (Klugmann et al., 2003; Madhavarao et al., 2004; Moffett et al., 2011). Elegant studies by Ledeen and colleagues (1984), using NAA radiolabeled on the acetate moiety, showed that when NAA was injected into the eye it was transported down the optic nerves and the radioactivity was incorporated into the ensheathing myelin lipids (Chakraborty et al., 2001). These findings indicate that NAA in neurons supplies acetyl groups for the synthesis of myelin lipids in oligodendrocytes. However, the current evidence indicates that NAA supplies only a portion of the requisite acetyl CoA for myelin lipid synthesis, with the majority coming from citrate produced in oligodendrocyte mitochondria. As such NAA appears to be a parallel pathway that may be more critical during the period of intensive myelination that begins shortly after birth. This is the time of suckling in mammals when glucose availability in the diet is low, and the brain relies more on ketone bodies for energy derivation.

It has been noted that it is unusual that oligodendrocytes would use NAA rather than exclusively using glucose for lipid synthesis during development (Ramos et al., 2011). In adult animals glucose is the primary energy deriving metabolite in the brain. However, it is well documented that during brain development ketone bodies are preferred over glucose as an energy source for neurons and oligodendrocytes (Edmond et al., 1987). It is also known that acetate is released from the liver along with ketone bodies to provide this substrate to other tissues of the body (Ballard, 1972; Yamashita et al., 2001). Using radiolabeled precursors Edmond and colleagues (1987) showed that ketone bodies were nine times more effective than glucose for supporting oligodendrocyte respiration during brain development. These findings indicate that ketone bodies and acetate are more critical energy metabolites for oligodendrocytes during brain development than in adults. This may help explain why NAA-derived acetate appears to be more critical for oligodendrocytes during postnatal myelination.

Acetate Deficiency and CD Pathogenesis

There is accumulating evidence that NAA is involved in lipid synthesis and myelination in the CNS (reviewed in Moffett et al., 2007). But the correlation with myelination is only partial because substantial brain and spinal cord vacuolation is observed in many gray matter areas with sparing of many white matter tracts in ASPA-deficient animal models of CD (Surendran et al., 2005). This gray matter vacuolation is first observed between postnatal days 14 and 21 in the *Nur7* ASPA-deficient mouse model coinciding with the peak of postnatal CNS myelination (Traka et al., 2008). Studies on the maturation of oligodendrocytes during postnatal myelination demonstrate the important role of histone acetylation and deacetylation in the epigenetic control of differentiation from oligodendrocyte precursor cells to mature oligodendrocytes (Ye et al., 2009; Copray et al., 2009; MacDonald & Roskams, 2009). We have proposed that NAA-derived acetate is an important source of acetyl CoA in oligodendrocytes for histone acetylation reactions that regulate chromatin structure and gene transcription (Arun et al., 2010; Ariyannur et al., 2010b). The dramatic reduction in acetate availability in oligodendrocytes

during brain development that results from ASPA deficiency may impact histone acetyltransferase reactions required for epigenetic gene regulation. The resultant disruption of oligodendrocyte differentiation and maturation would explain the observed loss of mature oligodendrocytes in the cerebellum and brainstem of *Nur7* ASPA-deficient mice (Traka et al., 2008), and the death of immature oligodendrocytes in ASPA − / − mice (Kumar et al., 2009). In addition, histone hyperacetylation has been reported during postnatal myelination in animal models of CD (Kumar et al., 2009; Mattan et al., 2010) suggesting that control over cellular differentiation is disrupted via ASPA deficiency. In preliminary studies we have also found that histone acetylation is substantially increased in the tremor rat model of CD, and that acetate supplementation with GTA significantly reverses these abnormalities (Fig. 2.1.3).

Free acetate cannot be metabolized until it is converted to acetyl CoA. Acetate derived from NAA hydrolysis is enzymatically converted to acetyl CoA by the enzyme acetyl coenzyme A synthase-1 (AceCS1). We observed that AceCS1 is present in the nuclei and cytoplasm of many oligodendrocytes during postnatal

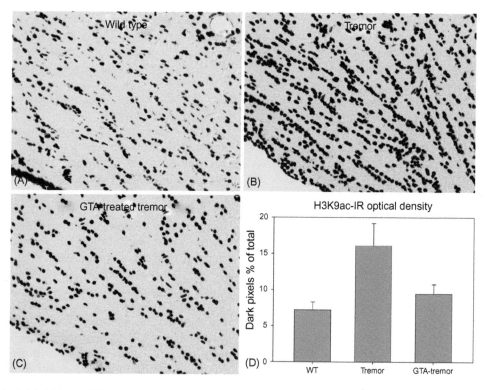

FIGURE 2.1.3 Acetylated histone H3 immunoreactivity (H3ac-IR) in the rat external capsule. Antibodies to histone H3 acetylated on the lysine-9 residue were used to examine histone acetylation in tremor and wild-type (WT) rats. (A) Shows H3ac-IR in the external capsule of a wild-type rat, with many oligodendrocyte cell nuclei expressing acetylated H3. (B) shows the same region of the external capsule from a tremor rat (∼70 days old). Many more oligodendrocyte nuclei express acetylated H3. (C) Shows the same region from a GTA-treated tremor rat (∼70 days old). The number of oligodendrocyte nuclei expressing acetylated H3 is reduced to near normal levels. (Methods: 20× objective; ChIP grade anti-H3K9ac antibodies, (Abcam#10812; 0.25 μg/ml). This figure is reproduced in color in the color plate section.

myelination in the rat (Ariyannur et al., 2010a). AceCS1 expression was upregulated in neurons and oligodendrocytes in adult tremor rats as compared with wild-type controls, and was returned to near-normal levels after acetate supplementation with GTA. AceCS1 has recently been shown to be one of the enzymes involved in histone acetylation reactions necessary for cell differentiation (Wellen et al., 2009) where citrate was the predominant source of acetyl CoA, but AceCS1 also provided some of the required substrate. The reduced substrate availability for AceCS1 in CD could negatively impact histone acetylation critical for proper oligodendrocyte maturation (Copray et al., 2009; Kumar et al., 2009). We propose that ASPA deficiency leads to improper regulation of histone acetylation in developing oligodendrocytes, preventing normal differentiation and leading to oligodendrocyte cell death, dysmyelination, neuronal injury, and inflammation and possibly even contributing to vacuole formation. The death of immature oligodendrocytes has been documented in ASPA-deficient mice (Kumar et al., 2009). These findings suggest that AceCS1 levels may be regulated in part by substrate availability whereby low acetate concentrations associated with ASPA deficiency result in upregulation of expression, and supplementation with exogenous acetate in ASPA deficiency leads to a normalization of expression. One important conclusion that can be drawn from these observations is that NAA-derived acetate is not only involved in brain myelination, but that it is also involved in providing some of the acetyl CoA required for histone acetylation and gene regulation associated with oligodendrocyte maturation during postnatal brain development.

Other Acetyl CoA Uses That May be Tied to NAA

Because NAA can act as a source of acetate groups for acetyl CoA synthesis (Burri et al., 1991; Mehta & Namboodiri, 1995), NAA can participate indirectly in many acetylation reactions, including not only nuclear histone acetylation, but also cytoplasmic protein acetylation reactions. Cytoplasmic and ER protein acetylation is becoming recognized as an important regulatory mechanism for controlling protein stability and function (Kouzarides, 2000; Costantini et al., 2007). We have proposed that another potential mechanism linking reduced acetyl CoA availability and the neuropathologies in CD could involve cytoplasmic acetylation reactions, including cotranslational and post-translational acetylation of proteins, particularly in oligodendrocytes (Arun et al., 2010). Oligodendrocytes have very active protein secretory pathways through the ER and are sensitive to disorders of protein misfolding. Recent work indicates that acetylation and deacetylation of certain nascent polypeptide chains in the ER secretory pathway of cells is required for stabilization and proper folding (Costantini et al., 2007; Spange et al., 2009; Guan & Xiong, 2010; Jonas et al., 2010). Acetyl CoA is required for the acetyltransferase reactions involved in acetylation at lysine sites on proteins, and the substantial drop in brain acetate levels that occurs in CD could have a negative impact on protein folding and stabilization, thus targeting proteins for ER-associated degradation. A dramatic loss of myelin basic protein and PLP/DM20 proteolipid proteins has been observed in the ASPA knockout mouse model combined with perinuclear retention of myelin protein staining. These findings indicate impairment in protein trafficking in oligodendrocytes (Kumar et al., 2009). Oligodendrocytes are highly susceptible to ER stress associated with disruptions in protein synthesis and trafficking (Lin & Popko, 2009). Recent studies in the newer mouse model of CD are consistent with the acetate/acetyl CoA deficiency hypothesis of CD (Francis et al., 2012).

Summary

Together, the currently available data suggest that NAA acts in part as a trophic support system for ensheathing oligodendrocytes, whereby neuronal axons supply NAA to oligodendrocytes, probably through a coordinated release-uptake system between neurons and oligodendrocytes. This trophic support appears to be most critical during the period of postnatal myelination when metabolic demands on oligodendrocytes are maximal, and when glucose supply is low. Despite the mounting evidence in favor of the trophic hypothesis, even this potential role for NAA requires further validation and experimental support before it becomes generally accepted. Additional roles in the nervous system such as osmoregulation await future studies.

NAAG

NAAG Synthesis

It has been postulated for some time that NAAG was synthesized non-ribosomally by the action of a peptide synthase enzyme, similar, for example, to how the tripeptide glutathione is synthesized. This conclusion was based on the observation that NAAG was synthesized in explanted neural tissue even in the presence of protein synthesis inhibitors (Cangro et al., 1987). NAAG synthesis in brain tissue was tentatively reported about 40 years ago (Reichelt and Kvamme 1973), but this area of research has progressed slowly in the ensuing years because most laboratories were unable to detect biosynthesis in broken cell preparations. Synthesis of NAAG from radiolabeled precursors has also been demonstrated in neuronal and glial cell culture systems (Arun et al., 2004, 2006, 2008; Gehl et al., 2004). However, until recently the identification and characterization of the synthetic enzyme remained elusive.

Recently, two members of the ATP grasp protein family were identified to be the NAAG synthetase enzymes. They are known as rimK-like family member B (*Rimklb*) and A (*Rimkla*) (Becker et al., 2010; Collard et al., 2010). The enzymes of this family (RIMK) are ATP-dependent glutamate ligases that ligate the α-amino group of glutamate to the carboxylic group of an acceptor. These ligases have been found to be specifically dependent upon NAA and ATP for their function and are inactive in the absence of either one. Both the enzymes have very high K_m values (1.48 mM NAA for RIMKLA) indicating that very high concentrations of NAA are required for enzyme activity (Collard et al., 2010). RIMKLB also has a low level of glutamate ligase activity toward citrate, forming β-citrylglutamate. RIMKLA was found to have about three times lower K_m value for NAA compared to RIMKLB, while the K_m values for citrate are comparable for both the enzymes. Both NAAG synthase enzymes share about 65% sequence identity. Also, RIMKLA was recently found to have an additional glutamate ligase activity to synthesize N-acetylaspartyl-glutamyl-glutamate (NAAG$_2$), a tripeptide. From the publically available database on protein localization, the newly identified RIMKLB and RIMKLA proteins have a primary neuronal localization with the highest expression levels in hindbrain and spinal cord. This expression pattern matches the expression levels observed using antibodies to protein-coupled NAAG (Moffett & Namboodiri, 1995, 2006). Future gene knockout studies should help to advance our understanding of the functional roles of NAAG in the CNS.

NAAG Localization

NAAG was first identified by Miyamoto and colleagues (1966) in bovine brain extracts in the mid-1960s. Using gas chromatography Miyake and Kakimoto (1981) found that NAAG increased in concentration in the brain and spinal cord from birth through adulthood in both rats and guinea pigs. Further studies showed that NAAG was most likely present in neurons, for example, the concentration of NAAG in gray matter was more than twice that

found in white matter, and the concentration in the CNS was over 100 times greater than the concentrations seen in peripheral organs (Miyake et al., 1981). In these studies NAAG was identified in the CNS of all mammalian, avian, reptilian, and amphibian species studied, with the lowest concentration noted in the CNS of fish. Further evidence for neuronal localization came from HPLC analyses of piriform cortex in the rat 3 days after unilateral olfactory bulbectomy showing a 22% drop in NAAG concentrations indicating that some of the NAAG in piriform cortex was associated with olfactory fibers or nerve endings (ffrench-Mullen et al., 1985). A number of evoked release studies showed that NAAG was released after depolarization in a calcium-dependent manner from terminals in the retina and retinal target areas in the brain (Tsai et al., 1988; Williamson et al., 1991; Williamson & Neale, 1992), as well as from tissue slices of striatum, cerebellum, and spinal cord (Zollinger et al., 1994). These and similar investigations demonstrated that NAAG is released synaptically from neurons in the same manner as classical neurotransmitters.

Development of antibodies and specialized fixation techniques permitted the visualization of NAAG in brain sections (Anderson et al., 1987; Cangro et al., 1987; Tieman et al., 1987). These studies showed that NAAG was present in neurons, axons, and synaptic terminals, but not in glia. Subsequent improvements to the methods provided very detailed neuroanatomical information on NAAG localization in the CNS of the rat (Moffett et al., 1993; Moffett et al., 1994; Moffett & Namboodiri, 1995, 2006; Moffett et al., 1993, 1994), cat (Tieman et al., 1987, 1991a), monkey (Tieman et al., 1991b; Moffett & Namboodiri, 2006), and human (Tieman & Tieman, 1996; Passani et al., 1997b). NAAG expression generally showed an increasing rostrocaudal concentration gradient, with lower levels in many forebrain areas, and higher levels in the medulla and spinal cord. However the visual system was an exception in the forebrain in that there were very high levels of NAAG expression in the optic nerve fibers and in synapses in visual target areas including the lateral geniculate, superior colliculus, suprachiasmatic nucleus, and accessory optic nuclei (Moffett et al., 1990; Moffett, 2003; Tieman, 2006). Ultrastructural studies have shown NAAG to be present in synaptic vesicles in the visual system and cerebellum (Williamson & Neale, 1988; Renno et al., 1997).

NAAG is not expressed in all neurons, as is apparently the case with NAA. NAAG expression is much more restricted than that of NAA. In some brain regions NAAG expression is relatively sparse, for example, only a relatively small percentage of

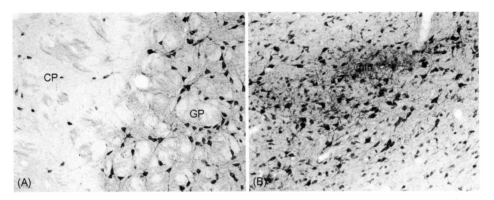

FIGURE 2.1.4 NAAG in rat striatum versus globus pallidus (GP) and in the lateral hypothalamus. NAAG expression was low in the striatum and accumbens, with only scattered neurons and axons of the internal capsule strongly stained (CP in A). In contrast, strong NAAG expression was observed in the majority of neurons in the GP along with strong staining in dendrites. Neurons of the lateral hypothalamus were intensely stained for NAAG, as were axons of the medial forebrain bundle (mfb; B) (10× objective in A and B). This figure is reproduced in color in the color plate section.

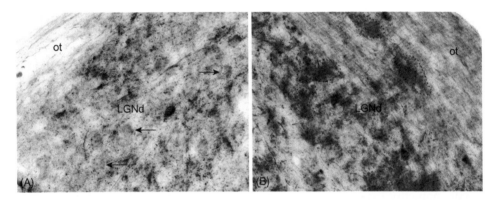

FIGURE 2.1.5 NAAG in the visual system. Some of the highest NAAG expression in the forebrain is associated with the visual pathways from retinal ganglion cells to the lateral geniculate nucleus, including the optic tracts (ot). NAAG-containing glomerular synapses (dotted outlines in B) are present throughout the dorsolateral geniculate nucleus (LGNd), and these contacts are lost upon optic nerve transection (A). The sections are double stained for NAAG (orange) and glutamic acid decarboxylase (purple) the enzyme that synthesizes the inhibitory neurotransmitter GABA. Arrows in A show NAAG expression in principle neurons of the lateral geniculate. This figure is reproduced in color in the color plate section.

neurons express NAAG in the rat striatum, whereas expression is very strong in the adjacent globus pallidus (Fig. 2.1.4). Other regions with notably high expression levels of NAAG in the rat forebrain include the hypothalamus (Fig. 2.1.4), the visual pathways and retinal target areas (Fig. 2.1.5), and the thalamic reticular nucleus. Therefore NAAG is present in both excitatory (visual pathways) and inhibitory neurons (globus pallidus and thalamic reticular nucleus). In fact NAAG has also been found in cholinergic, noradrenergic, and serotonergic neuronal groups (Forloni et al., 1987; Moffett & Namboodiri, 2006). These findings place NAAG in most neuronal types in the CNS, which is in good agreement with its proposed role as a neuromodulatory agent involved in neurotransmitter release regulation. NAAG is expressed at exceptionally high levels in the medulla and spinal cord in

the rat, suggesting an important role in somatosensory and motor functions, possibly including regulation of neurotransmitter release. NAAG expression also exhibits some species specificity. For example, large pyramidal neurons in neocortex typically express low levels of NAAG in the rat, but high levels of NAAG in the rhesus monkey (Fig. 2.1.6).

NAAG Catabolism

In 1987, Robinson and colleagues (1987) demonstrated NAAG hydrolyzing enzymatic activity by measuring hydrolysis of several radiolabeled NAAG substrates in lysed synaptosomal membrane preparations from rat forebrain. They assigned this activity the name *N*-acetylated α-linked acidic dipeptidase, or

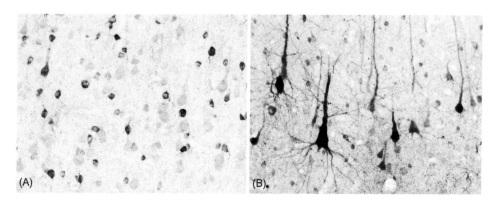

FIGURE 2.1.6   NAAG expression in layer V of neocortex. NAAG expression in rat neocortex was strong in interneurons and weak or absent in large pyramidal neurons (A). In contrast, in rhesus monkey large pyramidal neurons and smaller interneurons were immunoreactive for NAAG (B) (20× objective A and B). This figure is reproduced in color in the color plate section.

NAALADase. The enzyme activity was found to require mono and divalent anions and was inhibited by the excitatory amino acid agonist, L-quisqualic acid, as well as polyvalent anions such as phosphate and sulfate. They demonstrated that the enzyme hydrolyzes the aspartate-glutamate peptide bond but does not remove the NH_2-terminal acetate group. The enzyme was subsequently identified as identical to glutamate carboxypeptidase II (GCPII; Blakely et al., 1988), as well as the prostate cancer marker prostate-specific membrane antigen (Carter et al., 1996). Using a cloned GCPII, Luthi-Carter and coworkers (1998) reported that NAAG is hydrolyzed by GCPII. Inhibitors of GCPII such as β-NAAG, quisqualic acid, and 2-(phosphonomethyl) pentanedioic acid (PMPA) significantly inhibited the hydrolysis of NAAG. Subsequent investigations using mice lacking GCPII indicated that there is another enzyme in the brain designated GCPIII, which can carry out the hydrolysis of NAAG in the absence of GCPII (Bacich et al., 2002; Bzdega et al., 2004). GCPII knockout mice did not show any neurological abnormalities indicating that GCPIII in the brain was sufficient for metabolizing NAAG. A comparative study showed that several inhibitors of GCPII also inhibited GCPIII, and the two enzymes showed different pH and salt concentration dependence and substrate specificities indicating that these homologs might play distinct biological roles in the CNS (Hlouchova et al., 2007). Studies using recombinant GCPII and GCPIII indicated that GCPII is responsible for the majority of NAAG hydrolysis in the human brain (Sacha et al., 2007). Immunohistochemical studies indicate that the cellular localization of GCPII in the brain is exclusively in astrocytes, but that it is not expressed in all astrocytes (Sacha et al., 2007). In addition to the CNS, GCPII is also expressed in peripheral organs including prostate, kidney, and intestine among others.

NAAG, GCPII Inhibitors, and Metabotropic Glutamate Receptors

Unlike classical neurotransmitters, application of NAAG to various regions of the brain often elicits no electrophysiological response, or mixed responses that include slow depolarization or slow hyperpolarization (Henderson & Salt, 1988; Riveros & Orrego, 1984; Jones & Sillito, 1992). Studying the actions of NAAG in the nervous system is confounded by the fact that the NAAG-hydrolyzing enzyme GCPII does not generate inert substances, but instead generates glutamate, the most prevalent excitatory neurotransmitter in the brain. This is very distinct from most extracellular neurotransmitter-inactivating enzymes such as acetylcholine esterase, which generate less active metabolites that can be taken up and recycled. Synaptically released NAAG is rapidly converted to NAA and glutamate, but it is still uncertain if the glutamate generated by GCPII localized on astrocytes is taken up by the astrocytes immediately, or if it is available for binding to cell-surface ionotropic or metabotropic glutamate receptors. This uncertainty has made the study of NAAG actions in the nervous system difficult, and this difficulty is exacerbated by the fact that it has been extremely difficult to determine what receptors NAAG acts on. Initially it was thought that NAAG acted on ionotropic glutamate receptors including the *N*-methyl-D-aspartate (NMDA) receptor (Westbrook et al., 1986), but the high levels required for activation called into question the physiological relevance. Subsequently NAAG was reported to act through metabotropic glutamate receptors (mGluR) to inhibit cyclic AMP production (Wroblewska et al., 1993). Over the ensuing years the connection to mGluR, particularly the mGluR3 subtype of metabotropic receptor, has been the primary focus of the majority of work on NAAG actions in the CNS. However, this connection has not been without controversy, again because NAAG hydrolysis generates glutamate, and also because commercially available NAAG preparations have been found to be contaminated with low levels of glutamate that could be responsible for some of the reported actions (Chopra et al., 2009). For a review of the physiology of metabotropic glutamate receptors see Niswender and Conn (2010).

Because of the confounding issue of the high potency of glutamate at all types of metabotropic and ionotropic glutamate receptors, it has become standard procedure to study the actions of NAAG by inhibition of the hydrolytic enzyme GCPII. Limiting hydrolysis of NAAG theoretically leads to prolonged NAAG occupation of mGluR and reduced production of NAAG-derived glutamate (Wozniak et al., 2012). This approach, using GCPII inhibitors in conjunction with mGluR 2/3 receptor antagonists to block NAAG action at these receptors, has led to many interesting findings about possible NAAG actions. For example, inhibition of GCPII has shown significant protection of motor neurons in both *in vitro* and *in vivo* models of familial amyotrophic lateral sclerosis, and it was proposed that the decrease in extracellular glutamate is the mechanism involved in these observations (Ghadge et al., 2003; Thomas et al., 2003). It has also been hypothesized that altered glutamate neurotransmission in the brainstem is involved in pain perception in different animal models of pain (Burchiel et al., 1985; Kawamata & Omote, 1996) and GCPII inhibitors have shown protection against neuropathic pain supporting the above notion (Zhang et al., 2002, 2006; Yamada et al., 2012). Inhibition of GCPII has also shown promising results in the treatment of brain injury. Post-injury administration of GCPII inhibitor significantly reduced neuronal and astrocytic cell death in the hippocampus in a rat model of traumatic brain injury combined with a secondary hypoxic insult (Feng et al., 2012). Moreover, mice lacking GCPII showed significant protection against peripheral neuropathy and reduced infarct volume in an animal model of middle cerebral artery occlusion indicating the role of NAAG hydrolysis in peripheral neuropathy and stroke (Bacich et al., 2005).

There are a number of controversies that surround the above observations (reviewed in Johnson, 2011; Neale, 2011). The first involves a debate over whether or not the effects of GCPII inhibition involve NAAG, or the inhibitors themselves. Another controversy centers on whether NAAG actually acts through mGluR3 receptors, or works via mGluR2 receptors, or some other type of receptor. A widely accepted conclusion is that GCPII inhibitors increase NAAG levels in the brain and most or all of the observed effects of NAAG peptidase inhibition involve NAAG binding to the mGluR3 receptor subtype (Olszewski et al., 2012a; Neale, 2011). The evidence supporting this conclusion is substantial; however, this view has been challenged by a number of studies. For example, a microdialysis study testing the effect of 2-PMPA, a GCPII inhibitor, in a model of chronic pain (Nagel et al., 2006) concluded that while the anti-allodynic effect of 2-PMPA was observed, the NAAG concentration in dialysate did not reach a sufficient concentration to have any impact on metabotropic glutamate receptors. Two research groups have questioned the validity of the experimental results involving direct effects of NAAG based on their observation that the effect of NAAG in *in vitro* systems disappears when glutamate contamination in the commercial NAAG preparation is removed by further purification (Chopra et al., 2009; Fricker et al., 2009; Johnson, 2011). According to these investigators the observed effects are due to glutamate contamination, as well as contamination with other unknown compounds in commercially available NAAG preparations, and are not related to NAAG activity at any type of glutamate receptor. A review of these controversies has been published noting that many of the studies on NAAG actions at mGluR3 utilized re-purified NAAG, and the review concludes that the majority of studies indicate that NAAG is active at these receptors (Neale, 2011). Now that these controversies have been better delineated, and the genes for NAAG synthase have been identified, it is likely that studies in the near future will be able to come to more definitive conclusions on the actions of NAAG in the CNS, and possible activity at the mGluR3 receptor.

NAAG, mGluR, and Neurotransmitter Release Modulation

Metabotropic glutamate receptors are a diverse class of G-protein-coupled neuromodulatory receptors found throughout the CNS that regulate various processes including neuronal activity and neurotransmitter release (Niswender & Conn, 2010). mGluR3 receptors are present on presynaptic endings where they are in a position to modulate neurotransmitter release. Because NAAG is colocalized with virtually all major neurotransmitters including glutamate, GABA, dopamine, serotonin, norepinephrine, and acetylcholine, it is also in a position to regulate their release from neurons. In fact, several studies based on inhibition of GCPII and exogenous NAAG application have indicated that NAAG can act by inhibiting the release of neurotransmitters including glutamate and GABA from presynaptic terminals, most likely by an mGluR3-mediated mechanism (Zhao et al., 2001; Zhong et al., 2006). It is noteworthy that NAAG inhibits both excitatory and inhibitory neurotransmitter release, and further that NAAG localization in GABAergic and glutamatergic neurons is distinct. In excitatory systems such as the visual pathways NAAG is present in neuronal cell bodies, dendrites, axons, and synaptic terminals, whereas in GABAergic systems such as the thalamic reticular nucleus and globus pallidus, NAAG is only present in neuronal cell bodies and dendrites, but not in axonal projections or synaptic terminals (Moffett, 2003). These findings suggest that NAAG is coreleased with glutamate from synaptic endings, but that it may only be released from somatic and dendritic compartments in GABAergic neurons. While the concentrations of NAAG used in earlier studies ranged from low to high micromolar, a recent study has shown that NAAG is extraordinarily potent in inhibiting KCl induced release of glycine from spinal cord synaptosomal preparations with a dose response in the 0.01 to 1.0 pmol range (Romei et al., 2012). Furthermore, this effect of NAAG was reversed by LY341495, an mGluR2/3 antagonist and also by β-NAAG, a structural analog of NAAG that blocks GCPII enzymatic activity. Also, glutamate was not very effective under the experimental conditions ruling out the possibility that glutamate contamination in the NAAG preparation was responsible for the effect. The extraordinary potency of NAAG in this system is difficult to explain. The authors are of the opinion that the relatively higher concentrations required in earlier studies have to do with the degradation of NAAG by GCPII located on astrocytes. However, the effective concentration of NAAG is so low in this system that this explanation is not entirely convincing. The authors further suggested that the NAAG receptors involved are most likely located in non-synaptic transmission areas where receptors generally exhibit higher affinity than receptors expressed in the areas of synaptic transmission. Clearly, future studies are required to establish this extraordinarily potent receptor mediated action of NAAG.

NAAG and Schizophrenia

One theory of schizophrenia involves dysregulated glutamate signaling in certain brain regions including prefrontal cortex. This theory was predicated on observations that so-called open-channel NMDA receptor antagonists including PCP, MK801, and ketamine, produce schizophrenia-like symptoms in animals, and exacerbate those symptoms in schizophrenia patients. Open-channel NMDA antagonists block the channel only when it has opened because they bind within the ion channel itself. It has been found that inhibition of NAAG hydrolysis using GCPII inhibitors has the ability to reverse the effects of PCP in experimental

animals, and therefore it is thought that this may represent a novel method of treating schizophrenia. GCPII inhibition has shown promise in reducing both positive and negative symptoms in the rat and mouse (Olszewski et al., 2004; Takatsu et al., 2011; Zuo et al., 2012). More recently, this was found to be true for the dopamine-based model of schizophrenia in mice as well (Olszewski et al., 2012b). There is currently no consensus on the underlying mechanisms involved with one theory pointing to agonistic activity on mGluR3 receptors that can inhibit glutamate release (Zhao et al., 2001; Flores & Coyle, 2003; Zhong et al., 2006), and another that the decrease in free glutamate formation from NAAG after inhibition of GCPII plays a significant role in properly regulating glutamate release in the prefrontal cortex (Ghadge et al., 2003; Cavaletti & Slusher, 2012). In a more recent study testing the effect two GCP inhibitors in an animal model of schizophrenia, there was little or no correlation between the observed effect on motor activation and inhibition of GCPII activity *in vivo*. Currently there is also no general consensus on which subtype of mGluR is involved in the effects of GCPII inhibitors, with some evidence pointing to mGluR3, and other evidence pointing to mGluR2 (Fell et al., 2008; Woolley et al., 2008). Therefore, future studies in different model systems are needed to establish the mechanisms by which GCPII inhibition can reverse the effects of open-channel NMDA antagonists.

NAAG as a "Pro-transmitter"

In light of the diverse and contradictory findings in multiple model systems, it is difficult to come to a consensus on the controversies surrounding the actions of NAAG. This is indicated by only a very brief mention of NAAG in a recent comprehensive review on metabotropic glutamate receptors (Nicoletti et al., 2011). It is possible that part of the controversy is due to the diverse nature of the model systems used and partly due to the complex but closely related nature of the different members of the metabotropic glutamate receptor family. However, it is also possible that the current views of NAAG and metabotropic receptor activation are incomplete. There is one view of NAAG that has the potential to explain some of the reported discrepancies; namely that a major function of NAAG is to generate glutamate (Tsukamoto et al., 2007). If NAAG is viewed as a "pro-transmitter" rather than a neurotransmitter modulator, then the release of NAAG would generate local increases in extracellular glutamate in specific brain systems where GCPII was active, for example, at presynaptic, glial, or extrasynaptic glutamate receptors. In this view GCPII is the activating enzyme, glutamate is the active agent, and NAAG is acting as a pro-transmitter. Therefore, blocking GCPII blocks a specific type of glutamate release, perhaps at specialized synapses that contain GCPII, or at extrasynaptic sites where synaptically released glutamate is excluded. Because glutamate is more potent than NAAG at all types of ionotropic and metabotropic glutamate receptors, this view has some logical appeal. This interpretation could explain how blocking NAAG hydrolysis could prevent pain transmission in the brainstem, and why preventing NAAG breakdown would reduce brain injury due to ischemia or motor neuron disease. Future studies will clarify these issues and advance our understanding of the functional roles of NAAG in the CNS. Availability of mice in which the biosynthetic enzyme for NAAG is knocked out will be instrumental in this regard. It is safe to say that research into NAAG actions in the CNS is still in its early stages, and that major discoveries await future studies.

References

Anandatheerthavarada, H. K., Sepuri, N. B., Biswas, G., & Avadhani, N. G. (2008). An unusual TOM20/TOM22 bypass mechanism for the mitochondrial targeting of cytochrome P450 proteins containing N-terminal chimeric signals. *Journal of Biological Chemistry, 283*, 19769–19780.

Anderson, K. J., Borja, M. A., Cotman, C. W., Moffett, J. R., Namboodiri, M. A., & Neale, J. H. (1987). N-acetylaspartylglutamate identified in the rat retinal ganglion cells and their projections in the brain. *Brain Research, 411*, 172–177.

Ariyannur, P. S., Madhavarao, C. N., & Namboodiri, A. M. (2008). N-acetylaspartate synthesis in the brain: mitochondria vs. microsomes. *Brain Research, 1227*, 34–41.

Ariyannur, P. S., Moffett, J. R., Madhavarao, C. N., Arun, P., Vishnu, N., Jacobowitz, D., et al. (2010a). Nuclear-cytoplasmic localization of acetyl coenzyme A synthetase-1 in the rat brain. *Journal of Comparative Neurology, 518*, 2952–2977.

Ariyannur, P. S., Moffett, J. R., Manickam, P., Pattabiraman, N., Arun, P., Nitta, A., et al. (2010b). Methamphetamine-induced neuronal protein NAT8L is the NAA biosynthetic enzyme: Implications for specialized acetyl coenzyme A metabolism in the CNS. *Brain Research, 1335*, 1–13.

Arun, P., Madhavarao, C. N., Hershfield, J. R., Moffett, J. R., & Namboodiri, M. A. (2004). SH-SY5Y neuroblastoma cells: a model system for studying biosynthesis of NAAG. *Neuroreport, 15*, 1167–1170.

Arun, P., Madhavarao, C. N., Moffett, J. R., Hamilton, K., Grunberg, N. E., Ariyannur, P. S., et al. (2010). Metabolic acetate therapy improves phenotype in the tremor rat model of Canavan disease. *Journal of Inherited Metabolic Disease, 33*, 195–210.

Arun, P., Madhavarao, C. N., Moffett, J. R., & Namboodiri, A. M. (2006). Regulation of N-acetylaspartate and N-acetylaspartylglutamate biosynthesis by protein kinase activators. *Journal of Neurochemistry, 98*, 2034–2042.

Arun, P., Madhavarao, C. N., Moffett, J. R., & Namboodiri, A. M. (2008). Antipsychotic drugs increase N-acetylaspartate and N-acetylaspartylglutamate in SH-SY5Y human neuroblastoma cells. *Journal of Neurochemistry, 106*, 1669–1680.

Arun, P., Moffett, J. R., & Namboodiri, A. M. (2009). Evidence for mitochondrial and cytoplasmic N-acetylaspartate synthesis in SH-SY5Y neuroblastoma cells. *Neurochemistry International, 55*, 219–225.

Avadhani, N. G., Sangar, M. C., Bansal, S., & Bajpai, P. (2011). Bimodal targeting of cytochrome P450s to endoplasmic reticulum and mitochondria: the concept of chimeric signals. *FEBS Journal, 278*, 4218–4229.

Bacich, D. J., Ramadan, E., O'Keefe, D. S., Bukhari, N., Wegorzewska, I., Ojeifo, O., et al. (2002). Deletion of the glutamate carboxypeptidase II gene in mice reveals a second enzyme activity that hydrolyzes N-acetylaspartylglutamate. *Journal of Neurochemistry, 83*, 20–29.

Bacich, D. J., Wozniak, K. M., Lu, X. C., O'Keefe, D. S., Callizot, N., Heston, W. D., et al. (2005). Mice lacking glutamate carboxypeptidase II are protected from peripheral neuropathy and ischemic brain injury. *Journal of Neurochemistry, 95*, 314–323.

Ballard, F. J. (1972). Supply and utilization of acetate in mammals. *American Journal of Clinical Nutrition, 25*, 773–779.

Baslow, M. H. (1997). A review of phylogenetic and metabolic relationships between the acylamino acids, N-acetyl-L-aspartic acid and N-acetyl-L-histidine, in the vertebrate nervous system. *Journal of Neurochemistry, 68*, 1335–1344.

Baslow, M. H. (1999). Molecular water pumps and the aetiology of Canavan disease: a case of the sorcerer's apprentice. *Journal of Inherited Metabolic Diseases, 22*, 99–101.

Baslow, M. H. (2002). Evidence supporting a role for N-acetyl-L-aspartate as a molecular water pump in myelinated neurons in the central nervous system. An analytical review. *Neurochemistry International, 40*, 295–300.

Baslow, M. H. (2003). Brain N-acetylaspartate as a molecular water pump and its role in the etiology of Canavan disease: a mechanistic explanation. *Journal of Molecular Neuroscience, 21*, 185–190.

Baslow, M. H., Hrabe, J., & Guilfoyle, D. N. (2007). Dynamic relationship between neurostimulation and N-acetylaspartate metabolism in the human visual cortex: evidence that NAA functions as a molecular water pump during visual stimulation. *Journal of Molecular Neuroscience, 32*, 235–245.

Baslow, M. H., Hu, C., & Guilfoyle, D. N. (2012). Stimulation-induced decreases in the diffusion of extra-vascular water in the human visual cortex: a window in time and space on mechanisms of brain water transport and economy. *Journal of Molecular Neuroscience, 47*, 639–648.

Becker, I., Lodder, J., Gieselmann, V., & Eckhardt, M. (2010). Molecular characterization of N-acetylaspartylglutamate synthetase. *Journal of Biological Chemistry, 285*, 29156–29164.

Benarroch, E. E. (2008). N-acetylaspartate and N-acetylaspartylglutamate: neurobiology and clinical significance. *Neurology, 70*, 1353–1357.

Blakely, R. D., Robinson, M. B., Thompson, R. C., & Coyle, J. T. (1988). Hydrolysis of the brain dipeptide N-acetyl-L-aspartyl-L-glutamate: subcellular and regional distribution, ontogeny, and the effect of lesions on N-acetylated-alpha-linked acidic dipeptidase activity. *Journal of Neurochemistry, 50*, 1200–1209.

Brugger, S., Davis, J. M., Leucht, S., & Stone, J. M. (2011). Proton magnetic resonance spectroscopy and illness stage in schizophrenia—a systematic review and meta-analysis. *Biological Psychiatry, 69*, 495–503.

Burchiel, K. J., Russell, L. C., Lee, R. P., & Sima, A. A. (1985). Spontaneous activity of primary afferent neurons in diabetic BB/Wistar rats. A possible mechanism of chronic diabetic neuropathic pain. *Diabetes, 34*, 1210–1213.

Burlina, A. P., Ferrari, V., Facci, L., Skaper, S. D., & Burlina, A. B. (1997). Mast cells contain large quantities of secretagoguesensitive N-acetylaspartate. *Journal of Neurochemistry*, *69*, 1314–1317.

Burri, R., Steffen, C., & Herschkowitz, N. (1991). N-acetyl-L-aspartate is a major source of acetyl groups for lipid synthesis during rat brain development. *Developmental Neuroscience*, *13*, 403–412.

Bzdega, T., Crowe, S. L., Ramadan, E. R., Sciarretta, K. H., Olszewski, R. T., Ojeifo, O. A., et al. (2004). The cloning and characterization of a second brain enzyme with NAAG peptidase activity. *Journal of Neurochemistry*, *89*, 627–635.

Canavan, M. M. (1931). Schilder's encephalitis perioxalis diffusa. *Neurology*, *15*, 299–308.

Cangro, C. B., Namboodiri, M. A., Sklar, L. A., Corigliano-Murphy, A., & Neale, J. H. (1987). Immunohistochemistry and biosynthesis of N-acetylaspartylglutamate in spinal sensory ganglia. *Journal of Neurochemistry*, *49*, 1579–1588.

Carter, R. E., Feldman, A. R., & Coyle, J. T. (1996). Prostate-specific membrane antigen is a hydrolase with substrate and pharmacologic characteristics of a neuropeptidase. *Proceedings of the National Academy of Sciences USA*, *93*, 749–753.

Cavaletti, G., & Slusher, B. (2012). Regulation of glutamate synthesis via inhibition of glutamate carboxypeptidase II (GCPII): an effective method to treat central and peripheral nervous system disorders. *Current Medicinal Chemistry*, *19*, 1259–1260.

Chakraborty, G., Mekala, P., Yahya, D., Wu, G., & Ledeen, R. W. (2001). Intraneuronal N-acetylaspartate supplies acetyl groups for myelin lipid synthesis: evidence for myelin-associated aspartoacylase. *Journal of Neurochemistry*, *78*, 736–745.

Choi, I. Y., & Gruetter, R. (2004). Dynamic or inert metabolism? Turnover of N-acetyl aspartate and glutathione from D-[1-13C] glucose in the rat brain in vivo. *Journal of Neurochemistry*, *91*, 778–787.

Chopra, M., Yao, Y., Blake, T. J., Hampson, D. R., & Johnson, E. C. (2009). The neuroactive peptide N-acetylaspartylglutamate (NAAG) is not an agonist at the mGluR3 subtype of metabotropic glutamate receptor. *Journal of Pharmacology and Experimental Therapeutics*, *330*, 212–219.

Clark, J. B. (1998). N-acetyl aspartate: a marker for neuronal loss or mitochondrial dysfunction. *Developmental Neuroscience*, *20*, 271–276.

Collard, F., Stroobant, V., Lamosa, P., Kapanda, C. N., Lambert, D. M., Muccioli, G. G., et al. (2010). Molecular identification of N-acetylaspartylglutamate synthase and beta-citrylglutamate synthase. *Journal of Biological Chemistry*, *285*, 29826–29833.

Copray, S., Huynh, J. L., Sher, F., Casaccia-Bonnefil, P., & Boddeke, E. (2009). Epigenetic mechanisms facilitating oligodendrocyte development, maturation, and aging. *Glia*, *57*, 1579–1587.

Costantini, C., Ko, M. H., Jonas, M. C., & Puglielli, L. (2007). A reversible form of lysine acetylation in the ER and Golgi lumen controls the molecular stabilization of BACE1. *Biochemical Journal*, *407*, 383–395.

D'Adamo, A. F., Jr., & Yatsu, F. M. (1966). Acetate metabolism in the nervous system. N-acetyl-L-aspartic acid and the biosynthesis of brain lipids. *Journal of Neurochemistry*, *13*, 961–965.

Demougeot, C., Marie, C., Giroud, M., & Beley, A. (2004). N-acetylaspartate: a literature review of animal research on brain ischaemia. *Journal of Neurochemistry*, *90*, 776–783.

Edden, R. A., Pomper, M. G., & Barker, P. B. (2007). In vivo differentiation of N-acetyl aspartyl glutamate from N-acetyl aspartate at 3 Tesla. *Magnetic Resonance in Medicine*, *57*, 977–982.

Edmond, J., Robbins, R. A., Bergstrom, J. D., Cole, R. A., & de, V. J. (1987). Capacity for substrate utilization in oxidative metabolism by neurons, astrocytes, and oligodendrocytes from developing brain in primary culture. *Journal of Neuroscience Research*, *18*, 551–561.

Fell, M. J., Svensson, K. A., Johnson, B. G., & Schoepp, D. D. (2008). Evidence for the role of metabotropic glutamate (mGlu)2 not mGlu3 receptors in the preclinical antipsychotic pharmacology of the mGlu2/3 receptor agonist (-)-(1R,4S,5S,6S)-4-amino-2-sulfonylbicyclo[3.1.0]hexane-4,6-dicarboxylic acid (LY404039). *Journal of Pharmacology and Experimental Therapeutics*, *326*, 209–217.

Feng, J. F., Gurkoff, G. G., Van, K. C., Song, M., Lowe, D. A., Zhou, J., et al. (2012). NAAG peptidase inhibitor reduces cellular damage in a model of TBI with secondary hypoxia. *Brain Research*, *1469*, 144–152.

ffrench-Mullen, J. M., Koller, K., Zaczek, R., Coyle, J. T., Hori, N., & Carpenter, D. O. (1985). N-Acetylaspartylglutamate: possible role as the neurotransmitter of the lateral olfactory tract. *Proceedings of the National Academy of Sciences USA*, *82*, 3897–3900.

Flores, C., & Coyle, J. T. (2003). Regulation of glutamate carboxypeptidase II function in corticolimbic regions of rat brain by phencyclidine, haloperidol, and clozapine. *Neuropsychopharmacology*, *28*, 1227–1234.

Forloni, G. L., Grzanna, R., Blakely, R. D., & Coyle, J. T. (1987). Co-localization of N-acetyl-aspartyl-glutamate in central cholinergic, noradrenergic, and serotonergic neurons. *Synapse*, *1*, 455–460.

Francis, J. S., Strande, L., Markov, V., & Leone, P. (2012). Aspartoacylase supports oxidative energy metabolism during myelination. *Journal of Cerebral Blood Flow and Metabolism*, *32*, 1736.

Fricker, A. C., Selina Mok, M. H., de la Flor, R., Shah, A. J., Woolley, M., Dawson, L. A., et al. (2009). Effects of N-acetylaspartylglutamate (NAAG) at group II mGluRs and NMDAR. *Neuropharmacology*, *56*, 1060–1067.

Gehl, L. M., Saab, O. H., Bzdega, T., Wroblewska, B., & Neale, J. H. (2004). Biosynthesis of NAAG by an enzyme-mediated process in rat central nervous system neurons and glia. *Journal of Neurochemistry*, *90*, 989–997.

Ghadge, G. D., Slusher, B. S., Bodner, A., Canto, M. D., Wozniak, K., Thomas, A. G., et al. (2003). Glutamate carboxypeptidase II inhibition protects motor neurons from death in familial amyotrophic lateral sclerosis models. *Proceedings of the National Academy of SciencesUSA*, *100*, 9554–9559.

Goldstein, F. B. (1959). Biosynthesis of N-acetyl-L-aspartic acid. *Biochimica Biophysica Acta*, *33*, 583–584.

Goldstein, F. B. (1969). The enzymatic synthesis of N-acetyl-L-aspartic acid by subcellular preparations of rat brain. *Journal of Biological Chemistry*, *244*, 4257–4260.

Gonzalez-Toledo, E., Kelley, R. E., & Minagar, A. (2006). Role of magnetic resonance spectroscopy in diagnosis and management of multiple sclerosis. *Neurological Research*, *28*, 280–283.

Guan, K. L., & Xiong, Y. (2010). Regulation of intermediary metabolism by protein acetylation. *Trends in Biochemical Science*, *36*, 108–116.

Gullans, S. R., & Verbalis, J. G. (1993). Control of brain volume during hyperosmolar and hypoosmolar conditions. *Annual Review. Medicine*, *44*, 289–301.

Hagenfeldt, L., Bollgren, I., & Venizelos, N. (1987). N-acetylaspartic aciduria due to aspartoacylase deficiency—a new aetiology of childhood leukodystrophy. *Journal of Inherited Metabolic Disease*, *10*, 135–141.

Harris, K., Lin, A., Bhattacharya, P., Tran, T., Wong, W., & Ross, B. D. (2006). Regulation of NAA-synthesis in the human brain *in vivo*: Canavan's disease, Alzheimer's disease and schizophrenia. In J. R Moffett, S. B. Tieman, D. R. Weinberger, J. T. Coyle, & M. A. Namboodiri (Eds.), *N-Acetylaspartate: A Unique Neuronal Molecule In The Central Nervous System* (pp. 263–273). New York: Springer Science + Business Media.

Henderson, Z., & Salt, T. E. (1988). The effects of N-acetylaspartylglutamate and distribution of N-acetylaspartylglutamate-like immunoreactivity in the rat somatosensory thalamus. *Neuroscience*, *25*, 899–906.

Hlouchova, K., Barinka, C., Klusak, V., Sacha, P., Mlcochova, P., Majer, P., et al. (2007). Biochemical characterization of human glutamate carboxypeptidase III. *Journal of Neurochemistry, 101*, 682–696.

Jalil, M. A., Begum, L., Contreras, L., Pardo, B., Iijima, M., Li, M. X., et al. (2005). Reduced N-acetylaspartate levels in mice lacking Aralar, a brain-and muscle-type mitochondrial aspartate-glutamate carrier. *Journal of Biological Chemistry, 280*, 31333–31339.

Janson, C., McPhee, S., Bilaniuk, L., Haselgrove, J., Testaiuti, M., Freese, A., et al. (2002). Clinical protocol. Gene therapy of Canavan disease: AAV-2 vector for neurosurgical delivery of aspartoacylase gene (ASPA) to the human brain. *Human Gene Therapy, 13*, 1391–1412.

Johnson, E. C. (2011). N-acetylaspartylglutamate is not demonstrated to be a selective mGlureceptor agonist. *Journal of Neurochemistry, 119*, 896–898.

Jonas, M. C., Pehar, M., & Puglielli, L. (2010). AT-1 is the ER membrane acetyl-CoA transporter and is essential for cell viability. *Journal of Cell Science, 123*, 3378–3388.

Jones, H. E., & Sillito, A. M. (1992). The action of the putative neurotransmitters N-acetylaspartylglutamate and L-homocysteate in cat dorsal lateral geniculate nucleus. *Journal of Neurophysiology, 68*, 663–672.

Kantarci, K., & Jack, C. R., Jr. (2003). Neuroimaging in Alzheimer disease: an evidence-based review. *Neuroimaging Clinics of North America, 13*, 197–209.

Kaul, R., Balamurugan, K., Gao, G. P., & Matalon, R. (1994a). Canavan disease: genomic organization and localization of human ASPA to 17p13-ter and conservation of the ASPA gene during evolution. *Genomics, 21*, 364–370.

Kaul, R., Gao, G. P., Aloya, M., Balamurugan, K., Petrosky, A., Michals, K., et al. (1994b). Canavan disease: mutations among Jewish and non-jewish patients. *American Journal of Human Genetics, 55*, 34–41.

Kaul, R., Gao, G. P., Balamurugan, K., & Matalon, R. (1993). Cloning of the human aspartoacylase cDNA and a common missense mutation in Canavan disease. *Nature Genetics, 5*, 118–123.

Kaul, R., Gao, G. P., Matalon, R., Aloya, M., Su, Q., Jin, M., et al. (1996). Identification and expression of eight novel mutations among non-Jewish patients with Canavan disease. *American Journal of Human Genetics, 59*, 95–102.

Kawamata, M., & Omote, K. (1996). Involvement of increased excitatory amino acids and intracellular Ca^{2+} concentration in the spinal dorsal horn in an animal model of neuropathic pain. *Pain, 68*, 85–96.

Kitada, K., Akimitsu, T., Shigematsu, Y., Kondo, A., Maihara, T., Yokoi, N., et al. (2000). Accumulation of N-acetyl-L-aspartate in the brain of the tremor rat, a mutant exhibiting absence-like seizure and spongiform degeneration in the central nervous system. *Journal of Neurochemistry, 74*, 2512–2519.

Klugmann, M., Leichtlein, C. B., Symes, C. W., Serikawa, T., Young, D., & During, M. J. (2005). Restoration of aspartoacylase activity in CNS neurons does not ameliorate motor deficits and demyelination in a model of Canavan disease. *Molecular Therapy, 11*, 745–753.

Klugmann, M., Symes, C. W., Klaussner, B. K., Leichtlein, C. B., Serikawa, T., Young, D., et al. (2003). Identification and distribution of aspartoacylase in the postnatal rat brain. *Neuroreport, 14*, 1837–1840.

Kouzarides, T. (2000). Acetylation: a regulatory modification to rival phosphorylation? *EMBO Journal, 19*, 1176–1179.

Kumar, S., Biancotti, J. C., Matalon, R., & de, V. J. (2009). Lack of aspartoacylase activity disrupts survival and differentiation of neural progenitors and oligodendrocytes in a mouse model of Canavan disease. *Journal of Neuroscience Research, 87*, 3415–3427.

Kumar, S., Mattan, N. S., & de, V. J. (2006a). Canavan disease: a white matter disorder. *Mental Retardation Developmental Disabilities Research Review, 12*, 157–165.

Kumar, S., Sowmyalakshmi, R., Daniels, S. L., Chang, R., Surendran, S., Matalon, R., et al. (2006b). Does ASPA gene mutation in Canavan disease alter oligodendrocyte development? A tissue culture study of ASPA KO mice brain. In J. R Moffett, S. B. Tieman, D. R. Weinberger, J. T. Coyle, & M. A. Namboodiri (Eds.), *N-Acetylaspartate: A Unique Neuronal Molecule in the Central Nervous System* (pp. 175–182). New York: Springer Science + Business Media.

Ledeen, R. W. (1984). Lipid-metabolizing enzymes of myelin and their relation to the axon. *Journal of Lipid Research, 25*, 1548–1554.

Leone, P., Shera, D., McPhee, S. W., Francis, J. S., Kolodny, E. H., Bilaniuk, L. T., et al. (2012). Long-term follow-up after gene therapy for canavan disease. *Science Translational Medicine, 4*. 165ra163.

Lin, W., & Popko, B. (2009). Endoplasmic reticulum stress in disorders of myelinating cells. *Nature Neuroscience, 12*, 379–385.

Lindner, H., Hopfner, S., Tafler-Naumann, M., Miko, M., Konrad, L., & Rohm, K. H. (2000). The distribution of aminoacylase I among mammalian species and localization of the enzyme in porcine kidney. *Biochimie, 82*, 129–137.

Luthi-Carter, R., Barczak, A. K., Speno, H., & Coyle, J. T. (1998). Hydrolysis of the neuropeptide N-acetylaspartylglutamate (NAAG) by cloned human glutamate carboxypeptidase II. *Brain Research, 795*, 341–348.

MacDonald, J. L., & Roskams, A. J. (2009). Epigenetic regulation of nervous system development by DNA methylation and histone deacetylation. *Progress in Neurobiology, 88*, 170–183.

Madhavarao, C. N., Arun, P., Moffett, J. R., Szucs, S., Surendran, S., Matalon, R., et al. (2005). Defective N-acetylaspartate catabolism reduces brain acetate levels and myelin lipid synthesis in Canavan's disease. *Proceedings of the National Academy of Sciences USA, 102*, 5221–5226.

Madhavarao, C. N., Chinopoulos, C., Chandrasekaran, K., & Namboodiri, M. A. (2003). Characterization of the N-acetylaspartate biosynthetic enzyme from rat brain. *Journal of Neurochemistry, 86*, 824–835.

Madhavarao, C. N., Moffett, J. R., Moore, R. A., Viola, R. E., Namboodiri, M. A., & Jacobowitz, D. M. (2004). Immunohistochemical localization of aspartoacylase in the rat central nervous system. *Journal of Comparative Neurology, 472*, 318–329.

Matalon, R., Michals, K., Sebesta, D., Deanching, M., Gashkoff, P., & Casanova, J. (1988). Aspartoacylase deficiency and N-acetylaspartic aciduria in patients with canavan disease. *American Journal of Medical Genetics, 29*, 463–471.

Matalon, R., & Michals-Matalon, K. (1998). Molecular basis of Canavan disease. *European Journal of Paediatric Neurology, 2*, 69–76.

Mattan, N. S., Ghiani, C. A., Lloyd, M., Matalon, R., Bok, D., Casaccia, P., et al. (2010). Aspartoacylase deficiency affects early postnatal development of oligodendrocytes and myelination. *Neurobiology of Disease, 40*, 432–443.

Mehta, V., & Namboodiri, M. A. (1995). N-acetylaspartate as an acetyl source in the nervous system. *Molecular Brain Research, 31*, 151–157.

Miyake, M., & Kakimoto, Y. (1981). Developmental changes of N-acetyl-L-aspartic acid, N-acetyl-alpha-aspartylglutamic acid and beta-citryl-L-glutamic acid in different brain regions and spinal cords of rat and guinea pig. *Journal of Neurochemistry, 37*, 1064–1067.

Miyake, M., Kakimoto, Y., & Sorimachi, M. (1981). A gas chromatographic method for the determination of N-acetyl-L-aspartic acid, N-acetyl-aspartylglutamic acid and beta-citryl-L-glutamic acid and their distributions in the brain and other organs of various species of animals. Journal of Neurochemistry, 36, 804–810.

Miyamoto, E., Kakimoto, Y., & Sano, I. (1966). Identification of N-acetylaspartylglutamic acid in the bovine brain. Journal of Neurochemistry, 13, 999–1003.

Mlynarik, V., Cudalbu, C., Xin, L., & Gruetter, R. (2008). ^{1}H NMR spectroscopy of rat brain in vivo at 14.1Tesla: improvements in quantification of the neurochemical profile. Journal of Magnetic Resonance, 194, 163–168.

Moffett, J. R. (2003). Reductions in N-acetylaspartylglutamate and the 67 kDa form of glutamic acid decarboxylase immunoreactivities in the visual system of albino and pigmented rats after optic nerve transections. Journal of Comparative Neurology, 458, 221–239.

Moffett, J. R., Arun, P., Ariyannur, P. S., Garbern, J. Y., Jacobowitz, D. M., & Namboodiri, A. M. (2011). Extensive aspartoacylase expression in the rat central nervous system. Glia, 59, 1414–1434.

Moffett, J. R., & Namboodiri, M. A. (1995). Differential distribution of N-acetylaspartylglutamate and N-acetylaspartate immunoreactivities in rat forebrain. Journal of Neurocytology, 24, 409–433.

Moffett, J. R., & Namboodiri, M. A. (2006). Expression of N-acetylaspartate and N-acetylaspartylglutamate in the nervous system. In J. R. Moffett, S. B. Tieman, D. R. Weinberger, J. T. Coyle, & M. A. Namboodiri (Eds.), N-Acetylaspartate: A Unique Neuronal Molecule in the Central Nervous System (pp. 7–26). New York: Springer Science + Business Media.

Moffett, J. R., Namboodiri, M. A., Cangro, C. B., & Neale, J. H. (1991). Immunohistochemical localization of N-acetylaspartate in rat brain. Neuroreport, 2, 131–134.

Moffett, J. R., Namboodiri, M. A., & Neale, J. H. (1993). Enhanced carbodiimide fixation for immunohistochemistry: Application to the comparative distributions of N-acetylaspartylglutamate and N-acetylaspartate immunoreactivities in rat brain. Journal of Histochemistry and Cytochemistry, 41, 559–570.

Moffett, J. R., Palkovits, M., Namboodiri, M. A., & Neale, J. H. (1994). Comparative distribution of N-acetylaspartylglutamate and GAD$_{67}$ immunoreactivities in the cerebellum and precerebellar nuclei of the rat utilizing enhanced carbodiimide fixation and immunohistochemistry. Journal of Comparative Neurology, 347, 598–618.

Moffett, J. R., Ross, B., Arun, P., Madhavarao, C. N., & Namboodiri, A. M. (2007). N-Acetylaspartate in the CNS: From neurodiagnostics to neurobiology. Progress in Neurobiology, 81, 89–131.

Moffett, J. R., Tieman, S. B., Weinberger, D. R., Coyle, J. T., & Namboodiri, M. A. (2006). N-Acetylaspartate: a unique neuronal molecule in the central nervous system (Vol. 576).). New York: Springer Science + Business Media.

Moffett, J. R., Williamson, L. C., Palkovits, M., & Namboodiri, M. A. (1990). N-acetylaspartylglutamate: a transmitter candidate for the retinohypothalamic tract. Proceedings of the National Academy of Sciences, USA, 87, 8065–8069.

Moreno, A., Ross, B. D., & Bluml, S. (2001). Direct determination of the N-acetyl-L-aspartate synthesis rate in the human brain by ^{13}C MRS and [1-^{13}C]glucose infusion. Journal of Neurochemistry, 77, 347–350.

Nadler, J. V., & Cooper, J. R. (1972a). Metabolism of the aspartyl moiety of N-acetyl-L-aspartic acid in the rat brain. Journal of Neurochemistry, 19, 2091–2105.

Nadler, J. V., & Cooper, J. R. (1972b). N-acetyl-L-aspartic acid content of human neural tumours and bovine peripheral nervous tissues. Journal of Neurochemistry, 19, 313–319.

Nagel, J., Belozertseva, I., Greco, S., Kashkin, V., Malyshkin, A., Jirgensons, A., et al. (2006). Effects of NAAG peptidase inhibitor 2-PMPA in model chronic pain—relation to brain concentration. Neuropharmacology, 5, 1163–1171.

Namboodiri, M. A., Corigliano-Murphy, A., Jiang, G., Rollag, M., & Provencio, I. (2000). Murine aspartoacylase: cloning, expression and comparison with the human enzyme. Molecular Brain Research, 77, 285–289.

Neale, J. H. (2011). N-Acetylaspartylglutamate is an agonist at mGluR3 in vivo and in vitro. Journal of Neurochemistry, 119, 891–895.

Neale, J. H., Bzdega, T., & Wroblewska, B. (2000). N-Acetyl-aspartyl-glutamate: the most abundant peptide neurotransmitter in the mammalian central nervous system. Journal of Neurochemistry, 75, 443–452.

Nicoletti, F., Bockaert, J., Collingridge, G. L., Conn, P. J., Ferraguti, F., Schoepp, D. D., et al. (2011). Metabotropic glutamate receptors: from the workbench to the bedside. Neuropharmacology, 60, 1017–1041.

Niswender, C. M., & Conn, P. J. (2010). Metabotropic glutamate receptors: physiology, pharmacology, and disease. Annual Review of Pharmacology and Toxicology, 50, 295–322.

Niwa, M., Nitta, A., Mizoguchi, H., Ito, Y., Noda, Y., Nagai, T., et al. (2007). A novel molecule "shati" is involved in methamphetamine-induced hyperlocomotion, sensitization, and conditioned place preference. Journal of Neuroscience, 27, 7604–7615.

Olszewski, R. T., Bukhari, N., Zhou, J., Kozikowski, A. P., Wroblewski, J. T., Shamimi-Noori, S., et al. (2004). NAAG peptidase inhibition reduces locomotor activity and some stereotypes in the PCP model of schizophrenia via group II mGluR. Journal of Neurochemistry, 89, 876–885.

Olszewski, R. T., Bzdega, T., & Neale, J. H. (2012a). mGluR3 and not mGluR2 receptors mediate the efficacy of NAAG peptidase inhibitor in validated model of schizophrenia. Schizophrenia Research, 136, 160–161.

Olszewski, R. T., Janczura, K. J., Ball, S. R., Madore, J. C., Lavin, K. M., Lee, J. C., et al. (2012b). NAAG peptidase inhibitors block cognitive deficit induced by MK-801 and motor activation induced by d-amphetamine in animal models of schizophrenia. Translational Psychiatry, 2, e145.

Passani, L. A., Vonsattel, J. P., Carter, R. E., & Coyle, J. T. (1997a). N-acetylaspartylglutamate, N-acetylaspartate, and N-acetylated alpha-linked acidic dipeptidase in human brain and their alterations in Huntington and Alzheimer's diseases. Molecular and Chemical Neuropathology, 31, 97–118.

Passani, L. A., Vonsattel, J. P., & Coyle, J. T. (1997b). Distribution of N-acetylaspartylglutamate immunoreactivity in human brain and its alteration in neurodegenerative disease. Brain Research, 772, 9–22.

Patel, T. B., & Clark, J. B. (1979). Synthesis of N-acetyl-L-aspartate by rat brain mitochondria and its involvement in mitochondrial/cytosolic carbon transport. Biochemical Journal, 184, 539–546.

Perrier, J., Durand, A., Giardina, T., & Puigserver, A. (2005). Catabolism of intracellular N-terminal acetylated proteins: involvement of acylpeptide hydrolase and acylase. Biochimie, 87, 673–685.

Ramos, M., Pardo, B., Llorente-Folch, I., Saheki, T., Del, A. A., & Satrustegui, J. (2011). Deficiency of the mitochondrial transporter of aspartate/glutamate aralar/AGC1 causes hypomyelination and neuronal defects unrelated to myelin deficits in mouse brain. Journal of Neuroscience Research, 89, 2008–2017.

Reichelt, K. L., & Kvamme, E. (1967). Acetylated and peptide bound glutamate and aspartate in brain. Journal of Neurochemistry, 14, 987–996.

Renno, W. M., Lee, J. H., & Beitz, A. J. (1997). Light and electron microscopic immunohistochemical localization of N-acetylaspartylglutamate (NAAG) in the olivocerebellar pathway of the rat. Synapse, 26, 140–154.

Riederer, F., Bittsansky, M., Schmidt, C., Mlynarik, V., Baumgartner, C., Moser, E., et al. (2006). ^{1}H magnetic resonance spectroscopy at 3 T in cryptogenic and mesial temporal lobe epilepsy. *NMR in Biomedicine, 19*, 544−553.

Rigotti, D., Gass, A., Achtnichts, L., Inglese, M., Babb, J., Naegelin, Y., et al. (2011a). Multiple sclerosis severity scale and whole-brain N-acetylaspartate concentration for patients' assessment. *Multiple Sclerosis, 18*, 98−107.

Rigotti, D. J., Inglese, M., Babb, J. S., Rovaris, M., Benedetti, B., Filippi, M., et al. (2007). Serial whole-brain N-acetylaspartate concentration in healthy young adults. *American Journal of Neuroradiology, 28*, 1650−1651.

Rigotti, D. J., Kirov, I. I., Djvadi, B., Perry, N., Babb, J. S., & Gonen, O. (2011b). Longitudinal whole-brain N-acetylaspartate concentration in healthy adults. *American Journal of Neuroradiology, 32*, 1011−1015.

Riveros, N., & Orrego, F. (1984). A study of possible excitatory effects of N-acetylaspartylglutamate in different in vivo and in vitro brain preparations. *Brain Research, 299*, 393−395.

Robinson, M. B., Blakely, R. D., Couto, R., & Coyle, J. T. (1987). Hydrolysis of the brain dipeptide N-acetyl-L-aspartyl-L-glutamate. Identification and characterization of a novel N-acetylated alpha-linked acidic dipeptidase activity from rat brain. *Journal of Biological Chemistry, 262*, 14498−14506.

Romei, C., Raiteri, M., & Raiteri, L. (2012). Glycine release is regulated by metabotropic glutamate receptors sensitive to mGluR2/3 ligands and activated by N-acetylaspartylglutamate (NAAG). *Neuropharmacology, 66*, 311−316.

Sacha, P., Zamecnik, J., Barinka, C., Hlouchova, K., Vicha, A., Mlcochova, P., et al. (2007). Expression of glutamate carboxypeptidase II in human brain. *Neuroscience, 144*, 1361−1372.

Sangar, M. C., Bansal, S., & Avadhani, N. G. (2010). Bimodal targeting of microsomal cytochrome P450s to mitochondria: implications in drug metabolism and toxicity. *Expert Opinion Drug Metabolism and Toxicology, 6*, 1231−1251.

Satrustegui, J., Contreras, L., Ramos, M., Marmol, P., Del, A. A., Saheki, T., et al. (2007). Role of aralar, the mitochondrial transporter of aspartate-glutamate, in brain N-acetylaspartate formation and Ca^{2+} signaling in neuronal mitochondria. *Journal of Neuroscience Research, 85*, 3359−3366.

Savic, I., Lekvall, A., Greitz, D., & Helms, G. (2000). MR spectroscopy shows reduced frontal lobe concentrations of N-acetyl aspartate in patients with juvenile myoclonic epilepsy. *Epilepsia, 41*, 290−296.

Savic, I., Osterman, Y., & Helms, G. (2004). MRS shows syndrome differentiated metabolite changes in human-generalized epilepsies. *Neuroimage, 21*, 163−172.

Signoretti, S., Lazzarino, G., Tavazzi, B., & Vagnozzi, R. (2011). The pathophysiology of concussion. *PM R, 3*, S359−S368.

Signoretti, S., Vagnozzi, R., Tavazzi, B., & Lazzarino, G. (2010). Biochemical and neurochemical sequelae following mild traumatic brain injury: summary of experimental data and clinical implications. *Neurosurgical Focus, 29*, E1.

Simmons, M. L., Frondoza, C. G., & Coyle, J. T. (1991). Immunocytochemical localization of N-acetyl-aspartate with monoclonal antibodies. *Neuroscience, 45*, 37−45.

Sistermans, E. A., de Coo, R. F., van Beerendonk, H. M., Poll-The, BT, Kleijer, W. J., & van Oost, B. A. (2000). Mutation detection in the aspartoacylase gene in 17 patients with Canavan disease: four new mutations in the non-Jewish population. *European Journal of Human Genetics, 8*, 557−560.

Soupart, A., Schroeder, B., & Decaux, G. (2007). Treatment of hyponatraemia by urea decreases risks of brain complications in rats. Brain osmolyte contents analysis. *Nephrology Dialysis Transplantation, 22*, 1856−1863.

Spange, S., Wagner, T., Heinzel, T., & Kramer, O. H. (2009). Acetylation of non-histone proteins modulates cellular signalling at multiple levels. *International Journal of Biochemistry and Cell Biology, 41*, 185−198.

Surendran, S., Campbell, G. A., Tyring, S. K., & Matalon, R. (2005). Aspartoacylase gene knockout results in severe vacuolation in the white matter and gray matter of the spinal cord in the mouse. *Neurobiology of Disease, 18*, 385−389.

Suwanwelaa, N., Phanuphak, P., Phanthumchinda, K., Suwanwela, N. C., Tantivatana, J., Ruxrungtham, K., et al. (2000). Magnetic resonance spectroscopy of the brain in neurologically asymptomatic HIV-infected patients. *Magnetic Resonance Imaging, 18*, 859−865.

Tahay, G., Wiame, E., Tyteca, D., Courtoy, P. J., & Van, S. E. (2012). Determinants of the enzymatic activity and the subcellular localization of aspartate N-acetyltransferase. *Biochemical Journal, 441*, 105−112.

Takatsu, Y., Fujita, Y., Tsukamoto, T., Slusher, B. S., & Hashimoto, K. (2011). Orally active glutamate carboxypeptidase II inhibitor 2-MPPA attenuates dizocilpine-induced prepulse inhibition deficits in mice. *Brain Research, 1371*, 82−86.

Tallan, H. H. (1957). Studies on the distribution of N-acetyl-L-aspartic acid in brain. *Journal of Biological Chemistry, 224*, 41−45.

Tallan, H. H., Moore, S., & Stein, W. H. (1956). N-Acetyl-L-aspartic acid in brain. *Journal of Biological Chemistry, 219*, 257−264.

Taylor, D. L., Davies, S. E., Obrenovitch, T. P., Doheny, M. H., Patsalos, P. N., Clark, J. B., et al. (1995). Investigation into the role of N-acetylaspartate in cerebral osmoregulation. *Journal of Neurochemistry, 65*, 275−281.

Taylor, D. L., Davies, S. E., Obrenovitch, T. P., Urenjak, J., Richards, D. A., Clark, J. B., et al. (1994). Extracellular N-acetylaspartate in the rat brain: in vivo determination of basal levels and changes evoked by high K + . *Journal of Neurochemistry, 62*, 2349−2355.

Thomas, A. G., Corse, A. M., Coccia, C. F., Bilak, M. M., Rothstein, J. D., & Slusher, B. S. (2003). NAALADase inhibition protects motor neurons against chronic glutamate toxicity. *European Journal of Pharmacology, 471*, 177−184.

Tieman, S. B. (2006). Cellular localization of NAAG. In J. R. Moffett, S. B. Tieman, D. R. Weinberger, J. T. Coyle, & M. A. Namboodiri (Eds.), *N-Acetylaspartate: A unique neuronal molecule in the central nervous system* (pp. 289−301). New York, NY: Springer Science + Business Media.

Tieman, S. B., Cangro, C. B., & Neale, J. H. (1987). N-acetylaspartylglutamate immunoreactivity in neurons of the cat's visual system. *Brain Research, 420*, 188−193.

Tieman, S. B., Moffett, J. R., & Irtenkauf, S. M. (1991a). Effect of eye removal on N-acetylaspartylglutamate immunoreactivity in retinal targets of the cat. *Brain Research, 562*, 318−322.

Tieman, S. B., Neale, J. H., & Tieman, D. G. (1991b). N-acetylaspartylglutamate immunoreactivity in neurons of the monkey's visual pathway. *Journal of Comparative Neurology, 313*, 45−64.

Tieman, S. B., & Tieman, D. G. (1996). N-acetylaspartylglutamate immunoreactivity in human retina. *Vision Research, 36*, 941−947.

Traeger, E. C., & Rapin, I. (1998). The clinical course of Canavan disease. *Pediatric Neurology, 18*, 207−212.

Traka, M., Wollmann, R. L., Cerda, S. R., Dugas, J., Barres, B. A., & Popko, B. (2008). Nur7 is a nonsense mutation in the mouse aspartoacylase gene that causes spongy degeneration of the CNS. *Journal of Neuroscience, 28*, 11537−11549.

Truckenmiller, M. E., Namboodiri, M. A., Brownstein, M. J., & Neale, J. H. (1985). N-Acetylation of L-aspartate in the nervous system: differential distribution of a specific enzyme. *Journal of Neurochemistry, 45*, 1658−1662.

Tsai, G., & Coyle, J. T. (1995). N-acetylaspartate in neuropsychiatric disorders. *Progress in Neurobiology, 46*, 531−540.

Tsai, G., Forloni, G. L., Robinson, M. B., Stauch, B. L., & Coyle, J. T. (1988). Calcium-dependent evoked release of N-[3H]acetylaspartylglutamate from the optic pathway. *Journal of Neurochemistry, 51,* 1956–1959.

Tsukamoto, T., Wozniak, K. M., & Slusher, B. S. (2007). Progress in the discovery and development of glutamate carboxypeptidase II inhibitors. *Drug Discovery Today, 12,* 767–776.

Urenjak, J., Williams, S. R., Gadian, D. G., & Noble, M. (1992). Specific expression of N-acetylaspartate in neurons, oligodendrocyte-type-2 astrocyte progenitors, and immature oligodendrocytes in vitro. *Journal of Neurochemistry, 59,* 55–61.

Vagnozzi, R., Signoretti, S., Cristofori, L., Alessandrini, F., Floris, R., Isgro, E., et al. (2010). Assessment of metabolic brain damage and recovery following mild traumatic brain injury: a multicentre, proton magnetic resonance spectroscopic study in concussed patients. *Brain, 133,* 3232–3242.

van Bogaert, L., & Bertrand, I. (1949). Sur une idiotie familiale avec degerescence sponglieuse de neuraxe (note preliminaire). *Acta Neurology, 49,* 572–587.

Verbalis, J. G. (2006). Control of Brain Volume During Hypoosmolality and Hyperosmolality. In J. R Moffett, S. B. Tieman, D. R. Weinberger, J. T. Coyle, & M. A. Namboodiri (Eds.), *N-Acetylaspartate: A unique neuronal molecule in the central nervous system* (pp. 113–129). New York, NY: Springer Science + Business Media.

Wang, J., Matalon, R., Bhatia, G., Wu, G., Li, H., Liu, T., et al. (2007). Bimodal occurrence of aspartoacylase in myelin and cytosol of brain. *Journal of Neurochemistry, 101,* 448–457.

Wardlaw, J. M., Marshall, I., Wild, J., Dennis, M. S., Cannon, J., & Lewis, S. C. (1998). Studies of acute ischemic stroke with proton magnetic resonance spectroscopy: relation between time from onset, neurological deficit, metabolite abnormalities in the infarct, blood flow, and clinical outcome. *Stroke, 29,* 1618–1624.

Watanabe, T., Shiino, A., & Akiguchi, I. (2010). Absolute quantification in proton magnetic resonance spectroscopy is useful to differentiate amnesic mild cognitive impairment from Alzheimer's disease and healthy aging. *Dementia and Geriatric Cognitive Disorders, 30,* 71–77.

Wellen, K. E., Hatzivassiliou, G., Sachdeva, U. M., Bui, T. V., Cross, J. R., & Thompson, C. B. (2009). ATP-citrate lyase links cellular metabolism to histone acetylation. *Science, 324,* 1076–1080.

Westbrook, G. L., Mayer, M. L., Namboodiri, M. A., & Neale, J. H. (1986). High concentrations of N-acetylaspartylglutamate (NAAG) selectively activate NMDA receptors on mouse spinal cord neurons in cell culture. *Journal of Neuroscience, 6,* 3385–3392.

Wiame, E., Tyteca, D., Pierrot, N., Collard, F., Amyere, M., Noel, G., et al. (2010). Molecular Identification of Aspartate N-acetyltransferase and its Mutation in Hypoacetylaspartia. *Biochemistry Journal, 425,* 127–136.

Wibom, R., Lasorsa, F. M., Tohonen, V., Barbaro, M., Sterky, F. H., Kucinski, T., et al. (2009). AGC1 deficiency associated with global cerebral hypomyelination. *New England Journal of Medicine, 361,* 489–495.

Williamson, L. C., Eagles, D. A., Brady, M. J., Moffett, J. R., Namboodiri, M. A., & Neale, J. H. (1991). Localization and synaptic release of N-acetylaspartylglutamate in the chick retina and optic tectum. *European Journal of Neuroscience, 3,* 441–451.

Williamson, L. C., & Neale, J. H. (1988). Ultrastructural localization of N-acetylaspartylglutamate in synaptic vesicles of retinal neurons. *Brain Research, 456,* 375–381.

Williamson, L. C., & Neale, J. H. (1992). Uptake, metabolism, and release of N-[3H]acetylaspartylglutamate by the avian retina. *Journal of Neurochemistry, 58,* 2191–2199.

Wittsack, H. J., Kugel, H., Roth, B., & Heindel, W. (1996). Quantitative measurements with localized 1H MR spectroscopy in children with Canavan's disease. *Journal of Magnetic Resonance Imaging, 6,* 889–893.

Woolley, M. L., Pemberton, D. J., Bate, S., Corti, C., & Jones, D. N. (2008). The mGlu2 but not the mGlu3 receptor mediates the actions of the mGluR2/3 agonist, LY379268, in mouse models predictive of antipsychotic activity. *Psychopharmacology (Berl), 196,* 431–440.

Wozniak, K. M., Rojas, C., Wu, Y., & Slusher, B. S. (2012). The role of glutamate signaling in pain processes and its regulation by GCP II inhibition. *Current Medicinal Chemistry., 19,* 1323–1334.

Wroblewska, B., Wroblewski, J. T., Saab, O. H., & Neale, J. H. (1993). N-acetylaspartylglutamate inhibits forskolin-stimulated cyclic AMP levels via a metabotropic glutamate receptor in cultured cerebellar granule cells. *Journal of Neurochemistry, 61,* 943–948.

Yamada, T., Zuo, D., Yamamoto, T., Olszewski, R. T., Bzdega, T., Moffett, J. R., et al. (2012). NAAG peptidase inhibition in the periaqueductal gray and rostral ventromedial medulla reduces flinching in the formalin model of inflammation. *Molecular Pain, 8,* 67.

Yamashita, H., Kaneyuki, T., & Tagawa, K. (2001). Production of acetate in the liver and its utilization in peripheral tissues. *Biochimica Biophysica Acta, 1532,* 79–87.

Ye, F., Chen, Y., Hoang, T., Montgomery, R. L., Zhao, X. H., Bu, H., et al. (2009). HDAC1 and HDAC2 regulate oligodendrocyte differentiation by disrupting the beta-catenin-TCF interaction. *Nature Neuroscience, 12,* 829–838.

Zano, S., Wijayasinghe, Y. S., Malik, R., Smith, J., & Viola, R. E. (2012). Relationship between enzyme properties and disease progression in Canavan disease. *Journal of Inherited Metabolic Disease, 36,* 1–6.

Zeng, B. J., Wang, Z. H., Ribeiro, L. A., Leone, P., De Gasperi, R., Kim, S. J., et al. (2002). Identification and characterization of novel mutations of the aspartoacylase gene in non-Jewish patients with Canavan disease. *Journal of Inherited Metabolic Disease, 25,* 557–570.

Zhang, W., Murakawa, Y., Wozniak, K. M., Slusher, B., & Sima, A. A. (2006). The preventive and therapeutic effects of GCPII (NAALADase) inhibition on painful and sensory diabetic neuropathy. *Journal of the Neurological Sciences, 247,* 217–223.

Zhang, W., Slusher, B., Murakawa, Y., Wozniak, K. M., Tsukamoto, T., Jackson, P. F., et al. (2002). GCPII (NAALADase) inhibition prevents long-term diabetic neuropathy in type 1 diabetic BB/Wor rats. *Journal of the Neurological Sciences, 194,* 21–28.

Zhao, J., Ramadan, E., Cappiello, M., Wroblewska, B., Bzdega, T., & Neale, J. H. (2001). NAAG inhibits KCl-induced [(3)H]-GABA release via mGluR3, cAMP, PKA and L-type calcium conductance. *European Journal of Neuroscience, 13,* 340–346.

Zhong, C., Zhao, X., Van, K. C., Bzdega, T., Smyth, A., Zhou, J., et al. (2006). NAAG peptidase inhibitor increases dialysate NAAG and reduces glutamate, aspartate and GABA levels in the dorsal hippocampus following fluid percussion injury in the rat. *Journal of Neurochemistry, 97,* 1015–1025.

Zollinger, M., Brauchli-Theotokis, J., Gutteck-Amsler, U., Do, K. Q., Streit, P., & Cuenod, M. (1994). Release of N-acetylaspartylglutamate from slices of rat cerebellum, striatum, and spinal cord, and the effect of climbing fiber deprivation. *Journal of Neurochemistry, 63,* 1133–1142.

Zuo, D., Bzdega, T., Olszewski, R. T., Moffett, J. R., & Neale, J. H. (2012). Effects of N-acetylaspartylglutamate (NAAG) peptidase inhibition on release of glutamate and dopamine in the prefrontal cortex and nucleus accumbens in the phencyclidine model of schizophrenia. *Journal of Biological Chemistry, 287,* 21773–21782.

The Biochemistry of Creatine

Clare E. Turner and Nicholas Gant

Centre for Brain Research, The University of Auckland, New Zealand

INTRODUCTION

Creatine is a naturally occurring guanidino compound that plays a vital role in the storage and transport of cellular energy. The creatine molecule is a fundamental component of high-energy phosphate metabolism, required for buffering, transport, and regulation of cellular energy. Creatine is abundant in metabolically active tissue such as muscle, heart, and brain. It is synthesized endogenously and absorbed from dietary sources, with the typical total creatine pool in a 70 kg human amounting to approximately 120 g (Walker, 1979). The majority of endogenous creatine is stored within muscle and is subject to continuous degradation to creatinine and replenishment by a combination of dietary intake and endogenous synthesis. Creatine is consumed in diets containing fresh meat and fish and, to a lesser extent, dairy products. Creatine is also consumed in large quantities as the dietary supplement creatine monohydrate, a practice popular among athletes striving to improve muscular energy turnover and prevent fatigue. Recently work has been directed toward examining the utility of supplemental creatine to treat cerebral creatine-deficiency syndromes and various neurological conditions. Information derived from creatine magnetic resonance (MR) spectra is valuable for quantifying this metabolite's abundance *in vivo* and as a reference for other major metabolite concentrations.

CREATINE AND HIGH-ENERGY PHOSPHATE METABOLISM

Adenosine triphosphate (ATP) is the universal currency for energy provision in all biological processes. The hydrolysis of ATP occurs at functional microcompartments around the cell to liberate energy from a high-energy phosphate bond. This is achieved by an energy transfer pathway known as the creatine kinase/phosphocreatine (CK/PCr) energy shuttle. Creatine (Cr) is a fundamental component of the CK/PCr energy shuttle. The energy pathway provides immediate replenishment of ATP via high-energy phosphate compounds. The synthesis of ATP is not possible without the high-energy PCr, a metabolically inert molecule that indirectly serves to meet the energy requirements of cells and tissues. Cr is converted to PCr by the enzyme CK at energy-producing sites in the cell. PCr becomes part of the intracellular PCr pool and is used to phosphorylate adenine compounds, specifically the conversion of adenosine diphosphate (ADP) into ATP. Subsequently, generated ATP contributes to cellular processes by another fraction of CK specifically located at sites of ATP utilization.

CK catalyzes the reversible Lohmann reaction (Lohmann, 1934), which describes the fundamental pathway of the CK/PCr system as follows:

$$PCr + ADP \overset{CK}{\leftrightarrow} ATP + Cr$$

The Lohmann reaction utilizes the high-energy phosphate bond stored in PCr to phosphorylate ATP from ADP for an immediate energy source when required, or equivalently captures the available energy from ATP and stores this within PCr. As a result, the PCr molecule allows for the rapid resynthesis of ATP when needed, in the absence of oxygen and glucose. Up to 10 times the amount of energy gained from the available ATP pool can be stored in the form of high-energy PCr (Wallimann et al., 2011); this represents considerable potential to store energy and requires a large free Cr pool when ATP is available for this purpose.

Functions of the CK/PCr System

The CK/PCr system serves three major functions that ensure efficient utilization of energy. The first is to

---

91

act as a temporal energy buffer, employing PCr and Cr to maintain intracellular ATP concentrations at a sufficient level via parallel diffusion pathways between ATP and ADP. Neuronal energy requirements fluctuate constantly as a wide range of firing rates are achieved by any given neuron. A typical cortical pyramidal cell has an average firing rate of 4 Hz in rats (Fanselow & Nicolelis, 1999; Schoenbaum et al., 1999) and 1 Hz in humans; however, firing rates can increase to well over 30 Hz during acute periods of energy-demanding function (Attwell & Laughlin, 2001). Given that the majority of energy consumption within neurons is associated with the generation of action potentials, this translates to an approximate increase of over six times the typical oxidative energy production. PCr is crucial to maintain metabolism at these firing rates as neurons do not have the capacity to store glycogen, as is available in muscle. The CK/PCr system stabilizes cellular ATP concentrations at approximately 3–6 mM, at the expense of the PCr concentration, which constantly fluctuates (Wallimann et al., 2011). This process ensures efficient use of ATP for all cellular functions, where the energy gained from each ATP molecule hydrolyzed is rapidly recovered (see Fig. 2.2.1).

A second putative function of the CK/PCr system is to act as a spatial energy buffer, or "energy transport" system. The presence of localized and specific subcellular isoforms of CK (Eppenberger et al., 1967) creates tightly coupled connections between ATP-producing and ATP-consuming processes within the cell. This precise delivery of energy, initially coined the "phosphorylcreatine shuttle" by Bessman and Geiger (1981), may enable energy to be transported via PCr and Cr between energy-producing sites, such as the mitochondria, to functional microcompartments of the cell containing ATPases. MR diffusion

techniques have shown intracellular PCr diffusion occurs effectively over large distances relative to mitochondria and energy utilization sites—in accordance with the energy transport hypothesis (Gabr et al., 2011). However, studies examining diffusion efficiencies of Cr and PCr compared with adenine molecules report equivocal findings (Yoshizaki et al., 1990; de Graaf et al., 2000). Evidence to date is restricted to diffusion rates calculated at relatively low energy expenditures in muscle tissue. The importance of the CK/PCr shuttle may become clearer once examined using in vivo brain tissue during periods of peak energy demand.

The third function of the CK/PCr system involves the regulation of metabolic pathways and cellular energetics. A rise in the intracellular concentration of free ADP and protons is prevented by the functioning CK/PCr system (Iyengar, 1984). Such changes in the intracellular environment that would occur in the absence of the CK/PCr system initiate various cellular proteins and enzymes, leading to a range of damaging outcomes. Such outcomes include the local and global acidification of cells and the inactivation of cellular ATPases. PCr and Cr are metabolically inert compounds and as such, do not interact with or influence other metabolic pathways within the cell. This allows for their accumulation without any interference to basic metabolism. Furthermore, the CK/PCr system supports the maintenance of appropriate ATP/ADP ratios in the vicinity of both ATP-consuming and ATP-producing sites, subsequently matching the flux of high-energy phosphates through the Lohmann reaction to cellular energy demands. The CK/PCr system also indirectly regulates metabolic pathways involved in glycogenolysis and glycolysis via the accumulation of inorganic phosphate, a product of PCr hydrolysis (Meyer et al., 1986).

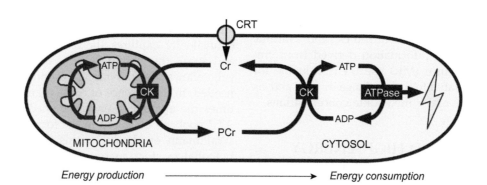

Energy production ⟶ *Energy consumption*

FIGURE 2.2.1   The CK/PCr system within a cell. Schematic representation of temporal and spatial energy buffering processes at key sites of energy production, storage, and liberation within a cell. Cr uptake occurs via the membrane-bound Cr transporter (CRT). Within the cell differing isotopes of CK utilize the Cr pool to shuttle energy between high-energy phosphate compounds. Examples of reversible PCr phosphorylation are shown for oxidative ATP production in mitochondria and energy liberation (via ATPase) in cytosolic ATP consumption. This figure is reproduced in color in the color plate section.

Cr Biosynthesis

Cr biosynthesis generates approximately 1.5–2 g of Cr per day, representing around 50% of the daily Cr requirement in humans (Wallimann et al., 2007). The biosynthesis of Cr involves two sequential steps. The transfer of an amidino group from arginine to glycine, catalyzed by L-arginine:glycine amidinotransferase (AGAT), yields the intermediate guanidinoacetate (GAA). In a second step GAA is then converted into Cr via the enzyme S-adenosyl-L-methionine:guanidinoacetate N-methyltransferase (GAMT; Walker, 1979; Wyss & Kaddurah-Daouk, 2000).

Exogenous synthesis of Cr is an interorgan process in which GAA is primarily produced in the kidney and methylated to Cr in the liver. However, Cr-synthesis enzymes have also been identified in other organs indicating Cr production may occur at numerous sites. Organs known to produce Cr include the pancreas (Wyss & Kaddurah-Daouk, 2000) and brain (Van Pilsum et al., 1972; Braissant et al., 2001).

Cr Transport and Storage

In general, tissues that contain the largest quantities of Cr have no capacity for its synthesis. As a result, once synthesized, Cr is transported via blood to target cells throughout the body, which have high or fluctuating energy needs through a *trans*-membrane spanning Cr transporter (CRT). The CRT is a member of the neurotransmitter transporter family. Transport of Cr through the CRT is highly specific, dependent on sodium and chloride ions, and saturable. Cr is cotransported across the membrane with two sodium ions and one chloride ion down their concentration gradients. This transport is electrogenic and is an example of secondary active transport driven by the sodium gradient established by the sodium/potassium-ATPase (Dai et al., 1999). The Michealis—Menton constant (K_m) for Cr within the systemic circulation has been determined as 15–77 μM (Loike et al., 1986; Nash et al., 1994; Sora et al., 1994; Dai et al., 1999). Serum concentrations of Cr are approximately 58 μM (Marescau et al., 1986), which shows that CRTs work close to saturation and therefore the density of transporters in the cell membrane may be the rate-limiting step for Cr accumulation in tissue. Furthermore, localization of transporter protein using immunohistochemical analysis has indicated that the CRT does not appear to be an abundant component of the plasma membrane, even in tissues containing high levels of Cr (Christie, 2007).

Localization of CRT mRNA levels show that the CRT is present in tissues with high-energy demands or significant absorptive functions (Guimbal & Kilimann, 1993; Gonzalez & Uhl, 1994; Schloss et al., 1994; Saltarelli et al., 1996; Peral et al., 2002). Transporter distribution appears to be related to CK activity, which in turn is associated to total tissue Cr concentration (Wyss & Kaddurah-Daouk, 2000). Muscle has the highest tissue Cr concentration with >90% of the body's total Cr concentration stored in skeletal muscle. Other tissues with substantial Cr concentrations are cardiac muscle, spermatozoa, and photoreceptors of the retina, while intermediate levels are found in the brain (Wyss & Kaddurah-Daouk, 2000). Cr uptake into tissue is regulated by intracellular Cr concentrations (Lukaszuk et al., 2002, 2005), the sodium gradient (Odoom et al., 1996), and the presence of insulin (Green et al., 1996; Steenge et al., 1998, 2000; Pittas et al., 2010) through the activation of sodium/potassium-ATPases.

Cr in the systemic circulation can be transported into the brain across the blood–brain barrier (BBB) via CRT in the microcapillary endothelial cells, but not astrocytes (Braissant et al., 2001). The K_m value for Cr at the BBB is 16.2 μM, 10- to 40-fold lower than values within the plasma (Ohtsuki et al., 2002). This suggests that the transport of Cr across the BBB is more than 90% saturated by endogenous plasma Cr and supplying Cr at a rate close to maximal capacity. In saying this, the BBB uptake pathway for Cr appears to be relatively inefficient (Ohtsuki et al., 2002; Perasso et al., 2003), particularly in adults, and therefore the central nervous system (CNS) must also rely on synthesis of Cr within the brain.

Cr Synthesis and Transport within the CNS

The expression of the CRT has been observed in microcapillary endothelial cells, but not astrocytes at the BBB, suggesting that the CNS is capable of importing Cr from the periphery, albeit with limited permeability to peripheral Cr (Braissant et al., 2001; Ohtsuki et al., 2002; Perasso et al., 2003). As such, the CNS must supply an important portion of its Cr needs from endogenous synthesis within the brain (Defalco & Davies, 1961). Although enzymatic activity necessary for brain Cr biosynthesis has been demonstrated for both AGAT (Van Pilsum et al., 1963) and GAMT (Van Pilsum et al., 1972), efforts to express enzyme mRNA to further localize AGAT and GAMT within neural tissue have produced conflicting results. *In situ* hybridization revealed ubiquitous expression of AGAT and GAMT mRNA in astrocytes, neurons, and oligodendrocytes, indicating that all cells in the CNS are able to synthesize Cr (Braissant et al., 2001). However, more recent immunohistochemistry work identifying the expression of GAMT in the mouse brain reports a more selective pattern suggesting that AGAT and GAMT are not coexpressed but rather are expressed in a dissociated way (Braissant et al., 2001; Schmidt et al.,

2004; Tachikawa et al., 2004; Nakashima et al., 2005). Expression of GAMT is strong in oligodendrocytes, moderate in astrocytes, and very low in neurons (Tachikawa et al., 2004). Enzyme localization evidence, together with that of distinct CK isoenzymes (see the section, CK within the CNS), offers strong support toward the role of neuronal support tissue, in particular oligodendrocytes, as a source of Cr in axonal mitochondria, neuronal cell bodies, dendrites, and synapses. Regardless of the specific location, the existence of enzymes involved in Cr biosynthesis, the apparent wide pattern of expression, and the presence of specific and localized CK isoforms emphasize the importance of the CK/PCr system to transport metabolic energy to highly active neural areas.

Cell types within the rodent and human CNS that depend on Cr for energy metabolism have been identified by localizing CRT mRNA and protein. Neurons appear to be the predominant cell type that contains the CRT, with smaller concentrations expressed in oligodendrocytes, while astrocytes do not express the CRT at all (Braissant et al., 2001; Ohtsuki et al., 2002; Tachikawa et al., 2004; Mak et al., 2009). These results perhaps further emphasize the reliance of neurons on support cells for Cr synthesis.

Distribution of the CRT throughout the CNS has been assessed through the localization of transporter mRNA and protein levels. CRT mRNA expression is high in the Purkinje and granule cell layers of the cerebellum, the pyramidal cell layer of the hippocampus, and some brainstem nuclei. Moderate levels have been detected in the cortex, globus pallidus, and most white matter tracts, while low levels have been detected in the striatum, nucleus accumbens, hippocampus molecular layer, and cerebellar molecular layer (Happe & Murrin, 1995).

The CRT has been observed to be particularly abundant in the major motor and sensory regions of the forebrain, brainstem and spinal cord, and forebrain regions associated with learning, memory, and limbic functions—congruent with areas responsible for symptoms observed in patients suffering from Cr-deficiency disorders (see the section, Treatment of cerebral Cr-deficiency syndromes). Regions with high CRT expression are suggested to have high metabolic requirements, further emphasizing the importance of the CK/PCr system in the CNS. Conversely, those with low expression are regions that are known to be particularly vulnerable to neurodegeneration.

CK WITHIN THE CNS

Two isotopes of CK have been discovered within neural tissue: ubiquitous mitochondrial CK (uCK-Mi)

and brain-type cytoplasmic CK (CK-B; Jacobs et al., 1964; Murone & Ogata, 1973; Friedman & Roberts, 1994; Kottke et al., 1994; Tachikawa et al., 2004). The presence of uCK-Mi is reported throughout the cell body but not in the nucleus of Golgi type I neurons of the mouse cerebral cortex (Friedman & Roberts, 1994), including excitatory and inhibitory neurons, where it is localized in the mitochondria (Tachikawa et al., 2004). This selective localization of uCK-Mi, which is bound to the outer surface of the inner mitochondrial membrane exclusively in neurons (Scholte, 1973), is assumed to mediate the transfer of high-energy phosphates coupled with ATP production in neuronal mitochondria. Cytoplasmic CKs such as CK-B, are thought to be involved in the resynthesis of ATP from PCr delivered from the mitochondria. Evidence suggests that CK-B is selectively expressed in astrocytes among the glial population, and present in excitatory and, at much higher concentrations, in inhibitory neurons of the neuronal population in mouse cerebral cortex (Tachikawa et al., 2004). Brain-type cytoplasmic CK is specifically located in neuronal processes and pyramidal cell dendrites (Friedman & Roberts, 1994) and is assumed to mediate the transfer of high-energy phosphates coupled with ATP utilization in functional sites throughout the cell. Inhibitory neurons, which possess higher levels of CK-B, are known to be extremely resistant to neurological insults that effect neuronal metabolism, suggesting that CK-B may function to maintain neuronal energy circuits when challenged with the deprivation of other metabolites.

THERAPEUTIC CR SUPPLEMENTATION

Oral Cr supplementation is used routinely by athletes and creatine monohydrate is one of the most widely purchased sports performance supplements. Oral supplementation of 20 g of Cr per day for one week can improve intramuscular Cr by up to 40% and as such improve the amount of work accomplished during dynamic high-intensity exercise (Balsom et al., 1993; Greenhaff et al., 1993; Birch et al., 1994; Earnest et al., 1995; Casey et al., 1996). Skeletal muscle fatigue develops rapidly during high-intensity exercise and is closely related to low intramuscular PCr content, with muscle PCr almost entirely depleted at the point of fatigue (Hultman et al., 1967; Katz et al., 1986). Cr supplementation offsets the characteristic decline in muscle power output conventionally experienced toward the end of strenuous bouts during intermittent exercise (Balsom et al., 1993; Greenhaff et al., 1993; Birch et al., 1994). Higher levels of intracellular Cr accelerate PCr resynthesis during recovery via an increased flux through the CK/PCr system, which in turn sustains ADP resphosphorylation and subsequently prolongs muscular work. Although it is impossible to ingest large doses of creatine naturally by diet alone, additional supplementation appears to pose no serious health risks and is capable of increasing Cr availability in other tissue, including the brain.

A standard muscle supplementation dose of 20 g of creatine monohydrate powder per day (in four divided doses) for a 4 week period can also produce a mean increase in neural Cr concentration of 8.7% (Dechent et al., 1999). Similar increases have also been achieved using an identical dose for shorter periods of time (Lyoo et al., 2003). Regional analysis of Cr-loaded humans shows cerebral Cr uptake is most pronounced in the thalamus (14.6%) and white matter tracts (11.5%), while lesser increases are evident in the cerebellum (5.4%) and cortical gray matter (4.7%).

Regionally dependent increases in total Cr concentration following excess Cr consumption appear to be related to a combination of factors including the distribution of the CRT throughout the brain and the initial concentration of Cr within the tissue prior to supplementation. Tissues with high presupplementation values (heart, brain, and skeletal muscle) experience low relative increases of total Cr (15–55% of presupplementation values), conversely tissue with low pre-supplementation values (liver, kidney, and lung) experience high relative increases in concentration (260–500%; Ipsiroglu et al., 2001). A major determinant of Cr uptake appears to be the metabolite concentration gradient between extracellular and intracellular environments, with larger concentration gradients driving greater relative increases from presupplementation values.

Treatment of Cerebral Cr-Deficiency Syndromes

The CK reaction and the transfer of high-energy phosphates shape a large metabolic network in the CNS that is highly versatile and involved in many physiological functions. The existence and necessity for the CK/PCr system in the CNS is functionally portrayed in cases where components of the CK/PCr system are deficient or absent. Primary Cr-deficiency syndromes manifest as a result of a deficiency in Cr biosynthesis enzymes, AGAT or GAMT, or the CRT, which leads to a complete absence or significant decrease in the Cr concentration of the CNS. Cr-deficiency syndromes are caused by mutations in AGAT, GAMT, or CRT genes (Stockler et al., 1994; Item et al., 2001; Salomons et al., 2001). The brain is the main organ affected in Cr-deficient patients

(Pyne-Geithman et al., 2004) who typically exhibit severe neurological symptoms in infancy.

During development, Cr is required to support regular axonal growth (Braissant et al., 2002), and deficiencies lead to underdeveloped axonal networks and reduced synaptic density—a morphological marker for mental retardation (Volpe, 2008). Microstructural defects suffered during development appear to be responsible for clinical symptoms that are not reversible upon Cr restoration after a deficiency syndrome has developed. In the mature brain, Cr deficiencies appear to cause a major disruption to cellular energy homeostasis. A reduction or absence of Cr results in diminished buffering capacity for peak ATP demand and transport capacity for high-energy phosphate compounds, which results in mitochondrial dysfunction.

Common clinical presentation in Cr-deficiency syndromes include delays in motor skill learning and speech acquisition, epilepsy, involuntary dyskinetic–dystonic movements, intellectual disability, and autistic behavior (Schulze et al., 1997; Battini et al., 2002; Rosenberg et al., 2004; Kleefstra et al., 2005; Mercimek-Mahmutoglu et al., 2006; Stockler et al., 2007). This diverse range of neurological symptoms emphasizes the importance of Cr for psychomotor function and cognition, is consistent with regions that express the CRT, and may in part be explained by the pattern of AGAT and GAMT expression and CRT distribution in the CNS.

Rodent knockout models have also been utilized to assess the importance of the CNS CK/PCr system, inducing comparable neurological deficits. Mice deficient in CK-B, an integral component of the CK/PCr system, present with morphological changes in hippocampal neurons and altered behavioral traits associated with deficits in hippocampal functioning (Jost et al., 2002; in 't Zandt et al., 2004; Streijger et al., 2005). Diminished habituation and spatial learning together with high-energy seizure susceptibility are thought to be caused by the lack of CK-B rendering the brain less efficient at coping with activity-related energy challenges.

Secondary Cr deficiencies are also observed in other pathological states of the brain, including stroke and hyperammonemia. Ischemic stroke is associated with a decrease in the total Cr concentration in the CNS (Gideon et al., 1994; Mathews et al., 1995; Lauriero et al., 1996; Lei et al., 2009), signifying failure of energy-dependent processes necessary for homeostatic cellular function. Excess ammonium can also be toxic within the CNS, causing irreversible damages to the developing brain through the alteration of neurotransmitter systems, axonal and dendritic growth, and signal transduction pathways (Cagnon & Braissant, 2007). Hyperammonemia generates a secondary Cr deficit in neural tissue that appears to modify the energy requirements of cells and eventually leads to cellular energy deficit, oxidative stress, and death (Braissant, 2002, 2010).

The restoration of cerebral Cr levels by oral Cr supplementation may be accompanied by significant improvement in clinical symptoms experienced in Cr-deficient patients suffering from AGAT and GAMT mutations (Stockler et al., 1994; Bianchi et al., 2000). Alleviation of involuntary movement disorders and a recovery in psychomental development and behavioral conditions have been associated with the replenishment of cerebral Cr; however, clinical improvements tend to be incomplete and developmental complications often remain (Stockler et al., 1997). Response to oral Cr supplementation is more pronounced for AGAT-deficient patients, believed to be a result of an accumulation in cerebral GAA concentrations associated with GAMT deficiency (Bianchi et al., 2000; Battini et al., 2002). Accumulation of GAA contributes to the pathophysiology in GAMT-deficient patients and cannot be completely normalized by Cr supplementation alone.

Presymptomatic treatment with Cr supplementation has been demonstrated to be effective in partial replenishment of brain Cr stores and prevents most Cr-deficiency outcomes in both AGAT-deficiency (Battini et al., 2006) and GAMT-deficiency disorders (Schulze et al., 2006; Schulze & Battini, 2007). This suggests that deficits associated with Cr-deficiency disorders are a result of irreversible brain impairment which, if addressed presymptomatically with treatment initiated before the occurrence of irreversible damage, may result in the prevention of clinical symptoms. Oral Cr supplementation is not effective in treating clinical symptoms in patients suffering from CRT mutations due to an inability to uptake Cr across the BBB, and for the case of endogenously synthesized Cr, across neuronal membranes within the brain (Poo-Arguelles et al., 2006).

Treatment of Other Neurological Disorders

Impaired energy metabolism also plays a critical role in the pathogenesis and progression of multiple neurological diseases, acting as a primary or secondary mechanism in the neuronal death cascade with reduced cellular energy states triggering both necrotic and apoptotic cell death (Green & Reed, 1998; Desagher & Martinou, 2000; Roy & Nicholson, 2000). Likewise, neurodegenerative diseases, characterized by a progressive loss of neurons within distinct areas of the brain, appear to share similar fundamental defective biochemical processes relating to mitochondrial

function and cellular bioenergetics that contribute to the pathogenesis of the disease. Maintaining ATP availability may play an important role in directly and indirectly ameliorating the severity of many pathologic mechanisms associated with neurological and neurodegenerative disorders and therefore represents a potential target for therapeutic intervention. The administration of oral Cr monohydrate has been investigated in a range of animal models of neurodegenerative disease in an attempt to enhance cellular bioenergetics and impede progression of the neurodegenerative process.

Parkinson's disease is a neurodegenerative disease that is characterized by movement disorders as a result of neuronal loss and dysfunction to dopaminergic neurons in the substantia nigra. Mitochondrial dysfunction and impaired energy metabolism appears to be central to the disease pathogenesis, with disruption to oxidative phosphorylation by inhibition of complex I in the electron transport chain (Nicklas et al., 1985; Bindoff et al., 1989), and impaired high-energy phosphate production (Beal, 2001) both reported. Administration of 1-methyl-4-phenyl-1,2,3,6-tetrahydropyridine (MPTP) produces parkinsonism in humans and animals and as such is used as an experimental model to mimic Parkinson's disease and investigate molecular mechanisms associated with the disease pathogenesis. Cr administration in mice has been reported to produce significant neuroprotection against MPTP-induced dopamine depletions and deterioration of substantia nigra neurons, suggesting that Cr supplementation aids in slowing the progression of Parkinson's disease (Matthews et al., 1999). The effectiveness of Cr has been tested in an initial clinical trial of Parkinson's disease patients (NINDS NET-PD Investigators, 2006, 2008). Results suggest that Cr was well tolerated in the patient population and further clinical testing may determine whether Cr supplementation is effective in slowing the progression of symptoms.

Huntington's disease causes selective degeneration of basal ganglia neurons and results in abnormal movements, lack of coordination, and altered mental ability and behavior. Huntington's disease is caused by a mutation to a gene in the huntingtin protein, which results in several toxic effects including metabolic and mitochondrial dysfunction (Gu et al., 1996; Beal, 2005; Ryu & Ferrante, 2005; van den Bogaard et al., 2011). Impaired energy metabolism and aberrant mitochondrial function play a prominent role in the pathogenesis of the disease evidenced by reduced cerebral glucose utilization (Kuhl et al., 1985; Mazziotta et al., 1987; Kuwert et al., 1990), decreases in mitochondria size and number in basal ganglia neurons (Ryu et al., 2005), decreases in muscular PCr to inorganic phosphate ratios, and increased neural lactate concentrations (Koroshetz et al., 1997). Cr administration has proven beneficial for both transgenic animal models of Huntington's disease (Ferrante et al., 2000; Andreassen et al., 2001) and clinical trials of Huntington's disease patients (Tabrizi et al., 2003, 2005). Dietary Cr supplementation in transgenic Huntington's disease mice improves neuronal survival and delays the development of brain atrophy, improving motor tasks and delaying the onset of weight loss (Ferrante et al., 2000; Andreassen et al., 2001). Interrupted deterioration of functional and neuropsychological capacity has also been reported in Cr-supplemented Huntington's disease patients (Tabrizi et al., 2003, 2005).

Amyotrophic lateral sclerosis (ALS) is a condition characterized by a range of progressive motor disabilities as a result of degeneration of motor neurons throughout the CNS. A number of the pathogenic mechanisms triggering cell death appear to converge with mitochondrial dysfunction (Okamoto et al., 1990; Sasaki & Iwata, 1996), in particular decreased mitochondrial respiratory chain activities (Borthwick et al., 1999), leading to subsequent cellular energy impairment. Several studies assessing the effectiveness of Cr supplementation in animal models of ALS report that oral administration delays the onset and slows progression of the clinical phenotype (Klivenyi et al., 1999, 2004; Ikeda et al., 2000; Zhang et al., 2003). Significant depletion of cortical ATP has been reported in ALS mice, which is partially ameliorated by Cr administration (Browne et al., 2006). Cr supplementation appears to be of no benefit to disease progression or survival in humans (Groeneveld et al., 2003; Shefner et al., 2004). The lack of positive outcomes may be a reflection of the Cr dosage administered, and it has been suggested that larger doses may be needed when treating rapidly progressing neurodegenerative disorders (Ferrante et al., 2005).

Stroke causes death and functional impairment resulting in long-term disability. The maintenance of ion gradients across neuronal membranes involves a significant amount of metabolic energy and is often impacted when challenged with a reduction in blood flow with stroke. Reduced blood flow induces a cascade of events resulting in the failure of sodium/potassium ion pumps, an influx of extracellular calcium ions, and resultant excitotoxicity that ultimately leads to the permanent loss of cellular integrity and eventual cell death. Neurons that are most severely affected by the hypoxic injury die rapidly by necrosis, and those that are less exposed to the metabolic failure in the penumbra succumb to programmed cell death via apoptosis (Tatsumi et al., 2003). Cr has been identified as a potential neuroprotective agent from the metabolic crisis that ensues during stroke. In animal models of ischemia, Cr-supplemented mice exhibit higher ATP and PCr concentrations during anoxic events (Wilken et al., 2000), increased PCr to inorganic phosphate ratios, reductions in the volume of brain edema (Adcock et al., 2002), and significantly lower cortical neuronal cell injury (Zhu et al., 2004). This Cr-mediated neuroprotection that appears to be due to a preservation of cellular bioenergetic status may also involve other mechanisms such as improved cerebrovascular function (Prass et al., 2007). Hypoxic energy failure may be prevented by Cr administered prior to ischemic events and oral Cr supplementation may offer a potential prophylactic option for patients with a high risk for stroke.

QUANTIFICATION OF BRAIN CR WITH MRS

A substantial amount of published work has assessed neural Cr concentrations in human participants *in vivo* using MR spectroscopy (MRS). Spectra are most commonly generated via ¹H MRS and easily resolved in most tissue types. With this method, the molecule produces two distinct singlets at 3.069 and 3.960 parts per million (ppm) representing the protons of the N-CH₃ group and the methylene protons of the acetate group, respectively (Fig. 2.2.2; Pischel & Gastner, 2007).

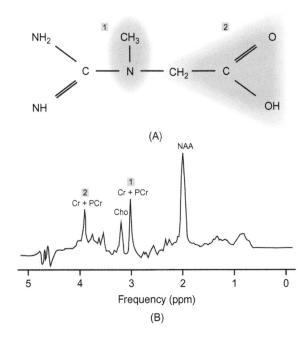

FIGURE 2.2.2 The Cr molecule: structure and spectra. Shaded areas highlight protons relative to the structural formula (A) that cause resonance within spectra (B) generated from ¹H MRS of human neural tissue. Two distinct resonances at 3.069 (1) and 3.960 ppm (2) represent protons of the N-CH₃ group and the methylene protons of the acetate group, respectively.

Resonance amplitudes are typically presented as ratios rather than absolute concentrations, with the understanding that most factors affecting resonance amplitude are homologous for all metabolite resonances in the spectrum (see Chapter 1.5). Frequently, Cr is used as the denominator in ratios of various resonance amplitudes (Chamard et al., 2012; Levin et al., 2012; Nie et al., 2012; Shu et al., 2013) under the premise that concentrations remain relatively stable in the brain, in normal and many pathologic states (De Stefano et al., 2002; Tartaglia et al., 2002; Condon, 2011). By expressing resonance amplitudes as ratios, any error obtained from imager and localization method differences, gain instabilities, regional susceptibility variations, and partial volume effects is assumed to be equal and therefore self-corrected when presented relative to another resonance of the same spectra (Li et al., 2003). The assumption in using a relative quantification method is that these benefits outweigh any cost associated with individual variation of each of the ratio components.

The previous assumption has been assessed by measuring absolute levels of N-acetylaspartate (NAA), Cho, and Cr and comparing these metabolites with relative NAA:Cr and Cho:Cr ratios in various regions throughout the brain (Li et al., 2003). These findings demonstrate that in >50% of the evaluated volumes of interest, relative ratio concentrations exhibited higher coefficients of variation than the absolute concentration counterparts. Furthermore, in 33% of the examined volumes of interest the ratio coefficient of variation exceeded the combined coefficient of variation from each of the constituents. Basing metabolite quantifications on ratios and assuming stable Cr concentrations may introduce more variability into spectra than it prevents. As such, the cost of relative quantification often exceeds any benefit and should therefore be approached with caution.

More accurate methods of metabolite quantification involve absolute quantification in combination with a structural analysis of the MRS volume of interest. Absolute quantification methods involve the calibration of resonance amplitudes with respect to an accurately defined external reference or brain-mimicking phantom relating to standard concentration units (Goodenough & Weaver, 1988; Woo et al., 2007). This strategy, known as the simulation phantom method, has been associated with highest accuracy and reproducibility of metabolite concentration estimates (Buchli & Boesiger, 1993; Buchli et al., 1994; Duc et al., 1998). Structural analysis of the MRS volume of interest is conducted to account for the variability in Cr storage across brain tissue. Due to the irregular distribution of the CRT, Cr is only stored and subsequently used for energy provision in gray and white matter. Because

MRS is typically performed on a macroscopic level, various brain compartments (gray matter, white matter, and cerebrospinal fluid, CSF) containing differing Cr concentrations may contribute to the resonance amplitude measured. Consequently, it can be difficult to determine precise Cr concentrations with spectra acquired from heterogeneous tissue (Jansen et al., 2006). As such, metabolite concentrations that are uncorrected for the contribution of CSF within the acquisition volume of interest are generally underestimated as the concentration of Cr in CSF tends to be low (Lynch et al., 1993). However, a structural analysis of the MRS volume of interest allows for the correction of the Cr resonance amplitude according to the proportion of tissue that is capable of storing Cr (Stagg et al., 2011) and should be considered when analyzing large volumes of interest that capture heterogeneous neural tissue.

CONCLUSIONS

The Cr molecule is a vital component of the CK/PCr energy shuttle, responsible for buffering, transporting, and regulating energy in tissues with a range of functional properties. The brain has fluctuating energy requirements and an efficient energy system is necessary to sustain a wide and dynamic range of neural firing rates. It is therefore not surprising that the brain appears capable of synthesizing and transporting Cr and relies on this metabolite for energy provision and transfer of high-energy phosphates to functional locations within neurons.

Progression of CNS diseases and deficiency syndromes are closely aligned with the capacity for Cr metabolism. Cr is thought to mediate neuroprotection by improving cellular bioenergetics and preserving cellular homeostasis. As such, supplementary Cr may offer potential therapeutic utility for disorders defined by impaired energy metabolism. High-energy phosphogens within the CNS and perturbations to cellular energetics are detectable in vivo by MRS. This technique provides a noninvasive diagnostic and powerful tool to study the role of Cr in health and neurological disease.

References

Adcock, K. H., Nedelcu, J., Loenneker, T., Martin, E., Wallimann, T., & Wagner, B. P. (2002). Neuroprotection of creatine supplementation in neonatal rats with transient cerebral hypoxia-ischemia. *Developmental Neuroscience*, 24(5), 382–388.

Andreassen, O. A., Dedeoglu, A., Ferrante, R. J., Jenkins, B. G., Ferrante, K. L., Thomas, M., et al. (2001). Creatine increase survival and delays motor symptoms in a transgenic animal model of Huntington's disease. *Neurobiology of Disease*, 8(3), 479–491.

Attwell, D., & Laughlin, S. B. (2001). An energy budget for signaling in the grey matter of the brain. *Journal of Cerebral Blood Flow and Metabolism, 21*(10), 1133–1145.

Balsom, P. D., Ekblom, B., Söerlund, K., Sjödln, B., & Hultman, E. (1993). Creatine supplementation and dynamic high-intensity intermittent exercise. *Scandinavian Journal of Medicine and Science in Sports, 3*(3), 143–149.

Battini, R., Alessandri, M. G., Leuzzi, V., Moro, F., Tosetti, M., Bianchi, M. C., et al. (2006). Arginine:glycine amidinotransferase (AGAT) deficiency in a newborn: early treatment can prevent phenotypic expression of the disease. *Journal of Pediatrics, 148*(6), 828–830.

Battini, R., Leuzzi, V., Carducci, C., Tosetti, M., Bianchi, M. C., Item, C. B., et al. (2002). Creatine depletion in a new case with AGAT deficiency: clinical and genetic study in a large pedigree. *Molecular Genetics and Metabolism, 77*(4), 326–331.

Beal, M. F. (2001). Mitochondria and oxidative damage in amyotrophic lateral sclerosis. *Functional Neurology, 16*(Suppl. 4), 161–169.

Beal, M. F. (2005). Mitochondria take center stage in aging and neurodegeneration. *Annals of Neurology, 58*(4), 495–505.

Bessman, S. P., & Geiger, P. J. (1981). Transport of energy in muscle: the phosphorylcreatine shuttle. *Science, 211*(4481), 448–452.

Bianchi, M. C., Tosetti, M., Fornai, F., Alessandri, M. G., Cipriani, P., De Vito, G., et al. (2000). Reversible brain creatine deficiency in two sisters with normal blood creatine level. *Annals of Neurology, 47*(4), 511–513.

Bindoff, L. A., Birch-Machin, M. A., Farnsworth, L., Gardner-Medwin, D., Lindsay, J. G., & Turnbull, D. M. (1989). Familial intermittent ataxia due to a defect of the E1 component of pyruvate dehydrogenase complex. *Journal of Neurological Sciences, 93*(2-3), 311–318.

Birch, R., Noble, D., & Greenhaff, P. L. (1994). The influence of dietary creatine supplementation on performance during repeated bouts of maximal isokinetic cycling in man. *European Journal of Applied Physiology and Occupational Physiology, 69*(3), 268–276.

Borthwick, G. M., Johnson, M. A., Ince, P. G., Shaw, P. J., & Turnbull, D. M. (1999). Mitochondrial enzyme activity in amyotrophic lateral sclerosis: implications for the role of mitochondria in neuronal cell death. *Annals of Neurology, 46*(5), 787–790.

Braissant, O. (2010). Ammonia toxicity to the brain: effects on creatine metabolism and transport and protective roles of creatine. *Molecular Genetics and Metabolism, 100*(Suppl. 1), S53–58.

Braissant, O., Henry, H., Loup, M., Eilers, B., & Bachmann, C. (2001). Endogenous synthesis and transport of creatine in the rat brain: an in situ hybridization study. *Brain Research Molecular Brain Research, 86*(1-2), 193–201.

Braissant, O., Henry, H., Villard, A. M., Zurich, M. G., Loup, M., Eilers, B., et al. (2002). Ammonium-induced impairment of axonal growth is prevented through glial creatine. *Journal of Neuroscience, 22*(22), 9810–9820.

Browne, S. E., Yang, L., DiMauro, J. P., Fuller, S. W., Licata, S. C., & Beal, M. F. (2006). Bioenergetic abnormalities in discrete cerebral motor pathways presage spinal cord pathology in the G93A SOD1 mouse model of ALS. *Neurobiology of Disease, 22*(3), 599–610.

Buchli, R., & Boesiger, P. (1993). Comparison of methods for the determination of absolute metabolite concentrations in human muscles by 31P MRS. *Magnetic Resonance in Medicine, 30*(5), 552–558.

Buchli, R., Martin, E., & Boesiger, P. (1994). Comparison of calibration strategies for the in vivo determination of absolute metabolite concentrations in the human brain by 31P MRS. *NMR in Biomedicine, 7*(5), 225–230.

Cagnon, L., & Braissant, O. (2007). Hyperammonemia-induced toxicity for the developing central nervous system. *Brain Research Reviews, 56*(1), 183–197.

Casey, A., Constantin-Teodosiu, D., Howell, S., Hultman, E., & Greenhaff, P. L. (1996). Creatine ingestion favorably affects performance and muscle metabolism during maximal exercise in humans. *American Journal of Physiology, 271*(1 Pt 1), E31–37.

Chamard, E., Theoret, H., Skopelja, E. N., Forwell, L. A., Johnson, A. M., & Echlin, P. S. (2012). A prospective study of physician-observed concussion during a varsity university hockey season: metabolic changes in ice hockey players. Part 4 of 4. *Neurosurgical Focus, 33*(6), E4.

Christie, D. L. (2007). Functional insights into the creatine transporter. *Subcellular Biochemistry, 46*, 99–118.

Condon, B. (2011). Magnetic resonance imaging and spectroscopy: how useful is it for prediction and prognosis? *EPMA Journal, 2*(4), 403–410.

Dai, W., Vinnakota, S., Qian, X., Kunze, D. L., & Sarkar, H. K. (1999). Molecular characterization of the human CRT-1 creatine transporter expressed in Xenopus oocytes. *Archives of Biochemistry and Biophysics, 361*(1), 75–84.

de Graaf, R. A., van Kranenburg, A., & Nicolay, K. (2000). In vivo (31)P-NMR diffusion spectroscopy of ATP and phosphocreatine in rat skeletal muscle. *Biophysics Journal, 78*(4), 1657–1664.

De Stefano, N., Narayanan, S., Francis, S. J., Smith, S., Mortilla, M., Tartaglia, M. C., et al. (2002). Diffuse axonal and tissue injury in patients with multiple sclerosis with low cerebral lesion load and no disability. *Archives of Neurology, 59*(10), 1565–1571.

Dechent, P., Pouwels, P. J., Wilken, B., Hanefeld, F., & Frahm, J. (1999). Increase of total creatine in human brain after oral supplementation of creatine-monohydrate. *American Journal of Physiology, 277*(3 Pt 2), R698–704.

Defalco, A. J., & Davies, R. K. (1961). The synthesis of creatine by the brain of the intact rat. *Journal of Neurochemistry, 7*, 308–312.

Desagher, S., & Martinou, J. C. (2000). Mitochondria as the central control point of apoptosis. *Trends in Cell Biology, 10*(9), 369–377.

Duc, C. O., Weber, O. M., Trabesinger, A. H., Meier, D., & Boesiger, P. (1998). Quantitative 1H MRS of the human brain in vivo based on the stimulation phantom calibration strategy. *Magnetic Resonance in Medicine, 39*(3), 491–496.

Earnest, C. P., Snell, P. G., Rodriguez, R., Almada, A. L., & Mitchell, T. L. (1995). The effect of creatine monohydrate ingestion on anaerobic power indices, muscular strength and body composition. *Acta Physiologica Scandinavica, 153*(2), 207–209.

Eppenberger, H. M., Dawson, D. M., & Kaplan, N. O. (1967). The comparative enzymology of creatine kinases. I. Isolation and characterization from chicken and rabbit tissues. *Journal of Biology and Chemistry, 242*(2), 204–209.

Fanselow, E. E., & Nicolelis, M. A. (1999). Behavioral modulation of tactile responses in the rat somatosensory system. *Journal of Neuroscience, 19*(17), 7603–7616.

Ferrante, K. L., Shefner, J., Zhang, H., Betensky, R., O'Brien, M., Yu, H., et al. (2005). Tolerance of high-dose (3,000 mg/day) coenzyme Q10 in ALS. *Neurology, 65*(11), 1834–1836.

Ferrante, R. J., Andreassen, O. A., Jenkins, B. G., Dedeoglu, A., Kuemmerle, S., Kubilus, J. K., et al. (2000). Neuroprotective effects of creatine in a transgenic mouse model of Huntington's disease. *Journal of Neuroscience, 20*(12), 4389–4397.

Friedman, D. L., & Roberts, R. (1994). Compartmentation of brain-type creatine kinase and ubiquitous mitochondrial creatine kinase in neurons: evidence for a creatine phosphate energy shuttle in adult rat brain. *Journal of Comparative Neurology, 343*(3), 500–511.

Gabr, R. E., El-Sharkawy, A. M., Schar, M., Weiss, R. G., & Bottomley, P. A. (2011). High-energy phosphate transfer in human muscle: diffusion of phosphocreatine. *American Journal of Physiology Cell Physiology*, 301(1), C234−241.

Gideon, P., Sperling, B., Arlien-Soborg, P., Olsen, T. S., & Henriksen, O. (1994). Long-term follow-up of cerebral infarction patients with proton magnetic resonance spectroscopy. *Stroke*, 25(5), 967−973.

Gonzalez, A. M., & Uhl, G. R. (1994). "Choline/orphan V8-2-1/creatine transporter" mRNA is expressed in nervous, renal and gastrointestinal systems. *Brain Research Molecular Brain Research*, 23 (3), 266−270.

Goodenough, D. J., & Weaver, K. E. (1988). Phantoms for specifications and quality assurance of MR imaging scanners. *Computerized Medical Imaging Graphics*, 12(4), 193−209.

Green, A. L., Hultman, E., Macdonald, I. A., Sewell, D. A., & Greenhaff, P. L. (1996). Carbohydrate ingestion augments skeletal muscle creatine accumulation during creatine supplementation in humans. *American Journal of Physiology*, 271(5 Pt 1), E821−826.

Green, D. R., & Reed, J. C. (1998). Mitochondria and apoptosis. *Science*, 281(5381), 1309−1312.

Greenhaff, P. L., Casey, A., Short, A. H., Harris, R., Soderlund, K., & Hultman, E. (1993). Influence of oral creatine supplementation of muscle torque during repeated bouts of maximal voluntary exercise in man. *Clinical Science (London)*, 84(5), 565−571.

Groeneveld, G. J., Veldink, J. H., van der Tweel, I., Kalmijn, S., Beijer, C., de Visser, M., et al. (2003). A randomized sequential trial of creatine in amyotrophic lateral sclerosis. *Annals of Neurology*, 53 (4), 437−445.

Gu, M., Gash, M. T., Mann, V. M., Javoy-Agid, F., Cooper, J. M., & Schapira, A. H. (1996). Mitochondrial defect in Huntington's disease caudate nucleus. *Annals of Neurology*, 39(3), 385−389.

Guimbal, C., & Kilimann, M. W. (1993). A Na(+)-dependent creatine transporter in rabbit brain, muscle, heart, and kidney. cDNA cloning and functional expression. *Journal of Biological Chemistry*, 268(12), 8418−8421.

Happe, H. K., & Murrin, L. C. (1995). In situ hybridization analysis of CHOT1, a creatine transporter, in the rat central nervous system. *Journal of Comparative Neurology*, 351(1), 94−103.

Hultman, E., Bergstrom, J., & Anderson, N. M. (1967). Breakdown and resynthesis of phosphorylcreatine and adenosine triphosphate in connection with muscular work in man. *Scandinavian Journal of Clinical Laboratory Investestigation*, 19(1), 56−66.

Ikeda, K., Iwasaki, Y., & Kinoshita, M. (2000). Oral administration of creatine monohydrate retards progression of motor neuron disease in the wobbler mouse. *Amyotrophic Lateral Sclerosis and Other Motor Neuron Disordorders*, 1(3), 207−212.

in 't Zandt, H. J., Renema, W. K., Streijger, F., Jost, C., Klomp, D. W., Oerlemans, F., et al. (2004). Cerebral creatine kinase deficiency influences metabolite levels and morphology in the mouse brain: a quantitative in vivo 1H and 31P magnetic resonance study. *Journal of Neurochemistry*, 90(6), 1321−1330.

Ipsiroglu, O. S., Stromberger, C., Ilas, J., Hoger, H., Muhl, A., & Stockler-Ipsiroglu, S. (2001). Changes of tissue creatine concentrations upon oral supplementation of creatine-monohydrate in various animal species. *Life Sciences*, 69(15), 1805−1815.

Item, C. B., Stockler-Ipsiroglu, S., Stromberger, C., Muhl, A., Alessandri, M. G., Bianchi, M. C., et al. (2001). Arginine:glycine amidinotransferase deficiency: the third inborn error of creatine metabolism in humans. *American Journal of Human Genetics*, 69(5), 1127−1133.

Iyengar, M. R. (1984). Creatine kinase as an intracellular regulator. *Journal of Muscle Research and Cell Motility*, 5(5), 527−534.

Jacobs, H., Heldt, H. W., & Klingenberg, M. (1964). High activity of creatine kinase in mitochondria from muscle and brain and evidence for a separate mitochondrial isoenzyme of creatine kinase. *Biochemical and Biophysical Research Communications*, 16(6), 516−521.

Jansen, J. F., Backes, W. H., Nicolay, K., & Kooi, M. E. (2006). 1H MR spectroscopy of the brain: absolute quantification of metabolites. *Radiology*, 240(2), 318−332.

Jost, C. R., Van Der Zee, C. E., In 't Zandt, H. J., Oerlemans, F., Verheij, M., Streijger, F., et al. (2002). Creatine kinase B-driven energy transfer in the brain is important for habituation and spatial learning behaviour, mossy fibre field size and determination of seizure susceptibility. *European Journal of Neuroscience*, 15(10), 1692−1706.

Katz, A., Sahlin, K., & Henriksson, J. (1986). Muscle ATP turnover rate during isometric contraction in humans. *Journal of Applied Physiology*, 60(6), 1839−1842.

Kleefstra, T., Rosenberg, E. H., Salomons, G. S., Stroink, H., van Bokhoven, H., Hamel, B. C., et al. (2005). Progressive intestinal, neurological and psychiatric problems in two adult males with cerebral creatine deficiency caused by an SLC6A8 mutation. *Clinical Genetics*, 68(4), 379−381.

Klivenyi, P., Calingasan, N. Y., Starkov, A., Stavrovskaya, I. G., Kristal, B. S., Yang, L., et al. (2004). Neuroprotective mechanisms of creatine occur in the absence of mitochondrial creatine kinase. *Neurobiology of Disease*, 15(3), 610−617.

Klivenyi, P., Ferrante, R. J., Matthews, R. T., Bogdanov, M. B., Klein, A. M., Andreassen, O. A., et al. (1999). Neuroprotective effects of creatine in a transgenic animal model of amyotrophic lateral sclerosis. *Nature Medicine*, 5(3), 347−350.

Koroshetz, W. J., Jenkins, B. G., Rosen, B. R., & Beal, M. F. (1997). Energy metabolism defects in Huntington's disease and effects of coenzyme Q10. *Annals of Neurology*, 41(2), 160−165.

Kottke, M., Wallimann, T., & Brdiczka, D. (1994). Dual electron microscopic localization of mitochondrial creatine kinase in brain mitochondria. *Biochemical Medicine and Metabolic Biology*, 51(2), 105−117.

Kuhl, D. E., Markham, C. H., Metter, E. J., Riege, W. H., Phelps, M. E., & Mazziotta, J. C. (1985). Local cerebral glucose utilization in symptomatic and presymptomatic Huntington's disease. *Research Publications Association for Research in Nervous and Mental Diseases*, 63, 199−209.

Kuwert, T., Lange, H. W., Langen, K. J., Herzog, H., Aulich, A., & Feinendegen, L. E. (1990). Cortical and subcortical glucose consumption measured by PET in patients with Huntington's disease. *Brain*, 113(Pt 5), 1405−1423.

Lauriero, F., Federico, F., Rubini, G., Conte, C., Simone, I., Inchingolo, V., et al. (1996). 99Tcm-HMPAO SPET and 1H-MRS (proton magnetic resonance spectroscopy) in patients with ischaemic cerebral infarction. *Nuclearl Medicine Communications*, 17(2), 140−146.

Lei, H., Berthet, C., Hirt, L., & Gruetter, R. (2009). Evolution of the neurochemical profile after transient focal cerebral ischemia in the mouse brain. *Journal of Cerebral Blood Flow and Metabolism*, 29 (4), 811−819.

Levin, B. E., Katzen, H. L., Maudsley, A., Post, J., Myerson, C., Govind, V., et al. (2012). Whole-Brain Proton MR Spectroscopic Imaging in Parkinson's Disease. *Journal of Neuroimaging*. Available from http://dx.doi.org/10.1111/j.1552-6569.2012.00733.x in press.

Li, B. S., Wang, H., & Gonen, O. (2003). Metabolite ratios to assumed stable creatine level may confound the quantification of proton brain MR spectroscopy. *Magnetic Resonance Imaging*, *21*(8), 923–928.

Lohmann, K. (1934). *Biochemische Zeitschrift*, *271*, 264.

Loike, J. D., Somes, M., & Silverstein, S. C. (1986). Creatine uptake, metabolism, and efflux in human monocytes and macrophages. *American Journal of Physiology*, *251*(1 Pt 1), C128–135.

Lukaszuk, J. M., Robertson, R. J., Arch, J. E., Moore, G. E., Yaw, K. M., Kelley, D. E., et al. (2002). Effect of creatine supplementation and a lacto-ovo-vegetarian diet on muscle creatine concentration. *International Journal of Sport Nutrition and Exerc Metabolism*, *12*(3), 336–348.

Lukaszuk, J. M., Robertson, R. J., Arch, J. E., & Moyna, N. M. (2005). Effect of a defined lacto-ovo-vegetarian diet and oral creatine monohydrate supplementation on plasma creatine concentration. *Journal of Strength and Conditioning Research*, *19*(4), 735–740.

Lynch, J., Peeling, J., Auty, A., & Sutherland, G. R. (1993). Nuclear magnetic resonance study of cerebrospinal fluid from patients with multiple sclerosis. *Canadian Journal of Neurological Sciences*, *20*(3), 194–198.

Lyoo, I. K., Kong, S. W., Sung, S. M., Hirashima, F., Parow, A., Hennen, J., et al. (2003). Multinuclear magnetic resonance spectroscopy of high-energy phosphate metabolites in human brain following oral supplementation of creatine-monohydrate. *Psychiatry Research*, *123*(2), 87–100.

Mak, C. S., Waldvogel, H. J., Dodd, J. R., Gilbert, R. T., Lowe, M. T., Birch, N. P., et al. (2009). Immunohistochemical localisation of the creatine transporter in the rat brain. *Neuroscience*, *163*(2), 571–585.

Marescau, B., De Deyn, P., Wiechert, P., Van Gorp, L., & Lowenthal, A. (1986). Comparative study of guanidino compounds in serum and brain of mouse, rat, rabbit, and man. *Journal of Neurochemistry*, *46*(3), 717–720.

Mathews, V. P., Barker, P. B., Blackband, S. J., Chatham, J. C., & Bryan, R. N. (1995). Cerebral metabolites in patients with acute and subacute strokes: concentrations determined by quantitative proton MR spectroscopy. *American Journal of Roentgenology*, *165*(3), 633–638.

Matthews, R. T., Ferrante, R. J., Klivenyi, P., Yang, L., Klein, A. M., Mueller, G., et al. (1999). Creatine and cyclocreatine attenuate MPTP neurotoxicity. *Experimental Neurology*, *157*(1), 142–149.

Mazziotta, J. C., Phelps, M. E., Pahl, J. J., Huang, S. C., Baxter, L. R., Riege, W. H., et al. (1987). Reduced cerebral glucose metabolism in asymptomatic subjects at risk for Huntington's disease. *New England Journal of Medicine*, *316*(7), 357–362.

Mercimek-Mahmutoglu, S., Stoeckler-Ipsiroglu, S., Adami, A., Appleton, R., Araujo, H. C., Duran, M., et al. (2006). GAMT deficiency: features, treatment, and outcome in an inborn error of creatine synthesis. *Neurology*, *67*(3), 480–484.

Meyer, R. A., Brown, T. R., Krilowicz, B. L., & Kushmerick, M. J. (1986). Phosphagen and intracellular pH changes during contraction of creatine-depleted rat muscle. *American Journal of Physiology*, *250*(2 Pt 1), C264–274.

Murone, I., & Ogata, K. (1973). Studies on creatine kinase of skeletal muscle and brain with special reference to subcellular distribution and isozymes. *Journal of Biochemistry*, *74*(1), 41–48.

Nakashima, T., Tomi, M., Tachikawa, M., Watanabe, M., Terasaki, T., & Hosoya, K. (2005). Evidence for creatine biosynthesis in Muller glia. *Glia*, *52*(1), 47–52.

Nash, S. R., Giros, B., Kingsmore, S. F., Rochelle, J. M., Suter, S. T., Gregor, P., et al. (1994). Cloning, pharmacological characterization, and genomic localization of the human creatine transporter. *Receptors Channels*, *2*(2), 165–174.

Nicklas, W. J., Vyas, I., & Heikkila, R. E. (1985). Inhibition of NADH-linked oxidation in brain mitochondria by 1-methyl-4-phenyl-pyridine, a metabolite of the neurotoxin, 1-methyl-4-phenyl-1,2,5,6-tetrahydropyridine. *Life Sciences*, *36*(26), 2503–2508.

Nie, K., Zhang, Y., Huang, B., Wang, L., Zhao, J., Huang, Z., et al. (2012). Marked N-acetylaspartate and choline metabolite changes in Parkinson's disease patients with mild cognitive impairment. *Parkinsonism and Related Disorders*, *19*(3), 329–334.

NINDS NET-PD Investigators (2006). A randomized, double-blind, futility clinical trial of creatine and minocycline in early Parkinson disease. *Neurology*, *66*(5), 664–671.

NINDS NET-PD Investigators (2008). A pilot clinical trial of creatine and minocycline in early Parkinson disease: 18-month results. *Clinical Neuropharmacology*, *31*(3), 141–150.

Odoom, J. E., Kemp, G. J., & Radda, G. K. (1996). The regulation of total creatine content in a myoblast cell line. *Molecular and Cellular Biochemistry*, *158*(2), 179–188.

Ohtsuki, S., Tachikawa, M., Takanaga, H., Shimizu, H., Watanabe, M., Hosoya, K., et al. (2002). The blood-brain barrier creatine transporter is a major pathway for supplying creatine to the brain. *Journal of Cerebral Blood Flow and Metabolism*, *22*(11), 1327–1335.

Okamoto, K., Hirai, S., Shoji, M., Senoh, Y., & Yamazaki, T. (1990). Axonal swellings in the corticospinal tracts in amyotrophic lateral sclerosis. *Acta Neuropathology*, *80*(2), 222–226.

Peral, M. J., Garcia-Delgado, M., Calonge, M. L., Duran, J. M., De La Horra, M. C., Wallimann, T., et al. (2002). Human, rat and chicken small intestinal Na + -Cl- -creatine transporter: functional, molecular characterization and localization. *Journal of Physiology*, *545* (Pt 1), 133–144.

Perasso, L., Cupello, A., Lunardi, G. L., Principato, C., Gandolfo, C., & Balestrino, M. (2003). Kinetics of creatine in blood and brain after intraperitoneal injection in the rat. *Brain Research*, *974*(1-2), 37–42.

Pischel, I., & Gastner, T. (2007). Creatine--its chemical synthesis, chemistry, and legal status. *Subcellular Biochemistry*, *46*, 291–307.

Pittas, G., Hazell, M. D., Simpson, E. J., & Greenhaff, P. L. (2010). Optimization of insulin-mediated creatine retention during creatine feeding in humans. *Journal of Sports Science*, *28*(1), 67–74.

Poo-Arguelles, P., Arias, A., Vilaseca, M. A., Ribes, A., Artuch, R., Sans-Fito, A., et al. (2006). X-Linked creatine transporter deficiency in two patients with severe mental retardation and autism. *Journal of Inherited Metabolic Disease*, *29*(1), 220–223.

Prass, K., Royl, G., Lindauer, U., Freyer, D., Megow, D., Dirnagl, U., et al. (2007). Improved reperfusion and neuroprotection by creatine in a mouse model of stroke. *Journal of Cerebral Blood Flow and Metabolism*, *27*(3), 452–459.

Pyne-Geithman, G. J., deGrauw, T. J., Cecil, K. M., Chuck, G., Lyons, M. A., Ishida, Y., et al. (2004). Presence of normal creatine in the muscle of a patient with a mutation in the creatine transporter: a case study. *Molecular and Cellular Biochemistry*, *262* (1-2), 35–39.

Rosenberg, E. H., Almeida, L. S., Kleefstra, T., deGrauw, R. S., Yntema, H. G., Bahi, N., et al. (2004). High prevalence of SLC6A8 deficiency in X-linked mental retardation. *American Journal of Human Genetics*, *75*(1), 97–105.

Roy, S., & Nicholson, D. W. (2000). Cross-talk in cell death signaling. *Journal of Experimental Medicine*, *192*(8), F21–25.

Ryu, H., & Ferrante, R. J. (2005). Emerging chemotherapeutic strategies for Huntington's disease. *Expert Opinion on Emerging Drugs*, *10*(2), 345–363.

Ryu, H., Rosas, H. D., Hersch, S. M., & Ferrante, R. J. (2005). The therapeutic role of creatine in Huntington's disease. *Pharmacology and Therapeutics, 108*(2), 193–207.

Salomons, G. S., van Dooren, S. J., Verhoeven, N. M., Cecil, K. M., Ball, W. S., Degrauw, T. J., et al. (2001). X-linked creatine-transporter gene (SLC6A8) defect: a new creatine-deficiency syndrome. *American Journal of Human Genetics, 68*(6), 1497–1500.

Saltarelli, M. D., Bauman, A. L., Moore, K. R., Bradley, C. C., & Blakely, R. D. (1996). Expression of the rat brain creatine transporter in situ and in transfected HeLa cells. *Developmental Neuroscience, 18*(5-6), 524–534.

Sasaki, S., & Iwata, M. (1996). Impairment of fast axonal transport in the proximal axons of anterior horn neurons in amyotrophic lateral sclerosis. *Neurology, 47*(2), 535–540.

Schloss, P., Mayser, W., & Betz, H. (1994). The putative rat choline transporter CHOT1 transports creatine and is highly expressed in neural and muscle-rich tissues. *Biochemical and Biophysical Research Communications, 198*(2), 637–645.

Schmidt, A., Marescau, B., Boehm, E. A., Renema, W. K., Peco, R., Das, A., et al. (2004). Severely altered guanidino compound levels, disturbed body weight homeostasis and impaired fertility in a mouse model of guanidinoacetate N-methyltransferase (GAMT) deficiency. *Human Molecular Genetics, 13*(9), 905–921.

Schoenbaum, G., Chiba, A. A., & Gallagher, M. (1999). Neural encoding in orbitofrontal cortex and basolateral amygdala during olfactory discrimination learning. *Journal of Neuroscience, 19*(5), 1876–1884.

Scholte, H. R. (1973). On the triple localization of creatine kinase in heart and skeletal muscle cells of the rat: evidence for the existence of myofibrillar and mitochondrial isoenzymes. *Biochimica Biophysica Acta, 305*(2), 413–427.

Schulze, A., & Battini, R. (2007). Pre-symptomatic treatment of creatine biosynthesis defects. *Subcellular Biochemistry, 46*, 167–181.

Schulze, A., Hess, T., Wevers, R., Mayatepek, E., Bachert, P., Marescau, B., et al. (1997). Creatine deficiency syndrome caused by guanidinoacetate methyltransferase deficiency: diagnostic tools for a new inborn error of metabolism. *Journal of Pediatrics, 131*(4), 626–631.

Schulze, A., Hoffmann, G. F., Bachert, P., Kirsch, S., Salomons, G. S., Verhoeven, N. M., et al. (2006). Presymptomatic treatment of neonatal guanidinoacetate methyltransferase deficiency. *Neurology, 67*(4), 719–721.

Shefner, J. M., Cudkowicz, M. E., Schoenfeld, D., Conrad, T., Taft, J., Chilton, M., et al. (2004). A clinical trial of creatine in ALS. *Neurology, 63*(9), 1656–1661.

Shu, X. J., Xue, L., Liu, W., Chen, F. Y., Zhu, C., Sun, X. H., et al. (2013). More vulnerability of left than right hippocampal damage in right-handed patients with post-traumatic stress disorder. *Psychiatry Research, 212*(3), 237–244.

Sora, I., Richman, J., Santoro, G., Wei, H., Wang, Y., Vanderah, T., et al. (1994). The cloning and expression of a human creatine transporter. *Biochemical and Biophysical Research Communications, 204*(1), 419–427.

Stagg, C. J., Bachtiar, V., & Johansen-Berg, H. (2011). The role of GABA in human motor learning. *Current Biology, 21*(6), 480–484.

Steenge, G. R., Lambourne, J., Casey, A., Macdonald, I. A., & Greenhaff, P. L. (1998). Stimulatory effect of insulin on creatine accumulation in human skeletal muscle. *American Journal of Physiology, 275*(6 Pt 1), E974–979.

Steenge, G. R., Simpson, E. J., & Greenhaff, P. L. (2000). Protein- and carbohydrate-induced augmentation of whole body creatine retention in humans. *Journal of Applied Physiology, 89*(3), 1165–1171.

Stockler, S., Holzbach, U., Hanefeld, F., Marquardt, I., Helms, G., Requart, M., et al. (1994). Creatine deficiency in the brain: a new, treatable inborn error of metabolism. *Pediatric Research, 36*(3), 409–413.

Stockler, S., Marescau, B., De Deyn, P. P., Trijbels, J. M., & Hanefeld, F. (1997). Guanidino compounds in guanidinoacetate methyltransferase deficiency, a new inborn error of creatine synthesis. *Metabolis, 46*(10), 1189–1193.

Stockler, S., Schutz, P. W., & Salomons, G. S. (2007). Cerebral creatine deficiency syndromes: clinical aspects, treatment and pathophysiology. *Subcellular Biochemistry, 46*, 149–166.

Streijger, F., Oerlemans, F., Ellenbroek, B. A., Jost, C. R., Wieringa, B., & Van der Zee, C. E. (2005). Structural and behavioural consequences of double deficiency for creatine kinases BCK and UbCKmit. *Behavioural Brain Research, 157*(2), 219–234.

Tabrizi, S. J., Blamire, A. M., Manners, D. N., Rajagopalan, B., Styles, P., Schapira, A. H., et al. (2003). Creatine therapy for Huntington's disease: clinical and MRS findings in a 1-year pilot study. *Neurology, 61*(1), 141–142.

Tabrizi, S. J., Blamire, A. M., Manners, D. N., Rajagopalan, B., Styles, P., Schapira, A. H., et al. (2005). High-dose creatine therapy for Huntington disease: a 2-year clinical and MRS study. *Neurology, 64*(9), 1655–1656.

Tachikawa, M., Fukaya, M., Terasaki, T., Ohtsuki, S., & Watanabe, M. (2004). Distinct cellular expressions of creatine synthetic enzyme GAMT and creatine kinases uCK-Mi and CK-B suggest a novel neuron-glial relationship for brain energy homeostasis. *European Journal of Neuroscience, 20*(1), 144–160.

Tartaglia, M. C., Narayanan, S., De Stefano, N., Arnaoutelis, R., Antel, S. B., Francis, S. J., et al. (2002). Choline is increased in prelesional normal appearing white matter in multiple sclerosis. *Journal of Neurology, 249*(10), 1382–1390.

Tatsumi, T., Shiraishi, J., Keira, N., Akashi, K., Mano, A., Yamanaka, S., et al. (2003). Intracellular ATP is required for mitochondrial apoptotic pathways in isolated hypoxic rat cardiac myocytes. *Cardiovascular Research, 59*(2), 428–440.

van den Bogaard, S. J., Dumas, E. M., Teeuwisse, W. M., Kan, H. E., Webb, A., Roos, R. A., et al. (2011). Exploratory 7-Tesla magnetic resonance spectroscopy in Huntington's disease provides in vivo evidence for impaired energy metabolism. *Journal of Neurology, 258*(12), 2230–2239.

Van Pilsum, J. F., Olsen, B., Taylor, D., Rozycki, T., & Pierce, J. C. (1963). Transamidinase activities, in vitro, of tissues from various mammals and from rats fed protein-free, creatine-supplemented and normal diets. *Archives of Biochemistry and Biophysics, 100*, 520–524.

Van Pilsum, J. F., Stephens, G. C., & Taylor, D. (1972). Distribution of creatine, guanidinoacetate and the enzymes for their biosynthesis in the animal kingdom. Implications for phylogeny. *Biochemical Journal, 126*(2), 325–345.

Volpe, J. J. (2008). *Neurology of the Newborn* (5th ed.). Philadelphia: Saunders.

Walker, J. B. (1979). Creatine: biosynthesis, regulation and function. In A. Meister (Ed.), *Advances in Enzymology and Related Areas of Molecular Biology* (Vol. 50, pp. 177–242). New York: John Wiley and Sons.

Wallimann, T., Tokarska-Schlattner, M., Neumann, D., Epand, R. H., Epand, R. F., Andres, R. H., et al. (2007). The phosphocreatine circuit: molecular and cellular physiology of creatine kinases, sensitivity to free readicals, and enhancement by creatine supplementation. In V. Saks (Ed.), *Molecular System Bioenergetics: Energy for Life*. Weinheim, Germany: Wiley-VCH.

Wallimann, T., Tokarska-Schlattner, M., & Schlattner, U. (2011). The creatine kinase system and pleiotropic effects of creatine. *Amino Acids, 40*(5), 1271–1296.

Wilken, B., Ramirez, J. M., Probst, I., Richter, D. W., & Hanefeld, F. (2000). Anoxic ATP depletion in neonatal mice brainstem is prevented by creatine supplementation. *Archives of Diseases in Childhood Fetal and Neonatal Edition, 82*(3), F224–227.

Woo, D. C., Kim, B. S., Jung, S. L., Park, H. J., Rhim, H. S., Jahng, G. H., et al. (2007). Development of a cone-shape phantom for multi-voxel MR spectroscopy. *Journal of Neurosciemce Methods, 162*(1-2), 101–107.

Wyss, M., & Kaddurah-Daouk, R. (2000). Creatine and creatinine metabolism. *Physiology Review, 80*(3), 1107–1213.

Yoshizaki, K., Watari, H., & Radda, G. K. (1990). Role of phosphocreatine in energy transport in skeletal muscle of bullfrog studied by 31P-NMR. *Biochimica Biophysica Acta, 1051*(2), 144–150.

Zhang, W., Narayanan, M., & Friedlander, R. M. (2003). Additive neuroprotective effects of minocycline with creatine in a mouse model of ALS. *Annals of Neurology, 53*(2), 267–270.

Zhu, S., Li, M., Figueroa, B. E., Liu, A., Stavrovskaya, I. G., Pasinelli, P., et al. (2004). Prophylactic creatine administration mediates neuroprotection in cerebral ischemia in mice. *Journal of Neuroscience, 24*(26), 5909–5912.

The Biochemistry of Choline

Joanne C. Lin and Nicholas Gant

Centre for Brain Research, The University of Auckland, New Zealand

INTRODUCTION

Choline (trimethyl-β-hydroxyethylammonium) is a quaternary ammonium compound with a complex role in various important neurochemical processes. It acts as a precursor for the neurotransmitter acetylcholine (Loffelholz et al., 1993) and other intracellular messaging molecules, it is involved in lipid transport and methyl-group metabolism, and is also an essential component of membrane phospholipids (Zeisel, 1999). Choline was recognized as an essential nutrient in 1998 (Food and Nutrition Board; Institute of Medicine, 1998) and is obtained from dietary sources or via *de novo* synthesis. Despite fairly large pools of total choline in the brain ($>20 \, \mu mol/g$), levels of free choline are very low; approximately 90% is bound in the phospholipids of cell membranes and a further 9% is present as hydrophilic metabolites such as phosphocholine and glycerophosphocholine (Klein et al., 1993). The breakdown of cellular membranes is a characteristic feature of neuronal degeneration in acute and chronic neurological disorders such as stroke and dementia, respectively (Klein, 2000), and is seen as an increase in the size of the choline peak. Furthermore, elevation of choline-containing metabolites can be a neurochemical hallmark of aberrant phospholipid metabolism in some cancers (Glunde & Serkova, 2006). The so-called choline peak at 3.2 parts per million (ppm) on a ^{1}H MRS spectrum is a heterogeneous peak representing a number of water soluble $-N(CH_3)_3$-containing compounds including free choline, phosphocholine, and glycerophosphocholine (Barker et al., 1994; Miller et al., 1996). These water-soluble breakdown products of membrane components are considered markers of cellular density and cell wall turnover, and can be used to investigate *in vivo* changes in metabolism associated with various disease states.

BIOSYNTHESIS

De novo synthesis of choline is carried out via sequential methylation of phosphatidylethanolamine (PE) to phosphatidylcholine (PC), catalyzed by phosphatidylethanolamine *N*-methyltransferase (PEMT) using *S*-adenosylmethionine (AdoMet) as a methyl-group donor (Bremer et al., 1960). Choline can then be generated from PC via the action of phospholipases. Choline is also released during the biosynthesis of phosphatidylserine (PS) from PC, catalyzed by PS synthase-1 (Kuge & Nishijima, 1997). The capacity of the brain for *de novo* synthesis is very low (Crews et al., 1980; Blusztajn & Wurtman, 1981; Andriamampandry et al., 1990); therefore, it is dependent on uptake of choline via a carrier present in the blood−brain barrier (Cornford et al., 1978).

De novo synthesis alone is not sufficient to meet human requirements. Dietary choline is absorbed from a variety of choline-containing food; milk, eggs, liver, and peanuts are especially rich in choline (Food and Nutrition Board; Institute of Medicine, 1998). PC (also known as lecithin) contains about 13% choline by weight (Canty & Zeisel, 1994). There are two distinct mechanisms for entry of choline into cells: a high-affinity (K_m or $K_t < 5 \, \mu M$) Na$^+$-dependent transporter' and a lower affinity ($K_i > 30 \, \mu M$) Na$^+$-independent transporter (Ishidate, 1989). The recommended adequate intake of choline is 550 mg/day for men and 425 mg/day for women (Food and Nutrition Board; Institute of Medicine, 1998). This value is estimated to be sufficient to prevent deficiency; however, inadequate data are available to support the determination of a more accurate estimated average requirement, i.e., the intake that meets the dietary requirement in 50% of the population. Dietary choline deficiency in humans is not recognized as lethal, but adults deprived of choline have been shown to develop fatty liver and muscle damage (Fischer et al., 2007). Furthermore, choline deficiency has been linked to other chronic conditions. When choline stores are inadequate, there is diminished capacity to methylate homocysteine to methionine and a consequent increase in plasma levels of homocysteine (da Costa et al., 2005). Elevated homocysteine levels have been associated with increased risk of heart disease and stroke (Homocysteine Studies Collaboration, 2002), cancer (Wu & Wu, 2002), cognitive decline (Seshadri et al., 2002), and osteoporotic fractures (van Meurs et al., 2004).

Pathways of Free Choline

In mammalian tissue, free choline participates in four enzyme-catalyzed pathways: oxidation, phosphorylation, acetylation, and base exchange.

Oxidation

Choline can be oxidized to betaine aldehyde, which is then converted to betaine by choline oxidase (choline dehydrogenase) in the liver and kidneys. The rate of hepatic betaine synthesis is faster than choline incorporation into phosphocholine (discussed later); however, betaine cannot be reduced to form choline. In the liver, betaine is an important donor of methyl groups for methionine biosynthesis from homocysteine (Vance & Vance, 2008).

Phosphorylation

Choline kinase catalyzes the phosphorylation of the hydroxyl group of choline by using ATP as the phosphate donor (Brophy et al., 1977), which is the first step in the generation of PC, the major fate of choline in the human brain (see the section, Phospholipid biosynthesis).

Acetylation

Despite only a small fraction of free choline undergoing acetylation (Cohen & Wurtman, 1975; Haubrich, 1975b), this pathway is vital as it produces the neurotransmitter acetylcholine. The reaction with acetyl coenzyme A is catalyzed by choline acetyltransferase (Nachmansohn & Machado, 1943), which is concentrated in cholinergic nerve terminals (Wajda et al., 1973). Systemically administered choline rapidly enters the brain (Haubrich et al., 1975a; Cornford et al., 1978) and results in elevation of serum choline concentration, brain choline concentration, and brain acetylcholine concentration (Cohen & Wurtman, 1975; Haubrich et al., 1975a).

Base Exchange

Base exchange pathways have been described in various tissue types, including the liver and brain (Porcellati et al., 1971; Salerno & Beeler, 1973; Orlando et al., 1977). PS is an essential phospholipid for the growth of mammalian cells (Kuge et al., 1986; Voelker & Frazier, 1986); its synthesis can occur through the exchange of serine with the choline moiety of PC or the ethanolamine moiety of PE (Kuge & Nishijima, 1997; Vance, 2008).

Phospholipid Biosynthesis

The main fate of choline is the synthesis of PC, the principal component of cell membranes. In mammalian cells, there are two pathways that synthesize PC *de novo*. The major pathway is the cytidine diphosphate (CDP)-choline pathway and occurs in all nucleated cells. It was originally described by Eugene Kennedy in the 1950s and is, therefore, referred to as the "Kennedy pathway" (Kennedy & Weiss, 1956). The CPD-choline pathway utilizes choline and consists of three enzymatic steps: (1) phosphorylation of choline to produce phosphocholine and ADP, catalyzed by choline kinase; (2) a reaction between phosphocholine and cytidine triphosphate (CTP) to produce CPD-choline, catalyzed by CTP:phosphocholine cytidylyltransferase, which is the rate-limiting step; and (3) the exchange of cytidine monophosphate for diacylglycerol to produce PC, catalyzed by CPD-choline:1,2-diacylglycerol cholinephosphotransferase. The second endogenous pathway for the generation of PC is catalyzed by PEMT; PE is converted to PC in a three-step sequential methylation using AdoMet as a methyl (Bremer & Greenberg, 1961). This pathway is only quantitatively significant within the liver where it contributes about 30% of total hepatic PC synthesis (Vance & Ridgway, 1988).

Phospholipid Catabolism

Phospholipids undergo rapid and continuous turnover in all tissues and cell types and are hydrolyzed by the phospholipase group of enzymes. Phospholipase subtypes (A_1, A_2, C, D) are diverse in the site of action on the phospholipid molecule, their function, mode of action, and regulation suggesting that the continued remodeling of cellular membranes and maintenance of homeostasis requires the action of more than one phospholipase (Wilton, 2008). The major degradative pathway for PC is PC to lyso-PC to glycerophosphocholine (GPC) to choline (Morash et al., 1988). Lyso-PC is a cell surfactant with potential for causing cellular toxicity; for this reason, it is rapidly converted to a fatty acid and GPC by lysophospholipase (Weltzien, 1979). GPC is quantitatively the major intracellular water-soluble catabolite of PC degradation; however, choline is the major product of PC degradation when both intracellular and extracellular metabolites are considered (Morash et al., 1988).

BIOLOGICAL FUNCTION

Choline is an integral component of several relevant neurochemical processes and its role in the body is complex. It is the major dietary source of labile methyl groups for AdoMet (Stead et al., 2006), and such methylation reactions play a major role in the biosynthesis of phospholipids and the regulation of metabolic processes. This section will outline the dietary requirement of choline in humans, and focus on the function of PC, the primary conversion product of choline, and the principal component of cell membranes.

Hepatic Phospholipids

PC biosynthesis is required for normal secretion of very low density lipoprotein (VLDL) secretion from hepatocytes; choline deficiency and, consequently, reduced levels of hepatic PC, attenuates secretion of VLDL from the liver (Yao & Vance, 1988; Verkade et al., 1993; Fast & Vance, 1995). The physiological importance of the relationship between hepatic PC biosynthesis and lipoprotein metabolism has recently been underscored in Pemt(−/−) mice, which develop non-alcoholic fatty liver disease but are protected from cardiovascular disease. Elevated VLDL is an established risk factor for heart disease (Lloyd-Jones et al., 2009); reduced hepatic levels of PC reduce the amount of VLDL particles in the circulation (Jacobs et al., 2004; Zhao et al., 2009). Conversely, animal models of impaired PC biosynthesis accumulate hepatic triglycerides as a result of attenuated VLDL secretion (Rinella et al., 2008; Jacobs et al., 2010). Therefore, PC-mediated regulation of VLDL secretion has the potential to alter the susceptibility to severe forms of non-alcoholic liver disease.

Neural Phospholipids

PC, PS, and PE are the most abundant phospholipids in mammalian cells (Kelly & Jacobs, 2011) and are structural components in cellular, mitochondrial, endoplasmic reticular, and lysosomal membranes (Tayebati & Amenta, 2013). Brain tissue contains relatively high amounts of phospholipids (~20–25%); among the different types of membranes in the brain, myelin contains the highest phospholipid content (Evans & Finean, 1965; Siakotos et al., 1969; Denisova, 1990). Phospholipids afford stability, fluidity, and permeability to neural membranes, and are also required for the proper function of integral membrane proteins, receptors, and ion channels (Farooqui & Horrocks, 1985).

INDICATORS OF MEMBRANE DAMAGE

Under normal circumstances, remodeling of phospholipids transiently generates low levels of intermediate lysophospholipids (Farooqui et al., 2000). However, neuronal trauma and neurodegenerative diseases can stimulate phospholipase activity and result in changes in phospholipid composition. One of the key pathological events during neurodegeneration is excitotoxicity, i.e., toxicity as a result of overstimulation of neurons by the excitatory neurotransmitter, glutamate (Klein, 2000). The postulated sequence of events in hypoxia suggests a reduction in ATP levels due to loss of energy production, followed by glutamate release, and excessive stimulation of glutamate receptors causing an influx of calcium (Rothman & Olney, 1995). Calcium overload can induce the pathological overactivation of catabolic enzymes, including proteases, nucleases, and phospholipases (Kristián & Siesjö, 1998). Pathological phospholipid breakdown is reflected in the appearance of PC breakdown products such as lyso-PC and GPC (Morash et al., 1988). Several neurological and metabolic conditions are characterized by accelerated phospholipid turnover. For example, in Alzheimer's disease, reported changes include reduced levels of PC and PE (Nitsch et al., 1992), and increased concentrations of metabolic breakdown products (Blusztajn et al., 1990; Nitsch et al., 1992). Loss of phospholipids and elevated choline-containing compounds are also observed in ischemic injury (Farber et al., 1981), neoplasms (Ackerstaff et al., 2003) and diseases of demyelination (van der Knaap & Pouwels, 2005).

THE Cho PEAK IN MRS

Conditions affecting the biosynthesis of phospholipids and/or cellular membrane integrity may be associated with changes detectable by MRS. Both ^{1}H and ^{31}P MRS have been used to identify and quantify metabolite dynamics in neurodegenerative and psychiatric diseases. Significant alterations in choline-containing compounds have been observed in studies of neoplasms, Alzheimer's disease, multiple sclerosis, and substance abuse.

^{1}H MRS

In ^{1}H MRS, the so-called choline peak (Cho) at 3.2 ppm is a heterogeneous peak due to the presence of nine spectroscopically identical protons on the trimethylammonium $(-N(CH_3)_3)$ moiety of choline containing-compounds including free choline, phosphocholine, and GPC (Barker et al., 1994; Miller et al., 1996). The majority of choline in the brain is bound in phospholipids, mainly as PC; however, membrane-bound choline is immobile and, therefore, invisible on a ^{1}H spectrum (Miller, 1991). Consequently, the Cho peak is usually composed to represent cytosolic choline and its putative breakdown products: phosphocholine ($\sim$400 nmol/g) and GPC ($\sim$600 nmol/g; Klein, 2000; Ross & Bluml, 2001). It should be noted that interpretation of phosphocholine and GPC levels is not straightforward. Unlike GPC, which is exclusively produced by phospholipase-induced PC breakdown, phosphocholine is both a catabolic and anabolic metabolite; therefore, an increase in the Cho signal may not necessarily reflect membrane breakdown but also phosphocholine formation from free choline and, thus, de novo PC biosynthesis.

^{1}H MRS has been widely used for the investigation of metabolites, and the Cho peak is considered a marker of cell density and cell wall turnover. Elevated levels of PC and total choline is one of the most widely established characteristics of cancer cells; increased choline levels have been detected in breast, prostate, and different types of brain tumors (Ackerstaff et al., 2003). The increased Cho peak in studies of tumors has been attributed to greater rates of membrane synthesis, increased cellularity, or rapid membrane turnover (Poptani et al., 1995). Elevated Cho ratios have not been consistently reported across all types of dementias (Valenzuela & Sachdev, 2001); however, it has been suggested that Cho levels may be elevated in dementias that are characterized by a profound cholinergic deficit, e.g., Alzheimer's disease and dementia with Lewy bodies (Kantarci et al., 2004). This may be a consequence of PC catabolism to provide free choline for the chronically deficient acetylcholine production (Wurtman et al., 1985). The pathological significance of elevated Cho within normal-appearing white matter (Bitsch et al., 1999; Tartaglia et al., 2002) and lesions (Arnold et al., 1992) in multiple sclerosis has been linked to active demyelination and inflammation (Arnold et al., 1992; Bitsch et al., 1999). Increments in the Cho peak is a commonly reported finding in studies of substance abuse, including alcohol (Ende et al., 2006), cocaine (Meyerhoff et al., 1999), and methamphetamine (Ernst et al., 2000; Nordahl et al., 2002), a change that has been attributed to increased membrane turnover and reactive gliosis. Detoxification and abstinence from drug use has also been associated with decreases in Cho levels (Nordahl et al., 2005; Ende et al., 2006), suggesting adaptive changes and/or metabolic recovery contributing to some degree of normalization of neuronal structure with drug cessation. Reports of Cho peak changes in schizophrenia have been inconsistent across studies, with some reporting no change (Bertolino et al., 1998) or reductions in the signal (Omori et al., 2000), which were attributed to structural abnormalities and volumetric reduction of white matter tracts (Andreasen et al., 1990).

^{31}P MRS

In comparison to ^{1}H MRS, ^{31}P MRS yields a higher resolution for the detection of phospholipid metabolites. It can detect several groups of signals, which represent inorganic phosphate, phosphomonoesters (PME), phosphodiesters (PDE), phosphocreatine, and others (Cady, 2012). The PME resonance has been suggested to represent phosphoethanolamine and, to a lesser extent, phosphocholine, while PDE peaks have been associated with GPC and glycerophosphoethanolamine (GPE), the catabolic breakdown product of PE. Due to its improved resolution for phosphoesters, ^{31}P MRS has been applied in the study of Alzheimer's disease; however, it has been less widely applied to other conditions.

The published data relating to phosphoesters in Alzheimer's disease are somewhat inconsistent. Increases in the PME signal have been reported in some studies of Alzheimer's disease (Brown et al., 1989; Cuenod et al., 1995) but not others (Bottomley et al., 1992; Murphy et al., 1993). Theoretically, the PDE peak, with signals from degradation products GPC and GPE, may be more easily interpreted as membrane degeneration than the PME signal; however, abnormalities in PDE have not been observed (Bottomley et al., 1992; Murphy et al., 1993). This may be due to GPC and GPE only representing minor proportions of the PDE peak in ^{31}P MRS (Klein, 2000).

CONCLUSIONS

Choline is an essential nutrient with a complex role in many important biochemical processes. It ensures structural integrity and signaling functions of cell membranes, it is a major source of methyl groups, it plays an important role as the precursor to neurotransmitter acetylcholine, and it is required for lipid transport and metabolism. The majority of choline in the body is found in phospholipids such as PC (the predominant phospholipid in mammalian cells). Chronic choline deficiency can result in hepatic dysfunction and is associated with increased risk of other diseases. Conditions affecting the metabolism and biosynthesis of phospholipids, or cellular membrane integrity may be detectable with MRS. Although there are some limitations with respect to the interpretation of MRS spectra, it is a valuable tool in identifying changes in choline-containing compounds as neurochemical hallmarks of disease.

References

Ackerstaff, E., Glunde, K., & Bhujwalla, Z. M. (2003). Choline phospholipid metabolism: A target in cancer cells? *Journal of Cellular Biochemistry, 90*(3), 525–533.

Andreasen, N. C., Ehrhardt, J. C., Swayze, V. W., II, Alliger, R. J., Yuh, W. T., Cohen, G., et al. (1990). Magnetic resonance imaging of the brain in schizophrenia. The pathophysiologic significance of structural abnormalities. *Archives of General Psychiatry, 47*(1), 35–44.

Andriamampandry, C., Massarelli, R., Freysz, L., & Kanfer, J. N. (1990). A rat brain cytosolic N-methyltransferase(s) activity converting phosphorylethanolamine into phosphorylcholine. *Biochemical and Biophysical Research Communications, 171*(2), 758–763.

Arnold, D. L., Matthews, P. M., Francis, G. S., O'Connor, J., & Antel, J. P. (1992). Proton magnetic resonance spectroscopic imaging for metabolic characterization of demyelinating plaques. *Annals of Neurology, 31*(3), 235–241.

Barker, P. B., Breiter, S. N., Soher, B. J., Chatham, J. C., Forder, J. R., Samphilipo, M. A., et al. (1994). Quantitative proton spectroscopy of canine brain: in vivo and in vitro correlations. *Magnetic Resonance in Medicine, 32*(2), 157–163.

Bertolino, A., Callicott, J. H., Elman, I., Mattay, V. S., Tedeschi, G., Frank, J. A., et al. (1998). Regionally specific neuronal pathology in untreated patients with schizophrenia: a proton magnetic resonance spectroscopic imaging study. *Biological Psychiatry, 43*(9), 641–648.

Bitsch, A., Bruhn, H., Vougioukas, V., Stringaris, A., Lassmann, H., Frahm, J., et al. (1999). Inflammatory CNS demyelination: Histopathologic correlation with in vivo quantitative proton MR spectroscopy. *American Journal of Neuroradiology, 20*(9), 1619–1627.

Blusztajn, J. K., Lopez Gonzalez-Coviella, I., Logue, M., Growdon, J. H., & Wurtman, R. J. (1990). Levels of phospholipid catabolic intermediates, glycerophosphocholine and glycerophosphoethanolamine, are elevated in brains of Alzheimer's disease but not of Down's syndrome patients. *Brain Research, 536*(1-2), 240–244.

Blusztajn, J. K., & Wurtman, R. J. (1981). Choline biosynthesis by a preparation enriched in synaptosomes from rat brain. *Nature, 290* (5805), 417–418.

Bottomley, P. A., Cousins, J. P., Pendrey, D. L., Wagle, W. A., Hardy, C. J., Eames, F. A., et al. (1992). Alzheimer dementia: quantification of energy metabolism and mobile phosphoesters with P-31 NMR spectroscopy. *Radiology, 183*(3), 695–699.

Bremer, J., Figard, P. H., & Greenberg, D. M. (1960). The biosynthesis of choline and its relation to phospholipid metabolism. *Biochimica et Biophysica Acta, 43*, 477–488.

Bremer, J., & Greenberg, D. M. (1961). Methyl transfering enzyme system of microsomes in the biosynthesis of lecithin (phosphatidylcholine). *Biochimica et Biophysica Acta, 46*(1), 205–216.

Brophy, P. J., Choy, P. C., Toone, J. R., & Vance, D. E. (1977). Choline kinase and ethanolamine kinase are separate, soluble enzymes in rat liver. *European Journal of Biochemistry, 78*(2), 491–495.

Brown, G. G., Levine, S. R., Gorell, J. M., Pettegrew, J. W., Gdowski, J. W., Bueri, J. A., et al. (1989). In vivo ^{31}P NMR profiles of Alzheimer's disease and multiple subcortical infarct dementia. *Neurology, 39*(11), 1423–1427.

Cady, E. (2012). In vivo cerebral ^{31}P magnetic resonance spectroscopy. In I. -Y. Choi, & R. Gruetter (Eds.), *Neural Metabolism in Vivo* (Vol. 4, pp. 149–179). New York: Springer.

Canty, D. J., & Zeisel, S. H. (1994). Lecithin and choline in human health and disease. *Nutrition Reviews, 52*(10), 327–339.

Cohen, E. L., & Wurtman, R. J. (1975). Brain acetylcholine: increase after systemic choline administration. *Life Sciences, 16*(7), 1095–1102.

Cornford, E. M., Braun, L. D., & Oldendorf, W. H. (1978). Carrier mediated blood-brain barrier transport of choline and certain choline analogs. *Journal of Neurochemistry, 30*(2), 299–308.

Crews, F. T., Hirata, F., & Axelrod, J. (1980). Identification and properties of methyltransferases that synthesize phosphatidylcholine in rat brain synaptosomes. *Journal of Neurochemistry, 34*(6), 1491–1498.

Cuenod, C. A., Kaplan, D. B., Michot, J. L., Jehenson, P., Leroy-Willig, A., Forette, F., et al. (1995). Phospholipid abnormalities in early Alzheimer's disease. In vivo phosphorus 31 magnetic resonance spectroscopy. *Archives of Neurology, 52*(1), 89–94.

da Costa, K. -A., Gaffney, C. E., Fischer, L. M., & Zeisel, S. H. (2005). Choline deficiency in mice and humans is associated with increased plasma homocysteine concentration after a methionine load. *American Journal of Clinical Nutrition, 81*(2), 440–444.

Denisova, N. A. (1990). Phospholipid composition of myelin and synaptosomal proteolipid from vertebrate brain. *International Journal of Biochemistry, 22*(5), 439–442.

Ende, G., Walter, S., Welzel, H., Demirakca, T., Wokrina, T., Ruf, M., et al. (2006). Alcohol consumption significantly influences the MR signal of frontal choline-containing compounds. *Neuroimage, 32* (2), 740–746.

Ernst, T., Chang, L., Leonido-Yee, M., & Speck, O. (2000). Evidence for long-term neurotoxicity associated with methamphetamine abuse: a ^{1}H MRS study. *Neurology, 54*(6), 1344–1349.

Evans, M. J., & Finean, J. B. (1965). The lipid composition of myelin from brain and peripheral nerve. *Journal of Neurochemistry, 12*(8), 729–734.

Farber, J. L., Chien, K. R., & Mittnacht, S., Jr. (1981). Myocardial ischemia: the pathogenesis of irreversible cell injury in ischemia. *American Journal of Pathology, 102*(2), 271–281.

Farooqui, A. A., & Horrocks, L. A. (1985). Metabolic and functional aspects of neural membrane phospholipids. *Phospholipids in the nervous system, 2*, 341–348.

Farooqui, A. A., Horrocks, L. A., & Farooqui, T. (2000). Deacylation and reacylation of neural membrane glycerophospholipids. *Journal of Molecular Neuroscience, 14*(3), 123–135.

Fast, D. G., & Vance, D. E. (1995). Nascent VLDL phospholipid composition is altered when phosphatidylcholine biosynthesis is inhibited: evidence for a novel mechanism that regulates VLDL secretion. *Biochimica et Biophysica Acta, 1258*(2), 159–168.

Fischer, L. M., daCosta, K. A., Kwock, L., Stewart, P. W., Lu, T. S., Stabler, S. P., et al. (2007). Sex and menopausal status influence human dietary requirements for the nutrient choline. *American Journal of Clinical Nutrition, 85*(5), 1275–1285.

Food and Nutrition Board; Institute of Medicine. (1998). Dietary reference intakes for thiamin, riboflavin, niacin, vitamin B6, folate, vitamin B12, pantothenic acid, biotin, and choline. Washington DC.

Glunde, K., & Serkova, N. J. (2006). Therapeutic targets and biomarkers identified in cancer choline phospholipid metabolism. *Pharmacogenomics, 7*(7), 1109–1123.

Haubrich, D. R., Wang, P. F., Clody, D. E., & Wedeking, P. W. (1975a). Increase in rat brain acetylcholine induced by choline or deanol. *Life Sciences, 17*(6), 975–980.

Haubrich, D. R., Wang, P. F., & Wedeking, P. W. (1975b). Distribution and metabolism of intravenously administered choline[methyl-^{3}H] and synthesis in vivo of acetylcholine in various tissues of guinea pigs. *Journal of Pharmacology and Experimental Therapeutics, 193*(1), 246–255.

Homocysteine Studies Collaboration (2002). Homocysteine and risk of ischemic heart disease and stroke: A meta-analysis. *JAMA, 288* (16), 2015–2022.

Ishidate, K. (1989). Choline transport and choline kinase. *Phosphatidylcholine Metabolism*9–32.

Jacobs, R. L., Devlin, C., Tabas, I., & Vance, D. E. (2004). Targeted deletion of hepatic CTP:phosphocholine cytidylyltransferase alpha in mice decreases plasma high density and very low density lipoproteins. *Journal of Biological Chemistry, 279*(45), 47402–47410.

Jacobs, R. L., Zhao, Y., Koonen, D. P., Sletten, T., Su, B., Lingrell, S., et al. (2010). Impaired de novo choline synthesis explains why phosphatidylethanolamine N-methyltransferase-deficient mice are protected from diet-induced obesity. *Journal of Biological Chemistry, 285*(29), 22403–22413.

Kantarci, K., Petersen, R. C., Boeve, B. F., Knopman, D. S., Tang-Wai, D. F., O'Brien, P. C., et al. (2004). ^{1}H MR spectroscopy in common dementias. *Neurology, 63*(8), 1393–1398.

Kelly, K., & Jacobs, R. (2011). Phospholipid biosynthesis. *AOCS Lipid Library.* <http://lipidlibrary.aocs.org/animbio/phospholipids/index.htm>.

Kennedy, E. P., & Weiss, S. B. (1956). The function of cytidine coenzymes in the biosynthesis of phospholipides. *Journal of Biological Chemistry, 222*(1), 193–214.

Klein, J. (2000). Membrane breakdown in acute and chronic neurodegeneration: focus on choline-containing phospholipids. *Journal of Neural Transmission, 107*(8-9), 1027–1063.

Klein, J., Gonzalez, R., Koppen, A., & Loffelholz, K. (1993). Free choline and choline metabolites in rat brain and body fluids: sensitive determination and implications for choline supply to the brain. *Neurochemistry International, 22*(3), 293–300.

Kristián, T., & Siesjö, B. K. (1998). Calcium in ischemic cell death. *Stroke, 29*(3), 705–718.

Kuge, O., & Nishijima, M. (1997). Phosphatidylserine synthase I and II of mammalian cells. *Biochimica et Biophysica Acta, 1348*(1-2), 151–156.

Kuge, O., Nishijima, M., & Akamatsu, Y. (1986). Phosphatidylserine biosynthesis in cultured Chinese hamster ovary cells. II. Isolation and characterization of phosphatidylserine auxotrophs. *Journal of Biological Chemistry, 261*(13), 5790–5794.

Lloyd-Jones, D., Adams, R., Carnethon, M., De Simone, G., Ferguson, T. B., Flegal, K., et al. (2009). Heart disease and stroke statistics–2009 update: a report from the American Heart Association Statistics Committee and Stroke Statistics Subcommittee. *Circulation, 119*(3), e21–181.

Loffelholz, K., Klein, J., & Koppen, A. (1993). Choline, a precursor of acetylcholine and phospholipids in the brain. *Progress in Brain Research, 98*, 197–200.

Meyerhoff, D. J., Bloomer, C., Schuff, N., Ezekiel, F., Norman, D., Clark, W., et al. (1999). Cortical metabolite alterations in abstinent cocaine and cocaine/alcohol-dependent subjects: proton magnetic resonance spectroscopic imaging. *Addiction Biology, 4*(4), 405–419.

Miller, B. L. (1991). A review of chemical issues in ^{1}H NMR spectroscopy: N-acetyl-L-aspartate, creatine and choline. *NMR in Biomedicine, 4*(2), 47–52.

Miller, B. L., Changl, L., Booth, R., Ernst, T., Cornford, M., Nikas, D., et al. (1996). In vivo ^{1}H MRS choline: correlation with in vitro chemistry/histology. *Life Sciences, 58*(22), 1929–1935.

Morash, S. C., Cook, H. W., & Spence, M. W. (1988). Phosphatidylcholine metabolism in cultured cells: catabolism via glycerophosphocholine. *Biochimica et Biophysica Acta, 961*(2), 194–202.

Murphy, D. G., Bottomley, P. A., Salerno, J. A., DeCarli, C., Mentis, M. J., Grady, C. L., et al. (1993). An in vivo study of phosphorus and glucose metabolism in Alzheimer's disease using magnetic resonance spectroscopy and PET. *Archives of General Psychiatry, 50* (5), 341–349.

Nachmansohn, D., & Machado, A. L. (1943). The formation of acetylcholine. A new enzyme: "Choline acetylase.". *Journal of Neurophysiology, 6*(5), 397–403.

Nitsch, R. M., Blusztajn, J. K., Pittas, A. G., Slack, B. E., Growdon, J. H., & Wurtman, R. J. (1992). Evidence for a membrane defect in Alzheimer disease brain. *Proceedings of the National Academy of Sciences USA, 89*(5), 1671–1675.

Nordahl, T. E., Salo, R., Natsuaki, Y., Galloway, G. P., Waters, C., Moore, C. D., et al. (2005). Methamphetamine users in sustained abstinence: a proton magnetic resonance spectroscopy study. *Archives of General Psychiatry, 62*(4), 444–452.

Nordahl, T. E., Salo, R., Possin, K., Gibson, D. R., Flynn, N., Leamon, M., et al. (2002). Low N-acetyl-aspartate and high choline in the anterior cingulum of recently abstinent methamphetamine-dependent subjects: a preliminary proton MRS study. Magnetic resonance spectroscopy. *Psychiatry Research Neuroimaging, 116* (1-2), 43–52.

Omori, M., Murata, T., Kimura, H., Koshimoto, Y., Kado, H., Ishimori, Y., et al. (2000). Thalamic abnormalities in patients with schizophrenia revealed by proton magnetic resonance spectroscopy. *Psychiatry Research Neuroimaging, 98*(3), 155–162.

Orlando, P., Arienti, G., Cerrito, F., Massari, P., & Porcellati, G. (1977). Quantitative evaluation of two pathways for phosphatidylcholine biosynthesis in rat brain in vivo. *Neurochemical Research, 2*(2), 191–201.

Poptani, H., Gupta, R. K., Roy, R., Pandey, R., Jain, V. K., & Chhabra, D. K. (1995). Characterization of intracranial mass lesions with in vivo proton MR spectroscopy. *American Journal of Neuroradiology, 16*(8), 1593–1603.

Porcellati, G., Arienti, G., Pirotta, M., & Giorgini, D. (1971). Base-exchange reactions for the synthesis of phospholipids in nervous tissue: The incorporation of serine and ethanolamine into the phospholipids of isolated brain microsomes. *Journal of Neurochemistry, 18*(8), 1395–1417.

Rinella, M. E., Elias, M. S., Smolak, R. R., Fu, T., Borensztajn, J., & Green, R. M. (2008). Mechanisms of hepatic steatosis in mice fed a lipogenic methionine choline-deficient diet. *Journal of Lipid Research, 49*(5), 1068–1076.

Ross, B., & Bluml, S. (2001). Magnetic resonance spectroscopy of the human brain. *Anatomical Record, 265*(2), 54–84.

Rothman, S. M., & Olney, J. W. (1995). Excitotoxicity and the NMDA receptor–still lethal after eight years. *Trends in Neurosciences, 18* (2), 57–58.

Salerno, D. M., & Beeler, D. A. (1973). The biosynthesis of phospholipids and their precursors in rat liver involving de novo methylation, and base-exchange pathways, in vivo. *Biochimica et Biophysica Acta, 326*(3), 325–338.

Seshadri, S., Beiser, A., Selhub, J., Jacques, P. F., Rosenberg, I. H., D'Agostino, R. B., et al. (2002). Plasma homocysteine as a risk factor for dementia and Alzheimer's disease. *New England Journal of Medicine, 346*(7), 476–483.

Siakotos, A. N., Rouser, G., & Fleischer, S. (1969). Phospholipid composition of human, bovine and frog myelin isolated on a large scale from brain and spinal cord. *Lipids, 4*(3), 239−242.

Stead, L. M., Brosnan, J. T., Brosnan, M. E., Vance, D. E., & Jacobs, R. L. (2006). Is it time to reevaluate methyl balance in humans? *American Journal of Clinical Nutrition, 83*(1), 5−10.

Tartaglia, M. C., Narayanan, S., De Stefano, N., Arnaoutelis, R., Antel, S. B., Francis, S. J., et al. (2002). Choline is increased in prelesional normal appearing white matter in multiple sclerosis. *Journal of Neurology, 249*(10), 1382−1390.

Tayebati, S. K., & Amenta, F. (2013). Choline-containing phospholipids: relevance to brain functional pathways. *Clinical Chemistry and Laboratory Medicine, 51*(3), 513−521.

Valenzuela, M. J., & Sachdev, P. (2001). Magnetic resonance spectroscopy in AD. *Neurology, 56*(5), 592−598.

van der Knaap, M. S., & Pouwels, P. J. W. (2005). *Magnetic resonance spectroscopy: basic principles and application in white matter disorders* (pp. 859-880). *Magnetic Resonance of Myelination and Myelin Disorders*. Berlin: Springer.

van Meurs, J. B., Dhonukshe-Rutten, R. A., Pluijm, S. M., van der Klift, M., de Jonge, R., Lindemans, J., et al. (2004). Homocysteine levels and the risk of osteoporotic fracture. *New England Journal of Medicine, 350*(20), 2033−2041.

Vance, D. E., & Ridgway, N. D. (1988). The methylation of phosphatidylethanolamine. *Progress in Lipid Research, 27*(1), 61−79.

Vance, J. E. (2008). Phosphatidylserine and phosphatidylethanolamine in mammalian cells: two metabolically related aminophospholipids. *Journal of Lipid Research, 49*(7), 1377−1387.

Vance, J. E., & Vance, D. E. (2008). Phospholipid biosynthesis in eukaryotes. In J. E. Vance, & D. E. Vance (Eds.), *Biochemistry of Lipids, Lipoproteins and Membranes* (Vol. 42, pp. 213−244). Amsterdam: Elsevier Science.

Verkade, H. J., Fast, D. G., Rusinol, A. E., Scraba, D. G., & Vance, D. E. (1993). Impaired biosynthesis of phosphatidylcholine causes a decrease in the number of very low density lipoprotein particles in the Golgi but not in the endoplasmic

reticulum of rat liver. *Journal of Biological Chemistry, 268*(33), 24990−24996.

Voelker, D. R., & Frazier, J. L. (1986). Isolation and characterization of a Chinese hamster ovary cell line requiring ethanolamine or phosphatidylserine for growth and exhibiting defective phosphatidylserine synthase activity. *Journal of Biological Chemistry, 261*(3), 1002−1008.

Wajda, I. J., Manigault, I., Hudick, J. P., & Lajtha, A. (1973). Regional and subcellular distribution of choline acetyltransferase in the brain of rats. *Journal of Neurochemistry, 21*(6), 1385−1401.

Weltzien, H. U. (1979). Cytolytic and membrane-perturbing properties of lysophosphatidylcholine. *Biochimica et Biophysica Acta, 559* (2-3), 259−287.

Wilton, D. C. (2008). Phospholipases. In E. V. Dennis, & E. V. Jean (Eds.), Biochemistry of lipids, lipoproteins and membranes (5th ed., pp. 305−330). San Diego, CA: Elsevier.

Wu, L. L., & Wu, J. T. (2002). Hyperhomocysteinemia is a risk factor for cancer and a new potential tumor marker. *Clinica Chimica Acta, 322*(1-2), 21−28.

Wurtman, R. J., Blusztajn, J. K., & Maire, J. C. (1985). "Autocannibalism" of choline-containing membrane phospholipids in the pathogenesis of Alzheimer's disease-A hypothesis. *Neurochemistry International, 7*(2), 369−372.

Yao, Z. M., & Vance, D. E. (1988). The active synthesis of phosphatidylcholine is required for very low density lipoprotein secretion from rat hepatocytes. *Journal of Biological Chemistry, 263*(6), 2998−3004.

Zeisel, S. H. (1999). Choline and phosphatidylcholine. In M. E. Shils (Ed.), *Modern Nutrition in Health and Disease* (pp. 513−523). Baltimore, MD: Lippincott Williams & Wilkins.

Zhao, Y., Su, B., Jacobs, R. L., Kennedy, B., Francis, G. A., Waddington, E., et al. (2009). Lack of phosphatidylethanolamine N-methyltransferase alters plasma VLDL phospholipids and attenuates atherosclerosis in mice. *Arteriosclerosis, Thrombosis, and Vascular Biology, 29*(9), 1349−1355.

Glutamate

Jun Shen

Molecular Imaging Branch, National Institute of Mental Health, Bethesda, Maryland, USA

INTRODUCTION

Glutamate, or glutamic acid, is a dicarboxylic acid with multiple biological roles. The amino acid glutamate carries a net negative charge. It is one of the five common amino acids (glutamate aspartate, D-serine, γ-aminobutyric acid (GABA), and glycine) that serve a neurotransmitter function. It is the primary excitatory neurotransmitter in the central nervous system (CNS) and can be found in all brain cell types, though its concentration is highest in neurons. In addition to its neurotransmitter role, glutamate also serves as a source of energy and ammonia, linking the metabolism of carbon and nitrogen (Erecinska & Silver, 1990).

Glutamate can be biosynthesized by rapid transamination with α-ketoglutarate via aspartate aminotransferase and, to a much lesser extent, from α-ketoglutarate and ammonium via glutamate dehydrogenase, a pyridine nucleotide-linked enzyme. Nerve terminals and their derived synaptosomes contain mitochondria that can generate glutamate from several substrates including pyruvate and glucose. The glutamate carbon skeleton is rapidly formed from glucose as is evident from numerous studies of the overall metabolism of isotope (^{13}C- or ^{14}C)-labeled glucose (Cerdan & Seelig, 1990; Cruz & Cerdan, 1999; Morris & Bachelard, 2003). In addition, glutamate is continuously formed by several other transamination reactions that use α-ketoglutarate as the receptor of the amino group, and during protein turnover. Rapid exchange between glutamate and α-ketoglutarate occurs in the ubiquitous malate-aspartate shuttle, which transfers reducing equivalents (NADH) from cytosol into mitochondria for oxidation (McKenna et al., 2006). In addition, glutamate is formed from glutamine by hydrolysis via a mitochondrial enzyme, glutaminase. Glutamate is an important component in the biosynthesis of many abundant molecules in brain such as N-acetylaspartylglutamate, glutathione, and proteins.

Glutamate is involved in glutamatergic neurotransmission through the glutamate–glutamine cycle between neurons and surrounding astrocytes (Hertz, 2004). The ^{1}H nuclear magnetic resonance (NMR) spectrum of glutamate is entirely composed of J-coupled resonances (de Graaf, 1998). At very high magnetic field strength, which is currently available for animal studies only, glutamate and glutamine can be spectrally resolved (see Fig. 2.4.1). Glutamate and glutamine, collectively, are often referred to as Glx because, at magnetic field strengths available in most clinical studies, MR signals of glutamate and glutamine overlap with each other at all of their resonant positions. Moreover, due to strong J-coupling effects, their ^{1}H spectra appear different at different echo times and different magnetic field strengths. These factors make their observation and quantification more difficult with ^{1}H MR spectroscopy (MRS) techniques than many other resonance signals such as those of N-acetylaspartate, creatine, and choline-containing compounds. The metabolic fluxes involving glutamate and glutamine are best studied using ^{13}C MRS by which their resonance signals can be unambiguously separated, even at relatively low magnetic field strengths.

ROLES OF GLUTAMATE IN BRAIN

Glutamate as a Neurotransmitter

Glutamate is the principal excitatory neurotransmitter in brain. At very low concentrations it excites essentially every neuron in the CNS. Glutamatergic pathways are involved in diverse processes and brain disorders such as depression, epilepsy, schizophrenia, ischemic brain damage, and learning. Most neurons that use glutamate as a neurotransmitter are projection neurons (e.g., the pyramidal neurons in the cerebral

111

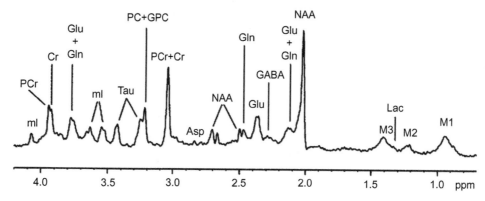

FIGURE 2.4.1 *In vivo* [1]H short-echo spectrum acquired from rat brain at 11.7 T (Yang & Shen, 2006). Asp, aspartate; Cr, creatine; GABA, γ-aminobutyric acid; Gln, glutamine; Glu, glutamate; GPC, glycerophosphocholine; Lac, lactate; M1, macromolecule at 0.92 ppm; M2, macromolecule at 1.21 ppm; M3, macromolecule at 1.39 ppm; mI, myo-inositol; NAA, *N*-acetylaspartate; PC, phosphocholine; PCr, phosphocreatine; Tau, taurine. Glutamate H4 and glutamine H4 are spectrally resolved.

cortex projecting to various subcortical regions and/or other cortical regions; ganglion neurons projecting from retina to the lateral geniculate) and somatic primary afferent sensory neurons. Glutamate and various glutamatergic pathways play important roles in the development of normal synaptic connections and memory in the brain (Shepherd, 1994).

Glutamate exerts powerful excitatory actions on a wide range of neurons in different brain regions. Neurotransmitter glutamate is stored in synaptic vesicles, which actively accumulate glutamate through an Mg^{2+}/ATP-dependent process. The concentration of glutamate within synaptic vesicles is believed to be very high, in excess of 20 mM (Erecinska & Silver, 1990). A large amount of experimental evidence demonstrates Ca^{2+}-dependent release of glutamate both *in vivo* and from isolated neural preparations. Glutamate-operated synapses and glutamate receptors are very widely distributed in the brain. Early experiments showed that sensitivity to iontophoresed glutamate is widespread in the brain because of the ubiquitous distribution of its receptors (Shepherd, 1994). For example, glutamate-operated synapses and glutamate receptors occur on neurons receiving inputs from many other neurotransmitter systems. Glutamate receptors are named after their most prominent neurotransmitter agonist. There are three classes of ionotropic glutamate receptors named after their selective agonists: *N*-methyl-D-aspartate (NMDA), α-amino-3-hydroxy-5-methyl-4-isoxazole propionic acid (AMPA), and kainite (KA). Metabotropic glutamate receptors (mGluRs) are linked by G-proteins to cytoplasmic enzymes. So far, the metabotropic receptors gene family has been shown to contain eight members, mGluR1–mGluR8. Both NMDA and AMPA receptors are present on most CNS neurons. Their activation underlies the vast majority of fast synaptic transmission. Ca^{2+} influx through NMDA and AMPA receptors also mediates synaptic plasticity.

Glutamate can become an excitoxin, especially when energy metabolism is impaired. Neurodegeneration results from excessive stimulation by glutamate. The mechanisms for this degeneration process are quite diverse and activation of all classes of ionotropic glutamate receptors has been implicated. For example, during ischemia, extracellular concentration of glutamate is markedly elevated (Rothman & Olney, 1986). In addition, depolarization-induced entry of Ca^{2+} stimulates the release of the vesicular glutamate neurotransmitter pool. At the same time, uptake of glutamate via Na^+-dependent glutamate transporters is impaired mainly due to cellular ion gradient discharge. Neuronal insult occurs due to AMPA receptor activation with concomitant NMDA receptor involvement and Ca^{2+} influx. The role of glutamate in epilepsy is also well documented in the literature (Coulter & Eid, 2012). Excessive stimulation of glutamatergic pathways and inhibition of glutamate transporters lead to glutamate receptor activation that can cause seizures. Numerous studies using animal models have shown that NMDA receptor antagonists can reduce the duration and intensity of seizures. Chronic glutamate receptor activation may also be involved in some neurodegenerative disorders such as amyotrophic lateral sclerosis and Huntington's chorea. Metabolic inhibition that leads to impaired energy production has been shown to predispose neurons to glutamate-mediated neurotoxicity (Greene & Greenamyre, 1996).

The Glutamate–Glutamine Cycle

Although glutamate is rapidly synthesized from glucose in neural tissues, the biochemical process for replenishing the neurotransmitter glutamate after glutamate release involves the glutamate–glutamine cycle (Erecinska & Silver, 1990). As a zwitterionic molecule glutamate cannot diffuse across cell membranes. It is now well understood that glutamate uptake plays important roles in regulating the extracellular concentration of glutamate in the brain. A major role for glutamate transporters is to limit the free concentration of glutamate in the extracellular space, preventing excessive stimulation of glutamate receptors (Rothstein et al., 1996). Excessive activation of glutamate receptors by glutamate can result in a number of pathological conditions and can lead to cell death. As with the catecholamines and serotonin, inactivation of released glutamate is primarily by reuptake via high-affinity, Na^+-dependent transport systems against its concentration gradient. Inactivation of glutamate is achieved once glutamate crosses the cell membrane. Both high-affinity ($K_m = 5-20\ \mu M$) and low-affinity ($K_m = 1-2\ mM$) transport systems exist (Gether et al., 2006). To date, many members of the Na^+-dependent glutamate transporter family have been cloned including glutamate transporter-1 (GLT-1) and the glutamate-aspartate transporter (GLAST). In the CNS, GLT-1 and GLAST are expressed primarily in glial cells and represent the primary transport carriers for glutamate uptake into astrocytes. Unlike other amine transporters the Na^+-dependent glutamate transporter family is not Cl^- dependent. The net transport of glutamate is increased by high intracellular K^+. With each transport cycle, two Na^+ ions accompany the movement of glutamate into the astrocytic intracellular compartment with one K^+ transported out, accompanied by either a bicarbonate ion or hydroxide ion.

Glutamate taken up by astroglial cells is either converted into glutamine by glutamine synthetase, which is exclusively located in glial cells (Hertz, 1979; Erecinska & Silver, 1990), or oxidized by assimilation into the Krebs cycle located in the mitochondria of glial cells. Once formed, the glutamine is readily discharged from astroglial cells by facilitated diffusion via Na^+ and H^+-coupled, electroneutral systems – N transporters. Glutamine readily enters nerve terminals by its low-affinity transport system or by diffusion. There, glutaminase converts it back into glutamate, which can be again used for neurotransmission or assimilated into the neuronal Krebs cycle. The existence of this glutamate–glutamine cycle was initially proposed based on the findings that isolated nerve terminals contain the majority of tissue content of glutaminase but no glutamine synthetase; the latter is found to be exclusively located in glial cells (Hertz, 1979). Numerous autoradiographic and biochemical studies clearly demonstrate that glutamate was selectively accumulated by glial cells and rapidly converted into glutamine. In contrast, glutamine preferentially entered neurons where it was converted in large proportions into glutamate (Duce & Keen, 1983). Although the glutamate–glutamine cycle was conceptualized many decades ago, it was not considered to be a significant metabolic flux. Only recently, because of the rapid advances of in vivo ^{13}C and ^{15}N MRS techniques, the glutamate–glutamine cycling flux was quantified in vivo in anesthetized rat brain (Sibson et al., 1997, 2001; Shen et al., 1998) and in human brain (Gruetter et al., 1998; Shen et al., 1999; Lebon et al., 2002). For an illustration of the glutamate–glutamine cycle and its relationship with astroglial and neuronal tricarboxylic acid (TCA) cycles, see Fig. 2.4.2. Using ^{13}C MRS techniques labeling kinetics of glutamate and glutamine can be measured during intravenous infusion of ^{13}C-labeled glucose. By quantitative analysis of the time courses of the ^{13}C MRS signals of glutamate and glutamine, the glutamate–glutamine cycling flux can be measured. Fig. 2.4.3 shows a typical glutamate C4 and glutamine C4 time course acquired during systemic infusion of [1-^{13}C]-glucose. The accumulated ^{13}C spectrum of the human brain is shown in Fig. 2.4.4. These and other in vivo MRS studies have established that the glutamate–glutamine cycle between glutamatergic neurons and glia is a major metabolic flux, reflecting synaptic glutamate release (Shen & Rothman, 2002). The glutamate–glutamine cycling flux is directly coupled to neuroenergetics (Sibson et al., 1998).

Glutamate as a Metabolite

Glutamate is an important metabolite linking the metabolism of carbon and nitrogen. The major reactions participated by glutamate in brain are detailed in the following list:

Aspartate aminotransferase reaction:
   glutamate + oxaloacetate ↔ α-ketoglutarate + aspartate
Glutamate dehydrogenase reaction:
   α-ketoglutarate + NH_3 + NADH + H^+ ↔ glutamate + NAD^+
Glutamic acid decarboxylase reaction:
   glutamate → GABA + CO_2
Glutaminase reaction:
   glutamine + H_2O → glutamate + NH_4^+
GABA transaminase reaction:
   GABA + α-ketoglutarate ↔ glutamate + succinic semialdehyde
Glutamine synthetase reaction:
   glutamate + NH_3 + ATP ↔ glutamine + ADP + P_i
γ-Glutamylcysteine synthetase reaction:
   glutamate + L-cysteine + ATP → γ-glutamylcysteine + ADP + P_i

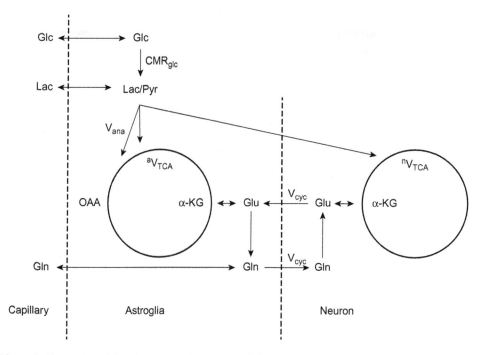

FIGURE 2.4.2   Schematic illustration of the glutamate–glutamine cycle between neurons and astroglia and glucose metabolism (adapted from Shen et al., 1999). Glutamate released from glutamatergic neurons is taken up from the synaptic cleft by surrounding astroglia. In astroglia, glutamate is converted into glutamine by glutamine synthetase. Glutamine is subsequently released by the astroglia, transported into the neurons, and converted back into glutamate by phosphate-activated glutaminase, which completes the glutamate–glutamine cycle. Glc, glucose; Pyr/Lac, pyruvate/lactate; OAA, oxaloacetate; α-KG, α-ketoglutarate; Glu, glutamate; Gln, glutamine; CMR_{glc}, cerebral metabolic rate of glucose utilization; V_{ana}, anaplerotic flux for *de novo* synthesis of oxaloacetate; $^aV_{TCA}$, astroglial TCA flux; V_{cyc}, glutamate–glutamine cycling flux; $^nV_{TCA}$, neuronal TCA cycle flux.

N-acetylated-α-linked-amino dipeptidase reaction:
  N-acetylaspartatylglutamate ↔
  N-acetylaspartate + glutamate
Alanine aminotransferase reaction:
  glutamate + pyruvate ↔ alanine + α-ketoglutarate
Ornithine aminotransferase reaction:
  ornithine + α-ketoglutarate ↔ glutamate
  + glutamic acid semialdehyde
Branched-chain amino acid aminotransferase reaction (an example):
  α-ketoisocaproate + glutamate ↔ leucine +
  α-ketoglutarate

A prominent difference between amino acid neurotransmitters and other neurotransmitters is their high concentration in neutral tissues. Unlike other neurotransmitters, amino acid neurotransmitters are ubiquitous and participate in numerous biochemical processes such as intermediary metabolism and protein turnover. Glutamate has been known to be one of the most abundant intracellular amino acids in mammals. The pool size of free glutamate in most brain regions is quite high (5–10 mM) (Erecinska & Silver, 1990). This is in contrast to other organs such as kidney and liver. Despite numerous efforts to understand the metabolism and neurotransmission of glutamate,

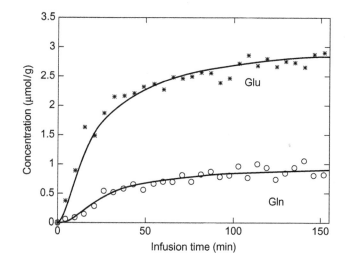

FIGURE 2.4.3   A time course of the concentrations of [4-^{13}C]-glutamate and [4-^{13}C]-glutamine for a human subject (Shen et al., 1999, with permission). The solid line represents the fit to the two-compartment model shown in Fig. 2.4.1. Asterisks, glutamate; open circles, glutamine.

the reason for maintaining a large glutamate pool in brain is still poorly understood.

It is possible that the high concentration of glutamate is a result of high metabolic demand in brain

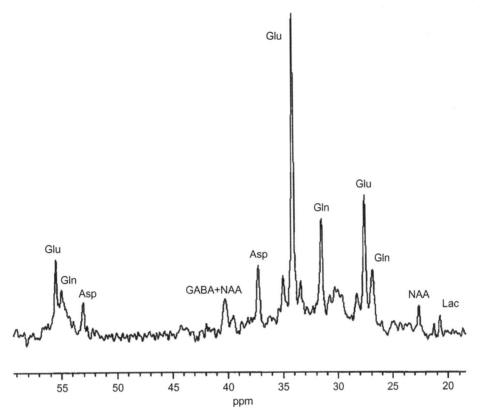

FIGURE 2.4.4 *In vivo* ^{13}C spectrum from the occipital/parietal lobes of a human subject using ^{1}H-localized adiabatic polarization transfer technique (Shen et al., 1999, with permission). The spectrum was an accumulation of 67.5 min of acquisition 60 min after the start of [1-^{13}]C-glucose infusion. Labeled resonances are [4-^{13}C]-glutamate (Glu4) and [4-^{13}C]-glutamine (Gln4), [3-^{13}C]-glutamate (Glu3), and [3-^{13}C]-gluta-mine (Gln3), respectively. Other resonances present in the spectrum include [3-^{13}C]-lactate at 21 ppm, the sum of the resonance of [2-^{13}C]-GABA, and the downfield resonance of the ^{13}C-^{13}C satellite of [4-^{13}C]-glutamate at 35 ppm, the sum of the resonance of [4-^{13}C]-GABA and *N*-acetyl aspartate at 41 ppm, and the resonance of [3-^{13}C]-aspartate at 37 ppm. Abbreviation definitions as in Figs. 2.4.1 and 2.4.2.

since glutamate, in addition to its neurotransmitter role, serves as a key component of intermediary metabolism, a precursor of many cellular components and a source of many other metabolites and neuro-transmitters such as GABA and *N*-acetylaspartylglu-tamate. The concentration of α-ketoglutarate is also relatively high, which could be due to the high K_m for its oxidation in the TCA cycle, leading to a large accu-mulation of α-ketoglutarate and subsequently enhanced transamination by aspartate aminotransfer-ase or enhanced animation by glutamate dehydroge-nase (Price & Stevens, 1999). Although the equilibrium of the glutamate dehydrogenase reaction is in favor of glutamate formation, rapid transamina-tion by aspartate aminotransferase predominates in the formation of glutamate in the CNS. Recent ^{13}C MRS experiments (Shen, 2005) have shown that there is a very rapid exchange between α-ketoglutarate and glutamate, which causes a sizable magnetization transfer effect on glutamate C-2 carbon at 55.7 parts per million (ppm) when the C-2 resonance of α-keto-glutarate at 206.0 ppm is saturated using radio

frequency pulses. The *in vivo* unidirectional glutamate→α-ketoglutarate flux, predominantly catalyzed by aspartate aminotransferase, has been determined to be 78 ± 9 μmol/g/min in anesthetized rat brain.

The rapid exchange between glutamate and the TCA cycle intermediate α-ketoglutarate intimately links glutamate with oxidative metabolism in both neuronal and glial cells. One of the most fruitful MRS techniques is *in vivo* ^{13}C MRS measurement of the rate of oxidative metabolism after administering ^{13}C-labeled substrates such as [1-^{13}C]-glucose or [1,6-^{13}C$_2$]-glucose (de Graaf et al., 2011). Because of the large brain glutamate pool predominantly located in gluta-matergic neurons, glutamate acts as an effective trap-ping pool for ^{13}C labels of the neuronal TCA cycle through exchange with mitochondrial α-ketoglutarate. The kinetics of the ^{13}C-label incorporation into neuro-nal glutamate contains the quantitative information of the TCA cycle flux. Therefore, *in vivo* ^{13}C MRS techni-ques allow noninvasive assessment of oxidative metabolism.

Glutamate is a precursor of the dipeptide neurotransmitter N-acetylaspartylglutamate, which plays a key role in glutamatergic signaling (Blakely & Coyle, 1988), most notably by antagonizing the effects of glutamate at NMDA receptors and regulating GABA receptor expression. N-acetylated-α-linked-amino dipeptidase catalyzes the formation and cleavage of N-acetylaspartylglutamate (Robinson et al., 1987; Luthi-Carter et al., 1998). In the proton MRS spectrum of brain the acetyl methyl proton peak of N-acetylaspartylglutamate partially overlaps with that of N-acetylaspartate. The N-acetylated-α-linked-amino dipeptidase reaction is much more rapid than the synthesis of N-acetylaspartate *per se* (Tyson & Sutherland, 1998; Xu et al., 2008). For more details, see Chapter 2.1.

α-Decarboxylation of glutamate via the action of glutamic acid decarboxylase converts glutamate into GABA. Glutamic acid decarboxylase is known to regulate the steady-state concentration of GABA. Glutamic acid decarboxylase is primarily, although not exclusively, localized to GABAergic neurons. As a result, the conversion of glutamate into GABA in the CNS occurs primarily in GABAergic neurons. In particular, axon terminals of GABAergic neurons possess a marked capacity for synthesizing GABA, which is then likely to be available for release into the synapse. The regulation of glutamic acid decarboxylase activity is linked to the interconversion between the cofactor-bound and free forms of the glutamic acid decarboxylase enzyme (for more details see Chapter 2.5).

Glutamate is also a precursor of the tripeptide antioxidant γ-glutamylcysteinylglycine (glutathione) which has a significant presence in brain tissue in millimolar concentrations. The production of glutathione is catalyzed first by the rate-limiting γ-glutamylcysteine synthetase and then by glutathione synthetase.

REGULATION OF GLUTAMATE CONCENTRATION

The "static" glutamate concentration measured by proton MRS (as opposed to its dynamic flux measurable using ^{13}C MRS) is a result of interplay between glutamate anabolism and its catabolism. The various enzymes involved in glutamate synthesis, degradation, and exchange with α-ketoglutarate control the overall concentration of glutamate. The activities of these enzymes are constantly adjusted by modulation of the concentration of various molecules including, when applicable, allosteric effectors. Coordination among different compartments, especially the neuronal and glial compartments via the glutamate–glutamine cycle, also regulates glutamate (and glutamine) concentrations (Stelmashook et al., 2011). Important metabolic

couplings exist between various cells and compartments through the use of common substrates and the exchange of several metabolic intermediates such as glutamate, glutamine, and GABA (Erecinska & Silver, 1990; Rothman et al., 2011). Because glutamate also acts as the major excitatory neurotransmitter in the CNS, the neurotransmission of glutamate is intimately related to its metabolism.

Glutamate is a nonessential amino acid. It does not cross the blood−brain barrier. Therefore it is synthesized from glucose and a variety of other precursors. Synthetic and metabolic enzymes for glutamate are localized to two main compartments of the brain: neurons and glial cells (Erecinska & Silver, 1990). There is no evidence of extracellular metabolism of glutamate in the CNS. Two precursors that exist in large quantities in the brain that give rise to glutamate are D-glucose and L-glutamine. When glucose is scarce, such as in hypoglycemia, glutamate can act as an important energy fuel due to its large pool size. Therefore, it is not surprising that glutamate level is reduced in hypoglycemia and many other pathophysiological conditions where normal oxidative metabolism is impaired. Glutamine is hydrolyzed by glutaminase into glutamate. Glutaminase is inhibited by glutamate and activated by phosphate and several other anions. Control of glutaminase activity appears to be mainly by product inhibition, with glutamate significantly attenuating its activity over the range of its concentrations found in the nerve terminal (Bradford et al., 1978). It was also observed in isolated synaptosomes and other preparations that inhibition of glutaminase is reduced after glutamate efflux from nerve terminals during neuronal activities to facilitate the synthesis of replacement neurotransmitter glutamate from glutaminase. Ammonium is a moderate inhibitor of glutaminase and also plays a role in regulating glutaminase activity. Furthermore, elevated ammonia level in the brain leads to excessive glutamine synthesis via glutamine synthetase for ammonia detoxification. The elevation of glutamine level in brain in hyperammonemia and hepatic encephalopathy is, in part, at the expense of reduced glutamate concentration (de Graaf et al., 1991).

Metabolic imbalance and changes in redox states in brain can lead to a shift in the rapid aspartate aminotransferase reaction, leading to altered glutamate concentration. Other possible routes of regulation of glutamate involve arginine, ornithine, and proline metabolism via arginase, ornithine aminotransferase, and proline oxidase reactions. The rates of glutamate synthesis in brain from these sources are very slow. As a result, their contribution to the overall glutamate concentration in brain is small (Shank & Campbell, 1983). Pharmaceutical agents that have profound influences on the CNS undoubtedly alter concentration of glutamate, among many other metabolites and neurotransmitters. For example, glutamate level in brain is elevated by amphetamines (Berntman et al., 1977). Deep anesthesia by phenobarbital has also been shown to reduce cerebral cortex glutamate concentration (Chapman et al., 1978).

INTERPRETATION OF CHANGES IN GLUTAMATE CONCENTRATION

Glutamate, like glutamine, aspartate, and GABA, exists in high concentration in brain tissue and represents a potentially important fuel source. Due to the multiple roles of glutamate and the many metabolic pathways it is involved with, interpretation of changes in glutamate concentration can be a difficult task in many complex situations. Since glutamate is also the primary excitatory neurotransmitter in the CNS, alteration in the overall glutamate level may affect the subtle balance between excitation and inhibition. In particular, caution is needed when attributing the chronic effects of brain disorders on the total concentrations of glutamate to changes in the glutamate—glutamine cycling flux. This is because many other factors could also contribute to or explain the observed alterations in the total concentrations of glutamate. For example, changes in aspartate aminotransferase and/or glutamate dehydrogenase activities could lead to altered total concentration of glutamate. In particular, most clinical MRS studies of neurological and psychiatric disorders only measured Glx, the unresolved glutamate and glutamine resonances. Due to the obvious connection between glutamate and glutamine via the glutamate—glutamine cycle and the related enzyme reactions, glutamate and glutamine levels can change in opposite directions (e.g., in hyperammonemia; de Graaf et al., 1991), resulting in a reduced sensitivity of Glx as a disease marker. Recently technological advances (Hurd et al., 2004) and the advent of high magnetic field MRI scanners (e.g., 7 T) have allowed spectral separation of glutamate from Glx. A more comprehensive characterization of the glutamatergic function can also be performed using ^{13}C MRS methods to measure the glutamate—glutamine cycling rate.

A recurring scenario in many pathophysiological situations where a decreased overall glucose consumption occurs (e.g., hypercapnia, barbiturate anesthesia, and hypoglycemia) is a reduced glutamate concentration. As summarized by Siesjö (1978) this can be attributed to a decreased delivery of glucose and subsequently an increase in oxidation of endogenous substrates including glutamate. Many studies have reported reduced glutamate level during hypercapnia (e.g., Shimizu et al., 1998). Barbiturate anesthesia (Betz & Gilboe, 1973; Chapman et al., 1978) was found to lower the concentration of most TCA cycle intermediates accompanied by a reduced glutamate concentration and an increased aspartate concentration. The combination of a decrease in glutamate and an increase in aspartate concentrations suggests that changes in amino acids are mainly due to a shift in the rapid aspartate aminotransferase reaction during barbiturate anesthesia. The aspartate aminotransferase reaction is driven toward the direction of aspartate formation. The overall effect is that more carbons are available for oxidation by the TCA cycle (α-ketoglutarate is reconverted into oxaloacetate by the TCA cycle), therefore, compensating for the reduced delivery of carbon skeletons from exogenous glucose caused by the administration of phenobarbital.

To further complicate the explanation of the changes in total glutamate concentration, because of the intricate connections between the many metabolic pathways involving glutamate, aspartate, and other amino acids as well as their high concentration (compared with oxaloacetate, α-ketoglutarate, and other TCA cycle intermediates), a shift of the aspartate aminotransferase to the direction of aspartate formation does not necessarily lead to a decrease in glutamate concentration and an increase in aspartate concentration. For example, upon global or focal ischemia (e.g., due to stroke) there is a rapid reduction in α-ketoglutarate and oxaloacetate concentrations resulting from a complete blockade of oxidative reactions (accompanied by an elevation in lactic acid concentration, a concomitant decrease in pH, and a marked reduction in energy storage molecules such as MRS-observable phosphocreatine and ATP (Weber et al., 2006). The decrease in α-ketoglutarate concentration is thought to be caused by a shift in the glutamate dehydrogenase reaction toward the formation of glutamate as expected from the increase in tissue concentrations of NH_3, NADH, and H^+. Due to the ubiquitous existence of the rapid aspartate aminotransferase reaction a decrease in α-ketoglutarate concentration is expected to cause a reduction in oxaloacetate concentration, leading to decreased glutamate concentration and increased aspartate concentration. But since these two amino acids occur at such high concentrations (compared with oxaloacetate and α-ketoglutarate) and because of the presence of other active pathways, no change in glutamate and aspartate concentrations were observed experimentally (Young & Lowry; 1966). Despite the insignificant change in total glutamate concentration (measured by proton MRS) there is rapid accumulation of glutamate in synapse and excessive glutamate release during ischemia, causing excessive activation of NMDA and AMPA receptors. As a consequence and due to the prevalence of NMDA and AMPA receptors, the intracellular accumulation of Ca^{2+} is greatly exacerbated. This pathological accumulation of Ca^{2+} leads to a cascade of events that can ultimately result in cell death (Kostandy, 2012).

It is known that brain tissue concentrations of lactate and pyruvate vary inversely with P_{CO2} of the arterial blood (Bain & Klein, 1949). Hypercapnia is associated with decreases in glutamate, α-ketoglutarate, and aspartate concentrations (Kazemi et al., 1973, 1976; van Leuven et al., 1974). It would be expected, at a first glance, that increases in tissue concentration of CO_2 should increase the rate of CO_2 fixation, therefore increasing the pool sizes of amino acids by anaplerotic activities. However, the concentrations of glutamate, aspartate, pyruvate, lactate, and all measurable TCA cycle intermediates have been found experimentally to decrease during hypercapnia. Due to hypercapnia, brain tissues become partially depleted of carbohydrate substrates. Consequently, endogenous fuel sources have to be mobilized to maintain energy production. Glutamate is made available for oxidation primarily by two mechanisms. First, an initial shift in the aspartate aminotransferase reaction toward aspartate formation produces carbon for oxidation by the TCA cycle. Second, oxidative deamination of glutamate by glutamate dehydrogenase consumes glutamate. Conversely, a decrease in blood P_{CO2} is associated with a progressive increase in α-ketoglutarate and glutamate concentration and a reduction in aspartate concentration (MacMillan & Siesjö, 1973). The metabolic changes associated with hypocapnia that affect carbohydrate metabolism are, to a large extent, opposite to those occurring in hypercapnia. The shift in the aspartate aminotransferase reaction during hypocapnia can be explained by a decrease in oxaloacetate concentration resulting from an increase in the $NADH/NAD^+$ ratio (Siesjö, 1978).

Tissue slices are known to respire with glutamate as substrate. During *in vivo* hypoglycemia consumption of glutamate (and other amino acids such as glutamine and GABA) occurs. The decrease in glutamate concentration during hypoglycemia is associated with an increase in aspartate concentration (Engelsen & Fonnum, 1983; Wong & Tyce, 1983). For example, in the brains of chronic hypoglycemic rats the concentrations of glutamate (as well as alanine and GABA) decreases and the concentration of aspartate is elevated. The concentration of pyridoxal-5'-phosphate, an enzyme cofactor in many reactions that generate several amino acids from TCA cycle intermediates, is also reduced. The above example provides evidence that glutamate, glutamine, aspartate, and GABA may serve as energy sources in brain during hypoglycemia. During acute hypoglycemia the brain can lose up to 10 μmol/g of glutamate and elevate aspartate concentration by up to 10 μmol/g (Lewis et al., 1974). Again, the concerted change in glutamate and aspartate during hypoglycemia can be explained by a massive shift in the aspartate aminotransferase reaction toward the direction of aspartate formation (Siesjo, 1978; Erecinska & Silver, 1990). This large shift in the aspartate aminotransferase reaction leads to increased production of α-ketoglutarate at the expense of oxaloacetate, bearing in mind that oxidative energy is released when α-ketoglutarate is reconverted to oxaloacetate in the TCA cycle. A simultaneous decrease in glutamine, GABA, and alanine during acute hypoglycemia suggests that the glutaminase, GABA transaminase, and alanine transaminase reactions all shift to the formation of glutamate to contribute additional glutamate for further conversion into α-ketoglutarate. The alanine transaminase reaction makes carbon skeletons available for oxidation in the TCA cycle via the pyruvate dehydrogenase reaction. In addition to the transaminase reactions and glutamine hydrolysis, oxidative deamination by glutamate dehydrogenase may also contribute to the reduction of tissue glutamate concentration during hypoglycemia, accompanied by an increase in ammonia level. This scenario agrees with the known shift of the redox state toward oxidation during hypoglycemia, which would shift the reversible glutamate dehydrogenase reaction to the formation of α-ketoglutarate (therefore reducing glutamate concentration).

In animal models of hibernation, the concentrations of glutamate and aspartate were decreased accompanied by an increase in GABA concentration and by an increase or decrease in glutamine concentration (Godin et al., 1967; Henry et al., 2007). The change in the overall amino acid profile is difficult to explain although it is quite likely that amino acids, including glutamate, are used as energy substrates during hibernation. It is also possible that anaplerosis activities are impaired during hibernation. Studies of the influence of hypothermia in anesthetized and artificially ventilated rats showed a decrease in cerebral cortex glutamate concentration and an increase in aspartate concentration (Hägerdal et al., 1975). Due to the release of ammonia from non-amino acid sources during hypothermia ammonia detoxification by animation of α-ketoglutarate would contribute to the depletion of α-ketoglutarate (there is no significant change in the brain glutamine level in the Hägerdal study; Hägerdal et al., 1975). The fall in α-ketoglutarate concentration could then cause a decrease in glutamate concentration and an increase in aspartate concentration by shifting the aspartate aminotransferase reaction toward the direction of aspartate formation. A simultaneous shift in the alanine aminotransferase could have also occurred as evidenced by the simultaneous increase in alanine concentration. This shift in alanine aminotransferase reaction also contributes to the decrease in glutamate concentration and provides additional α-ketoglutarate molecules for ammonia detoxification (Siesjö, 1978).

Changes in amino acids, glutamate in particular, may cause cell dysfunction during severe hypoxic stress because of its role as a powerful excitatory neurotransmitter. During hypoxic hypoxia increases in glutamate and GABA as well as a decrease in aspartate are observed (Siesjö et al., 1976). This change in glutamate concentration can be explained by a mismatch between the rate of glycolysis and the rate of oxidative metabolism, leading to accumulation of pyruvate and a reduction of both cytoplasmic and mitochondrial NAD^+, and subsequently causing a redox-dependent rise in the malate/oxaloacetate ratio. The rise in the malate/oxaloacetate ratio triggers a shift of the aspartate aminotransferase reaction in the direction of glutamate formation and aspartate consumption (Siesjö et al., 1976; Siesjö, 1978; Erecinska & Silver, 1990).

Glutamate and glutamatergic systems are implicated in many brain disorders. For example, abnormality in glutamate regulation is considered to be a major factor in the initiation, spread, and maintenance of seizure activities in many types of epilepsy. Topiramate, an effective antiepileptic drug, exerts its anticonvulsant action by selectively antagonizing AMPA and KA receptors (Costa et al., 2011). Animal studies have repeatedly shown that glutamate release is increased during seizure activities. Many patients with complex partial epilepsy or temporal lobe epilepsy have neuronal loss and sclerosis, especially in the mesial hippocampus. A recent study using in vitro ^{13}C MRS analysis of epileptogenic hippocampal tissue excised from patients infused with [2-^{13}C]-glucose found that the glutamate–glutamine cycling flux rate was significantly reduced in epilepsy patients with hippocampal sclerosis compared with those with minimal neuronal loss (Petroff et al., 2002). It was suggested that the measured low rate of glutamate–glutamine cycling, resulting from a failure in glial glutamate uptake, could account for slow glutamate clearance from the synaptic cleft, which causes excitotoxicity. Excitotoxicity by extracellular glutamate in turn causes cell damage and/or death, leading to a reduction in intracellular metabolic pools. This mechanism could explain why the total concentration of glutamate (and that of N-acetylaspartate, a putative neuronal marker) measured from human epileptic cortex excised for neurosurgical therapy of focal epilepsy is reduced, rather than elevated (Sherwin, 1999).

Dysfunction of glutamate and glutamate hyperactivity are involved in many brain disorders such as schizophrenia, major depression, Alzheimer's diseases, Parkinson's disease, amyotrophic lateral sclerosis, and dementia (e.g., Moghaddam & Adams, 1998). Although tissue-specific defects in glial transporter genes leading to impaired glutamate uptake and abnormal activation of glutamatergic pathways have been identified, in some cases it is unclear what role the total concentration of glutamate plays in these disorders. While in vivo ^{13}C MRS holds the promise of noninvasive measurement of glutamatergic abnormalities and their responses to therapeutic interventions in many brain disorders, most in vivo ^{13}C MRS studies of human brain so far have been limited to normal volunteers (Shen & Rothman, 2002). Few clinical applications of in vivo ^{13}C MRS to brain disorders have been performed and all of them were performed on a small number of patients (Bluml et al., 2001; Lin et al., 2003; Ross et al., 2003). Although there is evidence of altered glutamate–glutamine cycle in schizophrenia from enzymology studies of postmortem brain (Burbaeva et al., 2003) and in epilepsy and Huntington's disease from in vivo proton MRS measurement of the total glutamate (Pfund et al., 2000; Bender et al., 2005), direct measurement of altered glutamate–glutamine cycling fluxes in those brain diseases using in vivo ^{13}C MRS have not been performed. As outlined above, many possible factors such as changes in redox states and the activities of enzymes involved in glutamate metabolism could lead to an altered total concentration of glutamate. Therefore, a better characterization of the glutamatergic function could be performed with dynamic ^{13}C spectroscopy methods to measure the turnover of glutamate and glutamine.

CONCLUSIONS

This chapter has outlined the roles of glutamate as the principal excitatory neurotransmitter in the CNS and a key metabolite linking carbon and nitrogen metabolism, the major enzymes and pathways participating in the metabolism of glutamate and the glutamate–glutamine cycle, factors/agents regulating the total concentration of the glutamate measured by proton MRS, and the interpretation of changes in total glutamate concentration. As described, glutamatergic excitation in the functions of the brain is intricately related to the metabolic and transport mechanisms of glutamate. The knowledge of the biochemical aspects of glutamate is crucial to the interpretation of MRS measures of glutamate concentration and the glutamate–glutamine cycling flux.

References

Bain, J. A., & Klein, J. R. (1949). Effect of carbon dioxide on brain glucose, lactate, pyruvate and phosphates. *American Journal of Physiology, 158*, 478−484.

Bender, A., Auer, D. P., Merl, T., Reilmann, R., Saemann, P., Yassouridis, A., et al. (2005). Creatine supplementation lowers brain glutamate levels in Huntington's disease. *Journal of Neurology, 252*, 36−41.

Berntman, L., Carlsson, C., & Siesjö, B. K. (1977). Cerebral blood flow and cerebral metabolic rate in arterial hypoxia and in immobilization stress. *Acta Neurologica Scandinavica Supplement, 64*, 96−97.

Betz, A. L., & Gilboe, D. D. (1973). Effect of pentobarbital on amino acid and urea flux in the isolated dog brain. *American Journal of Physiology, 224*, 580−587.

Blakely, R. D., & Coyle, J. T. (1988). The neurobiology of N-acetylaspartylglutamate. *International Review of Neurobiology, 30*, 39−100.

Bluml, S., Moreno, A., Hwang, J. H., & Ross, B. D. (2001). 1-13C glucose magnetic resonance spectroscopy of pediatric and adult brain disorders. *NMR in Biomedicine, 14*, 19−32.

Bradford, H. . F, Ward, H. K., & Thomas, A. J. (1978). Glutamine−a major substrate for nerve endings. *Journal of Neurochemistry, 30*, 1453−1459.

Burbaeva, G. S., Boksha, I. S., Turishcheva, M. S., Vorobyeva, E. A., Savushkina, O. K., & Tereshkina, E. B. (2003). Glutamine synthetase and glutamate dehydrogenase in the prefrontal cortex of patients with schizophrenia. *Progress in Neuro-psychopharmacology and Biological Psychiatry, 27*, 675−680.

Cerdan, S., & Seelig, J. (1990). NMR studies of metabolism. *Annual Review of Biophysics and Biochemistry, 19*, 43−67.

Chapman, A. G., Nordström, C. H., & Siesjö, B. K. (1978). Influence of phenobarbital anesthesia on carbohydrate and amino acid metabolism in rat brain. *Anesthesiology, 48*, 175−182.

Costa, J., Fareleira, F., Ascenção, R., Borges, M., Sampaio, C., & Vaz-Carneiro, A. (2011). Clinical comparability of the new antiepileptic drugs in refractory partial epilepsy: a systematic review and meta-analysis. *Epilepsia, 52*, 1280−1291.

Coulter, D. A., & Eid, T. (2012). Astrocytic regulation of glutamate homeostasis in epilepsy. *Glia, 60*(8), 1215−1226.

Cruz, F., & Cerdan, S. (1999). Quantitative 13C NMR studies of metabolic compartmentation in the adult mammalian brain. *NMR in Biomedicine, 12*, 451−462.

de Graaf, A. A., Deutz, N. E., Bosman, D. K., Chamuleau, R. A., de Haan, J. G., & Bovee, W. M. (1991). The use of in vivo proton NMR to study the effects of hyperammonemia in the rat cerebral cortex. *NMR in Biomedicine, 4*, 31−37.

de Graaf, R. A, Rothman, D. L., & Behar, K. L. (2011). State of the art direct 13C and indirect 1H-[13C] NMR spectroscopy in vivo. A practical guide. *NMR in Biomedicine, 24*, 958−972.

de Graaf, R. A. (1998). *In vivo NMR spectroscopy*. Chichester, UK: John Wiley & Sons.

Duce, I. R., & Keen, P. (1983). Selective uptake of [3H]glutamine and [3H]glutamate into neurons and satellite cells of dorsal root ganglia in vitro. *Neuroscience, 8*, 861−866.

Engelsen, B., & Fonnum, F. (1983). Effects of hypoglycemia on the transmitter pool and the metabolic pool of glutamate in rat brain. *Neuroscience Letters, 42*, 317−322.

Erecinska, M., & Silver, I. A. (1990). Metabolism and role of glutamate in mammalian brain. *Progress in Neurobiology, 35*, 245−296.

Gether, U., Andersen, P. H., Larsson, O. M., & Schousboe, A. (2006). Neurotransmitter transporters: molecular function of important drug targets. *Trends in Pharmacological Science, 27*, 375−383.

Godin, Y., Mark, J., & Kayser, C. (1967). Ammonia and urea in the brain of garden dormice during hibernation. *Journal of Neurochemistry, 14*, 142−144.

Greene, J. G., & Greenamyre, J. T. (1996). Bioenergetics and glutamate excitotoxicity. *Progress in Neurobiology, 48*, 613−634.

Gruetter, R., Seaquist, E. R., Kim, S., & Ugurbil, K. (1998). Localized in vivo 13C-NMR of glutamate metabolism in the human brain: initial results at 4 Tesla. *Developmental Neuroscience, 20*, 380−388.

Hägerdal, M., Harp, J., & Siesjö, B. K. (1975). Effect of hypothermia upon organic phosphates, glycolytic metabolites, citric acid cycle intermediates and associated amino acids in rat cerebral cortex. *Journal of Neurochemistry, 24*, 743−748.

Henry, P. G., Russeth, K. P., Tkac, I., Drewes, L. R., Andrews, M. T., & Gruetter, R. (2007). Brain energy metabolism and neurotransmission at near-freezing temperatures: in vivo (1)H MRS study of a hibernating mammal. *Journal of Neurochemistry, 101*, 1505−1515.

Hertz, L. (1979). Functional interactions between neurons and astrocytes I. Turnover and metabolism of putative amino acid transmitters. *Progress in Neurobiology, 13*, 277−323.

Hertz, L. (2004). Intercellular metabolic compartmentation in the brain Past, present and future. *Neurochemistry International, 45*, 285−296.

Hurd, R., Sailasuta, N., Srinivasan, R., Vigneron, D. B., Pelletier, D., & Nelson, S. J. (2004). Measurement of brain glutamate using TE-averaged PRESS at 3T. *Magnetic Resonance in Medicine, 51*, 435−440.

Kazemi, H., Shore, N. S., Shih, V. E., & Shannon, D. C. (1973). Brain organic buffers in respiratory acidosis and alkalosis. *Journal of Applied Physiology, 34*, 478−482.

Kazemi, H., Wyen, J., van Leuven, F., & Leusen, I. (1976). The CSF HCO3 increase in hypercapnia relationship to HCO3, glutamate, glutamine and NH3 in brain. *Respiratory Physiology, 28*, 387−401.

Kostandy, B. B. (2012). The role of glutamate in neuronal ischemic injury: the role of spark in fire. *Neurological Sciences, 33*, 223−237.

Lebon, V., Petersen, K. F., Cline, G. W., Shen, J., Mason, G. F., Dufour, S., et al. (2002). Astroglial contribution to brain energy metabolism in humans revealed by 13C nuclear magnetic resonance spectroscopy. Elucidation of the dominant pathway for neurotransmitter glutamate repletion and measurement of astrocytic oxidative metabolism. *Journal of Neuroscience, 22*, 1523−1531.

Lewis, L. D., Ljunggren, B., Norberg, K., & Siesjö, B. K. (1974). Changes in carbohydrate substrates, amino acids and ammonia in the brain during insulin-induced hypoglycemia. *Journal of Neurochemistry, 23*(4), 659−671.

Lin, A. P., Shic, F., Enriquez, C., & Ross, B. D. (2003). Reduced glutamate neurotransmission in patients with Alzheimer's disease−an in vivo 13C magnetic resonance spectroscopy study. *MAGMA, 16*, 29−42.

Luthi-Carter, R., Berger, U. V., Barczak, A. K., Enna, M., & Coyle, J. T. (1998). Isolation and expression of a rat brain cDNA encoding glutamate carboxypeptidase II. *Proceedings of the National Academy of Sciences USA, 95*, 3215−3220.

MacMillan, V., & Siesjö, B. K. (1973). The influence of hypocapnia upon intracellular pH and upon some carbohydrate substrates, amino acids and organic phosphates in the brain. *Journal of Neurochemistry, 21*, 1283−1299.

McKenna, M. C., Waagepetersen, H. S., Schousboe, A., & Sonnewald, U. (2006). Neuronal and astrocytic shuttle mechanisms for cytosolic-mitochondrial transfer of reducing equivalents: current evidence and pharmacological tools. *Biochemistry and Pharmacology, 71*, 399−407.

Moghaddam, B., & Adams, B. W. (1998). Reversal of phencyclidine effects by a group II metabotropic glutamate receptor agonist in rats. *Science, 281*, 1349−1352.

Morris, P., & Bachelard, H. (2003). Reflections on the application of 13C-MRS to research on brain metabolism. *NMR in Biomedicine, 16*, 303−312.

Petroff, O. A., Errante, L. D., Rothman, D. L., Kim, J. H., & Spencer, D. D. (2002). Glutamate-glutamine cycling in the epileptic human hippocampus. *Epilepsia, 43*, 703–710.

Pfund, Z., Chugani, D. C., Juhasz, C., Muzik, O., Chugani, H. T., Wilds, I. B., et al. (2000). Evidence for coupling between glucose metabolism and glutamate cycling using FDG PET and 1H magnetic resonance spectroscopy in patients with epilepsy. *Journal of Cerebral Blood Flow and Metabolism, 20*, 871–878.

Price, N. C., & Stevens, L. (1999). *Fundamentals of Enzymology* (3rd ed.). Oxford, UK: Oxford University Press.

Robinson, M. B., Blakely, R. D., Couto, R., & Coyle, J. T. (1987). Hydrolysis of the brain dipeptide N-acetyl-L-aspartyl-L-glutamate. Identification and characterization of a novel N-acetylated alpha-linked acidic dipeptidase activity from rat brain. *Journal of Biological Chemistry, 262*, 14498–14506.

Ross, B. D., Lin, A., Harris, K., Bhattacharya, P., & Schweinsburg, B. (2003). Clinical experience with 13C MRS in vivo. *NMR in Biomedicine, 16*, 358–369.

Rothman, D. L., De Feyter, H. M., de Graaf, R. A., Mason, G. F., & Behar, K. L. (2011). 13C MRS studies of neuroenergetics and neurotransmitter cycling in humans. *NMR in Biomedicine, 24*, 943–957.

Rothman, S. M., & Olney, J. W. (1986). Glutamate and the pathophysiology of hypoxic–ischemic brain damage. *Annals of Neurology, 19* (2), 105–111.

Rothstein, J. D., Dykes-Hoberg, M., Pardo, C. A., Bristol, L. A., Jin, L., Kuncl, R. W., et al. (1996). Knockout of glutamate transporters reveals a major role for astroglial transport in excitotoxicity and clearance of glutamate. *Neuron, 16*(3), 675–686.

Shank, R. P., & Campbell, G. L. M. (1983). In (2nd ed.A. Lajitha (Ed.), *Handbook of Neurochemistry* (Vol. 3New York: Plenum Press.

Shen, J. (2005). In vivo carbon-13 magnetization transfer effect. Detection of aspartate aminotransferase reaction. *Magnetic Resonance in Medicine, 54*, 1321–1326.

Shen, J., Petersen, K. F., Behar, K. L., Brown, P., Nixon, T. W., Mason, G. F., et al. (1999). Determination of the rate of the glutamate/glutamine cycle in the human brain by in vivo 13C NMR. *Proceedings of the National Academy of Sciences USA, 96*, 8235–8240.

Shen, J., & Rothman, D. L. (2002). Magnetic resonance spectroscopic approaches to studying neuronal: glial interactions. *Biological Psychiatry, 52*, 694–700.

Shen, J., Sibson, N. R., Cline, G., Behar, K. L., Rothman, D. L., & Shulman, R. G. (1998). 15N-NMR spectroscopy studies of ammonia transport and glutamine synthesis in the hyperammonemic rat brain. *Development in Neuroscience, 20*, 434–443.

Shepherd, G. M (1994). *Neurobiology* (3rd ed.). Oxford, UK: Oxford University Press.

Sherwin, A. L. (1999). Neuroactive amino acids in focally epileptic human brain: a review. *Neurochemical Research, 24*, 1387–1395.

Shimizu, A., Kusagaya, H., & Issiki, A. (1998). Acidosis and neuroprotection in two types of acidosis model rats under isoflurane anesthesia: evaluation of blood flow, pH and amino acid levels in the cortex. *Masui, 47*, 1173–1182.

Sibson, N. R., Dhankhar, A., Mason, G. F., Behar, K. L., Rothman, D. L., & Shulman, R. G. (1997). In vivo 13C NMR measurements of cerebral glutamine synthesis as evidence for glutamate-glutamine cycling. *Proceedings of the National Academy of Sciences USA, 18*(94), 2699–2704.

Sibson, N. R., Dhankhar, A., Mason, G. F., Rothman, D. L., Behar, K. L., & Shulman, R. G. (1998). Stoichiometric coupling of brain glucose metabolism and glutamatergic neuronal activity. *Proceedings of the National Academy of Sciences USA, 95*, 316–321.

Sibson, N. R., Mason, G. F., Shen, J., Cline, G. W., Herskovits, A. Z., Wall, J. E., et al. (2001). In vivo 13C NMR measurement of neurotransmitter glutamate cycling, anaplerosis and TCA cycle flux in rat brain during. *Journal of Neurochemistry, 76*, 975–989.

Siesjö, B. K. (1978). *Brain Energy Metabolism*. Chichester, UK: John Wiley & Sons.

Siesjö, B. K., Borgström, L., Jóhannsson, H., Nilsson, B., Norberg, K., & Quistorff, B. (1976). Cerebral oxygenation in arterial hypoxia. *Advances in Experimental Medicine and Biology, 75*, 335–342.

Stelmashook, E. V., Isaev, N. K., Lozier, E. R., Goryacheva, E. S., & Khaspekov, L. G. (2011). Role of glutamine in neuronal survival and death during brain ischemia and hypoglycemia. *International Journal of Neuroscience, 121*, 415–422.

Tyson, R. L., & Sutherland, G. R. (1998). Labeling of N-acetylaspartate and N-acetylaspartylglutamate in rat neocortex, hippocampus and cerebellum from [1-13C]glucose. *Neuroscience Letters, 251*, 181–184.

van Leuven, F., Weyne, J., & Leusen, I. (1974). Influence of PCO2 on amino acids in the brain of the rat. *Archives Internationales de Physiologie et de Biochimie, 82*, 419–421.

Weber, R., Ramos-Cabrer, P., & Hoehn, M. (2006). Present status of magnetic resonance imaging and spectroscopy in animal stroke models. *Journal of Cerebral Blood Flow and Metabolism, 26*, 591–604.

Wong, K. L., & Tyce, G. M. (1983). Glucose and amino acid metabolism in rat brain during sustained hypoglycemia. *Neurochemical Research, 8*, 401–415.

Xu, S., Yang, J., & Shen, J. (2008). Measuring N-acetylaspartate synthesis in vivo using proton magnetic resonance spectroscopy. *Journal of Neuroscience Methods, 172*, 8–12.

Yang, J., & Shen, J. (2006). Increased oxygen consumption in the somatosensory cortex of alpha-chloralose anesthetized rats during forepaw stimulation determined using MRS at 11.7 Tesla. *Neuroimage, 32*, 1317–1325.

Young, R. L., & Lowry, O. H. (1966). Quantitative methods for measuring the histochemical distribution of alanine, glutamate and glutamine in brain. *Journal of Neurochemistry, 13*, 785–793.

Other Significant Metabolites: Myo-Inositol, GABA, Glutamine, and Lactate

Jonathan G. Best, Charlotte J. Stagg and Andrea Dennis

Oxford Centre for Functional MRI of the Brain (FMRIB), Department of Clinical
Neurosciences, University of Oxford, UK

INTRODUCTION

Alongside the most commonly acquired metabolites discussed in previous chapters, it is possible to quantify a number of other neurochemicals using magnetic resonance spectroscopy (MRS). Accurate quantification of these may only be possible at particular echo times, or with the use of edited sequences, and therefore they are somewhat less commonly described in the literature than those metabolites discussed in previous chapters. However, as the availability of more advanced MRS techniques increases, the potential utility of these neurochemicals for a wide range of neuro-scientific and clinical applications is becoming clear.

In this chapter we review four of these neurochemicals in some depth: myo-inositol, γ-aminobutyric acid (GABA), glutamine, and lactate. This should not be taken as an exhaustive list; many other metabolites can be quantified using MRS and their potential utility has yet to be fully explored.

MYO-INOSITOL

Inositol is a cyclic molecule consisting of a six-carbon ring and six hydroxyl groups, one arising from each carbon atom. Nine isomers have been described, of which myo-inositol is the most abundant in human tissue, representing ~90% of total inositol content. Scyllo-inositol accounts for much of the remaining fraction, and neo-inositol has been detected in trace amounts (Fisher et al., 2002). Myo-inositol can be measured *in vivo* using ^{1}H MRS, appearing as a pair of resonances at 3.52 and 3.61 parts per million (ppm) at short echo times. It has been proposed as a marker of

glial cell proliferation, and has also attracted interest as a precursor of intracellular second messengers formed by the phosphoinositol cycle, and as a major osmolyte in central nervous system tissue.

Physiology

Myo-inositol is obtained both from dietary sources and *de novo* synthesis. Grains and plant fibers are a particularly rich source of inositol, as inositol hexakis-phosphate. Synthesis predominantly takes place in the kidney. D-Glucose-6-phosphate, formed from glucose in the first step of glycolysis, is converted to D-myo-inositol-3-phosphate, then inositol-1-phosphate, which undergoes dephosphorylation within the brain to form free myo-inositol. The brain and cerebrospinal fluid (CSF) are relatively enriched in myo-inositol compared to plasma, with estimated typical concentrations of 6 mM in brain, 0.2 mM in CSF, and 0.03 mM in plasma (Fisher et al., 2002). Myo-inositol breakdown also occurs within the kidney, in which cleavage of the carbon ring yields D-glucuronate, which undergoes further breakdown in the liver, and is ultimately converted to carbon dioxide and water through carbohydrate metabolism.

Within the brain, myo-inositol is predominantly an intracellular molecule. It is taken up into cells via two sodium-myo-inositol cotransporters, SMIT1 and SMIT2, and a hydrogen-myo-inositol symporter, HMIT. The first of these to be identified, SMIT1, is a high-affinity transporter with a K_m for myo-inositol of 55 μM (Kwon et al., 1992; Hager et al., 1995). It takes up two sodium ions for each myo-inositol molecule, generating a net inward current. Its activity is increased by more negative membrane potentials, and decreased by extracellular acidification, although under physiological conditions, both these effects are relatively small (Hager et al., 1995; Matskevitch et al., 1998). SMIT2 is a similar transporter with a stoichiometry of 2:1 and a K_m of 120 μM (Coady et al., 2002). Within the brain, SMIT1 and SMIT2 are expressed by both neurons and glia, although SMIT1 is predominantly astrocytic and SMIT2 predominantly neuronal (Fu et al., 2012). HMIT is mainly expressed by astrocytes, and is structurally unrelated to either SMIT. It has a K_m of approximately 100 μM, and transports hydrogen ions and myo-inositol in a 1:1 ratio. Unlike SMIT1/2, it is stimulated by extracellular acidification, and is close to inactive at pH 7.5 or higher (Uldry et al., 2001).

Efflux of myo-inositol from neurons and glia occurs via a volume-sensitive organic osmolyte channel, also known as the volume-regulated anion channel (Jackson & Strange, 1993). This channel mediates the efflux of organic osmolytes, such as myo-inositol and taurine, in response to cell swelling. This is consistent with the role of myo-inositol in the cellular response of the brain to osmotic stress. The acute response to extracellular hypo-osmolality is primarily efflux of intracellular electrolytes, but during sustained stress, organic osmolytes are lost from affected tissue to regulate tissue osmolarity. For example, Videen and colleagues (1995) used MRS to demonstrate a 49% mean reduction in myo-inositol in the occipital cortex of patients with chronic hyponatremia. Conversely, chronic hypernatremia significantly increases brain myo-inositol content (Lien et al., 1990). Increased SMIT1 expression and SMIT1-mediated myo-inositol uptake have been demonstrated in rat cortical astrocytes subjected to hyperosmolar conditions (Strange et al., 1994). This upregulation appears to be mediated by the tonicity-sensitive transcription factor, tonicity-responsive enhancer binding protein (TonEBP). SMIT2 expression also increases, but this is not mediated by TonEBP (Bissonnette et al., 2008). Additionally, the cell volume-sensitive protein kinase, SGK1, is upregulated, stabilizing SMIT1 in the cell membrane (Klaus et al., 2008). A role for HMIT in cell volume regulation has not been established.

A proportion of intracellular myo-inositol participates in the phosphoinositol cycle Fig. 2.5.1), which generates the signaling molecules inositol-1,4,5-trisphosphate (IP$_3$), phosphatidylinositol-3,4-bisphosphate (PI(3,4)P$_2$), and phosphatidylinositol-3,4,5-trisphosphate (PI(3,4,5)P$_3$). IP$_3$ is formed by cleavage of the inositol head group-containing phospholipid, phosphatidylinositol-4,5-bisphosphate (PI(4,5)P$_2$) by phospholipase C (PLC) in response to activation of Gq-coupled receptors. IP$_3$ subsequently mediates calcium release from endoplasmic reticulum, and is inactivated by stepwise

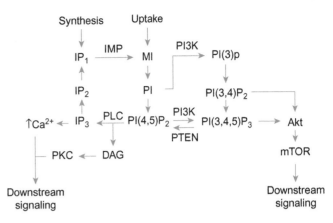

FIGURE 2.5.1 Formation of intracellular signaling molecules from myo-inositol through the phosphoinositol cycle (see text for key). IMP, inositol monophosphatase; PKC, protein kinase C; PI3K, phosphatidylinositol-3-kinase; PLC, phospholipase C. This figure is reproduced in color in the color plate section.

dephosphorylation to free inositol. Diacylglycerol is also produced from PI(4,5)P$_2$, activating protein kinase C (PKC), and is ultimately utilized for resynthesis of phosphatidylinositol from myo-inositol. PI(3,4)P$_2$ and PI(3,4,5)P$_3$ are produced from phosphatidylinositol by PI-3-kinase, the first step in the PI3K/Akt/mTOR pathway, which transduces signals from insulin-like growth factor receptors. Dephosphorylation of PI(3,4,5)P$_3$ to PI(4,5)P$_2$ occurs by PTEN, an important tumor suppressor.

Changes in myo-inositol level have been interpreted as indicating alterations in these fluxes in the phosphatidylinositol cycle; however, the proportion of intracellular myo-inositol, which participates in the PI cycle appears to be low, as even severe inositol depletion by means of genetic knockout of SMIT1 does not alter phosphoinositide levels significantly (Berry et al., 2004).

Applications

Glial Cell Marker

Myo-inositol is widely studied using MRS as a marker of glial cell proliferation, and increased myo-inositol concentrations have been detected in many neurological disorders, including neurodegenerative diseases, multiple sclerosis, and some brain tumors (Bitsch et al., 1999; Castillo et al., 2000; Duarte et al., 2012). The role of myo-inositol as a glial cell marker was first proposed by Brand and colleagues (1993), who used MRS to compare levels in cultured cells of neuronal and glial origin. Myo-inositol was present in rat astrocytes and glioma cells at approximately 6 mM concentration, but was undetectable in neurons. It was therefore concluded that myo-inositol is mainly contained within glia, and that neuronal levels must be less than 0.5 mM, the lower limit for detection by the MRS protocol used. Selective concentration within glia was supported by earlier work using radiolabeled myo-inositol, which showed significantly greater uptake by glial cells compared to neurons, and demonstrated a large cytosolic pool of myo-inositol present in glia, but not neurons (Glanville et al., 1989). However, neither study showed myo-inositol to be an exclusively glial molecule, and subsequent studies have shown myo-inositol to be present at high concentrations within some types of neuron, including the NTN-2 neuronal and 5H-SY5Y neuroblastoma cell lines, and the giant neurons of Dieter's nucleus in the rabbit (for a full review, see Fisher et al., 2002). It has also been noted that the neuronal cultures used in the study performed by Brand and colleagues (1993) were immature and lacked some of the physiological properties of neurons *in vivo*, notably containing very little *N*-acetylaspartate, a well established neuronal marker (Maddock & Buonocore, 2012). The assumption that myo-inositol is a specific glial marker should therefore be treated with caution.

The correlation between myo-inositol and gliosis *in vivo* has also been questioned. A few studies combining MRS with histological methods suggest that this relationship is complex. In macaques infected with the Simian Immunodeficiency Virus, J. P. Kim and colleagues (2005) found that marked frontal astrogliosis occurs as viral load rises during the acute phase of the infection. High-field postmortem MRS showed no accompanying changes in myo-inositol levels, failing to replicate previous work with *in vivo* spectroscopy at 1.5 T showing a 14% increase in the mI:Cr ratio. This suggests that glial cells can proliferate without increasing myo-inositol, and raises the possibility that at least part of the increase in the myo-inositol resonance observed with gliosis at low field strength actually corresponds to another, as yet uncharacterized, metabolite, separable from myo-inositol at high field strength only.

There is also evidence that myo-inositol can increase in neurological disease in the absence of gliosis. In a mouse model of spinocerebellar ataxia type 1 (SCA-1) overexpressing mutant ataxin 1, increased cerebellar myo-inositol occurs and correlates with histological evidence of disease progression, but little gliosis is observed on glial fibrillary acidic protein (GFAP) immunostaining (Oz et al., 2010b). Myo-inositol is also increased in the cerebellum and brainstem of humans with SCA-1, but CSF GFAP immunoreactivity is not increased, although this is a less sensitive measure of gliosis (Oz et al., 2010a).

In summary, myo-inositol concentrations appear generally to be higher in glia than neurons, and glial

uptake of myo-inositol exceeds that of neurons, possibly due to expression of the HMIT transporter. However, neurons also take up and use myo-inositol, and levels within some neurons equal those in glia. The myo-inositol resonance is increased in many conditions in which gliosis occurs, but this is not a specific change. Other mechanisms including osmoregulatory effects, local pH changes, altered intracellular metabolism of inositol and phosphoinositols, and contributions from other metabolites to the myo-inositol resonance, including glycine and inositol phosphates, should be considered.

Neurodegenerative Disease

Elevated myo-inositol levels have been observed in Alzheimer's dementia, Huntington's disease, and inherited ataxias. There is interest in whether this might represent a sensitive early marker of neurodegenerative disease, or a biomarker for monitoring disease progression and response to treatment. In Alzheimer's disease, myo-inositol shows promise in the diagnosis of amnestic mild cognitive impairment (MCI), a state in which memory is reduced without impairment of overall cognitive function. MCI progresses to dementia in some patients, and it is hoped that early treatment could prevent this. However, the distinction between patients with MCI and subjects with low-normal memory function is difficult. Myo-inositol is increased within the hippocampi of patients with Alzheimer's disease, and there is some evidence that smaller increases in myo-inositol may occur in MCI patients compared to controls (Watanabe et al., 2012). The ratio of *N*-acetylaspartate (NAA), a well-recognized neuronal marker, to myo-inositol in the posterior cingulate cortex can distinguish MCI from normal aging with a sensitivity of 0.75 and specificity of 0.8 (Wang et al., 2012).

In Alzheimer's disease, there is a relatively weak, but statistically significant, correlation between myo-inositol levels and reduced performance on tests of certain aspects of memory, particularly visual and verbal memory (Watanabe et al., 2012). A much stronger correlation has been described in one of the inherited ataxias, SCA-1. In human patients with SCA-1, cerebellar myo-inositol concentration measured with MRS correlates significantly with the clinical severity score on a standardized ataxia rating scale, with an R^2 of 0.59 (Oz et al., 2010a). Moreover, in the ataxin-1 mouse model, a similar correlation between myo-inositol concentration and neuropathological indicators of severity has been observed (Oz et al., 2010b). In both cases, correlations with NAA and glutamate were also observed, suggesting that the usefulness of myo-inositol as a biomarker might be increased by using it in conjunction with other central nervous system (CNS) metabolites.

Psychiatric Disease

MRS measurement of myo-inositol levels has been used to investigate the pathogenesis of psychiatric disorders, particularly bipolar disorder (BPD). Lithium, the first line treatment for acute mania and chronic mood stabilization in BPD, is a noncompetitive inhibitor of inositol monophosphatase, blocking resynthesis of inositol from inositol 1-phosphate. This is thought to slow activity of the phosphoinositol cycle, and therefore it has been inferred that overactivity of this cycle participates in the pathogenesis of BPD (Berridge et al., 1989). This hypothesis predicts that myo-inositol levels will be elevated in BPD, inositol monophosphates (detectable with ^{31}P MRS as part of the phosphomonoester peak) reduced, and these changes should be corrected by lithium treatment (Silverstone & McGrath, 2009). Additionally, lithium administration in healthy controls should lead to myo-inositol depletion and inositol monophosphate accumulation.

Administration of lithium in rats has been shown to rapidly increase inositol 1-phosphate and decrease myo-inositol concentrations, consistent with inhibition of inositol monophosphatase (Allison & Stewart, 1971; Allison et al., 1976). However, this finding has not been replicated in healthy human subjects. In their comprehensive review, Silverstone and McGrath (2009) identified four studies using MRS to measure myo-inositol and phosphomonoester levels after lithium administration. Of these, one showed an increase in phosphomonoesters in the frontal cortex (Yildiz et al., 2001). The others, one assessing the prefrontal cortex, and two the temporal lobe, found no change in either resonance (Silverstone & McGrath, 2009).

Relatively little evidence is available regarding inositol levels in unmedicated BPD, particularly in manic patients, who present practical and ethical difficulties in scanning prior to treatment. However, a study of 23 depressed BPD patients, 18 of whom had not been treated with lithium, showed no change in myo-inositol levels compared to controls (Frye et al., 2007). Further studies failed to find any change in myo-inositol in the anterior cingulate cortex of depressed and mixed-mood BPD patients (Dager et al., 2004), or the frontal lobes of a mixed group of manic and depressed patients (Port et al., 2008). However, the latter study did show an increase in the left caudate nucleus. Finally, a study of 10 children with mania found raised levels within the anterior cingulate cortex compared to controls, although the extent to which this finding can be extrapolated to adults is not certain (Davanzo et al., 2003). Overall, these results do not indicate that myo-inositol is consistently increased in BPD.

Two studies have provided limited evidence that lithium treatment may reduce myo-inositol levels in bipolar patients. Moore and colleagues (1999) assessed depressed bipolar patients prior to starting lithium treatment, and again at 5–7 days and 3–4 weeks. A significant decrease occurred within the frontal cortex within days of starting lithium, and persisted at 4 weeks. However, clinical improvement did not occur until 4 weeks, showing that reducing inositol levels is not in itself sufficient to improve symptoms. No changes occurred within temporal, occipital, or parietal cortex (Moore et al., 1999). In children with mania or hypomania, lithium treatment reduced myo-inositol in the anterior cingulate cortex within 1 week (Davanzo et al., 2001). The difference between these findings and studies of lithium administration in healthy controls is surprising. A possible explanation is that lithium noncompetitively binds the inositol monophosphatase enzyme substrate complex, so inhibition is thought to be greatest when the phosphoinositol cycle is most active. However, as discussed earlier, in vivo evidence for this hypothesis is limited.

Overall, the role of myo-inositol in BPD and the response to lithium treatment remains uncertain, and any changes in myo-inositol that do occur may be more associated with mania than depression. Many studies are confounded by medication use and heterogeneity in the clinical condition of the study population. Given that the hypothesis for the role of myo-inositol in BPD is based primarily on the efficacy of lithium in its treatment, it is perhaps unsurprising that consistent changes in myo-inositol have not been reported in other psychiatric disorders, notably schizophrenia and major depressive disorder (H. Kim et al. 2005).

Myo-Inositol and Neuronal Activity

Acute changes in myo-inositol concentrations have been observed within cortex exposed to electrical stimulation using MRS. In anaesthetized rats, continuous electrical forepaw stimulation was associated with a small, but statistically significant, decrease in myo-inositol within the contralateral somatosensory cortex (Xu et al., 2005). Cortical myo-inositol is also modified by anodal transcranial direct current stimulation, a subthreshold stimulation technique thought to increase local neuronal discharge rate (Rango et al., 2008), although, interestingly, a decrease, not an increase, was observed. Both of these results have been interpreted as indicating changes in PI cycle activity secondary to changes in synaptic activity. However, given the pH dependence of the HMIT transporter, and the association between neuronal activity, lactate release, and extracellular acidification (Chesler & Kaila, 1992;

Pellerin & Magistretti, 1994), myo-inositol uptake may also be affected. Confirmation of these preliminary observations could suggest a new role for myo-inositol as a noninvasive marker of neuronal activity.

GABA

GABA was first discovered in the brain the 1950s (Roberts & Frankel, 1950) and its role as the primary inhibitory neurotransmitter within the CNS was first demonstrated in the 1960s in the lobster; technical difficulties meant that confirmation of its role in the mammalian CNS came somewhat later (Saito et al., 1974). Now recognized as the primary inhibitory neurotransmitter within the brain, GABA appears to have important roles in disease states such as epilepsy, as well in influencing interindividual differences in behavior and in various types of synaptic plasticity.

Physiology

In humans, GABA is primarily produced by the decarboxylation of L-glutamate via the enzyme glutamate decarboxylase (GAD). GAD is found only within GABAergic interneurons within the cortex and is present as both an inactive apoenzyme (apoGAD) and an active holoenzyme form (holoGAD). GAD is activated by binding of the coenzyme pyridoxal 5'-phosphate (PLP), which is derived from vitamin B_6. The necessary role of PLP for activating GAD has been demonstrated in rats who were fed a vitamin B_6-deficient diet, who had normal levels of apoGAD but decreased levels of holoGAD and reduced GABA activity (Roberts & Frankel, 1951; Roberts et al., 1951).

Evidence also exists that GABA can also be catabolized from glucose directly, without needing to be metabolized via glutamate (Preece & Cerdán, 1996), or from putrescine, via formation of acetyl-putrescine and its subsequent oxidation by monoamine oxidase (Seiler, 1980). However, given $GAD - / -$ knockout mice have only $\sim 0.02\%$ of normal GABA levels (Ji et al., 1999), it is not clear to what extent these alternative pathways play a significant in GABA metabolism *in vivo*.

GABA has two primary distinct roles within the brain: it acts as a metabolite and as a neurotransmitter. Within GABAergic neurons, GABA appears to be highly compartmentalized into at least two metabolically active pools, one distributed throughout the cytoplasm and one limited to the synaptic vesicles. Meaningful estimates of the relative sizes of the two pools have been difficult to establish to date as tissue extracts contain many different types of GABAergic interneurons, and each type may differ greatly in their relative distribution of the two pools (Martin & Tobin, 2000). However, as described later based on selective knockout of the two isoforms of glutamic acid decarboxylase, the majority of GABA is associated with the metabolic pool, but that pool may have an important role in modulating cortical excitability.

GAD

Two distinct isoforms of GAD are found in the human CNS with differing molecular weights of 65 and 67 kDa. Derived from two separate genes, the two GAD isoforms have different amino acid sequences, enzymatic properties, and intracellular distributions (Erlander et al., 1991).

There is also increasing evidence that the two GAD isoforms have different roles within the brain. Cytoplasmic GABA, which makes up at least half of all GABA found in the cortex (Martin & Rimvall, 1993), appears to be produced via the constituently active GAD_{67}, which is found throughout the cytosol. GAD_{65}, conversely, is membrane-bound and found, in the main, closely associated with synaptic vesicles, suggesting that it is the primary enzyme for vesicular GABA production. In the developmental period, the ratio of GAD_{65} to GAD_{67} increases dramatically during synaptogenesis, strongly suggesting a specific role for GAD_{65} in neurotransmission (Greif et al., 1991, 1992). In line with this hypothesis, in adult mammals GAD_{65} activity inducible as a significant proportion is found in the inactive apoGAD form. In addition, GAD_{65}, but not GAD_{67}, forms complexes with the vesicular GABA transporter VGAT, allowing GABA uptake into synaptic vesicles ready for release at synaptic terminals (Wu et al., 2007). However, there is some evidence that in $GAD_{65} - / -$ knockout mice, GAD_{67} is able, to at least some degree, take over this role, suggesting a putative role for GAD_{67} in synaptic GABA production in disease states (Wu et al., 2007). $GAD_{67} - / -$ knockout mice are more difficult to study as they die from a cleft palate early in life, but have been shown to be reduced to approximately 7% of normal, supporting the existence of a relatively larger cytosolic pool of GABA compared with the synaptic GABA (Asada et al., 1997).

GABA Catabolism

GABA is primarily broken down by the mitochondrial enzyme GABA-transaminase (GABA-T) to succinic semialdehyde (SSA). SSA can be further converted into succinate within the tricarboxylic acid (TCA) cycle, therefore allowing a route by which the TCA cycle can function without α-ketoglutarate dehydrogenase, which accounts for approximately 10−20% of total TCA cycle flux, although that fraction is activity dependent (Martin & Rimvall, 1993; Patel et al., 2005; J. Yang et al., 2007;Van Eijsden et al., 2010).

This "GABA shunt" consists of four distinct steps: (1) conversion of α-ketoglutarate to glutamate, (2) conversion of glutamate to GABA by GAD, (3) catabolism of GABA to SSA by GABA-T, and (4) oxidation of SSA to succinate by succinic semialdehyde dehydrogenase (SSADH; Martin et al., 2000).

GABA is broken down in GABAergic neurons and in some astrocytes, though the astrocytic route is probably much less metabolically significant than neuronal degradation (Hyde & Robinson, 1976; Medina-Kauwe et al., 1994), and only ~20% of GABA released at synaptic terminals is taken up by the surrounding astrocytes (Schousboe, 2000). A number of antiepileptic drugs have been developed with the aim of inhibiting GABA-T, and thereby indirectly increasing synaptic GABA concentration; the most common is vigabatrin (see Chapter 3.3).

GABA as a Neurotransmitter and a Neuromodulator

As discussed previously, GABA has two major, distinct roles within the brain. It has an important role in metabolism, acting via the "GABA shunt" in the TCA cycle. In addition it has roles as a neurotransmitter and as a neuromodulator. There are two major families of GABA receptors, $GABA_A$ and $GABA_B$, which have distinct biophysical properties that lend themselves to their distinct roles in GABAergic inhibition within the cortex.

GABA_A Synapses

$GABA_A$ receptors mediate the bulk of fast inhibitory neurotransmission in the CNS. $GABA_A$ receptors are ligand-gated pentameric chloride channels and at least 19 related subtypes exist in mammals, composed from a variety of subunits that include α (subtypes 1–6), β (1–4), γ (1–3), δ, ε, π, and ρ. These different subunits have different sensitivities to GABA and to modulatory drugs, thereby allowing for a range of response across anatomical locations and cell types within the CNS.

In addition to $GABA_A$ receptors located at the $GABA_A$ synapse, extrasynaptic $GABA_A$ receptors exist that underpin the so-called extrasynaptic GABAergic "tone." GABA spillover from the synaptic cleft activates extrasynaptic $GABA_A$ receptors. The $GABA_A$ receptors found extrasynaptically are comprised of relatively rare subunits, particularly $\alpha 4$, $\alpha 6$, and δ. In particular, it is generally true that δ-subunit-containing $GABA_A$ receptors are extrasynaptic, but not all

extrasynaptic $GABA_A$ receptors contain δ-subunits (Belelli et al., 2009).

The unusual conformation of extrasynaptic $GABA_A$ receptors confers on them a series of properties, which are important in understanding their function. In particular, the δ-subunit confers on receptors a slower macroscopic current amplitude, increased outward rectification, and slower desensitization (Saxena & Macdonald, 1994; J. Fisher & Macdonald, 1997; Haas & Macdonald, 1999), making them ideal candidates for slow, tonic, GABAergic inhibition. In addition, the difference in physical properties between extrasynaptic $GABA_A$ receptors and synaptic $GABA_A$ receptors means that they have different pharmacological properties. They are not bound by classical benzodiazepines, but are highly modulated by neurosteroids and ethanol, and are exploited as novel therapeutic targets for a range of disorders including epilepsy, menstrual disorders, and stress (for a full review, see Belelli et al., 2009).

Extracellular GABA and intracellular GABA concentrations are closely related, with extracellular GABA concentration increasing rapidly and in proportion to intracellular GABA concentration when GABA breakdown is impaired by the acute application of vigabatrin (Piérard et al., 1999). It is likely that GABA levels as assessed by MRS reflect, at least to some extent, GABA neuromodulation as MRS-assessed GABA has been shown to be closely related to CSF GABA levels (Petroff & Rothman, 1998), and to extrasynaptic GABAergic tone (Stagg et al., 2011).

GABA_B Synapses

$GABA_B$ receptors are metabotropic receptors linked to potassium channels. They are found throughout the CNS both presynaptically and postsynaptically and are linked to inwardly rectifying potassium channels. Synaptically released GABA can activate presynaptic $GABA_B$ receptors on GABA neurons, reducing GABA release, or presynaptically on local glutamatergic neurons, decreasing glutamatergic release. Postsynaptic $GABA_B$ receptors are also present. In general $GABA_B$ receptors inhibit neuronal activity by local shunting and generate slow (100–500 ms) inhibitory potentials that hyperpolarize the membrane. Although $GABA_B$ receptors can be stimulated from a single synaptic release of GABA, they are more commonly stimulated via the release of GABA from several neurons simultaneously, and hence $GABA_B$ receptors are often thought of as acting as a paracrine signaling for the GABAergic system. (For a full review of $GABA_B$ receptors, see Gassmann & Bettler, 2012.)

The clinical implications of abnormalities in GABA signaling in epilepsy are discussed in Chapter 3.3. For a discussion of the role of GABA in behavior and plasticity, see Chapter 3.8.

GLUTAMINE

Glutamine is an abundant amino acid in the CNS, structurally similar to the neurotransmitter glutamate. It is an important intermediate in neurotransmitter metabolism and ammonia detoxification. At field strengths of 3 T and below, its resonance, at 2.45 ppm, overlaps substantially with that of glutamate, at 2.35 ppm. They have therefore traditionally been measured together, as the composite Glx peak. Until recently, MR imaging (MRI) scanners with sufficient field strength to reliably resolve these metabolites have only been available for small animal studies. The increasing availability of high-field human scanners, and the development of advanced pulse sequences (S. Yang et al., 2008; C. Choi et al., 2010), allows independent measurement of glutamate and glutamine in man, and offers new possibilities for studying neuronal metabolism and function.

Physiology

The overall content of glutamine in human brain is similar to that of other amino acids. However, its concentration in extracellular fluid is significantly higher, at approximately 0.4 mM (Kanamori and Ross, 2004). This approximates the plasma concentration of glutamine; therefore, little net glutamine exchange occurs across the blood–brain barrier under physiological conditions. Instead, most brain glutamine is synthesized by the amidation of glutamate by glutamine synthetase, an enzyme almost entirely restricted to astrocytes (Martinez-Hernandez et al., 1977). Two sources of glutamate exist for glutamine synthesis: first, *de novo* synthesis from the TCA cycle intermediates via α-ketoglutarate; second, uptake of glutamate released by glutamatergic neurons during synaptic transmission. Within astrocytes, glutamate synthetase is particularly expressed around glutamatergic synapses (Derouiche & Frotscher, 1991), and evidence from ^{13}C MRS studies indicates that uptake of synaptic glutamate provides up to 80–90% of the substrate for glutamine synthesis (Shen et al., 1999; see Chapters 3.11 and 4.2 for more details).

Glutamine degradation occurs mainly within neurons. Phosphate-activated glutaminase catalyzes its deamidation to glutamate, which is then used for neurotransmission or energy metabolism through the TCA cycle. Within GABAergic neurons, glutamate is also used for GABA synthesis by glutamic acid decarboxylase. Although neurons are able to synthesize glutamate from α-ketoglutarate, they are unable to replenish the TCA cycle intermediates used for this, as they lack pyruvate carboxylase, which links glycolysis to the TCA cycle by catalyzing the synthesis of oxaloacetate (Shank et al., 1985). As a consequence of this, neuronal glutamate synthesis is dependent on the uptake of glutamine released by astrocytes. The concept of the glutamate–glutamine cycle has therefore been developed, in which glutamate is synthesized within astrocytes from TCA cycle intermediates generated through glycolysis, converted to glutamine, and released into the extracellular space. Following uptake by neurons, it is used for glutamate synthesis, and released during neurotransmission. Astrocytes then use glutamate cleared from the synaptic space to resynthesize glutamine. A similar GABA–glutamine cycle is believed to operate at GABAergic synapses. (see Chapter 3.11 for more details.)

As the main source for glutamine synthesis is glutamate released during neurotransmission, the rate of the glutamate–glutamine cycle is proportional to the activity of glutamatergic neurons. However, because the cycle requires the active transport of glutamate and glutamine against a concentration gradient, an increase in the rate of the cycle must be matched by an increased energy supply. Studies using MRS to track the metabolism of ^{13}C-labeled glucose show that changes in the cycle rate are closely matched by changes in the rate of astrocytic glycolysis (Sibson et al., 1997, 1998), apparently in response to activation of the Na^+/K^+-ATPase following Na^+-coupled uptake of glutamate. The resulting increase in glycolysis generates ATP, to support glutamate uptake, and lactate, which may be released by astrocytes for use by neurons as an energy source (Pellerin & Magistretti, 1994). Since this metabolic cooperation is required to maintain glutamate uptake, and thus glutamine synthesis, changes in glutamine level in neurological disease may reflect metabolic dysfunction, as well as changes in glutamatergic synaptic activity.

As the brain lacks a urea cycle, it cannot detoxify ammonia by producing urea. Using ^{13}N labeling, it has instead been shown that glutamine synthesis from glutamate is the main fate for ammonia in the CNS (Cooper, 2012). Under physiological conditions, the main source of ammonia in the brain is the conversion of glutamine to glutamate within neurons, which is balanced by glutamine synthesis in astrocytes. However, during hyperammonemia, for example in liver failure, brain ammonia levels are increased by diffusion of ammonia from the blood. This can be compensated for by increased synthesis of glutamine, which then acts as a shuttle, transporting ammonia to the liver, where urea synthesis can occur. Consistent with this, both increased glutamine synthesis and TCA cycle activity have been demonstrated during hyperammonemia *in vivo* using ^{13}C MRS (Sibson et al., 2001). The resulting increase in brain glutamine may contribute to the pathogenesis of hyperammonemic encephalopathy (Tofteng et al., 2006).

Applications

The composite *Glx* peak has been widely used as a marker of glutamatergic neuronal activity, on the rationale that increased glutamatergic neurotransmission increases the rate of the glutamate–glutamine cycle, and thus synthesis of glutamate and glutamine from TCA cycle intermediates. With the availability of high-field MRI scanners, there is interest in the additional information gained by measuring glutamine and glutamate separately. In particular, changes in the ratio of these metabolites may indicate impairment of neurotransmitter cycling, through metabolic dysfunction of neurons or astrocytes. For example, a meta-analysis of MRS studies of the frontal cortex in schizophrenia showed no overall change in the *Glx* peak, but a significant reduction in glutamate and increase in glutamine (Marsman et al., 2013). Although abnormal glutamate signaling is thought to occur in schizophrenia, these results are more consistent with a failure of neuronal glutamate resynthesis, which would not be detected by measuring *Glx* alone. The same pattern of metabolic abnormalities has been shown in animal models of the neurodegenerative conditions, Alzheimer's dementia and Huntington's disease (Jenkins et al., 2000; J. K. Choi et al., 2010). Mitochondrial dysfunction has been suggested as a common theme in neurodegenerative disease, and given the mitochondrial location of phosphate-activated glutaminase, accumulation of glutamine, and an increase in the glutamine:glutamate ratio may represent a spectroscopic marker of this process.

Glutamine has also been investigated as a biomarker of metabolic dysfunction following stroke. In animal models of transient cerebral ischemia, a rise in glutamine has been shown to occur within 3 h of the ischemic insult, and to persist for up to 24 h (Lei et al., 2009). The size of the increase depends on the duration of ischemia, but an increase does not occur if ischemia is permanent. Raised glutamine appears therefore to be an indicator of recent reperfused ischemia (Berthet et al., 2011). A possible mechanism for this is excitotoxic glutamate release by neurons, which provides substrate for glutamine synthesis when reperfusion occurs. As a decrease in glutamate also occurs, reduced neuronal glutamine metabolism may also contribute, particularly as neurons are more vulnerable to hypoxia than glia. As these changes occur quickly following ischemia, and occur even in the absence of a structural lesion detectable by MRI, measurement of brain glutamine may have a clinical application in the diagnosis of transient ischemic attacks.

Although the increase in brain glutamine, which occurs during hyperammonemia, was originally thought to be neuroprotective, it is now accepted that this contributes to the development of encephalopathy during severe or prolonged hyperammonemia. Methionine sulfoximine, an inhibitor of glutamine synthetase, reduces metabolic abnormalities, astrocyte swelling, and mortality in hyperammonemic rats (Warren & Schenker, 1964). Glutamine accumulation within astrocytes may lead to brain edema by acting as an osmolyte; however, this seems to be balanced by efflux of other osmolytes, particularly myo-inositol and taurine. An alternative "Trojan horse" hypothesis has been proposed, whereby increased mitochondrial glutamine transport and metabolism leads to intramitochondrial ammonia accumulation, generation of reactive oxygen species, and mitochondrial permeability transition (Albrecht & Norenberg, 2006). Consistent with this, inhibition of mitochondrial glutamine uptake with L-histidine reduces brain edema in animal models (Rama Rao et al., 2010). Irrespective of the mechanism, glutamine has potential as a spectroscopic marker of hepatic encephalopathy and chronic liver disease. Kreis and colleagues (1990) first used MRS to demonstrate increased brain glutamine and reduced myo-inositol in a patient with hepatic encephalopathy, also observing smaller changes in two less severely affected patients. This finding has been confirmed in larger populations, with the size of the change in glutamine correlating both with the clinical grading of encephalopathy, and with MRI measures of brain edema (Laubenberger et al., 1997; Córdoba et al., 2001). Glutamine is increased in patients with subclinical encephalopathy compared to controls, suggesting that metabolic abnormalities occur early in liver disease. Given recent advances in MRS, it may soon be possible to detect subtle changes in glutamine in pre-encephalopathic patients, providing diagnostic and prognostic information. As abnormalities in glutamine are corrected by liver transplantation, it may also be useful as a biomarker for response to treatment (Córdoba et al., 2001).

LACTATE

Lactate is a three-carbon product ($CH_3CH(OH)COO^-$) of the glycolytic metabolism of glucose and is an essential intermediate of energy metabolism. Brain lactate can be measured *in vivo* using proton MRS. The three methyl-hydrogen groups give rise to a doublet signal at 1.32 ppm when measured using conventional ^{1}H MRS methods, as well as an additional quartet at 4.10 ppm, although this smaller resonance is rarely detected *in vivo* samples due to overlapping resonances from more concentrated metabolites. Brain lactate is elevated in conditions involving increased neural activation, in proportion to the degree of glutamatergic activity (Hu & Wilson, 1997; Pellerin et al., 1997). However, elevated brain lactate in the absence of increased activation is believed to be a marker of major pathology.

Physiology

Glycolysis

Glycolysis is the process that describes the breakdown of glucose (sugar) or glycogen (stored carbohydrate). Glucose and glycogen are the substrates for aerobic and anaerobic glycolysis. Glucose is transported into the cell via transporter proteins in the plasma membranes (e.g., GLUT-4 in skeletal muscle, GLUT-1 in the brain). During glycolysis the carboxylic acid, nicotinamide adenine dinucleotide (NAD+), is reduced to NADH, but this must be regenerated for glycolysis to continue. In the presence of oxygen, the NADH is oxidized to NAD+ within the mitochondria, producing pyruvate. This pyruvate is then transported into the mitochondria for complete oxidation by the Krebs cycle and the ultimate production of 36 ATP molecules through aerobic glycolysis. In cells that lack mitochondria or during hypoxia, NADH is oxidized to NAD+ in a reaction in which pyruvate is reduced to lactate, catalyzed by lactate dehydrogenase, yielding two ATP per glucose molecule (three from glycogen) while also producing protons (a process known as anaerobic glycolysis). Thus, the number of ATP molecules generated by glycolysis depends on both the substrate and the eventual fate of the pyruvate.

The lactate and protons produced in skeletal muscle during anaerobic glycolysis are removed from the cells via the Cori cycle in the liver, after which they are reconverted to glucose via gluconeogenesis. However, in the heart and brain they appear to be fully oxidized to CO_2 (Siesjo, 1978) suggesting a role for glycolysis, and thus lactate, as a major fuel in cerebral activation.

Cerebral Metabolic Ratio

At rest, the brain consumes ~20% of total body oxygen and 15% total body glucose, in stoichiometric amounts close to a 6:1 ratio, which represents complete oxidation of glucose to synthesis high energy phosphate bonds (ATP).

$$6O_2 + C_6H_{12}O_6 (glucose) \rightarrow 6H_2O + 6CO_2$$

Metabolic activity causes increases in cerebral blood flow, increased cerebral metabolic rate (CMR) for glucose (CMR_{glc}), and increased cerebral metabolic rate for oxygen (CMR_{O_2}). There is, however, a decoupling between CMR_{glc} and CMR_{O_2} during physiological activation (Fox et al., 1988). Studies using PET imaging (Mintun et al., 2002) and, more recently, using blood oxygenation level-dependent functional MRI (A. Lin et al., 2010) observed the CMR_{glc} to increases within the region of ~30–50% with visual stimulation, greatly out of proportion to a ~12–17% increase in CMR_{O2}. For a review of a wider range of stimuli see Shulman et al. (2002).

$$CMR = O_2 / (glucose + \tfrac{1}{2} \, lactate)$$

The decrease in the uptake ratio indicates a surplus of nonoxidative carbohydrate uptake by the activated brain, which suggests that energy is being produced under "anaerobic" conditions, resulting in the production of lactate. This is supported by ^{1}H MRS studies, which have shown transient lactate production in the brain to occur during mental activity (Madsen et al., 1999); on exposure to a reversing checkerboard stimulus (Fox et al., 1988); on exposure to a stressful situation (such as intravenous catheterization or placement in a confined environment such as a scanner; Fox et al., 1988); and during prolonged exercise (when plasma lactate is low; Nybo et al., 2002). Lactate, however, does not accumulate in the brain, the concentration is rarely greater than 1 mM, nor is it detected in high levels in the blood leaving the brain or in CSF. This may be due to a transient production and consumption of lactate within the active brain that occurs due to an initial glycolytic processing of glucose in the astrocytes, followed by a recoupling phase during which lactate is oxidized by the neurons. The brain's lactate level does therefore appear related to activity (Prichard et al., 1991; Hu & Wilson, 1997; Shulman et al., 2001; Mintun et al., 2002; Patel et al., 2005) and one hypothesis is that during excitatory, glutamatergic activity, nonoxidative glycolysis, and thus lactate production, fuel neuronal activity. This may be explained by the astrocyte-lactate shuffle (ANLS), although other hypotheses have been proposed and at present this is a highly active research area (Dienel, 2012) and will be discussed further in the following section.

Lactate as a Neuronal Metabolite

Observations following stimulation of an excitatory brain pathway have reported a rapid reduction in the extracellular lactate concentration, followed by a rapid rise, and finally a subsequent fall toward the resting value (Hu & Wilson, 1997). This initial drop has been hypothesized to be due to the rapid uptake of lactate by the neurons. The subsequent rise is a result of glycolysis within the astrocytes, driven by the energy demand caused by the uptake of synaptically released glutamate. One potential explanation for this behavior is ANLS (Pellerin & Magistretti, 1994), but alternate explanations that are equally consistent with this data and the *in vivo* MRS data have been proposed (see Mangia et al., 2009).

The ANLS theory suggests that glucose is taken up and lactate is produced within the astrocytes, with subsequent lactate release used to "feed" the neurons during activation. This is believed to occur due to the astrocyte end feet abutting on the cerebral blood vessels (Kacem et al., 1998) and also having a high affinity for specific glucose transporters (GLUT-1; Morgello et al., 1995; Yu & Ding, 1998), thus presenting an efficient uptake site for glucose. Exposure of astrocytes to glutamate directly enhances glucose transport. In contrast, glucose uptake in the neurons is reduced by the presence of glutamate. Once taken up into the astrocytes the glucose is not oxidized, but is converted into lactate via glycolysis. This is facilitated by the key characteristic of astrocytes—they lack a mitochondrial aspartate/glutamate carrier, which decreases their capacity to reduce NADH to NAD +. To maintain glycolytic flux, cytosolic NADH is converted to NAD + through a reaction catalyzed by the lactate dehydrogenase isoform LDH5, which is preferentially expressed in astrocytes. The lactate formed is then released in the extracellular space and then taken up by the neurons, facilitated by the preferential expression on the neuron of the lactate dehydrogenase isoform LDH1. The ANLS model proposes that once in the neurons, the lactate is then fully oxidized into CO_2, fueling neuronal activity.

While the astrocytes play many functions during neurotransmission, the hypothesis about their major "feeding role" as providers of lactate to neurons remains controversial. It is still under debate whether or not lactate is the preferential substrate of neurons for neurotransmissions-related energy needs. In a revision to the ANLS model proposed by Pellerin and Magistretti in 1994, Hyder et al., 2006 used the results from *in vivo* ^{13}C and ^{14}C MRS tracer studies to further explore the coupling between synaptic activity and glucose metabolism. Based on the findings from such studies, their model proposed that glucose uptake is not specific to the astrocytes but is in fact ubiquitous, and glucose oxidation can occur in the glia. In fact, it is estimated that ~26% of glucose uptake is by the neurons and ~74% is by the glia, of which ~15–30% is oxidized. Astrocytic lactate production is still generated through some glycolysis; however, flow to

neurons is less than in the ANLS model, with a small amount being effluxed into the blood.

Lactate produced via glycolysis within astrocytes can diffuse into the neuron for oxidation without being released into the circulation (van Hall, 2010). The specific mechanism, which permits the transport of lactate across cell membranes, is provided by the monocarboxylate transporters (MCT). Fourteen different MCTs have been identified, each of which transport lactate at different K_m values (Wilson et al., 1998). The MCT2 has the highest affinity for lactate with a K_m value of ~0.7 mM, whereas the MCT4 has a lower affinity a K_m of ~35 mM. The low-affinity MCT4 is suited for export of lactate by glycolytic fibers, and in the presence of LDH5 provides optimal settings to favor lactate production and release. MCT4 is in high affinity in the astrocytes, whereas the MCT2 suited for import are found exclusively in neurones. The MCT2 in the neurons are specifically found in the postsynaptic density at glutamatergic synapses in the cerebellum (Bergersen et al., 2001) and hippocampus (Bergersen et al., 2005), suggesting that the role of the MCT2 in the brain is linked to glutamatergic synaptic transmission (Bergersen, 2007), thus neuronal activation.

The presence of the key enzyme, LDH5, and transporter, MCT4, in the astrocytes may represent an example of metabolic compartmentation in favor of glycolytic activity. Of note is the fact the glial cells produce lactate, which in turn is oxidized to carbon dioxide and water in the neurons (Pellerin, 2005), does not qualify as *anaerobic metabolism* for the brain as a whole but may reflect compartmentation of glucose/glycogen metabolism as proposed within the ANLS model. It is important to stress, however, that this remains a theory as definitive proof of nonoxidative glial glucose uptake has not yet been shown at this stage.

Lactate and Neurotransmitter Recycling

Glutamate is the main excitatory neurotransmitter of the cerebral cortex. Glutamate is released from the presynaptic neuron and crosses the synapse to bind to the postsynaptic receptor. To terminate the action of glutamate, it is transported out of the synapse into the astrocytes, where it is converted back into glutamine. The glutamine is released and taken up by the presynaptic neuron where it is converted back to glutamate. Once in the astrocytes, glutamate is converted to glutamine through an ATP-requiring reaction catalyzed by the astrocyte specific enzyme glutamate synthase (Martinez-Hernandez et al., 1977). Glutamate is then released by the astrocytes and taken up by the neurons to replenish the neurotransmitter pool of glutamate. Since glutamate uptake is driven by the electrochemical gradient of sodium ions (Na^+), which is cotransported into the astrocytes with glutamate, activation of the Na^+/K^+-ATPase is required to maintain intracellular Na^+ levels. This process is therefore energetically demanding as recycling one molecule of the neurotransmitter between the astrocytes and neurons requires the oxidation of one glucose molecule by the neuron. Thus, until further evidence is provided to the contrary, the process which provides the ATP needed to restore Na^+ gradients due to neurotransmitter cycling and glutamine synthesis is glial glycolysis (Magistretti & Pellerin, 1999; Hyder et al., 2006). This process stimulates an increase in glucose uptake within the astrocytes and thus glycolytic energy production and lactate release. The increased lactate concentration under conditions of increased brain activity (Prichard et al., 1991) and in the presence of plentiful oxygen suggests that the rapid energy requirements for the removal of glutamate from the extracellular space cannot be met by normal oxidative metabolism (which proceeds more slowly; Shulman et al., 2001). The essential hypothesis is that only glycolytic ATP (in glia) is produced rapidly enough to clear glutamate from the extracellular space in the time needed to prepare the synapse for the next synaptic event. Interestingly, proposed mathematical models of compartmentalized metabolism of glucose (Aubert & Costalat, 2005; Aubert et al., 2005) have estimated that the astrocyte release, and neuronal uptake of lactate should occur within the first 30 s of neurotransmission. When considering the transient increase in tissue lactate during prolonged stimulation (Frahm et al., 1996) this may be providing support for the ANLS only during the early response to stimulation (Mangia et al., 2009). Based on this assumption, and data to suggest that the astrocytes oxidize the pyruvate produced during glycolysis (Hyder et al., 2006), it may appear that the relative uptake of glucose by the glia is to support functional activity (Oz et al., 2004; Cruz et al., 2005) as well as neurotransmitter cycling and glutamate synthesis.

MRS Applications

Although the concentration of lactate in the brain is at the low end of the MRS sensitivity range, ^{1}H MRS procedures at low fields (using spectral editing methods; Hanstock et al., 1988; Star-Lack et al., 1998; Maddock et al., 2009) and at high fields (Mangia et al., 2007b; Mekle et al., 2009) can reliably measure lactate levels in the brain both at rest and in response to metabolic challenges (Prichard et al., 1991; Dager et al., 1997; Mangia et al., 2007a). The methyl groups (CH3) give rise to a "doublet" 1.32 ppm, which can be detected in a clinical ^{1}H MRS platform. The methylene resonances detected by lipids, however, are centered very close the lactate resonance (1.3 ppm), which

means that some adjustments to standard clinical MRS sequencing are required in order to distinguish between them (Garcia-Martin et al., 2001; Drost et al., 2002). Large voxel sizes and long acquisition times are often used in order to optimize the lactate signal (Maddock & Buonocore, 2012). Changes in the lactate signal intensity at long TE, however, may correspond to the lactate changes predominantly in the extracellular space and/or changes in its relaxation properties rather than to changes in total lactate concentration per se. This can be overcome by using ultrashort TE sequencing with brain macromolecule suppression (Behar et al., 1994) at high resolution, which offers the benefits of more precise metabolite quantification including those with short T_2 relaxation times and increased signal-to-noise ratio (SNR; Mekle et al., 2009). Thus the best conditions to optimize the lactate signal with ^{1}H MRS is the use of specialized lipid suppression pulses with short TE at high fields or long TE with spectral editing at lower fields where less spectral resolution is available. Other considerations to optimize the sensitivity are to use larger voxel sizes, to increase the SNR, and, when scanning at high resolution (4 T or greater), to use surface or half-volume radiofrequency (RF) coils that will allow greater signal sensitivity (Maddock & Buonocore, 2012).

As it is technically challenging to accurately quantify metabolite concentration using MRS, brain lactate, like other metabolites, is usually reported in relation to the phospho-creatine and/or creatine MRS peaks, of which lactate is usually around 10% at rest. A recent study of spectra acquired at 7T however attempted metabolite quantification and reported an absolute brain lactate value of around 0.7 μMol.g^{-1}·min^{-1} at rest (Mekle et al., 2009).

MRS in Pathology

The concentration of lactate within the brain is rarely greater than 1 mM, thus when independent of an experimental paradigm designed to activate a specific brain region, an elevated lactate to creatine ratio observed during MRS is indicative of pathology. The appearance of an obvious lactate peak may suggest ischemia (Bruhn et al., 1989; Duijn et al., 1992), tumor (Alger et al., 1990; Herholz et al., 1992; Sijens et al., 1994), trauma (Chen et al., 2012), infection (Dusak et al., 2012), epilepsy (A. Lin et al., 2005), mitochondrial disease (A. Lin et al., 2005), or other pathological processes (Maddock & Buonocore, 2012). In fact, both lipids and lactate are released with cell destruction and necrosis (Lindskog et al., 2005; Sibtain et al., 2007). Lactate and lipids peaks are generally present in aggressive disease processes (Wirt, 2003).

In neuropsychology, patients with panic disorder exhibit an exaggerated visual cortex lactate response to visual stimulation. It is hypothesized that during the temporary accumulation of lactate in the extracellular fluid as occurs during activation, when the lactate produced in the astrocytes is transferred to the neurons, lactate accumulation in the brain regions that mediate fear and arousal may play a role in triggering spontaneous panic attacks (Maddock et al., 2009).

MRS during Neural Activation

^{1}H MRS studies of visual stimulation have shown increases of 25–100% in brain lactate levels with a decline to baseline during prolonged visual stimulation (Prichard et al., 1991; Sappey-Marinier et al., 1992; Frahm et al., 1996). Mangia and colleagues (Mangia, et al., 2007a) set out to quantify the time course of metabolite concentration in the human visual cortex during sustained visual stimulation. Using high-resolution 7 T imaging and a half-volume RF coil with increased local sensitivity to the visual cortex, two paradigms of continued visual stimulation (~5 and 10 min) resulted in lactate increases by 0.2 μmol/g (~30%) within first minutes of activation, reaching a new steady state and returned to baseline only after the end of the stimulation period. In a similar paradigm, Lin and colleagues (2012) also observed an increased lactate of ~26% after ~6 min of stimulation, this, however, returned to baseline after this time period despite continued stimulation. The authors suggested that the differences between these two studies may reflect differences in the task, the scanning sequence, or the neurons excited, but also hypothesized that, because of the permeability of the blood–brain barrier to lactate; the increase observed during stimulation could also lead to an increased efflux of lactate to the blood. This would account for decreased brain lactate levels recorded during continued visual stimulation. Lactate export to the extracellular compartment is believed to occur ~30–60s after onset of stimulation (de Boer et al., 1991). The observed peak thus represents a balance between production and efflux for metabolism. It is also possible that changes in brain lactate observed with visual stimulation reflect changes in its utilization as energy substrate by neurons (Hu & Wilson, 1997). While the exact time course of an increase in brain lactate during visual stimulation, the attainment of a new "steady state," exists is still under debate, ^{1}H MRS has been shown to be a powerful tool for investigated brain metabolism during mental activity in vivo.

MRS following Exercise

The brain at rest exhibits a net efflux of lactate, and the venous concentration is higher than the arterial. Net cerebral lactate uptake can occur, however, in conditions when arterial lactate is increased, e.g., during hypoglycemia (Lubow et al., 2006), high-intensity exercise (Ide et al., 2000), or during experimental intravenous infusion of sodium lactate (Dager et al., 1992, 1994). Thus, like skeletal muscle, the brain may consume plasma lactate when it is in ample supply, as has been shown recently using ^{13}C MRS (Boumezbeur et al., 2010). Boumezbeur and coworkers also showed that plasma lactate is metabolized by neurons and glia similarly to glucose and that the brain transport capacity was sufficient for lactate to supply over 60% of brain oxidative needs. Under such conditions, lactate is included in the CMR, as it is taken up by the neurons to fuel brain function (van Hall et al., 2009).

During high-intensity exercise cerebral carbohydrate delivery exceeds demand, but glucose uptake does not depend on arterial glucose concentration. Brain lactate uptake, however, does appear to be driven proportionally to arterial concentration, in the presence of elevated adrenaline (Seifert et al., 2009), which doubles both cerebral blood flow and CMR_{O_2} and also facilitates the transport of lactate across the blood–brain barrier (Seifert et al., 2009). Thus under certain conditions, lactate uptake from the blood may be preferential to glucose, possibly "sparing" brain glucose metabolism (Kemppainen et al., 2005; Rasmussen et al., 2008). The increase in brain lactate, however, is far smaller ($\sim 0.7–1.3$ mM.L.min^{-1}) than the increase in blood lactate (Maddock et al., 2011). It also returns to baseline much more quickly; however, no net release of lactate is observed even during very late recovery. The small increase in brain lactate following vigorous exercise, despite the large increase in plasma lactate, represents substantial clearance of lactate by the brain during exercise (van Hall et al., 2009). The low CMR, however, indicates that a large surplus of carbohydrates is taken up by the brain, which is likely to be more than can be oxidized within neurons to pyruvate (Dalsgaard, 2006; Volianitis et al., 2008).

A possible fate for the excess lactate taken up by the brain during vigorous exercise not used for neuronal metabolism (Hertz & Fillenz, 1999; Dalsgaard, 2006; Secher et al., 2006) may be a net shift between the catabolism and synthesis of amino acids. Animal studies have suggested that exercise has a major effect on brain glutamatergic systems (van Praag, 2009) and that whole-brain levels of glutamate and glutamine are significantly increased after vigorous exercise (Guezennec et al., 1998; Miyazaki et al., 2003). An MRS study at 1.5 T examined the change in lactate and a combined measure of glutamate and glutamine (Glx) following vigorous exercise. Using an edited ^{1}H MRS method with a voxel placed in the visual cortex, the authors reported a sustained increase in brain lactate (19%) following exercise and a transient 18% increase in brain in Glx. The change in lactate, however, was too small to account for the excess nonoxidized CHO typically taken up during exercise, but the increase in Glx may represent an activity-dependent increase in glutamate. The authors acknowledged that the results may, in part, also be due to neural activation from the visual cortex. Exercise has been shown to produce widespread cerebral metabolic activation (Fukuyama et al., 1997; Delp et al., 2001) possibly reflecting the "mental effort" to exercise, thus the effect of the increased lactate availability and the increased lactate demand are difficult to distinguish.

CONCLUSIONS

The number of neurochemicals visible via MRS approaches is increasing with the increasing availability of advanced editing approaches or ultrahigh field MR systems. As these are increasingly investigated for both clinical and neuroscientific applications, their utility as markers of specific processes within the CNS is increasing.

References

Albrecht, J., & Norenberg, M. D. (2006). Glutamine: a Trojan horse in ammonia neurotoxicity. *Hepatology, 44*(4), 788–794.

Alger, J. R., Frank, J. A., Bizzi, A., Fulham, M. J., DeSouza, B. X., Duhaney, M. O., et al. (1990). Metabolism of human gliomas: assessment with H-1 MR spectroscopy and F-18 fluorodeoxyglucose PET. *Radiology, 177*(3), 633–641.

Allison, J. H., Blisner, M. E., Holland, W. H., Hipps, P. P., & Sherman, W. R. (1976). Increased brain myo-inositol 1-phosphate in lithium-treated rats. *Biochemical Biophysical Research Communications, 71*(2), 664–670.

Allison, J. H., & Stewart, M. A. (1971). Reduced brain inositol in lithium-treated rats. *Nature New Biology, 233*(43), 267–268.

Asada, H., Kawamura, Y., Maruyama, K., Kume, H., Ding, R. G., Kanbara, N., et al. (1997). Cleft palate and decreased brain gamma-aminobutyric acid in mice lacking the 67-kDa isoform of glutamic acid decarboxylase. *Proceedings of the National Academy of Sciences USA, 94*(12), 6496–6499.

Aubert, A., & Costalat, R. (2005). Interaction between astrocytes and neurons studied using a mathematical model of compartmentalized energy metabolism. *Journal of Cerebral Blood Flow and Metabolism, 25*(11), 1476–1490.

Aubert, A., Costalat, R., Magistretti, P. J., & Pellerin, L. (2005). Brain lactate kinetics: Modeling evidence for neuronal lactate uptake upon activation. *Proceedings of the National Academy of Sciences USA, 102*(45), 16448–16453.

Behar, K. L., Rothman, D. L., Spencer, D. D., & Petroff, O. A. (1994). Analysis of macromolecule resonances in 1H NMR spectra of human brain. *Magnetic Resonance in Medicine, 32*(3), 294–302.

Belelli, D., Harrison, N. L., Maguire, J., Macdonald, R. L., Walker, M. C., & Cope, D. W. (2009). Extrasynaptic GABAA receptors: form, pharmacology, and function. *Journal of Neuroscience, 29*(41), 12757–12763.

Bergersen, L., Waerhaug, O., Helm, J., Thomas, M., Laake, P., Davies, A. J., et al. (2001). A novel postsynaptic density protein: the monocarboxylate transporter MCT2 is co-localized with delta-glutamate receptors in postsynaptic densities of parallel fiber-Purkinje cell synapses. *Experimental Brain Research, 136*(4), 523–534.

Bergersen, L. H. (2007). Is lactate food for neurons? Comparison of monocarboxylate transporter subtypes in brain and muscle. *Neuroscience, 145*(1), 11–19.

Bergersen, L. H., Magistretti, P. J., & Pellerin, L. (2005). Selective postsynaptic co-localization of MCT2 with AMPA receptor GluR2/3 subunits at excitatory synapses exhibiting AMPA receptor trafficking. *Cerebral Cortex, 15*(4), 361–370.

Berridge, M. J., Downes, C. P., & Hanley, M. R. (1989). Neural and developmental actions of lithium: a unifying hypothesis. *Cell, 59*(3), 411–419.

Berry, G., Buccafusca, R., Greer, J., & Eccleston, E. (2004). Phosphoinositide deficiency due to inositol depletion is not a mechanism of lithium action in brain. *Molecular Genetics and Metabolism, 82*(1), 87–92.

Berthet, C., Lei, H., Gruetter, R., & Hirt, L. (2011). Early predictive biomarkers for lesion after transient cerebral ischemia. *Stroke, 42*(3), 799–805.

Bissonnette, P., Lahjouji, K., Coady, M. J., & Lapointe, J. Y. (2008). Effects of hyperosmolarity on the Na+ -myo-inositol cotransporter SMIT2 stably transfected in the Madin-Darby canine kidney cell line. *American Journal of Physiology Cell Physiology, 295*(3), C791–799.

Bitsch, A., Bruhn, H., Vougioukas, V., Stringaris, A., Lassmann, H., Frahm, J., et al. (1999). Inflammatory CNS demyelination: histopathologic correlation with in vivo quantitative proton MR spectroscopy. *American Journal of Neuroradiology, 20*(9), 1619–1627.

Boumezbeur, F., Petersen, K. F., Cline, G. W., Mason, G. F., Behar, K. L., Shulman, G. I., et al. (2010). The contribution of blood lactate to brain energy metabolism in humans measured by dynamic 13C nuclear magnetic resonance spectroscopy. *Journal of Neuroscience, 30*(42), 13983–13991.

Brand, A., Richter-Landsberg, C., & Leibfritz, D. (1993). Multinuclear NMR studies on the energy metabolism of glial and neuronal cells. *Developmental Neuroscience, 15*(3–5), 289–298.

Bruhn, H., Frahm, J., Gyngell, M. L., Merboldt, K. D., Hanicke, W., & Sauter, R. (1989). Cerebral metabolism in man after acute stroke: new observations using localized proton NMR spectroscopy. *Magnetic Resonance in Med, 9*(1), 126–131.

Castillo, M., Smith, J. K., & Kwock, L. (2000). Correlation of myo-inositol levels and grading of cerebral astrocytomas. *American Journal of Neuroradiology, 21*(9), 1645–1649.

Chen, J., Jin, H., Zhang, Y., Liang, Q., Liao, H., Guo, Z., et al. (2012). MRS and diffusion tensor image in mild traumatic brain injuries. *Asian Pacific Journal of Tropical Medicine, 5*(1), 67–70.

Chesler, M., & Kaila, K. (1992). Modulation of pH by neuronal activity. *Trends in Neuroscience, 15*(10), 396–402.

Choi, C., Dimitrov, I. E., Douglas, D., Patel, A., Kaiser, L. G., Amezcua, C. A., et al. (2010). Improvement of resolution for brain coupled metabolites by optimized (1)H MRS at 7T. *NMR in Biomedicine, 23*(9), 1044–1052.

Choi, J. K., Jenkins, B. G., Carreras, I., Kaymakcalan, S., Cormier, K., Kowall, N. W., et al. (2010). Anti-inflammatory treatment in AD mice protects against neuronal pathology. *Experimental Neurology, 223*(2), 377–384.

Coady, M. J., Wallendorff, B., Gagnon, D. G., & Lapointe, J. Y. (2002). Identification of a novel Na+ /myo-inositol cotransporter. *Journal of Biology and Chemistry, 277*(38), 35219–35224.

Cooper, A. J. (2012). The role of glutamine synthetase and glutamate dehydrogenase in cerebral ammonia homeostasis. *Neurochemical Research, 37*(11), 2439–2455.

Córdoba, J., Alonso, J., Rovira, A., Jacas, C., Sanpedro, F., Castells, L., et al. (2001). The development of low-grade cerebral edema in cirrhosis is supported by the evolution of (1)H-magnetic resonance abnormalities after liver transplantation. *Journal of Hepatology*, 35(5), 598–604.

Cruz, N., Lasater, A, Zielke, HR, & Dienel, GA. (2005). Activation of astrocytes in brain of conscious rats during acoustic stimulation: acetate utilisation in working brain. *Journal of Neurochemistry*, 92, 934–947.

Dager, S. R., Friedman, S. D., Parow, A., Demopulos, C., Stoll, A. L., Lyoo, I. K., et al. (2004). Brain metabolic alterations in medication-free patients with bipolar disorder. *Archives of General Psychiatry*, 61(5), 450–458.

Dager, S. R., Marro, K. I., Richards, T. L., & Metzger, G. D. (1992). MRS detection of whole brain lactate rise during 1 M sodium lactate infusion in rats. *Biological Psychiatry*, 32(10), 913–921.

Dager, S. R., Marro, K. I., Richards, T. L., & Metzger, G. D. (1994). Preliminary application of magnetic resonance spectroscopy to investigate lactate-induced panic. *American Journal of Psychiatry*, 151(1), 57–63.

Dager, S. R., Richards, T., Strauss, W., & Artru, A. (1997). Single-voxel 1H-MRS investigation of brain metabolic changes during lactate-induced panic. *Psychiatry Research*, 76(2-3), 89–99.

Dalsgaard, M. K. (2006). Fuelling cerebral activity in exercising man. *Journal of Cerebral Blood Flow and Metabolism*, 26(6), 731–750.

Davanzo, P., Thomas, M. A., Yue, K., Oshiro, T., Belin, T., Strober, M., et al. (2001). Decreased anterior cingulate myo-inositol/creatine spectroscopy resonance with lithium treatment in children with bipolar disorder. *Neuropsychopharmacology*, 24(4), 359–369.

Davanzo, P., Yue, K., Thomas, M. A., Belin, T., Mintz, J., Venkatraman, T. N., et al. (2003). Proton magnetic resonance spectroscopy of bipolar disorder versus intermittent explosive disorder in children and adolescents. *American Journal of Psychiatry*, 160(8), 1442–1452.

de Boer, J., Postema, F., Plijter-Groendijk, H., & Korf, J. (1991). Continuous monitoring of extracellular lactate concentration by microdialysis lactography for the study of rat muscle metabolism in vivo. *Pflugers Archiv*, 419(1), 1–6.

Delp, M. D., Armstrong, R. B., Godfrey, D. A., Laughlin, M. H., Ross, C. D., & Wilkerson, M. K. (2001). Exercise increases blood flow to locomotor, vestibular, cardiorespiratory and visual regions of the brain in miniature swine. *Journal of Physiology*, 533(Pt 3), 849–859.

Derouiche, A., & Frotscher, M. (1991). Astroglial processes around identified glutamatergic synapses contain glutamine synthetase: evidence for transmitter degradation. *Brain Research*, 552(2), 346–350.

Dienel, G. A. (2012). Brain lactate metabolism: the discoveries and the controversies. *Journal of Cerebral Blood Flow and Metabolism*, 32(7), 1107–1138.

Drost, D. J., Riddle, W. R., & Clarke, G. D. (2002). Proton magnetic resonance spectroscopy in the brain: report of AAPM MR Task Group #9. *Medical Physics*, 29(9), 2177–2197.

Duarte, J. M., Lei, H., Mlynárik, V., & Gruetter, R. (2012). The neurochemical profile quantified by in vivo 1H NMR spectroscopy. *Neuroimage*, 61(2), 342–362.

Duijn, J. H., Matson, G. B., Maudsley, A. A., Hugg, J. W., & Weiner, M. W. (1992). Human brain infarction: proton MR spectroscopy. *Radiology*, 183(3), 711–718.

Dusak, A., Hakyemez, B., Kocaeli, H., & Bekar, A. (2012). Magnetic resonance spectroscopy findings of pyogenic, tuberculous, and Cryptococcus intracranial abscesses. *Neurochemical Research*, 37(2), 233–237.

Erlander, M. G., Tillakaratne, N. J., Feldblum, S., Patel, N., & Tobin, A. J. (1991). Two genes encode distinct glutamate decarboxylases. *Neuron*, 7(1), 91–100.

Fisher, J. L., & Macdonald, R. L. (1997). Single channel properties of recombinant GABAA receptors containing gamma 2 or delta subtypes expressed with alpha 1 and beta 3 subtypes in mouse L929 cells. *Journal of Physiology*, 505(Pt 2), 283–297.

Fisher, S., Novak, J., & Agranoff, B. (2002). Inositol and higher inositol phosphates in neural tissues: homeostasis, metabolism and functional significance. *Journal of Neurochemistry*, 82(4), 736–754.

Fox, P. T., Raichle, M. E., Mintun, M. A., & Dence, C. (1988). Nonoxidative glucose consumption during focal physiologic neural activity. *Science*, 241(4864), 462–464.

Frahm, J., Kruger, G., Merboldt, K. D., & Kleinschmidt, A. (1996). Dynamic uncoupling and recoupling of perfusion and oxidative metabolism during focal brain activation in man. *Magnetic Resonance in Medicine*, 35(2), 143–148.

Frye, M. A., Watzl, J., Banakar, S., O'Neill, J., Mintz, J., Davanzo, P., et al. (2007). Increased anterior cingulate/medial prefrontal cortical glutamate and creatine in bipolar depression. *Neuropsychopharmacology*, 32(12), 2490–2499.

Fu, H., Li, B., Hertz, L., & Peng, L. (2012). Contributions in astrocytes of SMIT1/2 and HMIT to myo-inositol uptake at different concentrations and pH. *Neurochemistry International*, 61(2), 187–194.

Fukuyama, H., Ouchi, Y., Matsuzaki, S., Nagahama, Y., Yamauchi, H., Ogawa, M., et al. (1997). Brain functional activity during gait in normal subjects: a SPECT study. *Neuroscience Letters*, 228(3), 183–186.

Garcia-Martin, M. L., Herigault, G., Remy, C., Farion, R., Ballesteros, P., Coles, J. A., et al. (2001). Mapping extracellular pH in rat brain gliomas in vivo by 1H magnetic resonance spectroscopic imaging: comparison with maps of metabolites. *Cancer Research*, 61(17), 6524–6531.

Gassmann, M., & Bettler, B. (2012). Regulation of neuronal GABAB receptor functions by subunit composition. *Nature Reviews Neuroscience*, 13(6), 380–394.

Glanville, N. T., Byers, D. M., Cook, H. W., Spence, M. W., & Palmer, F. B. (1989). Differences in the metabolism of inositol and phosphoinositides by cultured cells of neuronal and glial origin. *Biochimica Biophysica Acta*, 1004(2), 169–179.

Greif, K. F., Erlander, M. G., Tillakaratne, N. J., & Tobin, A. J. (1991). Postnatal expression of glutamate decarboxylases in developing rat cerebellum. *Neurochemical Research*, 16(3), 235–242.

Greif, K. F., Tillakaratne, N. J., Erlander, M. G., Feldblum, S., & Tobin, A. J. (1992). Transient increase in expression of a glutamate decarboxylase (GAD) mRNA during the postnatal development of the rat striatum. *Developmental Biology*, 153(1), 158–164.

Guezennec, C. Y., Abdelmalki, A., Serrurier, B., Merino, D., Bigard, X., Berthelot, M., et al. (1998). Effects of prolonged exercise on brain ammonia and amino acids. *International Journal of Sports Medicine*, 19(5), 323–327.

Haas, K. F., & Macdonald, R. L. (1999). GABAA receptor subunit gamma2 and delta subtypes confer unique kinetic properties on recombinant GABAA receptor currents in mouse fibroblasts. *Journal of Physiology*, 514(Pt 1), 27–45.

Hager, K., Hazama, A., Kwon, H. M., Loo, D. D., Handler, J. S., & Wright, E. M. (1995). Kinetics and specificity of the renal Na + / myo-inositol cotransporter expressed in Xenopus oocytes. *Journal of Membrane Biology*, 143(2), 103–113.

Hanstock, C. C., Rothman, D. L., Prichard, J. W., Jue, T., & Shulman, R. G. (1988). Spatially localized 1H NMR spectra of metabolites in the human brain. *Proceedings of the National Academy of Sciences USA*, 85(6), 1821–1825.

Herholz, K., Heindel, W., Luyten, P. R., denHollander, J. A., Pietrzyk, U., Voges, J., et al. (1992). In vivo imaging of glucose consumption and lactate concentration in human gliomas. *Annals of Neurology*, 31(3), 319–327.

Hertz, L., & Fillenz, M. (1999). Does the 'mystery of the extra glucose' during CNS activation reflect glutamate synthesis? *Neurochemistry International*, 34(1), 71–75.

Hu, Y., & Wilson, G. S. (1997). A temporary local energy pool coupled to neuronal activity: fluctuations of extracellular lactate levels in rat brain monitored with rapid-response enzyme-based sensor. *Journal of Neurochemistry, 69*(4), 1484−1490.

Hyde, J. C., & Robinson, N. (1976). Electron cytochemical localization of gamma-aminobutyric acid catabolism in rat cerebellar cortex. *Histochemistry, 49*(1), 51−65.

Hyder, F., Patel, A. B., Gjedde, A., Rothman, D. L., Behar, K. L., & Shulman, R. G. (2006). Neuronal-glial glucose oxidation and glutamatergic-GABAergic function. *Journal of Cerebral Blood Flow and Metabolism, 26*(7), 865−877.

Ide, K., Schmalbruch, I. K., Quistorff, B., Horn, A., & Secher, N. H. (2000). Lactate, glucose and O2 uptake in human brain during recovery from maximal exercise. *Journal of Physiology, 522*(Pt 1), 159−164.

Jackson, P. S., & Strange, K. (1993). Volume-sensitive anion channels mediate swelling-activated inositol and taurine efflux. *American Journal of Physiology, 265*(6 Pt 1), C1489−1500.

Jenkins, B. G., Klivenyi, P., Kustermann, E., Andreassen, O. A., Ferrante, R. J., Rosen, B. R., et al. (2000). Nonlinear decrease over time in N-acetyl aspartate levels in the absence of neuronal loss and increases in glutamine and glucose in transgenic Huntington's disease mice. *Journal of Neurochemistry, 74*(5), 2108−2119.

Ji, F., Kanbara, N., & Obata, K. (1999). GABA and histogenesis in fetal and neonatal mouse brain lacking both the isoforms of glutamic acid decarboxylase. *Neuroscience Research, 33*(3), 187−194.

Kacem, K., Lacombe, P., Seylaz, J., & Bonvento, G. (1998). Structural organization of the perivascular astrocyte endfeet and their relationship with the endothelial glucose transporter: a confocal microscopy study. *Glia, 23*(1), 1−10.

Kanamori, K., & Ross, B. D. (2004). Quantitative determination of extracellular glutamine concentration in rat brain, and its elevation in vivo by system A transport inhibitor, α-(methylamino) isobutyrate. *Journal of Neurochemistry, 90*(1), 203−210.

Kemppainen, J., Aalto, S., Fujimoto, T., Kalliokoski, K. K., Langsjo, J., Oikonen, V., et al. (2005). High intensity exercise decreases global brain glucose uptake in humans. *Journal of Physiology, 568*(Pt 1), 323−332.

Kim, H., McGrath, B. M., & Silverstone, P. H. (2005). A review of the possible relevance of inositol and the phosphatidylinositol second messenger system (PI-cycle) to psychiatric disorders−focus on magnetic resonance spectroscopy (MRS) studies. *Human Psychopharmacology, 20*(5), 309−326.

Kim, J. P., Lentz, M. R., Westmoreland, S. V., Greco, J. B., Ratai, E. M., Halpern, E., et al. (2005). Relationships between astrogliosis and 1H MR spectroscopic measures of brain choline/creatine and myo-inositol/creatine in a primate model. *American Journal of Neuroradiology, 26*(4), 752−759.

Klaus, F., Palmada, M., Lindner, R., Laufer, J., Jeyaraj, S., Lang, F., et al. (2008). Up-regulation of hypertonicity-activated myo-inositol transporter SMIT1 by the cell volume-sensitive protein kinase SGK1. *Journal of Physiology, 586*(6), 1539−1547.

Kreis, R., Farrow, N., & Ross, B. D. (1990). Diagnosis of hepatic encephalopathy by proton magnetic resonance spectroscopy. *Lancet, 336*(8715), 635−636.

Kwon, H. M., Yamauchi, A., Uchida, S., Preston, A. S., Garcia-Perez, A., Burg, M. B., et al. (1992). Cloning of the cDNa for a Na + / myo-inositol cotransporter, a hypertonicity stress protein. *Journal of Biological Chemistry, 267*(9), 6297−6301.

Laubenberger, J., Häussinger, D., Bayer, S., Gufler, H., Hennig, J., & Langer, M. (1997). Proton magnetic resonance spectroscopy of the brain in symptomatic and asymptomatic patients with liver cirrhosis. *Gastroenterology, 112*(5), 1610−1616.

Lei, H., Berthet, C., Hirt, L., & Gruetter, R. (2009). Evolution of the neurochemical profile after transient focal cerebral ischemia in the mouse brain. *Journal of Cerebral Blood Flow and Metabolism, 29*(4), 811−819.

Lien, Y. H., Shapiro, J. I., & Chan, L. (1990). Effects of hypernatremia on organic brain osmoles. *Journal of Clinical Investigation, 85*(5), 1427−1435.

Lin, A., Ross, B. D., Harris, K., & Wong, W. (2005). Efficacy of proton magnetic resonance spectroscopy in neurological diagnosis and neurotherapeutic decision making. *NeuroRx, 2*(2), 197−214.

Lin, A. L., Fox, P. T., Hardies, J., Duong, T. Q., & Gao, J. H. (2010). Nonlinear coupling between cerebral blood flow, oxygen consumption, and ATP production in human visual cortex. *Proceedings of the National Academy of Sciences USA, 107*(18), 8446−8451.

Lin, Y., Stephenson, M. C., Xin, L., Napolitano, A., & Morris, P. G. (2012). Investigating the metabolic changes due to visual stimulation using functional proton magnetic resonance spectroscopy at 7 T. *Journal of Cerebral Blood Flow and Metabolism, 32*(8), 1484−1495.

Lindskog, M., Spenger, C., Klason, T., Jarvet, J., Graslund, A., Johnsen, J. I., et al. (2005). Proton magnetic resonance spectroscopy in neuroblastoma: current status, prospects and limitations. *Cancer Letters, 228*(1−2), 247−255.

Lubow, J. M., Pinon, I. G., Avogaro, A., Cobelli, C., Treeson, D. M., Mandeville, K. A., et al. (2006). Brain oxygen utilization is unchanged by hypoglycemia in normal humans: lactate, alanine, and leucine uptake are not sufficient to offset energy deficit. *American Journal of Physiology, Endocrinology and Metabolism, 290* (1), E149−E153.

Maddock, R. J., & Buonocore, M. H. (2012). MR Spectroscopic Studies of the Brain in Psychiatric Disorders. *Current Topics in Behavioral Neuroscience*in press

Maddock, R. J., Buonocore, M. H., Copeland, L. E., & Richards, A. L. (2009). Elevated brain lactate responses to neural activation in panic disorder: a dynamic 1H-MRS study. *Molecular Psychiatry, 14* (5), 537−545.

Maddock, R. J., Casazza, G. A., Buonocore, M. H., & Tanase, C. (2011). Vigorous exercise increases brain lactate and Glx (glutamate + glutamine): a dynamic 1H-MRS study. *Neuroimage, 57*(4), 1324−1330.

Madsen, P. L., Cruz, N. F., Sokoloff, L., & Dienel, G. A. (1999). Cerebral oxygen/glucose ratio is low during sensory stimulation and rises above normal during recovery: excess glucose consumption during stimulation is not accounted for by lactate efflux from or accumulation in brain tissue. *Journal of Cerebral Blood Flow and Metabolism, 19*(4), 393−400.

Magistretti, P. J., & Pellerin, L. (1999). Cellular mechanisms of brain energy metabolism and their relevance to functional brain imaging. *Philosophical Transactions of the Royal Society London B Biological Sciences, 354*(1387), 1155−1163.

Mangia, S., Giove, F., Tkac, I., Logothetis, N. K., Henry, P. G., Olman, C. A., et al. (2009). Metabolic and hemodynamic events after changes in neuronal activity: current hypotheses, theoretical predictions and in vivo NMR experimental findings. *Journal of Cerebral Blood Flow and Metabolism, 29*(3), 441−463.

Mangia, S., Tkac, I., Gruetter, R., Van de Moortele, P. F., Maraviglia, B., & Ugurbil, K. (2007a). Sustained neuronal activation raises oxidative metabolism to a new steady-state level: evidence from 1H NMR spectroscopy in the human visual cortex. *Journal of Cerebral Blood Flow and Metabolism, 27*(5), 1055−1063.

Mangia, S., Tkac, I., Logothetis, N. K., Gruetter, R., Van de Moortele, P. F., & Ugurbil, K. (2007b). Dynamics of lactate concentration and blood oxygen level-dependent effect in the human visual cortex during repeated identical stimuli. *Journal of Neuroscience Research, 85*(15), 3340−3346.

Marsman, A., van den Heuvel, M. P., Klomp, D. W., Kahn, R. S., Luijten, P. R., & Hulshoff Pol, H. E. (2013). Glutamate in schizophrenia: a focused review and meta-analysis of 1H-MRS studies. *Schizophrenia Bulletin, 39*(1), 120−129.

Martin, D. L., & Rimvall, K. (1993). Regulation of gamma-aminobutyric acid synthesis in the brain. *Journal of Neurochemistry, 60*(2), 395–407.

Martin, D. L., & Tobin, A. (2000). Mechanisms controlling GABA synthesis and degradation in the brain. In D. L. Martin, & D. L. Olsen (Eds.), *GABA in the Nervous System: The View at Fifty Years* (pp. 25–41). Philadelphia: Lippincott, Williams and Wilkins.

Martinez-Hernandez, A., Bell, K. P., & Norenberg, M. D. (1977). Glutamine synthetase: glial localization in brain. *Science, 195* (4284), 1356–1358.

Matskevitch, J., Wagner, C. A., Risler, T., Kwon, H. M., Handler, J. S., Waldegger, S., et al. (1998). Effect of extracellular pH on the myo-inositol transporter SMIT expressed in *Xenopus* oocytes. *Pflugers Archiv, 436*(6), 854–857.

Medina-Kauwe, L. K., Tillakaratne, N. J., Wu, J. Y., & Tobin, A. J. (1994). A rat brain cDNA encodes enzymatically active GABA transaminase and provides a molecular probe for GABA-catabolizing cells. *Journal of Neurochemistry, 62*(4), 1267–1275.

Mekle, R., Mlynarik, V., Gambarota, G., Hergt, M., Krueger, G., & Gruetter, R. (2009). MR spectroscopy of the human brain with enhanced signal intensity at ultrashort echo times on a clinical platform at 3T and 7T. *Magnetic Resonance in Medicine, 61*(6), 1279–1285.

Mintun, M. A., Vlassenko, A. G., Shulman, G. L., & Snyder, A. Z. (2002). Time-related increase of oxygen utilization in continuously activated human visual cortex. *Neuroimage, 16*(2), 531–537.

Miyazaki, T., Matsuzaki, Y., Karube, M., Bouscarel, B., Miyakawa, S., & Tanaka, N. (2003). Amino acid ratios in plasma and tissues in a rat model of liver cirrhosis before and after exercise. *Hepatology Research, 27*(3), 230–237.

Moore, G. J., Bebchuk, J. M., Parrish, J. K., Faulk, M. W., Arfken, C. L., Strahl-Bevacqua, J., et al. (1999). Temporal dissociation between lithium-induced changes in frontal lobe myo-inositol and clinical response in manic-depressive illness. *American Journal of Psychiatry, 156*(12), 1902–1908.

Morgello, S., Uson, R. R., Schwartz, E. J., & Haber, R. S. (1995). The human blood-brain barrier glucose transporter (GLUT1) is a glucose transporter of gray matter astrocytes. *Glia, 14*(1), 43–54.

Nybo, L., Nielsen, B., Pedersen, B. K., Moller, K., & Secher, N. H. (2002). Interleukin-6 release from the human brain during prolonged exercise. *Journal of Physiology, 542*(Pt 3), 991–995.

Oz, G., Berkich, DA, Henry, PG, Xu, Y, LaNoue, K, Hutson, SM, et al. (2004). Neuroglial metabolism in the awake rat brain: CO₂ fixation increases with brain activity. *Journal of Neuroscience, 24*, 11273–11279.

Oz, G., Hutter, D., Tkác, I., Clark, H. B., Gross, M. D., Jiang, H., et al. (2010a). Neurochemical alterations in spinocerebellar ataxia type 1 and their correlations with clinical status. *Movement Disorders, 25*(9), 1253–1261.

Oz, G., Nelson, C. D., Koski, D. M., Henry, P. G., Marjanska, M., Deelchand, D. K., et al. (2010b). Noninvasive detection of presymptomatic and progressive neurodegeneration in a mouse model of spinocerebellar ataxia type 1. *Journal of Neuroscience, 30* (10), 3831–3838.

Patel, A. B., De Graaf, R. A., Mason, G. F., Rothman, D. L., Shulman, R. G., & Behar, K. L. (2005). The contribution of GABA to glutamate/glutamine cycling and energy metabolism in the rat cortex in vivo. *Proceedings of the National Academy of Sciences USA, 102* (15), 5588–5593.

Pellerin, L. (2005). How astrocytes feed hungry neurons. *Molecular Neurobiology, 32*(1), 59–72.

Pellerin, L., & Magistretti, P. (1994). Glutamate uptake into astrocytes stimulates aerobic glycolysis: a mechanism coupling neuronal activity to glucose utilization. *Proceedings of the National Academy of Sciences USA, 91*(22), 10625–10629.

Pellerin, L., Stolz, M., Sorg, O., Martin, J. L., Deschepper, C. F., & Magistretti, P. J. (1997). Regulation of energy metabolism by neurotransmitters in astrocytes in primary culture and in an immortalized cell line. *Glia, 21*(1), 74–83.

Petroff, O. A., & Rothman, D. L. (1998). Measuring human brain GABA in vivo: effects of GABA-transaminase inhibition with vigabatrin. *Molecular Neurobiology, 16*(1), 97–121.

Piérard, C., Pérès, M., Satabin, P., Guezennec, C. Y., & Lagarde, D. (1999). Effects of GABA-transaminase inhibition on brain metabolism and amino-acid compartmentation: an in vivo study by 2D 1 H-NMR spectroscopy coupled with microdialysis. *Experimental Brain Research, 127*(3), 321–327.

Port, J. D., Unal, S. S., Mrazek, D. A., & Marcus, S. M. (2008). Metabolic alterations in medication-free patients with bipolar disorder: a 3T CSF-corrected magnetic resonance spectroscopic imaging study. *Psychiatry Research, 162*(2), 113–121.

Preece, N. E. N., & Cerdán, S. S. (1996). Metabolic precursors and compartmentation of cerebral GABA in vigabatrin-treated rats. *Journal of Neurochemistry, 67*(4), 1718–1725.

Prichard, J., Rothman, D., Novotny, E., Petroff, O., Kuwabara, T., Avison, M., et al. (1991). Lactate rise detected by 1H NMR in human visual cortex during physiologic stimulation. *Proceedings of the National Academy of Sciences USA, 88*(13), 5829–5831.

Rama Rao, K. V., Reddy, P. V., Tong, X., & Norenberg, M. D. (2010). Brain edema in acute liver failure: inhibition by L-histidine. *American Journal of Pathology, 176*(3), 1400–1408.

Rango, M., Cogiamanian, F., Marceglia, S., Barberis, B., Arighi, A., Biondetti, P., et al. (2008). Myoinositol content in the human brain is modified by transcranial direct current stimulation in a matter of minutes: a 1H-MRS study. *Magnetic Resonance in Medicine, 60* (4), 782–789.

Rasmussen, P., van Hall, G., Gam, C., Jans, O., Zaar, M., Secher, N. H., et al. (2008). Human brain is oxidizing substantial quantities of lactate under basal and hyperlactatemic conditions. *FASEB Journal, 22*(1b96).

Roberts, E., & Frankel, S. (1950). gamma-Aminobutyric acid in brain: its formation from glutamic acid. *Journal of Biological Chemistry, 187*(1), 55–63.

Roberts, E., & Frankel, S. (1951). Glutamic acid decarboxylase in brain. *Journal of Biological Chemistry, 188*(2), 789–795.

Roberts, E., Younger, F., & Frankel, S. (1951). Influence of dietary pyridoxine on glutamic decarboxylase activity of brain. *Journal of Biological Chemistry, 191*(1), 277–285.

Saito, K., Barber, R., Wu, J., Matsuda, T., Roberts, E., & Vaughn, J. E. (1974). Immunohistochemical localization of glutamate decarboxylase in rat cerebellum. *Proceedings of the National Academy of Sciences USA, 71*(2), 269–273.

Sappey-Marinier, D., Calabrese, G., Fein, G., Hugg, J. W., Biggins, C., & Weiner, M. W. (1992). Effect of photic stimulation on human visual cortex lactate and phosphates using 1H and 31P magnetic resonance spectroscopy. *Journal of Cerebral Blood Flow and Metabolism, 12*(4), 584–592.

Saxena, N. C., & Macdonald, R. L. (1994). Assembly of GABAA receptor subunits: role of the delta subunit. *Journal of Neuroscience, 14*(11 Pt 2), 7077–7086.

Schousboe, A. (2000). Pharmacological and functional characterization of astrocytic GABA transport: a short review. *Neurochemical Research, 25*(9-10), 1241–1244.

Secher, N. H., Quistorff, B., & Dalsgaard, M. K. (2006). [The muscles work, but the brain gets tired]. *Ugeskrft Laeger, 168*(51), 4503–4506.

Seifert, T. S., Brassard, P., Jorgensen, T. B., Hamada, A. J., Rasmussen, P., Quistorff, B., et al. (2009). Cerebral non-oxidative carbohydrate consumption in humans driven by adrenaline. *Journal of Physiology, 587*(Pt 1), 285–293.

Seiler, N. N. (1980). On the role of GABA in vertebrate polyamine metabolism. *Physiological Chemistry and Physics*, 12(5), 411–429.

Shank, R. P., Bennett, G. S., Freytag, S. O., & Campbell, G. L. (1985). Pyruvate carboxylase: an astrocyte-specific enzyme implicated in the replenishment of amino acid neurotransmitter pools. *Brain Research*, 329(1-2), 364–367.

Shen, J., Petersen, K. F., Behar, K. L., Brown, P., Nixon, T. W., Mason, G. F., et al. (1999). Determination of the rate of the glutamate/glutamine cycle in the human brain by in vivo 13C NMR. *Proceedings of the National Academy of Sciences USA*, 96(14), 8235–8240.

Shulman, R. G., Hyder, F., & Rothman, D. L. (2001). Lactate efflux and the neuroenergetic basis of brain function. *NMR in Biomedicine*, 14(7-8), 389–396.

Shulman, R. G., Hyder, F., & Rothman, D. L. (2002). Biophysical basis of brain activity: implications for neuroimaging. *Quarterly Review of Biophysics*, 35(3), 287–325.

Sibson, N. R., Dhankhar, A., Mason, G. F., Behar, K. L., Rothman, D. L., & Shulman, R. G. (1997). In vivo 13C NMR measurements of cerebral glutamine synthesis as evidence for glutamate-glutamine cycling. *Proceedings of the National Academy of Sciences USA*, 94(6), 2699–2704.

Sibson, N. R., Dhankhar, A., Mason, G. F., Rothman, D., Behar, K., & Shulman, R. G. (1998). Stoichiometric coupling of brain glucose metabolism and glutamatergic neuronal activity. *Proceedings of the National Academy of Sciences USA*, 95, 316–321.

Sibson, N. R., Mason, G. F., Shen, J., Cline, G. W., Herskovits, A. Z., Wall, J. E., et al. (2001). In vivo (13)C NMR measurement of neurotransmitter glutamate cycling, anaplerosis and TCA cycle flux in rat brain during. *Journal of Neurochemistry*, 76(4), 975–989.

Sibtain, N. A., Howe, F. A., & Saunders, D. E. (2007). The clinical value of proton magnetic resonance spectroscopy in adult brain tumours. *Clinical Radiology*, 62(2), 109–119.

Siesjo, B. K. (1978). *Brain Energy Metabolism*. New York: John Wiley and Sons.

Sijens, P. E., van Dijk, P., & Oudkerk, M. (1994). Correlation between choline level and Gd-DTPA enhancement in patients with brain metastases of mammary carcinoma. *Magnetic Resonance in Medicine*, 32(5), 549–555.

Silverstone, P. H., & McGrath, B. M. (2009). Lithium and valproate and their possible effects on the myo-inositol second messenger system in healthy volunteers and bipolar patients. *International Review of Psychiatry*, 21(4), 414–423.

Stagg, C., Bestmann, S., Constantinescu, A. O., Moreno, L. M., Allman, C., Mekle, R., et al. (2011). Relationship between physiological measures of excitability and levels of glutamate and GABA in the human motor cortex. *Journal of Physiology*, 589(Pt 23), 5845–5855.

Star-Lack, J., Spielman, D., Adalsteinsson, E., Kurhanewicz, J., Terris, D. J., & Vigneron, D. B. (1998). In vivo lactate editing with simultaneous detection of choline, creatine, NAA, and lipid singlets at 1.5 T using PRESS excitation with applications to the study of brain and head and neck tumors. *Journal of Magnetic Resonance*, 133(2), 243–254.

Strange, K., Emma, F., Paredes, A., & Morrison, R. (1994). Osmoregulatory changes in myo-inositol content and Na + /myo-inositol cotransport in rat cortical astrocytes. *Glia*, 12(1), 35–43.

Tofteng, F., Hauerberg, J., Hansen, B. A., Pedersen, C. B., Jørgensen, L., & Larsen, F. S. (2006). Persistent arterial hyperammonemia increases the concentration of glutamine and alanine in the brain and correlates with intracranial pressure in patients with fulminant hepatic failure. *Journal of Cerebral Blood Flow and Metabolism*, 26(1), 21–27.

Uldry, M., Ibberson, M., Horisberger, J. D., Chatton, J. Y., Riederer, B. M., & Thorens, B. (2001). Identification of a mammalian H (+)-myo-inositol symporter expressed predominantly in the brain. *EMBO Journal*, 20(16), 4467–4477.

Van Eijsden, P., Behar, K., Mason, G., Braun, K., & De Graaf, R. (2010). In vivoneurochemical profiling of rat brain by 1H-[13C] NMR spectroscopy: cerebral energetics and glutamatergic/GABAergic neurotransmission. *Journal of Neurochemistry*, 112(1), 24–33.

van Hall, G. (2010). Lactate kinetics in human tissues at rest and during exercise. *Acta Physiologica (Oxford)*, 199(4), 499–508.

van Hall, G., Stromstad, M., Rasmussen, P., Jans, O., Zaar, M., Gam, C., et al. (2009). Blood lactate is an important energy source for the human brain. *Journal of Cereb Blood Flow and Metabolism*, 29(6), 1121–1129.

van Praag, H. (2009). Exercise and the brain: something to chew on. *Trends in Neuroscience*, 32(5), 283–290.

Videen, J. S., Michaelis, T., Pinto, P., & Ross, B. D. (1995). Human cerebral osmolytes during chronic hyponatremia. A proton magnetic resonance spectroscopy study. *Journal of Clinical Investigation*, 95(2), 788–793.

Volianitis, S., Fabricius-Bjerre, A., Overgaard, A., Stromstad, M., Bjarrum, M., Carlson, C., et al. (2008). The cerebral metabolic ratio is not affected by oxygen availability during maximal exercise in humans. *Journal of Physiology*, 586(1), 107–112.

Wang, T., Xiao, S., Li, X., Ding, B., Ling, H., Chen, K., et al. (2012). Using proton magnetic resonance spectroscopy to identify mild cognitive impairment. *International Psychogeriatrics*, 24(1), 19–27.

Warren, K. S., & Schenker, S. (1964). Effect of an inhibitor of glutamine synthesis (methionine sulfoxime) on ammonia toxicity and metabolism. *Journal of Laboratory and Clinical Medicine*, 64, 442–449.

Watanabe, T., Shiino, A., & Akiguchi, I. (2012). Hippocampal metabolites and memory performances in patients with amnestic mild cognitive impairment and Alzheimer's disease. *Neurobiology of Learning and Memory*, 97(3), 289–293.

Wilson, M. C., Jackson, V. N., Heddle, C., Price, N. T., Pilegaard, H., Juel, C., et al. (1998). Lactic acid efflux from white skeletal muscle is catalyzed by the monocarboxylate transporter isoform MCT3. *Journal of Biological Chemistry*, 273(26), 15920–15926.

Wirt, M. D. A. P., & Petermann, G. W. (2003). Magnetic resonance spectroscopy: A basic guide to data acquisition and interpretation. *Applied Radiology* 25–30.

Wu, H., Jin, Y., Buddhala, C., Osterhaus, G., Cohen, E., Jin, H., et al. (2007). Role of glutamate decarboxylase (GAD) isoform, GAD65, in GABA synthesis and transport into synaptic vesicles—Evidence from GAD65-knockout mice studies. *Brain Research*, 1154, 80–83.

Xu, S., Yang, J., Li, C. Q., Zhu, W., & Shen, J. (2005). Metabolic alterations in focally activated primary somatosensory cortex of alpha-chloralose-anesthetized rats measured by 1H MRS at 11.7 T. *Neuroimage*, 28(2), 401–409.

Yang, J., Li, S. S., Bacher, J., & Shen, J. (2007). Quantification of cortical GABA-glutamine cycling rate using in vivo magnetic resonance signal of [2-13C]GABA derived from glia-specific substrate [2-13C]acetate. *Neurochemistry International*, 50(2), 371–378.

Yang, S., Hu, J., Kou, Z., & Yang, Y. (2008). Spectral simplification for resolved glutamate and glutamine measurement using a standard STEAM sequence with optimized timing parameters at 3, 4, 4.7, 7, and 9.4T. *Magnetic Resonance in Medicine*, 59(2), 236–244.

Yildiz, A., Demopulos, C. M., Moore, C. M., Renshaw, P. F., & Sachs, G. S. (2001). Effect of lithium on phosphoinositide metabolism in human brain: a proton decoupled (31)P magnetic resonance spectroscopy study. *Biological Psychiatry*, 50(1), 3–7.

Yu, S., & Ding, W. G. (1998). The 45 skDa form of glucose transporter 1 (GLUT1) is localized in oligodendrocyte and astrocyte but not in microglia in the rat brain. *Brain Research*, 797(1), 65–72.

APPLICATIONS OF PROTON-MRS

Usefulness of Proton Magnetic Resonance Spectroscopy in the Clinical Management of Brain Tumors

Carles Majós[1,2], Margarida Julià-Sapé[2,3,4] and Carles Arús[3,2,4]

[1]Institut de Diagnòstic per la Imatge (IDI), L'Hospitalet de Llobregat, Barcelona, Spain [2]Centro de Investigación Biomédica en Red en Bioingeniería, Biomateriales y Nanomedicina (CIBER-BBN), Cerdanyola del Vallès, Spain [3]Departament de Bioquímica i Biologia Molecular, Unitat de Bioquímica de Biociències, Edifici Cs, Universitat Autònoma de Barcelona (UAB) and [4]Institut de Biotecnologia i de Biomedicina (IBB), Universitat Autònoma de Barcelona (UAB), Cerdanyola del Vallès, Spain

INTRODUCTION

Magnetic resonance (MR) is a powerful technique that benefits from the properties of nuclei with an odd quantum number (an odd number of protons or neutrons), which are known as MR-active nuclei. When these are placed in an external magnetic field, they are able to absorb radiofrequency (RF) energy and to re-emit it during the transition to their original state. The hydrogen nucleus (^{1}H) is the most frequently studied nucleus since it has almost 100% natural abundance. This chapter will therefore concentrate on the utility of proton MR spectroscopy (^{1}H MRS). Other MR-active nuclei, such as the ^{13}C and ^{31}P stable isotopes, are not used as widely as ^{1}H, and are therefore not covered here (see the section, Proton MRS in the classification of brain tumors). The use of ^{31}P and ^{13}C may well increase in the near future thanks to novel techniques such as hyperpolarization, which increases signal-to-noise ratio (SNR) of detection by several orders of magnitude of, for instance, ^{13}C-labeled substances (Ardenkjaer-Larsen et al., 2003; Harzstark et al., 2012).

^{1}H MRS provides a kind of "metabolic fingerprint" of the tissue studied, thanks to the signals from protons of those molecules that are in solution in the millimolar range of concentration. In this way, several metabolites can be detected noninvasively using ^{1}H MRS: lactate, lipids, alanine, creatine, and choline, among others (for details see the section, ^{1}H MRS

acquisition and normal values). This information can be relevant in the clinical management of brain tumoral masses as it has long been recognized that different tumor types have different metabolic fingerprints (Negendank, 1992; Burtscher et al., 2000; McKnight et al., 2002; Galanaud et al., 2006; Fellows et al., 2009).

^{1}H MRS has therefore long been seen as a potentially useful adjunct to conventional MR imaging (MRI), which provides morphologic information of the brain. In some cases the diagnostic information provided by MRI can be nonspecific (Julià-Sape et al., 2006a), and therefore the additional information provided by MRS can be useful to reinforce a clinical suspicion, or to specify a wide differential diagnosis. The advantage ^{1}H MRS has over other potential techniques is that it can be gathered with most commercially available magnets, often during the same scan as the MRI.

This chapter considers three distinct scenarios in which ^{1}H MRS may be of utility in a clinical setting. First, when an abnormal mass is found in the brain, MRS can help in the differentiation between tumor and pseudotumoral pathology. Second, when the mass has been identified as a tumor, MRS can be of help in suggesting a specific diagnosis before a tumor sample can be analyzed by the pathologist. Finally, after treatment, MRS can be of help in the assessment of new lesions, by distinguishing between tumor progression and post-treatment changes. In this chapter, we will assess the role of ^{1}H MRS in each one of these situations from a clinical point of view.

^{1}H MRS ACQUISITION AND NORMAL VALUES

How to Obtain ^{1}H MRS Data

An in-depth review of the details of ^{1}H MRS acquisition is beyond the scope of this chapter. The reader is advised to consult other sources for essential background information, as well as Section 1 of this book (Danielsen & Ross, 1999; Kwock et al., 2006; McLean & Cross 2009; van der Graaf, 2010).

An MR spectrum can be summarily described as a "graph with peaks" (Fig. 3.1.1), where the x-axis is plotted in adimensional units of parts per million (ppm) and the y-axis, depicting amplitude, is characteristically given in arbitrary units. The ppm units are relative to a reference frequency, for example, unsuppressed water at 4.75 ppm. Peaks appear at constant frequencies and are characteristic of the specific resonance frequency of the MR-visible ^{1}H in different molecules, for example, the signal reflected by the three protons of the methyl group of creatine at approximately 3.03 ppm. The amplitude of the peak is directly proportional to the number of resonating protons available and thereby, indirectly, to the concentration of the substance (see Chapter 1.5).

For MRS applications, MR signal is localized, or generated from a prespecified volume, and the methods for doing this can be divided into single volume (voxel) (SV), when the signal comes from a volume of tissue defined by the intersection of three selected orthogonal planes, and multivoxel techniques (MV), where phase-encoding gradients in one, two, or three directions are used so that the signal comes from a grid of small voxels (Fig. 3.1.2), in a manner similar to MR imaging (see the section, Introduction). This chapter will deal with SV MRS. Further information regarding the use of MV MRS for tumor management can be obtained from various sources (Preul et al., 1996; De Stefano et al., 1998; De Edelenyi et al., 2000; Pirzkall et al., 2001; McKnight et al., 2002; Nelson, 2003; Raizer et al., 2005).

In addition to the strength of the magnetic field, a number of other acquisition parameters are also relevant in the acquisition of ^{1}H MRS signals. In particular, the echo time (or time of echo, TE), which is usually measured in milliseconds (ms), is probably the single most influential parameter determining the quantifiable neurochemicals in a given spectrum. Acquisitions at long TE (TE > 45 ms) come with less baseline distortion, at the cost of fewer observable metabolites, particularly those with a short T_2

relaxation time (i.e., lipids, macromolecules) with lower signal intensity at longer TEs, and those with phase modulation (i.e., myo-inositol; mI). T_2 decay or relaxation time in the transversal plane relates to the magnetic interaction that occurs between adjacent nuclei and the length of time for which this interaction takes place in different types of molecules or tissues, which causes the signal to decay. Typically, water has a long T_2 and fat/lipids have short T_2.

Once an MR spectrum has been obtained it has to be processed and analyzed. This usually requires assigning the contribution of a specific biochemical substance to each of the peaks or signals observed in the spectrum, i.e., peak identification. This is feasible as the frequency of resonance of each functional group is mostly constant at physiological pH. Assignment is usually performed using readily available chemical shift (resonance frequency) information from high-resolution MRS performed at high field intensities with model solutions and biopsies or extracts and from phantoms, which are solutions of known substances at known concentrations, placed in the same 1.5 T magnets as those used for *in vivo* studies. Lately, high-resolution magic angle spinning (HRMAS) of tissue biopsies (Andrew et al., 1959; Martinez-Bisbal et al., 2004), particularly after focused microwave irradiation (Davila et al., 2012; Simões et al., 2013), is also used for assignments of peak contributors. The HRMAS data acquisition methodology allows for the analysis of brain tumor biopsy patterns at high resolution without resorting to tissue extraction and with a resolution comparable to liquid state NMR (Beckonert et al., 2010). Andrew and collaborators (1959) demonstrated that rapid spinning of a sample at a specific angle (the magic angle, 54.7°) relative to the applied magnetic field reduced the line-broadening effects, caused by dipolar couplings or chemical shift anisotropy.

At the time of starting a patient MR study, if the clinicians have a suspicion that the symptoms are caused by an abnormal brain mass, the first decision required is where to localize the voxel. If the abnormal brain mass looks like a tumor upon MRI—in particular if there is mass effect—the choice can be between placing the voxel or volume of interest (VOI) for the MRS in the solid-proliferative region or in the necrotic-cystic area. If the diagnostic question to be answered is whether the mass is a tumor or an abscess, then the VOI should be placed over the cystic region, to check with MRS for the presence of endogenous and secreted bacterial metabolism byproducts in the cyst. If the abnormality is mostly cystic and the solid component is very small, so that it is difficult to place a small VOI that yields sufficient signal, then the VOI has to be placed in the cyst, but the spectrum should not be compared for diagnostic purposes to those obtained from solid regions (Poptani et al., 1995;

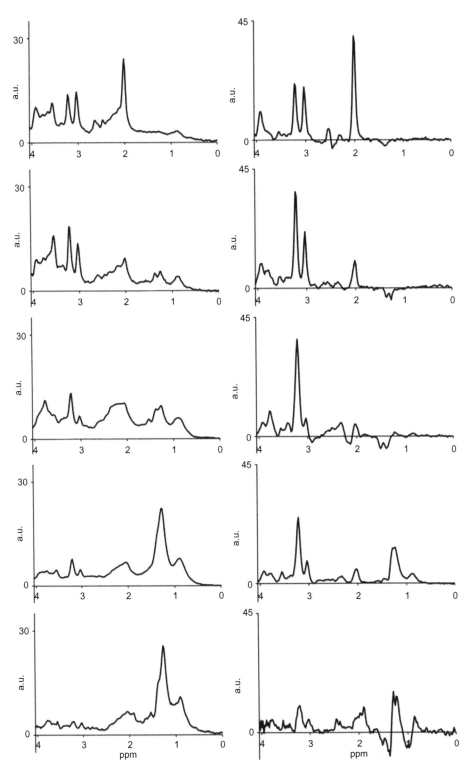

FIGURE 3.1.1 Mean ^{1}H MRS acquired from human brain tumors and other brain masses, using SV spectroscopy at 1.5 T. (adapted from Tate et al., 2006). Left column, short TE; right column, long TE (see text in the section, How to obtain ^{1}H MRS data, for the SV and TE abbreviation). X-axis, ppm; y-axis, a.u. arbitrary units. Top to bottom, normal brain tissue (short TE, $n = 22$, long TE, $n = 15$), astrocytoma WHO grade II (short TE, $n = 22$, long TE, $n = 20$), meningioma WHO grade I (short TE, $n = 58$, long TE, $n = 62$), glioblastoma (short TE, $n = 86$, long TE, $n = 79$), and abscess (short TE, $n = 8$, long TE, $n = 8$).

Candiota et al., 2004). In most cases, however, it will be advisable to place the VOI in the most active region of the tumor, from the metabolic point of view, and usually, therefore, this will inform the order in which the MRI and MRS studies are performed, with the MRI to be performed first, with contrast administration, to identify the most active region, which is usually contrast enhancing.

In order to use MRS as a clinical diagnostic tool, an MR spectrum must be obtained with sufficient SNR. In general, the larger the VOI the better the SNR, except when tumors are heterogeneous, or when the tumor is

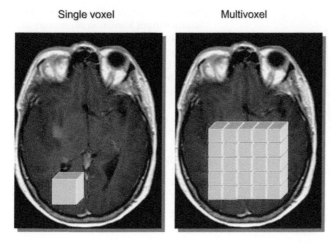

FIGURE 3.1.2   Left, SV volume. Right, MV, overlaid on an MRI. The information gathered from each voxel is a spectrum, such as those in Fig. 3.1.1.

near the skull base, which may pose field homogeneity problems. Most commonly, SV MRS within a tumor utilizes a $2 \times 2 \times 2 \, cm^3$ voxel. It is important to note that SNR increases proportionally with volume, then small changes in voxel size have a dramatic impact in SNR. For example, increasing from $2 \times 2 \times 2 \, cm^3$ to $2.5 \times 2.5 \times 2.5 \, cm^3$ almost doubles the volume from which the spectrum is acquired and therefore the theoretical SNR of the recorded signal. In this respect, a general rule would be to use VOIs as large as possible only restricted by the heterogeneity or actual size of the lesion.

If only a small VOI can be accommodated, time averaging may also be employed to increase the SNR. Time averaging consists of recording the signal multiple times and summing together all the acquisitions. This approach minimizes noise, which decreases with the square root of the repeated number of measurements. As an example, doubling the number of spectra acquired may increase SNR up to 1.4-fold. Nonetheless, it must be taken into account that longer scan durations are likely to result in more artifacts caused by involuntary movement. Therefore, VOI size and placing will always be a compromise between tumor size and location and available recording time: it is recommended that an experienced neuroradiologist with training in MRS decides on both parameters for each patient.

In order to be able to compare the results of any individual MRS examination with the literature or to analyze them statistically, it is advisable to use a set of acquisition parameters that are as standard as possible. Recently, a multicenter project called INTERPRET (Tate et al., 2006) resulted in a publicly available database of brain tumor spectra (Julià-Sape et al., 2006b)

and in a decision-support system for abnormal brain mass diagnosis (Tate et al., 2006; Perez-Ruiz et al., 2010), using the following guidelines:

1. RF coils: Use the standard head coil for send and receive, or body coil for exciting and head coil (standard CP or multi-array) for receiving. Magnetic field, 1.5 T; VOI size, between $1.5 \times 1.5 \times 1.5$ and $2 \times 2 \times 2 \, cm^3$.
2. Short-echo time Point RESolved Spectroscopy (PRESS) acquisition. TE (30−32) ms; TR (1600−2000) ms; number of acquisitions with no water suppression (8−16); number of acquisitions with water suppression 128−192; dummy scans, 4.
3. Short-echo time STimulated Echo Acquisition Mode (STEAM) acquisition (this is an alternative to protocol 2). TE (20−32) ms; TR (1600−2000) ms; number of acquisitions with no water suppression (8−32); number of acquisitions with water suppression 256; dummy scans 4.
4. Long-echo time PRESS acquisition. TE, (135−144) ms; TR, (1600−2000) ms; number of acquisitions, no water suppression (8−16); number of acquisitions, suppressed water, (128−192); dummy scans, 4.

Which Neurochemicals can be Identified in a ^1H MR Spectrum?

As stated previously, the MRS signal is derived from protons contained in different metabolites in solution, which are found inside cells or in extracellular space at millimolar concentrations. Each proton in every different molecular environment has a characteristic resonance frequency, expressed in Hertz or more frequently in *in vivo* data, in ppm. Table 3.1.1 summarizes some of the metabolites that will be discussed in the following paragraphs.

Beginning with the lower frequencies, there is the methyl (CH_3) of lactate (LAC), which produces a doublet centered at 1.33 ppm, pointing downward (inverted) at a TE of 135−144 ms with STEAM or PRESS sequences due to J-coupling phase modulation. The doublet points upward at short TE (20−35 ms) or at longer TE (272−288 ms). The CH_3 of alanine (ALA) produces another doublet centered at 1.47 ppm. It is also inverted at long TE (135−144 ms) and upright at short TE (20−35 ms) or at longer TE (272−288 ms). The CH_3 of fatty acids and the $(CH_2)_n$ of fatty acids, usually contained in triglycerides inside intracellular or extracellular lipid droplets (necrotic cores), result in major peaks at 0.9 and 1.3 ppm, which are known as NMR-visible mobile lipids (ML), which are more intense at short TE sequences due to their T_2 (the spin−spin relaxation).

TABLE 3.1.1 The Most Common Metabolites Found in MR Spectra of Brain and Brain Tumors

TABLE 3.1.1 The Most Common Metabolites Found in MR Spectra of Brain and Brain Tumors

Metabolite	Abbreviation	Resonance frequency(ppm)	Apparent multiplicity
Lipids (CH_3)	ML	0.9	Singlet
Lipids (CH_2)$_n$	ML	1.3	Singlet
Lactate	LAC	1.33	Doublet
Alanine	ALA	1.47	Doublet
Acetate	Ac	1.92	Singlet
N-acetyl aspartate	NAA	2.02	Singlet
Glutamate	GLU	2.10	Multiplet
Glutamine	GLN	2.14	Multiplet
Glutamate	GLU	2.35	Triplet
Succinate	SUC	2.42	Singlet
Glutamine	GLN	2.46	Triplet
N-acetyl aspartate	NAA	2.50	Quadruplet
Creatine	CR	3.03	Singlet
Choline	CHO	3.21	Singlet
Scyllo-inositol	sI	3.35	Singlet
Taurine	TAU	3.43	Triplet
Choline	CHO	3.52	Triplet
Myo-inositol	mI	3.55	Quadruplet
Glycine	GLY	3.56	Singlet
Glutamate	GLU	3.77	Triplet
Glutamine	GLN	3.78	Triplet
Alanine	ALA	3.79	Quadruplet
Creatine	CR	3.93	Singlet

The CH_3 group of N-acetyl compounds, is found at 2.02 ppm. This signal primarily reflects the contribution of N-acetylaspartate (NAA) in normal or peritumoral brain tissue, although it can also contain contributions from other N-acetylated substances in tumoral tissue, for example, in cystic tumors (Candiota et al., 2004). There is also an additional methylene (CH_2) group of NAA, which resonates at 2.61 ppm.

Near the major N-acetyl compound resonance at 2.02 ppm there are the resonances of glutamine (GLN) and glutamate (GLU), which are difficult to separate at lower field strengths and therefore commonly referred to, in combination, as GLX. Their β-CH_2 and γ-CH_2 moieties produce multiple peaks in the 2.0−2.46 ppm frequency range and the α-CH group does so in the 3.6−3.8 ppm range.

The CH_3 of creatine (CR) and phosphocreatine (PCR), usually given as total CR, gives one strong signal at 3.03 ppm. Their CH_2 resonates at 3.93 ppm. CR at 3.03 ppm is regarded as the least variable of all resonances in brain tissue and tumors, and is therefore usually employed as internal reference: for example, to give a NAA/CR ratio.

γ-Aminobutyric acid (GABA) has several peaks: 1.9 ppm (β-CH_2), 2.3 ppm (α-CH_2), and 3.00 ppm (γ-CH_2) with the latter usually obscured by the CR signal at 3.03 ppm. Choline (CHO) and other trimethylamine-containing compounds such as phosphocholine and glycerophosphocholine give a signal centered at 3.21 ppm due to nine protons in their (CH_3)$_3$ group. Taurine (TAU) has two CH_2 groups, which give two triplets at 3.25 and 3.42 ppm, but at 1.5 T partially overlap with the CHO, mI, and glucose signals.

The C2−C6 protons of glucose (GLUC) resonate in the 3.43−3.80 ppm range, but at 1.5 T the signals are low, and therefore difficult to separate from noise, except in certain pathologies like diabetes or low-grade glial tumors (Bruhn et al., 1991; Moreno-Torres et al., 2004). The two CH_2 protons of glycine (GLY) and the CH protons on C1, C3, C4, and C6 of mI coresonate at 3.55 ppm, and there is an additional mI resonance at 4.06 ppm. GLY can be distinguished from mI at 3.55 ppm if MRS is acquired twice: one spectrum at short TE and the other at long TE (for example, 30 and 136 ms). The mI signal is significantly reduced at longer TEs such as 136 ms (Barba et al., 2001), but the GLY is not.

TO BE OR NOT TO BE A TUMOR, THAT IS THE QUESTION

When a patient presents with a progressive neurologic deficit, seizures, or symptoms of raised intracranial pressure, a radiological exam (CT scan or MRI) is indicated to rule out a brain mass. If, unfortunately, the radiological examination shows a brain mass, the first question to address is whether the mass can be tumoral or not. A possible flow diagram for establishing a preliminary hypothesis on the nature of the mass, based on MRS, is shown in Fig. 3.1.3. This first assessment is highly important, and the management of the patient will strongly depend on this first evaluation. Two different scenarios may be envisaged, depending on the solid or necrotic aspect of the mass.

Discrimination between Tumor and Pseudotumor when a Necrotic Mass is Found

If a necrotic mass is found in the brain, the main differential diagnosis should include a necrosis-containing tumor (glioblastoma or metastasis) and abscess.

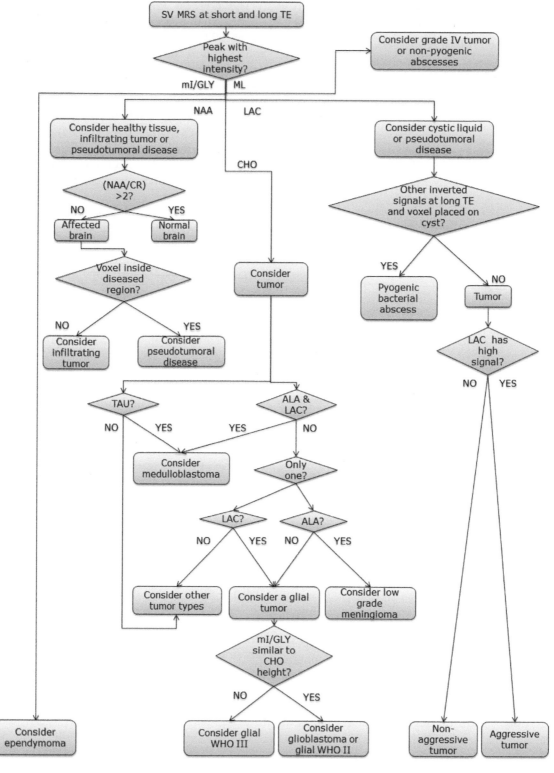

FIGURE 3.1.3   Suggested flow chart to aid reporting of an SV MRS result.

The standard treatment of an aggressive, malignant, primary brain tumor includes maximal surgical resection, while treatment of an abscess requires urgent surgical drainage. Accordingly, a suspicion of abscess requires an urgent surgical procedure of relatively low invasiveness (trephine craniotomy and drainage), but a suspicion of tumor requires a planned invasive surgical procedure. Therefore it is essential that the radiological assessment is as accurate as possible, to the point that the evaluation of a brain mass, which has characteristics suspicious of an abscess, has been suggested to be the only indication for urgent MRS. Diffusion-weighted MRI (DWI) also plays a relevant role in the radiological assessment of necrotic focal brain masses. Possibly due to bacterial cell infiltration and proteinaceous fluid, Brownian motion of free water is restricted in abscesses and, accordingly, they show hyperintensity on DWI, and low apparent diffusion coefficient (ADC). This is a highly sensitive finding, but not totally specific, as some tumors show a similar radiological appearance. Therefore a technique that, in combination with DWI can improve the specificity of MR in the diagnosis of brain abscess can be of help. This is the role that proton MRS can play in the clinical management of a suspected abscess. Proton MRS is highly specific for the diagnosis of abscess, although has a low sensitivity. Accordingly, an MRS examination compatible with abscess increases the diagnostic certainty. The reason for the high specificity of MRS is the capability of MRS to detect metabolites that are produced by bacterial metabolism that cannot be found in brain parenchyma (either normal or tumoral).

There are two main characteristics in the spectral pattern of brain abscesses: the loss of the normal spectral pattern of brain parenchyma, and the appearance of specific abscess markers. The typical spectral pattern of brain parenchyma, consisting on CHO, CR, and NAA peaks in different, but relatively consistent proportions, disappears in abscesses because the tissue studied no longer corresponds to such brain parenchyma. Moreover, some specific markers of bacterial metabolism appear, in particular acetate (a singlet centered at 1.92 ppm) and succinate (a singlet centered at 2.42 ppm). Other compounds that appear due to the bacterial metabolism are LAC, ALA, and various free amino acids (AA; these are seen as a broad peak centered at 0.9 ppm, which is inverted at intermediate TE) (Kim et al., 1997; Martinez-Perez et al., 1997; Burtscher & Holtas, 1999). An example of abscess is shown in Fig. 3.1.4, which can be compared to a necrotic tumor seen in Fig. 3.1.5 that showed similar features to the abscess on MRI and DWI.

Nevertheless, three additional confounding factors should be taken into account at this point. The specific markers of abscess disappear fast when treatment starts, due to the early arrest of bacterial metabolism (Burtscher & Holtas, 1999), which justifies the need to perform spectroscopy before starting treatment with antibiotic therapy. Another consideration is that the MRS pattern usually described within abscess tissue, with acetate and succinate peaks, is typical of brain abscesses caused by anaerobic bacteria and, accordingly, is not seen when abscesses are produced by other agents (Pal et al., 2010). In addition, abscesses from intracellular pathogens such as *Toxoplasma gondii* or *Listeria monocytogenes* display a spectral pattern that is fairly similar to that of necrotic brain tumors (Kosaric & Carroll 1971; Chinn et al., 1995; Simone et al., 1998; Lai et al., 2002; Barcelo et al., 2010) and this has to be taken into account in HIV-positive patients presenting with a focal brain lesion. In those cases, either lymphoma or a brain infection such as *Toxoplasma* should be considered as possibilities. Accordingly, a joint multi-modal MR evaluation with perfusion MRI and MRS has better potential for distinguishing these types of lesions (Barcelo et al., 2010).

Discrimination between Tumor and Pseudotumor in a Solid Mass

When a solid mass is found in the brain, the main diagnoses that should be considered are tumors without necrosis (World Health Organization (WHO) grades I–III) and pseudotumoral diseases such as demyelinating disease, subacute ischemic lesions, and inflammatory processes. There are also a non-negligible number of cases in which pathologic examination is absent or indeterminate and the lesion spontaneously regresses on follow-up. Only an unspecific diagnosis of "benign pseudotumoral lesion" can be established in these cases, but it is important to include them in the pseudotumoral group for improved clinical applicability.

Clinical management is largely different for tumors and pseudotumors. Stereotactic biopsy or surgical resection should be considered in tumors, while laboratory tests and/or follow-up have to be indicated in pseudotumors.

In many cases, reliable differentiation of neoplastic from non-neoplastic brain masses by conventional MRI is difficult, or even impossible. Proton MRS can bring additional biochemical information useful for this discrimination. Elevated CHO levels and reduced NAA have been reported in acute multiple sclerosis lesions and have been explained by reactive astrogliosis, inflammation, and early axonal degeneration (Arnold et al., 1992; Ernst et al., 1998; Bitsch et al., 1999; Narayana, 2005). In a recent study, we evaluated the application of these findings in the differentiation of tumors and pseudotumors. We found that the peak height ratio between mI and NAA at short echo time and the peak height ratio between CHO and NAA at long echo time were the ones that better discriminated between entities. Accordingly, an mI:NAA > 0.9 at short TE would suggest tumor, and the same for a ratio CHO:NAA > 1.9 at long TE

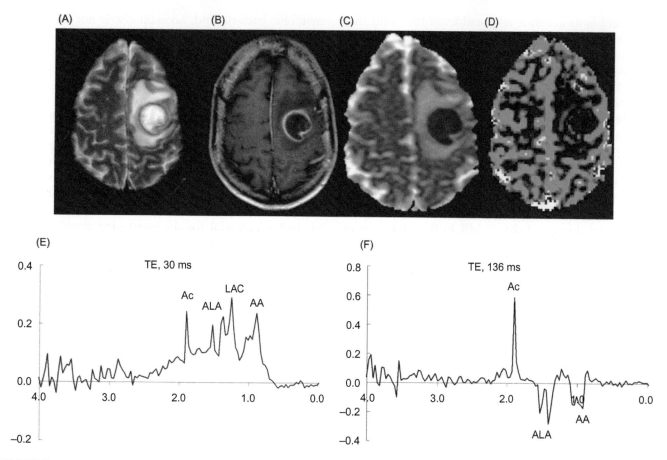

FIGURE 3.1.4   MR study at 1.5 T of a left frontal necrotic mass confirmed to be an abscess after drainage. The conventional MR exam shows a necrotic mass in the T_2-weighted images with a thin wall of low intensity signal (A). Smooth enhancement in the wall without nodularities (B) is seen on T_1-weighted images after contrast. The ADC map of a DWI study shows reduced diffusion in the mass (C). No significant areas of increased cerebral blood volume are found in the perfusion-weighted MR study (D). The spectra of the cystic mass content obtained at short (E) and long TE (F) shows a loss of the pattern of normal brain parenchyma, with no NAA, CR. and CHO resonances identifiable above the level of noise, and some characteristic resonances of abscess such as acetate (Ac), alanine (ALA), lactate (LAC), and amino acids (AA). All spectra shown in this figure and all subsequent figures in this chapter were obtained at IDI Bellvitge on a Philips 1.5 T scanner, with SV short (30 ms) or long (136 ms) TE PRESS acquisition.

(Majós et al., 2009a; (Figs. 3.1.6 and 3.1.7).The performance of these rules was evaluated in new cases not included in the first study. We found that 30/32 cases (94%) were correctly classified at short TE, 25/33 cases (76%) at long TE, and 21/21 cases (100%) when both acquisitions agreed on the same diagnosis (Majós et al., 2010). These findings suggest that a larger decrease in neuron function (reflected by a NAA decrease) and a greater membrane turnover (seen as a CHO increase) are characteristic of tumors as opposed to pseudotumors. Figs. 3.1.7 and 3.1.8 show two examples of the utility of MRS in this respect. Furthermore, the classifier developed by Majós and collaborators (2009a) is accessible through a freely available decision support system (DSS) at http://gabrmn.uab.es/dss (Tate et al., 2006; Perez-Ruiz et al., 2010).

PROTON MRS IN THE CLASSIFICATION OF BRAIN TUMORS

Is this Tumor Intraparenchymatous or Extraparenchymatous? MRS in the Differential Diagnosis of Radiologically Atypical Meningiomas

Intracranial meningiomas usually have typical radiological appearances and diagnosis by conventional imaging is relatively accurate in most cases (Julià-Sape et al., 2006a). Nevertheless, a small percentage of up to 10% of meningiomas are seen to be atypical on imaging alone and, therefore, their diagnosis may not be confidently suggested by MRI (Guo, 1988; Osborn, 1994; Ginsberg, 1996). On the other hand, some intra-axial tumors such as glioblastoma or

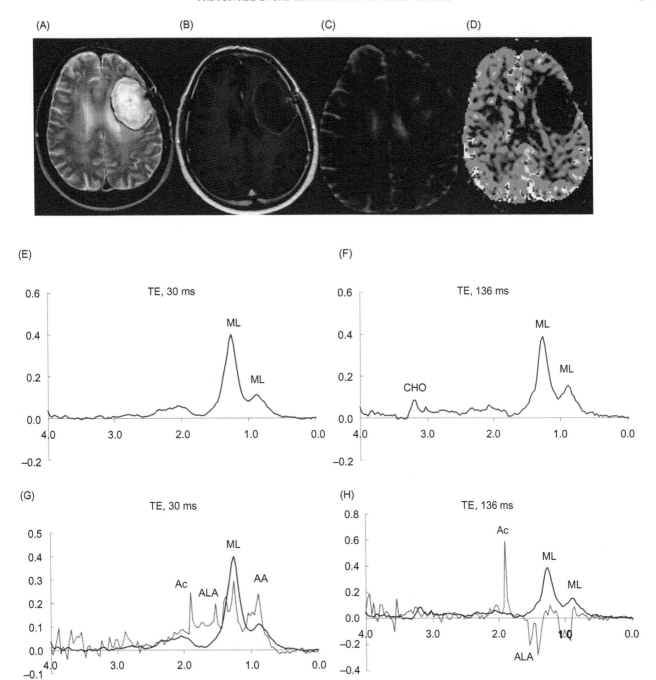

FIGURE 3.1.5 MR study of a left frontal necrotic mass corresponding to residual glioblastoma after treatment. The conventional and physiological MR exam is very similar to Fig. 3.1.4. There is a necrotic mass with a thin wall of low intensity signal on T_2-weighted imaging (A) and smooth enhancement on T_1-weighted image after contrast (B). The ADC map shows reduced diffusion in the mass (C) and no significant areas of increased cerebral blood volume are found (D). The spectra are useful to differentiate this case from the pathology of the case in Fig. 3.1.4. Spectral pattern of brain parenchyma is mostly lost in this case too due to the predominance of necrosis. Nevertheless, the spectra at short (E) and long TE (F) shows predominance of ML (necrosis) without markers of bacterial metabolism. Small peaks of CHO and CR can be identified at long TE. (G) and (H) show the spectra of Fig. 3.1.4 (red) and (E) and (F) (black) overlapped to highlight the differences between both pathologies on MRS.

metastasis, may be in contact with brain surfaces and produce an extra-axial presentation, making diagnosis difficult. In both cases an additional effort has to be made to assess the intraparenchymal or extraparenchymal origin of the mass. Accurate presurgical diagnosis in such cases may have important implications for the management of meningiomas, suggesting preoperative endovascular embolization, or

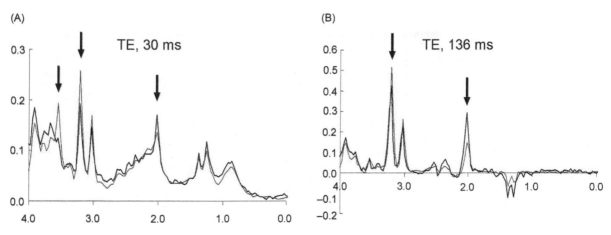

FIGURE 3.1.6 Mean spectra of solid tumors ($n = 48$) (red) and pseudotumoral masses ($n = 8$) (black) overlapped at short (A) and long (B) TE. The main differences at short TE are found in mI, CHO, and NAA (arrows). At long TE, differences are found in NAA and CHO (arrows). (Adapted from Majós et al., 2009a).

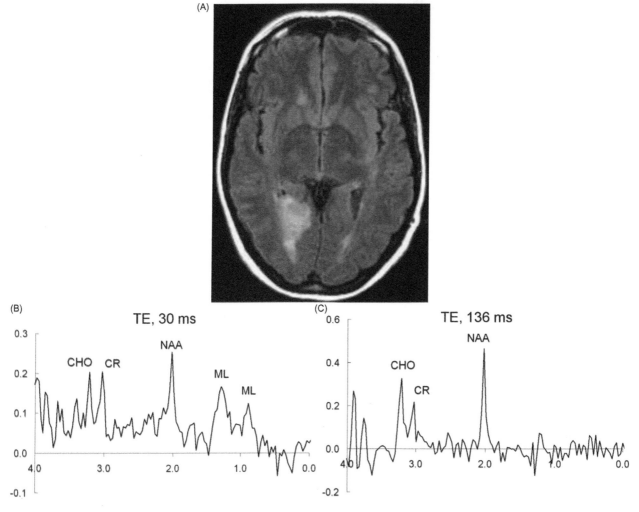

FIGURE 3.1.7 Differentiation between tumor and pseudotumoral mass in solid brain lesions. (A) The FLAIR MRI shows a solid intraparenchymatous mass in the medial parieto-occipital area. The lesion produces mass effect to the occipital horn of the ventricle. No other lesions were found. A low-grade tumor was suspected. Proton MRS at short (B) and long (C) echo time shows a non-tumoral pattern, according to the quantitative criteria described in Majós et al., 2009a. Multiple sclerosis was diagnosed by means of laboratory tests and follow-up.

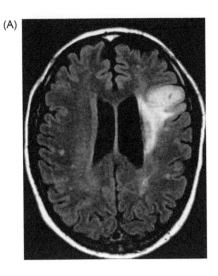

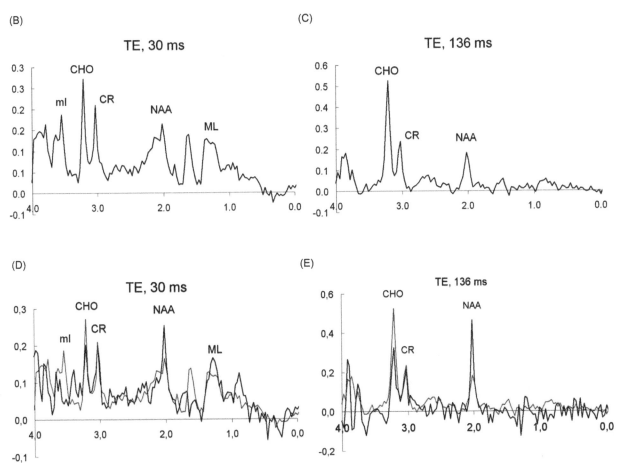

FIGURE 3.1.8 Intraparenchymatous brain tumor exploration. Axial FLAIR image (A) that shows an area of hyperintensity in the inferior left frontal lobe. There is mass effect over the cortical sulci, but lateral retraction of the body of the lateral ventricle. A low-grade tumor was suspected by imaging. The suspicion was reinforced by the spectra obtained at short (B) and long (C) echo times, both showing a tumoral pattern according to the quantitative criteria described in Majós et al., 2009a). Surgical resection resulted in an oligoastrocytoma grade II. (D) and (E) show MR spectra overlapped for a better analysis of the differences found between cases (black, Fig. 3.1.7B and C; red, B and C, and Fig. 3.1.8).

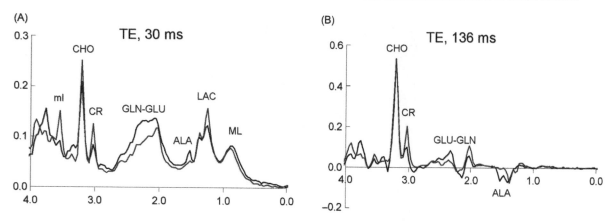

FIGURE 3.1.9   Mean spectra of meningiomas (black line) at short (A) and long (B) echo time. Anaplastic astrocytoma is the tumor type that shows the spectral pattern more similar to meningioma. Mean spectra of anaplastic astrocytoma are shown in red for comparison.

indicating follow-up by imaging instead of surgical resection. Additionally, surgery of intracranial tumors requires an accurate planning and localization of eloquent areas of the brain prior to surgery. Proton MRS may play a role in identifying those radiologically atypical meningiomas and intraparenchymatous tumors with extraparenchymatous appearance.

Meningiomas show a characteristic pattern on MRS consisting of high CHO, low CR and NAA, high GLX, and the presence of ALA. Fig. 3.1.9 shows a characteristic mean spectrum from a meningioma. In a study performed in 37 meningiomas and 93 other intracranial brain tumors, we found that the more discriminative findings of meningioma were ALA, GLX, CHO, and CR (Majós et al., 2003). Finding a tumor with high ALA, GLX, and CHO, and low CR is quite pathognomonic of meningioma, even when a meningeal origin cannot be clearly demonstrated. Figs. 3.1.10 and 3.1.11 illustrate some examples of the utility of MRS for the identification of an intraparenchymatous or extraparenchymatous origin in brain tumors. See also the INTERPRET DSS and Julià-Sape et al. (2012) for pattern recognition-based classifiers for differential meningioma discrimination.

Is this Tumor Really a Benign Meningioma? Spectroscopy in High-Grade Extraparenchymatous Tumors

Most extraparenchymatous tumors are benign meningiomas. Accordingly, treatment is not considered urgent if no critical signs are found, and follow-up by imaging can be the option suggested for these cases. Nevertheless, we must take into account that a small proportion of meningeal tumors are not benign, but rather WHO grade II (atypical meningioma) and grade III (anaplastic meningioma) meningeal tumors. Additionally, other more aggressive tumoral types, such as hemangiopericytomas or metastases, can appear close to the meninges. These tumors need early treatment due to their malignant evolution. Moreover, they have a higher tendency to bleed during resection and intra-arterial embolization may be needed prior to surgery.

It has been traditionally considered that tumors with large edema and mass effect could be malignant, but this rule is not 100% effective. Proton MRS can also play a role in narrowing this differential diagnosis. To this end, (Garcia-Gomez et al., 2008; Vellido et al., 2009) demonstrated that malignant meningiomas show increased lipids at both long and short TEs and, accordingly, a diagnosis of malignancy should be suspected in a tumor that shows high lipid content provided they are not related to subcutaneous fat contamination (Fig. 3.1.12).

Hemangiopericytomas are rare tumors (between 0.4 and 1% of all central nervous system lesions; (Guthrie et al., 1989; Kleihues & Cavenee, 2000) that are usually confused during an MRI evaluation with more common tumors arising from or located close to the meninges, such as meningiomas. Barba and collaborators (2001) found that when high mI is found in an extraparenchymatous tumor a hemangiopericytoma can be suggested. Hemangiopericytomas show a high peak at 3.55 ppm at short TE (20–32 ms), which at long TE (135–144 ms) decreases drastically in intensity, in agreement with an origin in the mI metabolite, whereas meningiomas do not show a high signal at 3.55 ppm at either a short or long TE (Fig. 3.1.13). This MRS pattern difference allows a clear discrimination between hemangiopericytoma and meningioma in the latent space screen of the INTERPRET DSS (Tate et al., 2006).

(A)

(B)

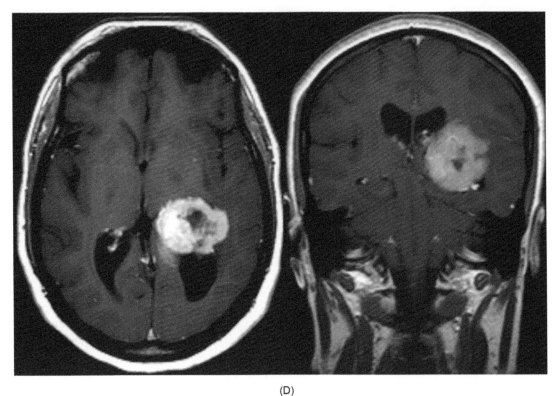

(C)

(D)

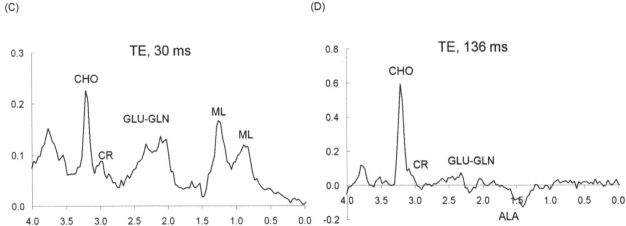

FIGURE 3.1.10 Intraventricular meningioma with intraparenchymatous radiological aspect. Abnormal brain mass with an extensive central area of no contrast enhancement on T_1-weighted image after contrast administration in axial (A) and coronal (B) planes, which suggest necrosis. A typical pattern of visible ALA with high GLX and CHO on MRS (C, D) jointly with absence of mobile lipids at long TE strongly suggest meningioma (Majos et al., 2009b).

Could this Tumor be a Lymphoma?

Primary central nervous system lymphoma (PCNSL) is an uncommon and aggressive tumor that represents only 2.3 % of all primary brain tumors. Median survival in untreated patients is low, only 2–3 months. Specific treatment can significantly improve this survival range, but it should be started as soon as possible in order to achieve optimal results.

Accordingly, early diagnosis is crucial in these patients. An additional point to be taken into account is that medication with steroids can alter the histological pattern of PCNSL and can obscure its diagnosis by the pathologist. Accordingly, a biopsy of the brain mass should be done always before starting treatment with steroids if a PCNSL is suspected. Additionally, PCNSL is highly sensitive to treatment with chemoradiotherapy, while the impact of the degree of surgical

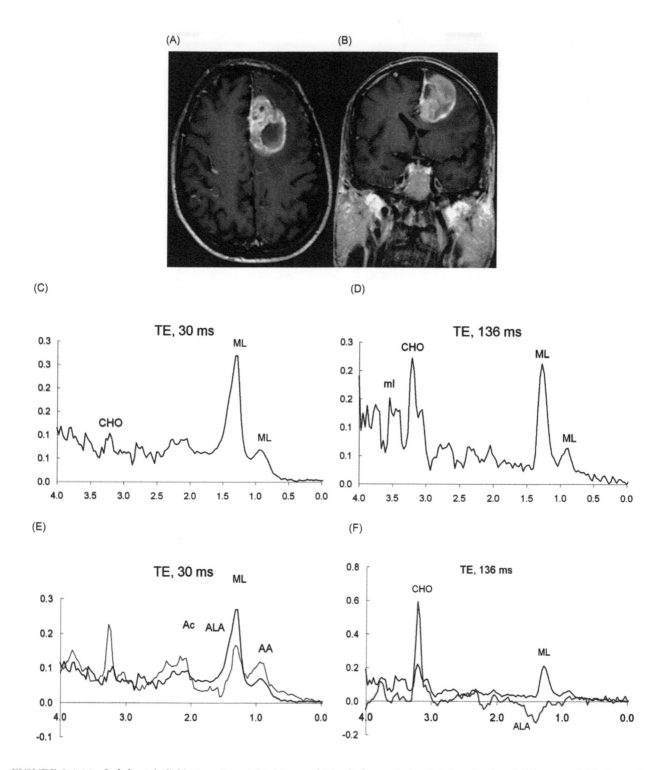

FIGURE 3.1.11   Left frontal glioblastoma. T$_1$-weighted image obtained after contrast administration in axial (A) coronal (B) planes show a heterogeneous mass with large contact with meninges and dural tail. An extraparenchymatous tumor can be suspected. Proton MRS (C and D) show MLs on both TE (short TE at left, long TE at right) attributable to necrosis. Note that the pattern clearly differs from case in Fig. 3.1.10. (E) and (F), the bottom rows show the spectra from Fig. 3.1.10 overlapped for a better assessment of differences between cases.

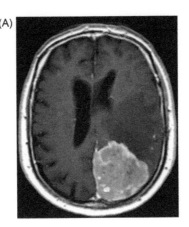

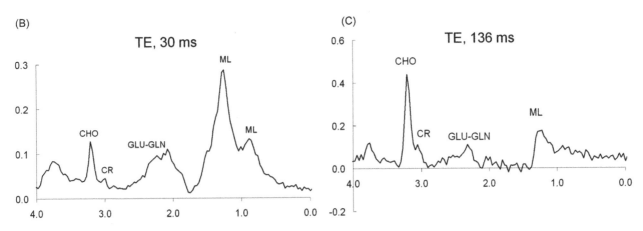

FIGURE 3.1.12   Atypical meningioma (WHO grade II). (A) Axial T$_1$-weighted image shows a large left parieto-occipital mass compatible with meningioma. There is large amount of edema in white matter and mass effect. Proton MRS shows MLs on both TE (B and C), which were not explained by subcutaneous fat contamination. There is also high CHO and GLX.

resection in survival is relatively low (Bellinzona et al., 2005). Therefore, a suspicion of PCNSL supported by noninvasive diagnostic tests such as MRS could be relevant in patient's management, by indicating the need of a brain biopsy before starting treatment with steroids, under the knowledge that maximal surgical resection could be unnecessary if a PCNSL is confirmed by histology. Proton MRS can help MRI in reinforcing the suspicion of lymphoma when a compatible mass is found by imaging (Kuker et al., 2005; Taillibert et al., 2008; Zacharia et al., 2008). Harting and collaborators (2003) found lipid peaks of significantly higher amplitudes in solid PCNSL than in solid low and high-grade astrocytomas. PCNSL cases also demonstrate raised CHO resonances relative to CR and NAA.

In our experience, anaplastic astrocytoma is the tumor type with the greatest degree of similarity to lymphoma on MRS examination (unpublished results). Fig. 3.1.14 shows the mean spectra from lymphoma and anaplastic astrocytoma. We found that the resonances that provide a better visual identification of lymphoma are low mI, low CHO, and presence of a

resonance shouldering the CHO peak at 3.3 that could be due to TAU.

Despite the fact that preoperative characterization of these tumors with MRS is challenging, there are hints for some potential utility of MRS as a complementary tool in the evaluation of response to therapy. A small follow-up study with multivoxel spectroscopy at long TE (135 ms) on 18 PCNSL patients (Raizer et al., 2005), showed that in responders, the CHO:CR ratio decreased while the NAA:CHO and NAA:CR increased. The opposite happened with the nonresponders. Kaplan—Meier curves also showed that those patients in whom ML and LAC resonances were not seen had a longer progression-free survival rate, albeit this was a nonsignificant result in this cohort. In addition, a case report (Taillibert et al., 2008) showed results in the same direction: decrease of the NAA:CR ratio and increase of CHO:CR when the volume of the lesion increased after failure of first-line methotrexate and CHO levels back to baseline as the lesion regressed after successful second-line treatment.

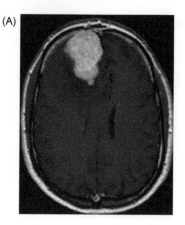

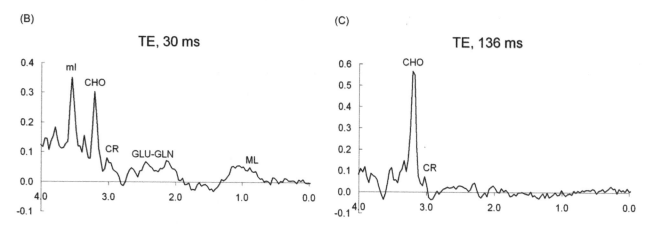

FIGURE 3.1.13   Hemangiopericytoma example case. (A) Axial T$_1$-weighted image after contrast administration shows a right frontal mass: The tumor shows homogeneous contrast enhancement. Proton MRS clearly depicts a high mI peak at short TE (B) that disappears at long TE (C), which cannot be seen in low-grade meningiomas (see Figs 3.1.9 and 3.1.10 for comparison).

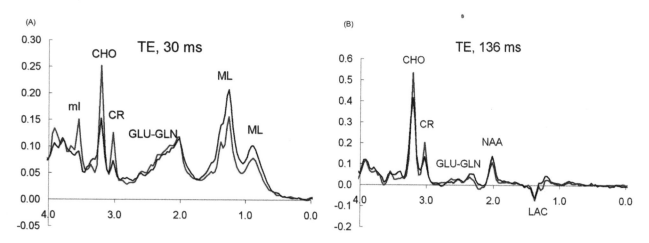

FIGURE 3.1.14   Mean spectra of lymphoma (red) and anaplastic astrocytoma (black) at short (A) and long (B) TE.

MRS IN THE ASSESSMENT OF GLIAL TUMOR GRADE

Glial tumors are the most common malignant primary tumors found in the brain. Their management and prognosis largely depends on their WHO grade. The spectroscopic findings that have been related to astrocytoma include decreased signal of NAA, increased CHO, and moderate reduction of CR. CHO has been reported to be directly correlated with tumor grade in glial tumors (Herminghaus et al., 2002). Nevertheless, there is no full consensus in a linear correlation relationship. It is commonly accepted that CHO is higher in anaplastic astrocytoma than in low-grade astrocytoma; nevertheless some studies have found CHO levels to be lower in glioblastoma than in anaplastic astrocytoma (Kinoshita & Yokota, 1997; Castillo & Kwock, 1998; Roda et al., 2000; Dowling et al., 2001; Howe et al., 2003). The discrepancy found between studies can be related to voxel positioning. Studies in which the main part of the tissue included in the VOI is solid can show high levels of CHO, while high CHO is not a common finding in VOIs that are predominantly necrotic, for which high levels of ML are clear markers. Accordingly, finding high levels of ML can be correlated to necrosis and would suggest a WHO grade IV tumor (Castillo & Kwock 1998; Kaminogo et al., 2001; Tzika et al., 2002). LAC has been also suggested to increase with tumor grade. This compound is thought to increase when the tumoral energetic requirements produce an activation of the glycolytic pathway. Some studies have shown that this finding is highly variable (Kugel et al., 1992). Our findings agree with this high variability for LAC detection and, accordingly reduced applicability in tumor classification.

mI and glycine (GLY) can also play a relevant role in glioma grading. These two resonances appear at the same position in the 1.5 T *in vivo* spectrum, centered at 3.5 ppm. mI is mainly found in short TE spectra, but largely disappears at long TE due to its short T_2 relaxation time and modulation pattern, (see the previous discussion of hemangiopericytomas). On the other hand, GLY is a singlet with long T_2 and remains identifiable on long TE spectra. Some studies have reported mI to be high in low-grade astrocytoma, and low in glioblastoma (Maxwell et al., 1998; Castillo et al., 2000; Roda et al., 2000; Howe et al., 2003). The opposite happens with GLY, in that it increases with tumoral WHO grade (Carpinelli et al., 1996; Roda et al., 2000). We (Candiota et al., 2011) developed an (mI + GLY):CR index to grade glial tumors based on 86 astrocytic tumor cases (astrocytoma WHO grade II, A2, III, A3, and IV, GBM) of the INTERPRET database (Julià-Sape et al., 2006b), for which the grade and type of tumor

had been established by agreement of a panel of three consulting pathologists. Voxel positioning for the MRS had also been performed using standard criteria, over the cellular part of the tumor (Tate et al., 2006). The (mI + GLY):CR index (Fig. 3.1.15) can be calculated as follows:

$$(mI + GLY)/CR \text{ index} = [(\text{peak height at 3.55 ppm},$$

$$\text{short TE})/(\text{peak height at 3.03 ppm}, \text{short TE})]/$$

$$[(\text{peak height at 3.55 ppm}, \text{long TE})/(\text{peak height at}$$

$$3.03 \text{ ppm}, \text{long TE})]$$

Fig. 3.1.16 also shows the mean spectra of low-grade astrocytoma, anaplastic astrocytoma, and glioblastoma at short and long echo time. Further details about using the whole MRS pattern for glioma grading purposes using a DSS can be obtained from Perez-Ruiz et al. (2010) and Julià-Sape et al. (2012).

Is this a Glioblastoma or a Metastasis?

It is difficult to differentiate between glioblastoma and solitary metastasis (Hagen et al., 1995; Ishimaru et al., 2001; Bell et al., 2002; Julià-Sape et al., 2006a).

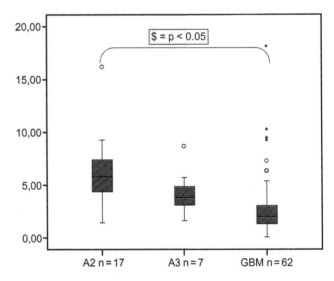

FIGURE 3.1.15 Boxplot for (mI + GLY):CR index automatically calculated from actual *in vivo* spectra. $, Significant differences using an ANOVA test between the A2 (astrocytoma WHO grade II), A3 (astrocytoma WHO grade III), and GBM (glioblastoma) groups. Number of cases for each group is given on the abscissa axis, Y-axis corresponds to (mI + GLY):CR index values. In the boxplots, upper and lower box limits represent 3rd and 1st quartiles, respectively. The central thick line is the median. Whiskers label maximum values comprised between the quartile and the product interquartile range (IQR) × 1.5. Outliers are represented as circles when value is within the 1.5 and 3.0 × IQR. *, Extreme outliers (higher than 3.0 × IQR). (Adapted from Candiota et al., 2011).

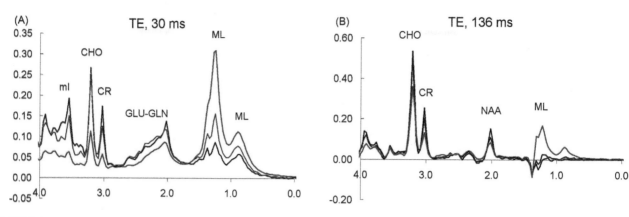

FIGURE 3.1.16 Mean spectra of glial tumors at short (A) and long (B) echo time. Low-grade (WHO grade II) astrocytoma in black, anaplastic astrocytoma (WHO grade III) in blue, and glioblastoma (red). mI is high in low-grade astrocytoma and low in glioblastoma at short TE. High lipids are a typical finding of glioblastomas at both TE. A high CHO:CR ratio is characteristic of anaplastic astrocytoma.

Since glioblastomas are infiltrative and metastases are not, in theory, the simplest approach would be to acquire one SV MRS inside the abnormal mass and another one in the peritumoral region, or outside the area of contrast enhancement (Burtscher et al., 2000): the expected finding would be abnormal spectra with necrotic ML in the contrast enhancement area for both tumor types, while in metastasis, the peri-enhancing region would be characteristic of normal brain, whereas in a glioblastoma it would be pathological, in concordance with results from perfusion and permeability MRI (Server et al., 2010).

In practice, the problem of distinguishing glioblastomas from metastases with MRS is recognized to be a challenging one (Ishimaru et al., 2001; Fan et al., 2004; Opstad et al., 2004; Garcia-Gomez et al., 2009): the spectrum in both pathologies is dominated by ML resonances (Auer et al., 2001), which result from necrosis (Negendank et al., 1996). The problem has therefore been bypassed in most statistical studies using MRS by considering glioblastomas and metastases as a superclass of "WHO grade IV malignant tumors" and solving other diagnostic discriminations (Devos et al., 2004; Lukas et al., 2004; Tate et al., 2006; Garcia-Gomez et al., 2008; Garcia-Gomez et al., 2009; Vellido et al., 2009).

In this respect, we developed a formula to separate both types (Vellido et al., 2012), using a multicentre dataset (Julià-Sapé, et al. 2006b) which included 78 glioblastomas and 31 metastases that had SV MRS at two echo times (short, 20–32 ms and long, 135–144 ms), coupled to a robust and exhaustive system for selecting features that were used for training a mathematical classifier for these two types of tumors. We also tested the classifiers with an additional multicenter testing dataset of 40 cases (30 glioblastomas and 10 metastases), obtaining a sensitivity of 90% and specificity of 83.3% with only five spectral features (2.32, 2.29, 2.02, and

3.01 ppm at long TE and 2.17 ppm at short TE). This simple classification formula is available for testing with new cases at http://gabrmn.uab.es/dss.

PROTON MRS IN THE FOLLOW-UP OF BRAIN TUMORS

MRI plays a pivotal role in the follow-up of intracranial tumors after oncologic treatment. Regular follow-up imaging is needed in order to identify regrowth as early as possible and to alter treatment when progressive disease is identified (see the section, Could this tumor be a lymphoma?). When a mass is found at follow-up, progressive disease has to be suspected. Nevertheless, in some cases the growth of the mass is not related to viable tumor, but to necrosis secondary to the oncologic treatment (radiation necrosis). Progressive disease means treatment failure and requires additional new treatment, while the treatment has to be maintained in radiation necrosis jointly with anti-edema treatment. Differentiation between both entities by conventional imaging is not unequivocal and proton MRS can provide additional useful information (Sundgren, 2009; Elias et al., 2011). Two different reports suggested that this differentiation can be carried out on the basis of the ratios between CHO, CR, and NAA. Weybright and collaborators (2004, 2005) reached 27/28 accuracy with the criterion "if CHO:CR > 1.8 or CHO:NAA > 1.8, then recurrent tumor." Zeng and collaborators (2007), with a similar criterion ("if CHO:CR > 1.71 or CHO:NAA > 1.71, then recurrent tumor"). reached 25/26 accuracy.

Nevertheless, the evaluation of focal brain masses after oncologic treatment remains challenging, and two additional aspects have to be taken into account. First, the degree of metabolic changes in spectroscopy (ratios CHO:CR and NAA:CHO) depends on the degree of the radiation injury (Chan et al., 1999). And second, there is some evolution in the changes in the spectroscopic pattern with time (Esteve et al., 1998). Accordingly, the evaluation in these cases has to be done in the context of a multidisciplinary team, pooling the knowledge of all clinical information that could be relevant in each particular case, including MRS (Matsusue et al., 2010).

Acknowledgments

Our research is partially supported by projects PHENOIMA (SAF2008-03323), from Ministerio de Ciencia e Innovación and MARESCAN (SAF2011-23870), from Ministerio de Economía y Competitividad, in Spain, and also partially funded by CIBER-BBN, which is an initiative of the VI National R&D&I Plan 2008–2011, CIBER Actions, and financed by the Instituto de Salud Carlos III with assistance from the European Regional Development Fund.

References

Andrew, E. R., Bradbury, A., et al. (1959). Removal of dipolar broadening of nuclear magnetic resonance spectra of solids by specimen rotation. *Nature, 183*(4678), 1802–1803.

Ardenkjaer-Larsen, J. H., Fridlund, B., et al. (2003). Increase in signal-to-noise ratio of >10,000 times in liquid-state NMR. *Proceedings of the National Academy of Sciences USA, 100*(18), 10158–10163.

Arnold, D. L., Matthews, P. M., et al. (1992). Proton magnetic resonance spectroscopic imaging for metabolic characterization of demyelinating plaques. *Annals of Neurology, 31*(3), 235–241.

Auer, D. P., Gössl, C., et al. (2001). Improved analysis of 1H-MR spectra in the presence of mobile lipids. *Magnetic Resonance in Medicine, 46*(3), 615–618.

Barba, I., Moreno, A., et al. (2001). Magnetic resonance spectroscopy of brain hemangiopericytomas: high myoinositol concentrations and discrimination from meningiomas. *Journal of Neurosurgery, 94*(1), 55–60.

Barcelo, C., Catalaa, I., et al. (2010). [Interest of MR perfusion and MR spectroscopy for the diagnostic of atypical cerebral toxoplasmosis]. *Journal of Neuroradiology, 37*(1), 68–71.

Beckonert, O., Coen, M., et al. (2010). High-resolution magic-angle-spinning NMR spectroscopy for metabolic profiling of intact tissues. *Nature Protocols, 5*(6), 1019–1032.

Bell, D., Grant, R., et al. (2002). How well do radiologists diagnose intracerebral tumour histology on CT? Findings from a prospective multicentre study. *British Journal of Neurosurgery, 16*(6), 573–577.

Bellinzona, M., Roser, F., et al. (2005). Surgical removal of primary central nervous system lymphomas (PCNSL) presenting as space occupying lesions: a series of 33 cases. *European Journal of Surgical Oncology, 31*(1), 100–105.

Bitsch, A., Bruhn, H., et al. (1999). Inflammatory CNS demyelination: histopathologic correlation with in vivo quantitative proton MR spectroscopy. *American Journal of Neuroradiology, 20*(9), 1619–1627.

Bruhn, H., Michaelis, T., et al. (1991). Monitoring cerebral glucose in diabetics by proton MRS. *Lancet, 337*(8743), 745–746.

Burtscher, I. M., & Holtas, S. (1999). In vivo proton MR spectroscopy of untreated and treated brain abscesses. *American Journal of Neuroradiology, 20*(6), 1049–1053.

Burtscher, I. M., Skagerberg, G., et al. (2000). Proton MR spectroscopy and preoperative diagnostic accuracy: an evaluation of intracranial mass lesions characterized by stereotactic biopsy findings. *American Journal of Neuroradiology, 21*(1), 84–93.

Candiota, A. P., Majos, C., et al. (2004). Assignment of the 2.03 ppm resonance in in vivo 1H MRS of human brain tumour cystic fluid: contribution of macromolecules. *MAGMA, 17*(1), 36–46.

Candiota, A. P., Majos, C., et al. (2011). Non-invasive grading of astrocytic tumours from the relative contents of myo-inositol and glycine measured by in vivo MRS. *JBR-BTR, 94*(6), 319–329.

Carpinelli, G., Carapella, C. M., et al. (1996). Differentiation of glioblastoma multiforme from astrocytomas by in vitro 1H MRS analysis of human brain tumors. *Anticancer Research, 16*(3B), 1559–1563.

Castillo, M., & Kwock, L. (1998). Proton MR spectroscopy of common brain tumors. *Neuroimaging Clinics of North America, 8*(4), 733–752.

Castillo, M., Smith, J. K., et al. (2000). Correlation of myo-inositol levels and grading of cerebral astrocytomas. *American Journal of Neuroradiology, 21*(9), 1645–1649.

Chan, Y. L., Yeung, D. K., et al. (1999). Proton magnetic resonance spectroscopy of late delayed radiation-induced injury of the brain. *Journal of Magnetic Resonance Imaging, 10*(2), 130–137.

Chinn, R. J., Wilkinson, I. D., et al. (1995). Toxoplasmosis and primary central nervous system lymphoma in HIV infection: diagnosis with MR spectroscopy. *Radiology, 197*(3), 649–654.

Danielsen, E. R., & Ross, B. (1999). *Magnetic Resonance Spectroscopy Diagnosis of Neurological Diseases*. New York: M. Dekker.

Davila, M., Candiota, A. P., et al. (2012). Minimization of spectral pattern changes during HRMAS experiments at 37 degrees Celsius by prior focused microwave irradiation. *MAGMA, 25*(5), 401–410.

De Edelenyi, F. S., Rubin, C., et al. (2000). A new approach for analyzing proton magnetic resonance spectroscopic images of brain tumors: nosologic images. *Nature Medicine, 6*(11), 1287–1289.

De Stefano, N., Caramanos, Z., et al. (1998). In vivo differentiation of astrocytic brain tumors and isolated demyelinating lesions of the type seen in multiple sclerosis using 1H magnetic resonance spectroscopic imaging. *Annals of Neurology, 44*(2), 273–278.

Devos, A., Lukas, L., et al. (2004). Classification of brain tumours using short echo time 1H MR spectra. *Journal of Magnetic Resonance, 170*(1), 164–175.

Dowling, C., Bollen, A. W., et al. (2001). Preoperative proton MR spectroscopic imaging of brain tumors: correlation with histopathologic analysis of resection specimens. *American Journal of Neuroradiology, 22*(4), 604–612.

Elias, A. E., Carlos, R. C., et al. (2011). MR spectroscopy using normalized and non-normalized metabolite ratios for differentiating recurrent brain tumor from radiation injury. *Academy of Radiology, 18*(9), 1101–1108.

Ernst, T., Chang, L., et al. (1998). Physiologic MRI of a tumefactive multiple sclerosis lesion. *Neurology, 51*(5), 1486–1488.

Esteve, F., Rubin, C., et al. (1998). Transient metabolic changes observed with proton MR spectroscopy in normal human brain after radiation therapy. *International Journal of Radiation Oncology Biology Physics, 40*(2), 279–286.

Fan, G., Sun, B., et al. (2004). In vivo single-voxel proton MR spectroscopy in the differentiation of high-grade gliomas and solitary metastases. *Clinical Radiology, 59*(1), 77–85.

Fellows, G., A. Wright, et al. (2009, April). Targeted use of ^{1}H-MRS is as accurate as histology in the diagnosis of glioblastoma multiforme. In: *Paper presented at the Proceedings 17th Scientific Meeting, International Society for Magnetic Resonance in Medicine*, Honolulu.

Galanaud, D., Nicoli, F., et al. (2006). Noninvasive diagnostic assessment of brain tumors using combined in vivo MR imaging and spectroscopy. *Magnetic Resonance in Medicine, 55*(6), 1236–1245.

Garcia-Gomez, J. M., Luts, J., et al. (2009). Multiproject-multicenter evaluation of automatic brain tumor classification by magnetic resonance spectroscopy. *MAGMA, 22*(1), 5–18.

Garcia-Gomez, J. M., Tortajada, S., et al. (2008). The effect of combining two echo times in automatic brain tumor classification by MRS. *NMR in Biomedicine*, 21(10), 1112–1125.

Ginsberg, L. E. (1996). Radiology of meningiomas. *Journal of Neuro-oncology*, 29(3), 229–238.

Guo, X. D. (1988). [Atypical computed tomographic features of intracranial meningioma (analysis of 20 cases)]. *Zhonghua Fang She Xue Za Zhi*, 22(5), 273–275.

Guthrie, B. L., Ebersold, M. J., et al. (1989). Meningeal hemangiopericytoma: histopathological features, treatment, and long-term follow-up of 44 cases. *Neurosurgery*, 25(4), 514–522.

Hagen, T., Nieder, C., et al. (1995). [Correlation of preoperative neuroradiologic with postoperative histologic diagnosis in pathological intracranial processes]. *Radiologe*, 35(0033-832X), 7 Print.

Harting, I., Hartmann, M., et al. (2003). Differentiating primary central nervous system lymphoma from glioma in humans using localised proton magnetic resonance spectroscopy. *Neuroscience Letters*, 342(3), 163–166.

Harzstark, A. L., Weinberg, V. K., et al. (2012). A first-in-human phase I imaging study using hyperpolarized 1c-13 pyruvate (h-Py) in patients (pts) with localized prostate cancer (l-PCa). 2012 ASCO Annual Meeting. Chicago, IL *Journal of Clinical Oncology*, 30. ((Suppl):1).

Herminghaus, S., Pilatus, U., et al. (2002). Increased choline levels coincide with enhanced proliferative activity of human neuroepithelial brain tumors. *NMR in Biomedicine*, 15(6), 385–392.

Howe, F. A., Barton, S. J., et al. (2003). Metabolic profiles of human brain tumors using quantitative in vivo 1H magnetic resonance spectroscopy. *Magnetic Resonance in Medicine*, 49(2), 223–232.

Ishimaru, H., Morikawa, M., et al. (2001). Differentiation between high-grade glioma and metastatic brain tumor using single-voxel proton MR spectroscopy. *European Radiology*, 11(9), 1784–1791.

Julia-Sape, M., Acosta, D., et al. (2006a). Comparison between neuroimaging classifications and histopathological diagnoses using an international multicenter brain tumor magnetic resonance imaging database. *Journal of Neurosurgery*, 105(1), 6–14.

Julia-Sape, M., Acosta, D., et al. (2006b). A multi-centre, web-accessible and quality control-checked database of in vivo MR spectra of brain tumour patients. *MAGMA*, 19(1), 22–33.

Julia-Sape, M., Coronel, I., et al. (2012). Prospective diagnostic performance evaluation of single-voxel 1H MRS for typing and grading of brain tumours. *NMR in Biomedicine*, 25(4), 661–673.

Kaminogo, M., Ishimaru, H., et al. (2001). Diagnostic potential of short echo time MR spectroscopy of gliomas with single-voxel and point-resolved spatially localised proton spectroscopy of brain. *Neuroradiology*, 43(5), 353–363.

Kim, S. H., Chang, K. H., et al. (1997). Brain abscess and brain tumor: discrimination with in vivo H-1 MR spectroscopy. *Radiology*, 204(1), 239–245.

Kinoshita, Y., & Yokota, A. (1997). Absolute concentrations of metabolites in human brain tumors using in vitro proton magnetic resonance spectroscopy. *NMR in Biomedicine*, 10(1), 2–12.

Kleihues, P., & Cavenee, W. K. (2000). *Pathology and Genetics of Tumours of The Nervous System*. Lyon, France: IARC Press.

Kosaric, N., & Carroll, K. K. (1971). Phospholipids of Listeria monocytogenes. *Biochimica et Biophysica Acta Lipids and Lipid Metabolism*, 239(3), 428–442.

Kugel, H., Heindel, W., et al. (1992). Human brain tumors: spectral patterns detected with localized H-1 MR spectroscopy. *Radiology*, 183(3), 701–709.

Kuker, W., Nagele, T., et al. (2005). Primary central nervous system lymphomas (PCNSL): MRI features at presentation in 100 patients. *Journal of Neuro-oncology*, 72(2), 169–177.

Kwock, L., Smith, J. K., et al. (2006). Clinical role of proton magnetic resonance spectroscopy in oncology: brain, breast, and prostate cancer. *Lancet Oncology*, 7(10), 859–868.

Lai, P. H., Ho, J. T., et al. (2002). Brain abscess and necrotic brain tumor: discrimination with proton MR spectroscopy and diffusion-weighted imaging. *American Journal of Neuroradiology*, 23(8), 1369–1377.

Lukas, L., Devos, A., et al. (2004). Brain tumor classification based on long echo proton MRS signals. *Artificial Intelligence in Medicine*, 31(1), 73–89.

Majos, C., Aguilera, C., et al. (2009a). Proton MR spectroscopy improves discrimination between tumor and pseudotumoral lesion in solid brain masses. *American Journal of Neuroradiology*, 30(3), 544–551.

Majos, C., Aguilera, C., et al. (2009b). In vivo proton magnetic resonance spectroscopy of intraventricular tumours of the brain. *European Radiology*, 19(8), 2049–2059.

Majos, C., Alonso, J., et al. (2003). Utility of proton MR spectroscopy in the diagnosis of radiologically atypical intracranial meningiomas. *Neuroradiology*, 45(3), 129–136.

Majós, C., Cos, M., Camins, A., et al. (2010). A retrospective study about the usefulness of proton MR spectroscopy in the discrimination between tumour and pseudotumoural lesion in solid brain masses. In: *Paper presented at the XXXIX Reunión anual Sociedad Española de Neurorradiología, Badajoz, Spain*.

Martinez-Bisbal, M. C., Marti-Bonmati, L., et al. (2004). 1H and 13C HR-MAS spectroscopy of intact biopsy samples ex vivo and in vivo 1H MRS study of human high grade gliomas. *NMR in Biomedicine*, 17(4), 191–205.

Martinez-Perez, I., Moreno, A., et al. (1997). Diagnosis of brain abscess by magnetic resonance spectroscopy. Report of two cases. *Journal of Neurosurgery*, 86(4), 708–713.

Matsusue, E., Fink, J., et al. (2010). Distinction between glioma progression and post-radiation change by combined physiologic MR imaging. *Neuroradiology*, 52(4), 297–306.

Maxwell, R. J., Martinez-Perez, I., et al. (1998). Pattern recognition analysis of 1H NMR spectra from perchloric acid extracts of human brain tumor biopsies. *Magnetic Resonance in Medicine*, 39(6), 869–877.

McKnight, T. R., von dem Bussche, M. H., et al. (2002). Histopathological validation of a three-dimensional magnetic resonance spectroscopy index as a predictor of tumor presence. *Journal of Neurosurgery*, 97(4), 794–802.

McLean, M. A., & Cross, J. J. (2009). Magnetic resonance spectroscopy: principles and applications in neurosurgery. *British Journal of Neurosurgery*, 23(1), 5–13.

Moreno-Torres, A., Martinez-Perez, I., et al. (2004). Taurine detection by proton magnetic resonance spectroscopy in medulloblastoma: contribution to noninvasive differential diagnosis with cerebellar astrocytoma. *Neurosurgery*, 55(4), 824–829 discussion 829.

Narayana, P. A. (2005). Magnetic resonance spectroscopy in the monitoring of multiple sclerosis. *Journal of Neuroimaging*, 15(Suppl. 4), 46S–57S.

Negendank, W. (1992). Studies of human tumors by MRS: a review. *NMR in Biomedicine*, 5(5), 303–324.

Negendank, W. G., Sauter, R., et al. (1996). Proton magnetic resonance spectroscopy in patients with glial tumors: a multicenter study. *Journal of Neurosurgery*, 84(3), 449–458.

Nelson, S. J. (2003). Multivoxel magnetic resonance spectroscopy of brain tumors. *Molecular Cancer Therapy*, 2(5), 497–507.

Opstad, K. S., Murphy, M. M., et al. (2004). Differentiation of metastases from high-grade gliomas using short echo time 1H spectroscopy. *Journal of Magnetic Resonance Imaging*, 20(2), 187–192.

Osborn, A. G. (1994). *Diagnostic Neuroradiology*. St. Louis, MO: Mosby.

Pal, D., Bhattacharyya, A., et al. (2010). In vivo proton MR spectroscopy evaluation of pyogenic brain abscesses: a report of 194 cases. *American Journal of Neuroradiology*, 31(2), 360–366.

Perez-Ruiz, A., Julia-Sape, M., et al. (2010). The INTERPRET Decision-Support System version 3.0 for evaluation of Magnetic Resonance Spectroscopy data from human brain tumours and other abnormal brain masses. *BMC Bioinformatics, 11*(1), 581.

Pirzkall, A., McKnight, T. R., et al. (2001). MR-spectroscopy guided target delineation for high-grade gliomas. *International Journal of Radiation Oncology Biology Physics, 50*(4), 915–928.

Poptani, H., Gupta, R. K., et al. (1995). Cystic intracranial mass lesions: possible role of in vivo MR spectroscopy in its differential diagnosis. *Magnetic Resonance Imaging, 13*(7), 1019–1029.

Preul, M. C., Caramanos, Z., et al. (1996). Accurate, noninvasive diagnosis of human brain tumors by using proton magnetic resonance spectroscopy. *Nature Medicine, 2*(3), 323–325.

Raizer, J. J., Koutcher, J. A., et al. (2005). Proton magnetic resonance spectroscopy in immunocompetent patients with primary central nervous system lymphoma. *Journal of Neuro-oncology, 71*(2), 173–180.

Roda, J. M., Pascual, J. M., et al. (2000). Nonhistological diagnosis of human cerebral tumors by 1H magnetic resonance spectroscopy and amino acid analysis. *Clinical Cancer Research, 6*(10), 3983–3993.

Server, A., Josefsen, R., et al. (2010). Proton magnetic resonance spectroscopy in the distinction of high-grade cerebral gliomas from single metastatic brain tumors. *Acta Radiology, 51*(3), 316–325.

Simões, R. V., Candiota, A. P., et al. (2013). In vivo magnetic resonance spectroscopic imaging and ex vivo quantitative neuropathology by high resolution magic angle spinning proton magnetic resonance spectroscopy. In R. Martínez Murillo, & A. Martínez (Eds.), *Animal Models of Brain Tumors* (Vol. 77, pp. 329–365). Totowa, NJ: Humana Press.

Simone, I. L., Federico, F., et al. (1998). Localised 1H-MR spectroscopy for metabolic characterisation of diffuse and focal brain lesions in patients infected with HIV. *Journal of Neurology, Neurosurgery & Psychiatry, 64*(4), 516–523.

Sundgren, P. C. (2009). MR spectroscopy in radiation injury. *American Journal of Neuroradiology, 30*(8), 1469–1476.

Taillibert, S., Guillevin, R., et al. (2008). Brain lymphoma: usefulness of the magnetic resonance spectroscopy. *Journal of Neuro-oncology, 86*(2), 225–229.

Tate, A. R., Underwood, J., et al. (2006). Development of a decision support system for diagnosis and grading of brain tumours using in vivo magnetic resonance single voxel spectra. *NMR in Biomedicine, 19*(4), 411–434.

Tzika, A. A., Cheng, L. L., et al. (2002). Biochemical characterization of pediatric brain tumors by using in vivo and ex vivo magnetic resonance spectroscopy. *Journal of Neurosurgery, 96*(6), 1023–1031.

van der Graaf, M. (2010). In vivo magnetic resonance spectroscopy: basic methodology and clinical applications. *European Biophysics Journal, 39*(4), 527–540.

Vellido, A., Romero, E., et al. (2009). Outlier exploration and diagnostic classification of a multi-centre 1H-MRS brain tumour database. *Neurocomputing, 72*(13-15), 3085–3097.

Vellido, A., Romero, E., et al. (2012). Robust discrimination of glioblastomas from metastatic brain tumors on the basis of single-voxel (1)H MRS. *NMR in Biomedicine, 25*(6), 819–828.

Weybright, P., Maly, P., et al. (2004). MR spectroscopy in the evaluation of recurrent contrast-enhancing lesions in the posterior fossa after tumor treatment. *Neuroradiology, 46*(7), 541–549.

Weybright, P., Sundgren, P. C., et al. (2005). Differentiation between brain tumor recurrence and radiation injury using MR spectroscopy. *American Journal of Roentgenology, 185*(6), 1471–1476.

Zacharia, T. T., Law, M., et al. (2008). Central nervous system lymphoma characterization by diffusion-weighted imaging and MR spectroscopy. *Journal of Neuroimaging, 18*(4), 411–417.

Zeng, Q. S., Li, C. F., et al. (2007). Multivoxel 3D proton MR spectroscopy in the distinction of recurrent glioma from radiation injury. *Journal of Neuro-oncology, 84*(1), 63–69.

Multiple Sclerosis and Inflammatory Diseases

Nicola De Stefano and Antonio Giorgio

Department of Medicine, Surgery and Neuroscience, University of Siena, Italy

INTRODUCTION

Over the past decades, magnetic resonance imaging (MRI) methodologies have been widely applied to the study of inflammatory/demyelinating disorders of the brain, providing important clues to the pathogenesis, course, and diagnostic workup of such conditions. Studies of proton MR spectroscopy (^{1}H MRS) have been particularly important in this setting. Indeed, by providing evidence of early neurodegeneration, based on levels of *N*-acetylaspartate (NAA), such studies led to a reassessment of the role of axonal damage in a primary demyelinating condition such as multiple sclerosis (MS). Further, by showing changes in brain metabolites such as choline (Cho) and myo-inositol (mI), ^{1}H MRS has confirmed the role of myelin damage and repair in MS.

This chapter covers the most relevant applications of ^{1}H MRS in this field, with an emphasis on MS.

MS

MS is a model of inflammatory autoimmune disorder of the central nervous system (CNS). The etiology of MS is still unknown, although it seems the result of an interaction between unspecific environmental factors and susceptibility genes. These factors activate a cascade of pathological events, which are apparent in the CNS as acute inflammation, focal demyelination, neurodegeneration, and partial remyelination.

MS is the major cause of neurological disability in young adults of Western countries. Clinically, it manifests more frequently with a relapsing–remitting (RR) course, which has a wide heterogeneity of symptoms, potentially involving any part of the CNS. The acute episodes (i.e., relapses) are characterized initially by a complete clinical recovery. However, over the years

recurrent relapses are followed by only partial recovery, leaving persistent neurological deficits. Then, a progression of clinical disability without relapses (secondary progressive form; SP) ensues. Rarely (10% of cases), the disease has a continuous worsening of neurological status from the onset, without superimposed bouts (primary progressive form; PP). The prognosis of MS is unpredictable, with a high degree of variability in the final outcome, but the disability progression is usually relentless.

Conventional MRI has a major role in the recently developed diagnostic criteria for MS (McDonald et al., 2001; Polman et al., 2011) because of its sensitivity in detecting MS lesions and their changes over time (Filippi et al., 2003b). MS lesions appear on conventional MRI as multiple white matter (WM) foci of various size, irregular shape, asymmetric distribution, and high signal intensity on T_2-weighted images. Signal hyperintensity on T_2-weighted images lacks pathological specificity as it may reflect edema, demyelination, axonal loss, gliosis, or remyelination (Filippi & Rocca, 2007). A subset of these lesions appears hypointense on T_1-weighted images, and more specifically represents axonal loss and severe tissue damage (van Waesberghe et al., 1998). On post-gadolinium T_1-weighted images, some MS lesions can appear hyperintense, reflecting intense inflammatory activity and mononuclear cell infiltration (Katz et al., 1993).

Despite the sensitivity of conventional MRI for detecting MS lesions, some important limitations exist. First, pathological specificity of the MRI-visible MS lesions is low. Second, conventional MRI is unable to detect and quantify the extent of damage in the normal-appearing brain (Peterson & Trapp, 2005). These drawbacks probably explain the limited association between the measures of conventional MRI and clinical status of MS patients (Barkhof, 2002; Filippi & Rocca, 2007). Against this background, modern

162

quantitative MRI techniques such as ^{1}H MRS have been developed and applied to the study of MS.

^{1}H MRS of MS Lesions

In the last decade, a plethora of ^{1}H MRS studies have provided *in vivo* chemical-pathological characterization of the MR-visible lesions and normal-appearing brain in MS (Arnold et al., 2000; Narayana, 2005). In demyelinating lesions large enough to allow the acquisition of spectra without significant partial volume effect, ^{1}H MRS at both short and long echo times (TE) shows an increase of Cho and sometimes of lactate since the early phases of the focal process (Davie et al., 1994; De Stefano et al., 1995b). Indeed, abnormalities in the resonance intensity of Cho reflect an increase in the steady-state levels of membrane phospholipids released during active myelin breakdown. Increase in lactate may be a primary sign of hypermetabolism of the inflammatory cells. In large acute demyelinating lesions, a decrease of creatine (Cr) can also be detected (De Stefano et al., 1995a). Short TE spectra show transient increase in visible lipids, released during myelin breakdown (Narayana et al., 1998), and more stable increase in mI (Fernando et al., 2004). All these changes are consistently accompanied by marked decrease in NAA, which is a measure of axonal injury reflecting metabolic or structural changes (Matthews et al., 1998). Glutamate levels were also found elevated in acute MS lesions, suggesting a relationship between axonal damage in active lesions and glutamate excitotoxicity (Srinivasan et al., 2005).

After the acute phase and during a period of days to weeks, there is a gradual return of raised lactate resonance intensities to normal levels (De Stefano et al., 1995a). Cr also returns to normal levels within a few days (De Stefano et al., 1995a) or, alternatively, may have a small residual increase, presumably related to gliosis (Caramanos et al., 2005). Persistent increase of mI signal in chronic MS lesions may be linked to microglial proliferation (Brex et al., 2000; Helms et al., 2000; Kapeller et al., 2002). Resonance intensities of Cho, lipids, and mI usually return to normal within few months (Brenner et al., 1993; De Stefano et al., 1995a). The signal intensity of NAA may remain low or show partial recovery, starting soon after the acute phase and lasting for many months (De Stefano et al., 1995b). The recovery of NAA within MS lesions may be caused by transient metabolic changes in neuronal mitochondria, resolution of edema, or modification of the relative partial volume of axons caused by increase in the diameter of previously shrunk axons secondary to remyelination (De Stefano et al., 1995b).

^{1}H MRS of the MS Normal-Appearing Brain

Early single-voxel ^{1}H MRS studies focused mainly on MR-visible lesions (Wolinsky et al., 1990; Arnold et al., 2000). However, more recent studies, taking advantage of a better ^{1}H MRS imaging methodology, have shown that metabolic changes are not confined to MS lesions but are present both close to and far from them (Husted et al., 1994; Davie et al., 1997; Narayanan et al., 1997; Fu et al., 1998; Narayana et al., 1998; Sarchielli et al., 1999).

The NAA decrease found in the normal-appearing white matter (NAWM) is usually ascribed to axonal damage (Matthews et al., 1998) and, albeit present at early stages (De Stefano et al., 2001), is more pronounced in advanced stages of MS (Falini et al., 1998; Fu et al., 1998; Matthews et al., 1998).

The diffuse axonal abnormalities seem to result from nonlesional abnormalities either associated with subtle myelin pathology that is not visible on conventional MRI or with subtle axonal pathology, possibly due to the action of diffusible factors associated with inflammation (Hohlfeld, 1997). However, results of other experimental studies reporting that axonal damage may partially occur, via a mechanism related to the presence of an abnormal glia—axonal interaction even with low or absent inflammation (Bitsch et al., 2000; Peterson et al., 2001; Garbern et al., 2002), suggest that a primary neurodegeneration also may have a role in MS.

The degree of such NAA reduction diminishes with its distance from the center of a lesion (Arnold, 2005; De Stefano et al., 1999), in line with the notion that the widespread abnormalities are partially linked to a dying back of transected axons within MS lesions (Trapp et al., 1998). However, lower levels of NAA are also present without any clear-cut relation with T_2-visible MS lesions (De Stefano et al., 2002), and thus independently of focal demyelination, as it occurs in RRMS patients with minimal lesion accrual and in those with PPMS, who usually have low brain T_2-lesion load.

Axonal damage is not the only pathological process occurring in the NAWM of MS brains. Indeed, a number of ^{1}H MRS studies in patients with both clinically isolated syndromes suggestive of MS (Fernando et al., 2004) and established MS (Kapeller et al., 2001; Chard et al., 2002) have demonstrated a large increase in mI remote from T_2-hyperintense lesions, suggesting a significant increase in glial cell activity in the NAWM of MS patients. In addition, some studies show that abnormal magnetization transfer ratio and increases in lipids and Cho resonance intensities can precede new MS lesion formation in the NAWM (Filippi et al., 1998; Goodkin et al., 1998; Pike et al., 2000). Thus, focal WM abnormalities probably develop well before the

MR appearance of gadolinium enhancement and T_2-hyperintense lesions, as a result of microscopic damage to myelin in a macroscopically normal WM.

^{1}H MRS data do confirm such relatively new concepts of MS pathology by showing signal from lipids (which become visible due to demyelination) in regions that later will develop new T_2-hyperintense lesions (Narayana et al., 1998). These data are in agreement with those of another ^{1}H MRS study, which found a focal increase in Cho preceding the development of new T_2-hyperintense lesions (Tartaglia et al., 2002), thus confirming that a low-grade, focal myelin pathology may predate the development of acute, severe inflammation.

More recent ^{1}H MRS studies have focused on metabolic abnormalities in the gray matter (GM), confirming the important contribution of GM pathology in MS (Filippi, 2001). Decrease in NAA in the cerebral cortex may be small or absent in the early stages, but seems to be marked in patients with progressive disease (Sharma et al., 2001; Sarchielli et al., 2002; Adalsteinsson et al., 2003; Filippi et al., 2003a). In contrast, NAA decrease in the deep GM is more consistently found from the early stages (Wylezinska et al., 2003; Inglese et al., 2004; Geurts et al., 2006). In some studies where both ^{1}H MRS and histopathological methods have been applied in RR and SPMS patients, the degree of *in vivo* NAA decrease and *ex vivo* loss of thalamic neurons was similar (Cifelli et al., 2002; Wylezinska et al., 2003). In contrast with this, however, a very recent 1H MRS study (Kirov et al., 2013) on early RRMS patients followed-up semi-annually for 3 years showed that WM glial abnormalities (Cr, Cho, and mI) were larger than axonal (NAA) abnormalities and progressed over time, whereas axonal values showed partial recovery and changes in the global GM were absent. This suggests that a neuronal dysfunction, rather than true damage, may occur in the early stage of MS.

^{1}H MRS of the Spinal Cord

The role of spinal cord damage in MS and its contribution to permanent disability is well known. Indeed, histopathological studies have demonstrated atrophy and axonal loss in the lateral columns of the cervical cord, although the correlation between these two measures is not particularly close. ^{1}H MRS can provide valuable information on true axonal damage in the spinal cord of MS patients.

Technical hurdles exist, however, in performing ^{1}H MRS of the spinal cord due to magnetic field inhomogeneities, physiological movements, and small cross-sectional area. This explains the paucity of ^{1}H MRS studies of the spinal cord performed thus far.

A recent study on a 3 T scanner showed in cervical MS lesions a significant decrease of NAA/Cho and an increase in Cho/Cr and mI/Cr in comparison with cervical spine tissue of healthy subjects (Marliani et al., 2010). In addition, normal-appearing cervical cord in MS patients showed a significant decrease in NAA when compared to healthy subjects (Kendi et al., 2004). In particular, a 32% reduction of NAA levels alongside a 15% volume loss was present in the cervical cord, indicating significant neuroaxonal injury. Importantly, spinal cord NAA showed a correlation with the cerebellar subscore of the Extended Disability Status Scale (EDSS) whereas no correlations were found with cord atrophy or brain lesion load (Blamire et al., 2007).

In another ^{1}H MRS study (Ciccarelli et al., 2007) on MS patients with cervical cord relapse and lesions, patients had reduced levels of NAA. Significant correlations were found between EDSS and mI, Cho and Cr, and between 9-hole peg test (9-HPT) and Cr. The concentration of mI was independently associated with the EDSS.

Interestingly, recovered patients from a cervical cord relapse showed a sustained increase in NAA after 1 month and a greater increase was associated with better recovery, especially in patients with short disease duration (Ciccarelli et al., 2010a). This was interpreted as the presence of a repair mechanism that may be driven by increased axonal mitochondrial metabolism.

NAA can be considered as a combination of axonal structural integrity and mitochondrial metabolism. Thus, by modeling NAA with imaging measures of axonal structural integrity (axial diffusivity and cross-sectional area) it was shown that lower residual variance in NAA, reflecting reduced mitochondrial metabolism, was associated with greater clinical disability, independently of structural damage (Ciccarelli et al., 2010b).

While the few ^{1}H MRS studies on MS cervical cord conducted thus far have offered useful information on tissue damage, this method, if further exploited, can potentially provide a more complete picture of neurodegeneration in the spinal cord of MS patients.

^{1}H MRS and Clinical Status in MS

Since the pathological mechanisms underpinning disability in MS are obvious targets for novel treatments, their understanding is crucial. ^{1}H MRS, by providing quantitative measures for noninvasively detecting axonal injury/loss in patients with MS, allows the exploration of dynamic relations between such measures and disability *in vivo*.

By and large, such correlation is explained by changes of NAA/Cr in the NAWM (Fu et al., 1998), in line with evidence of widespread pathology gleaned from other MRI methodologies.

Thus, a number of longitudinal ^{1}H MRS studies have demonstrated highly significant associations between changes in NAA/Cr and worsening of clinical disability in patients with isolated acute demyelinating lesions (De Stefano et al., 1995a) and in those with established MS and RR (Davie et al., 1995; De Stefano et al., 1997, 1998). It must be stressed, however, that the relationship of NAA/Cr with disability is far from perfect, probably due to a number of important factors. First, to determine the total axonal loss based on the measure of the NAA per unit volume (NAA density), it is necessary to correct for the axonal loss associated with brain atrophy. Second, although the location of axonal damage/loss in the NAWM is relatively homogeneous across the brain, the contribution of spinal cord pathology is not strongly reflected by changes in brain NAA. Third, the brain has plasticity mechanisms that can be recruited in order to mask axonal damage/loss at early stage of MS. Indeed, axonal injury occurs in MS even in the absence of clinical disability and becomes clinically relevant only when a "threshold" of axonal loss is reached and mechanisms of compensatory reserve in the CNS are exhausted.

In addition to NAA and Cr, other metabolites seem to have clinical relevance. Indeed, Cho and lipid signals show good prediction toward development of acute and severe inflammation. Further, widespread mI increase in patients with the different disease forms suggests the presence of glial proliferation in MS brains and its relevance to clinical disability. In contrast, increases of glutamate in lesions and normal-appearing brain seem to be related, at least in part, to ongoing neurodegenerative processes.

Alongside physical disability, ^{1}H MRS has also shown a good sensitivity for the cognitive status of patients with MS, especially in the normal-appearing brain, enabling the differentiation between MS patients with and without cognitive impairment. Level of NAA/Cr showed a closer correlation with cognitive scores in the right than in the left hemisphere (Christodoulou et al., 2003). A recent study on genotype–phenotype association in MS showed that human leukocyte antigen (HLA) DRB1*1501 allele is linked to an NAA decrease within NAWM and to an impairment of cognition as measured by the paced auditory serial addition test performance (Okuda et al., 2009). Moreover, in early stage MS MRS-derived axonal damage of the right locus ceruleus in the pons was associated with selective attention deficit, as measured

by a dichotic listening paradigm (Gadea et al., 2004). ^{1}H MRS has also revealed a relation between integrity of frontal lobe and memory function in MS, by demonstrating a significant correlation of NAA/Cr in the frontal cingulate gyrus with the Wechsler Memory Scale (Staffen et al., 2005).

Recent studies demonstrated the use of MRS for monitoring therapy in MS patients, highlighting that MRS seems to be accurate and reproducible in longitudinal studies. A standardized MRS protocol has been used in a substudy of a multicenter phase III clinical trial that involved a homogeneous acquisition procedure of single-voxel MRS and a centralized analysis of the MRS data. Preliminary results of this trial, which failed to show evidence of therapeutic efficacy (Narayanan et al., 2005), showed no NAA/Cr change over time in either the treated group or the placebo group. However, the study established the feasibility of brain metabolite levels, particularly NAA, as an outcome measure in clinical trials. Because pathologic specificity of MRS measures toward MS pathology is attractive for multicenter clinical trials, guidelines suggesting simple and robust MRS protocols applicable in this setting on a wide range of commercial MR scanners have been provided (De Stefano et al., 2007).

Using MRS to Distinguish MS from Other Inflammatory Diseases

Intracranial infection, inflammation, and demyelination are pathogenic mechanisms that underlie a wide range of disorders in CNS. In this context, MRI plays a key role in the diagnostic workup and therapeutic decisions and, in recent years, advanced MR methods, in particular ^{1}H MRS, have provided a valuable contribution. For instance, ^{1}H MRS findings in conditions as different as bacterial abscesses, tuberculomas, herpes simplex encephalitis, and human immunodeficiency virus (HIV)-related infections have demonstrated specific metabolic profiles that turned out to be useful in differential diagnosis.

Overall, there is evidence that ^{1}H MRS can be employed for supporting diagnosis in individual cases of infectious, inflammatory, or demyelinating disease.

Intracranial Infections

Infections of the CNS are often life-threatening conditions that may have a rapid progression. The prognosis often depends on the prompt recognition of both the pathogen and site of inflammation. Significant morbidity or mortality occurs, especially in bacterial infections, if appropriate therapies are not started promptly.

The clinical presentation of these conditions may vary significantly. The clinical involvement of the CNS usually includes heterogeneous focal deficits (due to the focal brain lesion) as well as altered mental status and, possibly, seizures (due to the diffuse inflammation). Analysis of cerebrospinal fluid (CSF), laboratory analysis, and, in selected cases, biopsy are the foundation for identifying the infectious agent. However, brain MRI is important as it clearly shows the inflammatory brain lesions, thus allowing a rapid diagnosis and subsequent therapeutic decisions.

In this context, ^{1}H MRS has been shown to be useful, since some brain lesions are difficult to interpret on conventional MRI and, in some cases, the infected brain tissue is characterized by specific spectroscopic patterns (Cecil & Lenkinski, 1998; Foerster et al., 2007).

Brain Abscess

Brain abscess is a focal suppurative process within the brain parenchyma, which is usually secondary to local extension from a contiguous source of infection (e.g., otitis, sinusitis, or mastoiditis) or to hematogenous dissemination of an extracranial infection. The clinical manifestations are usually fever and signs of raised intracranial pressure. However, in some cases, these signs of infection may be subtle or absent, with serious difficulties in interpreting the clinical picture. Conventional MRI is the main noninvasive tool for a diagnosis of brain abscess, revealing a ring-enhancing lesion with perifocal edema, although this also occurs in other necrotic masses (i.e., glioblastoma and metastasis; Haimes et al., 1989; Kastrup et al., 2005). In the case of hematogenous abscess, the MRI lesions are usually multiple and almost all pyogenic abscesses have markedly hyperintense signal on diffusion-weighted imaging, secondary to restricted water diffusion (Kastrup et al., 2005; Kingsley et al., 2006). However, diagnosis of pyogenic brain abscess remains difficult and, in many cases, the biopsy is inevitable. In uncertain cases, additional information can be gleaned from ^{1}H MRS, which enables a better lesion characterization (Poptani et al., 1995b, 1999). Several in vivo ^{1}H MRS studies have demonstrated the presence, in the center of the pyogenic lesion, of specific resonances such as succinate (2.40 ppm), acetate (1.92 ppm), alanine (a doublet centered at 1.47 ppm), and amino acids (valine, leucine, and isoleucine resonating together at 0.90 ppm) as well as lipids and lactate. This metabolic pattern has been confirmed in several in vitro studies and might show small differences in case of aerobic or anaerobic infections (Garg et al., 2004).

In particular, ^{1}H MRS has shown to be beneficial in differentiating a brain abscess from other cystic lesions (Poptani et al., 1995a). In these cases, the resonances of succinate, acetate, alanine, and amino acids can be found in untreated bacterial abscesses or soon after the initiation of treatment, but are not detected in normal or sterile pathologic human tissue (Gupta et al., 2001; Kingsley et al., 2006; Foerster et al., 2007; Lai et al., 2007). Spectra of arachnoid cysts, for example, typically show lactate signal and no other metabolites, easily allowing a differential diagnosis with a pyogenic mass (Kingsley et al., 2006). In the latter, the presence of succinate and acetate resonance intensity is probably the result of increased glycolysis (Garg et al., 2004). The detection of valine, leucine, and isoleucine signals should be related to the massive necrosis of neutrophils within the lesion producing a massive release of proteolytic enzymes that hydrolyze the proteins into amino acids (Mendz et al., 1989). In a brain mass, the resonance intensities of acetate, succinate, and amino acids can be considered as markers of infection, since they are not usually found in spectra from intracranial tumors (Grand et al., 1996; Dev et al., 1998; Poptani et al., 1999; Lai et al., 2002). Moreover, while lactate, alanine, and lipid resonance intensities can be often found in both meningiomas and brain abscesses, a raised Cho peak can be found only in conditions of increased cell proliferation and density, as occurs in a neoplastic tissue (Tedeschi et al., 1997; Foerster et al., 2007; McKnight et al., 2007). Overall, these data suggest that ^{1}H MRS provides useful information for differentiating an abscess from brain masses. However, it should be taken into account that the distinctive ^{1}H MRS pattern of a brain abscess changes a few days after starting the antibiotic treatment, which leads to a loss of the resonances related to the infectious process (i.e., acetate, succinate, and amino acids; Burtscher & Holtas, 1999).

Herpes Simplex and Other Viral Encephalitides

The most common cause of encephalitis is herpes simplex virus (HSV) infection. Brain invasion occurs after reactivation of a latent virus in the ganglia of cranial nerves. Patients present often with hyperpyrexia, altered mental status, focal neurological deficits, and seizures. The clinical course and prognosis are usually severe. The gold standard for diagnosis of HSV encephalitis is the detection of HSV DNA in the CSF. However, as treatment with antiviral therapy should be initiated as early as possible, MRI (or CT) can be important to support diagnosis. High signal is usually found on T_2-weighted and fluid attenuated inversion recovery (FLAIR) images, especially in temporal and inferior frontal lobes (Schroth et al., 1987; Tien et al., 1993). Mass effect on the lateral ventricles can sometimes be present. ^{1}H MRS studies have shown metabolic alterations of the HSV lesion, which is characterized by reduced NAA/Cr, elevated Cho/Cr, and the presence of lactate. There is a marked reduction of NAA/Cr, probably in relation to the severe neuronal loss caused by the infection (Salvan et al., 1999). An increase of the Cr signal due to astrocytosis is also probable (Salvan et al., 1999). The lactate signal, not always present, is probably due to the activity of macrophages and other inflammatory cells (Menon et al., 1990b; Takanashi et al., 1997). The Cho/Cr ratio is usually lower than in malignant tumors (Kingsley et al., 2006). However, the spectroscopic pattern of HSV infection is nonspecific and the use of ^{1}H MRS in this context is limited. The use of ^{1}H MRS to chart disease evolution could be more useful.

HIV Encephalopathy

This HIV-induced encephalopathy has been well characterized. It generally occurs in the late disease stage, when immunodepression becomes more severe, leading to the HIV-related dementia. This is a subcortical dementia characterized by progressive loss of cognitive functions, often later accompanied by motor impairment (Nath et al., 2008). Cortical/subcortical atrophy is usually present on conventional MRI. The primary infection from HIV may lead also to variable focal abnormalities of the deep WM (Trotot & Gray, 1997; Offiah &Turnbull, 2006). In severe cases, diffuse symmetric hyperintensity is present in the supratentorial WM, predominantly in the frontal and parietal lobes. There have been several ^{1}H MRS studies showing metabolic abnormalities in the brain of patients with HIV (Menon et al., 1990a; Jarvik et al., 1993; Meyerhoff et al., 1993; Chong et al., 1994; Wilkinson et al., 1997; Salvan et al., 1999; Tarasow et al., 2003; Yiannoutsos et al., 2004) such as reduction in NAA and increase in Cho and mI in both lesions and normal-appearing brain. Decreased NAA is present in virtually all cases. The Cho signal likely increases when the immunodepression becomes more important. The increase of mI should be related to the glial reaction observed in the brain parenchyma (Meyerhoff et al., 1999; Moller et al., 1999; Salvan et al., 1999). The brain metabolic pattern provided by ^{1}H MRS is not disease specific and does not help significantly in the diagnostic workup. However, there is compelling evidence that ^{1}H MRS reveals abnormalities in neurologically asymptomatic subjects and therefore it may be of particular value in documenting early CNS involvement when both neurological examination and conventional MRI are normal. Several other studies have shown that the ^{1}H MRS patterns have a good correlation with clinical status (Chong et al., 1993; Meyerhoff et al., 1999; Salvan et al., 1997; Chang et al., 2002; Paul et al., 2007). Furthermore, ^{1}H MRS has been successfully used in HIV multicenter trials to monitor brain changes after therapy (Salvan et al., 1997). This has

become particularly important given the availability of highly active antiretroviral therapy in HIV.

Progressive Multifocal Leukoencephalopathy

Patients with depletion of the immune system may develop progressive multifocal leukoencephalopathy (PML). This is a potentially life-threatening demyelinating disease caused by the JC virus, a polyomavirus. Primary infection is usually not associated with clinical symptoms and the virus resides quiescently in the kidney, CNS, and peripheral lymphocytes (Ferrante et al., 1995). The immune deficiency presumably leads to the reactivation of JC virus. The use of the monoclonal antibody natalizumab (an $\alpha4\beta1$ integrin inhibitor) to treat rapidly evolving severe RRMS has been associated with development of PML, especially in patients with high anti-JCV antibody titer, long exposure to the drug, and prior use of immunosuppressive therapies (Kleinschmidt-DeMasters et al., 2012).

Definitive diagnosis of PML is based on pathologic examination of brain tissue, but less invasive diagnostic methods are more often utilized in clinical practice. Conventional MRI shows multiple, asymmetric foci of hyperintense signal on T_2-weighted and FLAIR images. They are mainly subcortical (with involvement of the U-fibers) and located almost exclusively in the WM (Yousry et al., 2006). The JC virus predominantly infects oligodendrocytes and astrocytes, resulting in severe demyelination and cell loss whereas the inflammatory reaction is usually moderate (von Einsiedel et al., 1993). The spectra pattern of PML lesions is characterized by increase of Cho (due to demyelination) and sometimes of Cr (due to astrocytosis). The lactate signal may be present, probably reflecting necrosis or macrophagic infiltration. The NAA resonance is often diminished, especially in the lesion center, where neuronal damage/loss secondary to demyelination is more evident. At short TE, large increase of the lipid signal may add to the lactate and, possibly, amino acid signals. The resonance of mI may be increased as well (Chang et al., 1997; Simone et al., 1998; Iranzo et al., 1999). Although these metabolic alterations are nonspecific, this pattern could be useful to differentiate this type of lesion (i.e., demyelinating) from other brain lesions (i.e., cystic, tumoral, etc.) occurring in immunodepleted individuals.

Acute Disseminated Encephalomyelitis

Acute disseminated encephalomyelitis (ADEM) is an acute, autoimmune, demyelinating disorder of the CNS. Common symptoms include altered consciousness and multiple focal neurological deficits. Diagnosis generally relies on the clinical features, CSF analysis, and neuroimaging. A differential diagnosis should be made with MS and, sometimes, with other less frequent conditions such as vasculitides and leukoencephalopathies. Clinical symptoms may guide diagnosis, as ADEM usually is monophasic and presents days after a viral illness or vaccination. On conventional MRI, lesions of ADEM are strikingly similar to other demyelinating conditions such as MS. Lesions include foci with variable T_1-weighted hypointensity, T_2-weighted hyperintensity, and contrast enhancement after gadolinium administration. The WM is primarily affected, but deep GM structures and brainstem may be affected as well. Early diagnosis might have implications for treatment, particularly in differentiating ADEM from MS (Kesselring et al., 1990). ^{1}H MRS can be useful for diagnosis and monitoring clinical outcome. Similarly to other demyelinating conditions, spectra of ADEM lesions show reduction in NAA, variable changes in Cho, and the presence of lactate during the acute phase (Gabis et al., 2004). Marked decrease in NAA can be the only abnormality in the acute or chronic phase. In a few cases, a partial recovery of NAA has been reported (Bizzi et al., 2001). The lack of Cho elevation may support the diagnosis of ADEM versus MS. Interestingly the metabolic pattern of the normal-appearing brain is usually normal (Bizzi et al., 2001), further assisting in the differential diagnosis between ADEM and MS.

CONCLUSIONS

^{1}H MRS can be used in clinical practice to characterize in individual patients the metabolic pattern of infectious, inflammatory, and demyelinating diseases, thus contributing to disentangling the diagnostic workup of these conditions.

The information provided by ^{1}H MRS enables a better knowledge of the pathological underpinnings of these disorders. In MS, ^{1}H MRS has been applied to chart progress over time, and in some cases to monitor treatment response.

Despite limitations, ^{1}H MRS can also be potentially implemented in large, multicenter MS clinical trials.

References

Adalsteinsson, E., Langer-Gould, A., Homer, R. J., Rao, A., Sullivan, E. V., Lima, C. A., et al. (2003). Gray matter N-acetyl aspartate deficits in secondary progressive but not relapsing-remitting multiple sclerosis. *American Journal of Neuroradiology, 24*, 1941–1945.

Arnold, D. L. (2005). Changes observed in multiple sclerosis using magnetic resonance imaging reflect a focal pathology distributed along axonal pathways. *Journal of Neurology, 252*(Suppl 5), v25–v29.

Arnold, D. L., De Stefano, N., Narayanan, S., & Matthews, P. M. (2000). Proton MR spectroscopy in multiple sclerosis. *Neuroimaging Clinics of North America, 10*, 789–798, ix–x.

Barkhof, F. (2002). The clinico-radiological paradox in multiple sclerosis revisited. *Current Opinion in Neurology, 15*, 239–245.

Bitsch, A., Schuchardt, J., Bunkowski, S., Kuhlmann, T., & Bruck, W. (2000). Acute axonal injury in multiple sclerosis. Correlation with demyelination and inflammation. *Brain, 123*(Pt 6), 1174–1183.

Bizzi, A., Ulug, A. M., Crawford, T. O., Passe, T., Bugiani, M., Bryan, R. N., et al. (2001). Quantitative proton MR spectroscopic imaging in acute disseminated encephalomyelitis. *American Journal of Neuroradiology, 22*, 1125–1130.

Blamire, A. M., Cader, S., Lee, M., Palace, J., & Matthews, P. M. (2007). Axonal damage in the spinal cord of multiple sclerosis patients detected by magnetic resonance spectroscopy. *Magnetic Resonance in Medicine, 58*, 880–885.

Brenner, R. E., Munro, P. M., Williams, S. C., Bell, J. D., Barker, G. J., Hawkins, C. P., et al. (1993). The proton NMR spectrum in acute EAE: the significance of the change in the Cho:Cr ratio. *Magnetic Resonance in Medicine, 29*, 737–745.

Brex, P. A., Parker, G. J., Leary, S. M., Molyneux, P. D., Barker, G. J., Davie, C. A., et al. (2000). Lesion heterogeneity in multiple sclerosis: a study of the relations between appearances on T1 weighted images, T1 relaxation times, and metabolite concentrations. *Journal of Neurology, Neurosurgery, and Psychiatry, 68*, 627–632.

Burtscher, I. M., & Holtas, S. (1999). In vivo proton MR spectroscopy of untreated and treated brain abscesses. *American Journal of Neuroradiology, 20*, 1049–1053.

Caramanos, Z., Narayanan, S., & Arnold, D. L. (2005). 1H-MRS quantification of tNA and tCr in patients with multiple sclerosis: a meta-analytic review. *Brain, 128*, 2483–2506.

Cecil, K. M., & Lenkinski, R. E. (1998). Proton MR spectroscopy in inflammatory and infectious brain disorders. *Neuroimaging Clinics in North America, 8*, 863–880.

Chang, L., Ernst, T., Tornatore, C., Aronow, H., Melchor, R., Walot, I., et al. (1997). Metabolite abnormalities in progressive multifocal leukoencephalopathy by proton magnetic resonance spectroscopy. *Neurology, 48*, 836–845.

Chang, L., Ernst, T., Witt, M. D., Ames, N., Gaiefsky, M., & Miller, E. (2002). Relationships among brain metabolites, cognitive function, and viral loads in antiretroviral-naive HIV patients. *Neuroimage, 17*, 1638–1648.

Chard, D. T., Griffin, C. M., McLean, M. A., Kapeller, P., Kapoor, R., Thompson, A. J., et al. (2002). Brain metabolite changes in cortical grey and normal-appearing white matter in clinically early relapsing-remitting multiple sclerosis. *Brain, 125*, 2342–2352.

Chong, W. K., Paley, M., Wilkinson, I. D., Hall-Craggs, M. A., Sweeney, B., Harrison, M. J., et al. (1994). Localized cerebral proton MR spectroscopy in HIV infection and AIDS. *American Jouranl of Neuroradiology, 15*, 21–25.

Chong, W. K., Sweeney, B., Wilkinson, I. D., Paley, M., Hall-Craggs, M. A., Kendall, B. E., et al. (1993). Proton spectroscopy of the brain in HIV infection: correlation with clinical, immunologic, and MR imaging findings. *Radiology, 188*, 119–124.

Christodoulou, C., Krupp, L. B., Liang, Z., Huang, W., Melville, P., Roque, C., et al. (2003). Cognitive performance and MR markers of cerebral injury in cognitively impaired MS patients. *Neurology, 60*, 1793–1798.

Ciccarelli, O., Altmann, D. R., McLean, M. A., Wheeler-Kingshott, C. A., Wimpey, K., Miller, D. H., et al. (2010a). Spinal cord repair in MS: does mitochondrial metabolism play a role? *Neurology, 74*, 721–727.

Ciccarelli, O., Toosy, A. T., De Stefano, N., Wheeler-Kingshott, C. A., Miller, D. H., & Thompson, A. J. (2010b). Assessing neuronal metabolism in vivo by modeling imaging measures. *Journal of Neuroscience, 30*, 15030–15033.

Ciccarelli, O., Wheeler-Kingshott, C. A., McLean, M. A., Cercignani, M., Wimpey, K., Miller, D. H., et al. (2007). Spinal cord spectroscopy and diffusion-based tractography to assess acute disability in multiple sclerosis. *Brain, 130,* 2220–2231.

Cifelli, A., Arridge, M., Jezzard, P., Esiri, M. M., Palace, J., & Matthews, P. M. (2002). Thalamic neurodegeneration in multiple sclerosis. *Annals of Neurology, 52,* 650–653.

Davie, C. A., Barker, G. J., Thompson, A. J., Tofts, P. S., McDonald, W. I., & Miller, D. H. (1997). 1H magnetic resonance spectroscopy of chronic cerebral white matter lesions and normal appearing white matter in multiple sclerosis. *Journal of Neurology, Neurosurgery, Psychiatry, 63,* 736–742.

Davie, C. A., Barker, G. J., Webb, S., Tofts, P. S., Thompson, A. J., Harding, A. E., et al. (1995). Persistent functional deficit in multiple sclerosis and autosomal dominant cerebellar ataxia is associated with axon loss. *Brain, 118*(Pt 6), 1583–1592.

Davie, C. A., Hawkins, C. P., Barker, G. J., Brennan, A., Tofts, P. S., Miller, D. H., et al. (1994). Serial proton magnetic resonance spectroscopy in acute multiple sclerosis lesions. *Brain, 117*(Pt 1), 49–58.

De Stefano, N., Filippi, M., Miller, D., Pouwels, P. J., Rovira, A., Gass, A., et al. (2007). Guidelines for using proton MR spectroscopy in multicenter clinical MS studies. *Neurology, 69,* 1942–1952.

De Stefano, N., Matthews, P. M., Antel, J. P., Preul, M., Francis, G., & Arnold, D. L. (1995a). Chemical pathology of acute demyelinating lesions and its correlation with disability. *Annals of Neurology, 38,* 901–909.

De Stefano, N., Matthews, P. M., & Arnold, D. L. (1995b). Reversible decreases in N-acetylaspartate after acute brain injury. *Magnetic Resonance in Medicine, 34,* 721–727.

De Stefano, N., Matthews, P. M., Fu, L., Narayanan, S., Stanley, J., Francis, G. S., et al. (1998). Axonal damage correlates with disability in patients with relapsing-remitting multiple sclerosis. Results of a longitudinal magnetic resonance spectroscopy study. *Brain, 121*(Pt 8), 1469–1477.

De Stefano, N., Matthews, P. M., Narayanan, S., Francis, G. S., Antel, J. P., & Arnold, D. L. (1997). Axonal dysfunction and disability in a relapse of multiple sclerosis: longitudinal study of a patient. *Neurology, 49,* 1138–1141.

De Stefano, N., Narayanan, S., Francis, G. S., Arnaoutelis, R., Tartaglia, M. C., Antel, J. P., et al. (2001). Evidence of axonal damage in the early stages of multiple sclerosis and its relevance to disability. *Archives of Neurology, 58,* 65–70.

De Stefano, N., Narayanan, S., Francis, S. J., Smith, S., Mortilla, M., Tartaglia, M. C., et al. (2002). Diffuse axonal and tissue injury in patients with multiple sclerosis with low cerebral lesion load and no disability. *Archives of Neurology, 59,* 1565–1571.

De Stefano, N., Narayanan, S., Matthews, P. M., Francis, G. S., Antel, J. P., & Arnold, D. L. (1999). In vivo evidence for axonal dysfunction remote from focal cerebral demyelination of the type seen in multiple sclerosis. *Brain, 122*(Pt 10), 1933–1939.

Dev, R., Gupta, R. K., Poptani, H., Roy, R., Sharma, S., & Husain, M. (1998). Role of in vivo proton magnetic resonance spectroscopy in the diagnosis and management of brain abscesses. *Neurosurgery, 42,* 37–42; discussion 42-43.

Falini, A., Calabrese, G., Filippi, M., Origgi, D., Lipari, S., Colombo, B., et al. (1998). Benign versus secondary-progressive multiple sclerosis: the potential role of proton MR spectroscopy in defining the nature of disability. *American Journal of Neuroradiology, 19,* 223–229.

Fernando, K. T., McLean, M. A., Chard, D. T., MacManus, D. G., Dalton, C. M., Miszkiel, K. A., et al. (2004). Elevated white matter myo-inositol in clinically isolated syndromes suggestive of multiple sclerosis. *Brain, 127,* 1361–1369.

Ferrante, P., Caldarelli-Stefano, R., Omodeo-Zorini, E., Vago, L., Boldorini, R., & Costanzi, G. (1995). PCR detection of JC virus DNA in brain tissue from patients with and without progressive

multifocal leukoencephalopathy. *Journal of Medical Virology, 47,* 219–225.

Filippi, M. (2001). Multiple sclerosis: a white matter disease with associated gray matter damage. *Journal of Neurological Science, 185,* 3–4.

Filippi, M., Bozzali, M., Rovaris, M., Gonen, O., Kesavadas, C., Ghezzi, A., et al. (2003a). Evidence for widespread axonal damage at the earliest clinical stage of multiple sclerosis. *Brain, 126,* 433–437.

Filippi, M., & Rocca, M. A. (2007). Conventional MRI in multiple sclerosis. *Journal of Neuroimaging, 17*(Suppl 1), 3S–9S.

Filippi, M., Rocca, M. A., & Comi, G. (2003b). The use of quantitative magnetic-resonance-based techniques to monitor the evolution of multiple sclerosis. *Lancet Neurology, 2,* 337–346.

Filippi, M., Rocca, M. A., Martino, G., Horsfield, M. A., & Comi, G. (1998). Magnetization transfer changes in the normal appearing white matter precede the appearance of enhancing lesions in patients with multiple sclerosis. *Annals of Neurology, 43,* 809–814.

Foerster, B. R., Thurnher, M. M., Malani, P. N., Petrou, M., Carets-Zumelzu, F., & Sundgren, P. C. (2007). Intracranial infections: clinical and imaging characteristics. *Acta Radiology, 48,* 875–893.

Fu, L., Matthews, P. M., De Stefano, N., Worsley, K. J., Narayanan, S., Francis, G. S., et al. (1998). Imaging axonal damage of normal-appearing white matter in multiple sclerosis. *Brain, 121*(Pt 1), 103–113.

Gabis, L. V., Panasci, D. J., Andriola, M. R., & Huang, W. (2004). Acute disseminated encephalomyelitis: an MRI/MRS longitudinal study. *Pediatric Neurology, 30,* 324–329.

Gadea, M., Martinez-Bisbal, M. C., Marti-Bonmati, L., Espert, R., Casanova, B., Coret, F., et al. (2004). Spectroscopic axonal damage of the right locus coeruleus relates to selective attention impairment in early stage relapsing-remitting multiple sclerosis. *Brain, 127,* 89–98.

Garbern, J. Y., Yool, D. A., Moore, G. J., Wilds, I. B., Faulk, M. W., Klugmann, M., et al. (2002). Patients lacking the major CNS myelin protein, proteolipid protein 1, develop length-dependent axonal degeneration in the absence of demyelination and inflammation. *Brain, 125,* 551–561.

Garg, M., Gupta, R. K., Husain, M., Chawla, S., Chawla, J., Kumar, R., et al. (2004). Brain abscesses: etiologic categorization with in vivo proton MR spectroscopy. *Radiology, 230,* 519–527.

Geurts, J. J., Reuling, I. E., Vrenken, H., Uitdehaag, B. M., Polman, C. H., Castelijns, J. A., et al. (2006). MR spectroscopic evidence for thalamic and hippocampal, but not cortical, damage in multiple sclerosis. *Magnetic Resonance in Medicine, 55,* 478–483.

Goodkin, D. E., Rooney, W. D., Sloan, R., Bacchetti, P., Gee, L., Vermathen, M., et al. (1998). A serial study of new MS lesions and the white matter from which they arise. *Neurology, 51,* 1689–1697.

Grand, S., Lai, E. S., Esteve, F., Rubin, C., Hoffmann, D., Remy, C., et al. (1996). In vivo 1 H MRS of brain abscesses versus necrotic brain tumors. *Neurology, 47,* 846–848.

Gupta, R. K., Vatsal, D. K., Husain, N., Chawla, S., Prasad, K. N., Roy, R., et al. (2001). Differentiation of tuberculous from pyogenic brain abscesses with in vivo proton MR spectroscopy and magnetization transfer MR imaging. *American Journal of Neuroradiology, 22,* 1503–1509.

Haimes, A. B., Zimmerman, R. D., Morgello, S., Weingarten, K., Becker, R. D., Jennis, R., et al. (1989). MR imaging of brain abscesses. *American Journal of Roentgenology, 152,* 1073–1085.

Helms, G., Stawiarz, L., Kivisakk, P., & Link, H. (2000). Regression analysis of metabolite concentrations estimated from localized proton MR spectra of active and chronic multiple sclerosis lesions. *Magnetic Resonance in Medicine, 43,* 102–110.

Hohlfeld, R. (1997). Biotechnological agents for the immunotherapy of multiple sclerosis. Principles, problems and perspectives. *Brain*, 120(Pt 5), 865–916.

Husted, C. A., Goodin, D. S., Hugg, J. W., Maudsley, A. A., Tsuruda, J. S., de Bie, S. H., et al. (1994). Biochemical alterations in multiple sclerosis lesions and normal-appearing white matter detected by in vivo 31 P and 1 H spectroscopic imaging. *Annals of Neurology*, 36, 157–165.

Inglese, M., Liu, S., Babb, J. S., Mannon, L. J., Grossman, R. I., & Gonen, O. (2004). Three-dimensional proton spectroscopy of deep gray matter nuclei in relapsing-remitting MS. *Neurology*, 63, 170–172.

Iranzo, A., Moreno, A., Pujol, J., Marti-Fabregas, J., Domingo, P., Molet, J., et al. (1999). Proton magnetic resonance spectroscopy pattern of progressive multifocal leukoencephalopathy in AIDS. *Journal of Neurology Neurosurgery Psychiatry*, 66, 520–523.

Jarvik, J. G., Lenkinski, R. E., Grossman, R. I., Gomori, J. M., Schnall, M. D., & Frank, I. (1993). Proton MR spectroscopy of HIV-infected patients: characterization of abnormalities with imaging and clinical correlation. *Radiology*, 186, 739–744.

Kapeller, P., Brex, P. A., Chard, D., Dalton, C., Griffin, C. M., McLean, M. A., et al. (2002). Quantitative 1 H MRS imaging 14 years after presenting with a clinically isolated syndrome suggestive of multiple sclerosis. *Multiple Sclerosis*, 8, 207–210.

Kapeller, P., McLean, M. A., Griffin, C. M., Chard, D., Parker, G. J., Barker, G. J., et al. (2001). Preliminary evidence for neuronal damage in cortical grey matter and normal appearing white matter in short duration relapsing-remitting multiple sclerosis: a quantitative MR spectroscopic imaging study. *Journal of Neurology*, 248, 131–138.

Kastrup, O., Wanke, I., & Maschke, M. (2005). Neuroimaging of infections. *NeuroRx*, 2, 324–332.

Katz, D., Taubenberger, J. K., Cannella, B., McFarlin, D. E., Raine, C. S., & McFarland, H. F. (1993). Correlation between magnetic resonance imaging findings and lesion development in chronic, active multiple sclerosis. *Annals of Neurology*, 34, 661–669.

Kendi, A. T., Tan, F. U., Kendi, M., Yilmaz, S., Huvaj, S., & Tellioglu, S. (2004). MR spectroscopy of cervical spinal cord in patients with multiple sclerosis. *Neuroradiology*, 46, 764–769.

Kesselring, J., Miller, D. H., Robb, S. A., Kendall, B. E., Moseley, I. F., Kingsley, D., et al. (1990). Acute disseminated encephalomyelitis. MRI findings and the distinction from multiple sclerosis. *Brain*, 113(Pt 2), 291–302.

Kingsley, P. B., Shah, T. C., & Woldenberg, R. (2006). Identification of diffuse and focal brain lesions by clinical magnetic resonance spectroscopy. *NMR in Biomedicine*, 19, 435–462.

Kirov, A., II, Tal, J. S., Babb, J., Herbert, & Gonen, O. (2013). Serial proton MR spectroscopy of gray and white matter in relapsing-remitting MS. *Neurology*, 80, 39–46.

Kleinschmidt-DeMasters, B. K., Miravalle, A., Schowinsky, J., Corboy, J., & Vollmer, T. (2012). Update on PML and PML-IRIS occurring in multiple sclerosis patients treated with natalizumab. *Journal of Neuropathology & Experimental Neurology*, 71, 604–617.

Lai, P. H., Ho, J. T., Chen, W. L., Hsu, S. S., Wang, J. S., Pan, H. B., et al. (2002). Brain abscess and necrotic brain tumor: discrimination with proton MR spectroscopy and diffusion-weighted imaging. *American Journal of Neuroradiology*, 23, 1369–1377.

Lai, P. H., Hsu, S. S., Ding, S. W., Ko, C. W., Fu, J. H., Weng, M. J., et al. (2007). Proton magnetic resonance spectroscopy and diffusion-weighted imaging in intracranial cystic mass lesions. *Surgical Neurology*, 68(Suppl 1), S25–S36.

Marliani, A. F., Clementi, V., Albini Riccioli, L., Agati, R., Carpenzano, M., Salvi, F., et al. (2010). Quantitative cervical spinal cord 3 T proton MR spectroscopy in multiple sclerosis. *American Journal of Neuroradiology*, 31, 180–184.

Matthews, P. M., De Stefano, N., Narayanan, S., Francis, G. S., Wolinsky, J. S., Antel, J. P., et al. (1998). Putting magnetic resonance spectroscopy studies in context: axonal damage and disability in multiple sclerosis. *Seminars in Neurology*, 18, 327–336.

McDonald, W. I., Compston, A., Edan, G., Goodkin, D., Hartung, H. P., Lublin, F. D., et al. (2001). Recommended diagnostic criteria for multiple sclerosis: guidelines from the International Panel on the diagnosis of multiple sclerosis. *Annals of Neurology*, 50, 121–127.

McKnight, T. R., Lamborn, K. R., Love, T. D., Berger, M. S., Chang, S., Dillon, W. P., et al. (2007). Correlation of magnetic resonance spectroscopic and growth characteristics within Grades II and III gliomas. *Journal of Neurosurgery*, 106, 660–666.

Mendz, G. L., McCall, M. N., & Kuchel, P. W. (1989). Identification of methyl resonances in the 1 H NMR spectrum of incubated blood cell lysates. *Journal of Biological Chemistry*, 264, 2100–2107.

Menon, D. K., Baudouin, C. J., Tomlinson, D., & Hoyle, C. (1990a). Proton MR spectroscopy and imaging of the brain in AIDS: evidence of neuronal loss in regions that appear normal with imaging. *Journal of Computer Assisted Tomography*, 14, 882–885.

Menon, D. K., Sargentoni, J., Peden, C. J., Bell, J. D., Cox, I. J., Coutts, G. A., et al. (1990b). Proton MR spectroscopy in herpes simplex encephalitis: assessment of neuronal loss. *Journal of Computer Assisted Tomography*, 14, 449–452.

Meyerhoff, D. J., Bloomer, C., Cardenas, V., Norman, D., Weiner, M. W., & Fein, G. (1999). Elevated subcortical choline metabolites in cognitively and clinically asymptomatic HIV+ patients. *Neurology*, 52, 995–1003.

Meyerhoff, D. J., MacKay, S., Bachman, L., Poole, N., Dillon, W. P., Weiner, M. W., et al. (1993). Reduced brain N-acetylaspartate suggests neuronal loss in cognitively impaired human immunodeficiency virus-seropositive individuals: in vivo 1 H magnetic resonance spectroscopic imaging. *Neurology*, 43, 509–515.

Moller, H. E., Vermathen, P., Lentschig, M. G., Schuierer, G., Schwarz, S., Wiedermann, D., et al. (1999). Metabolic characterization of AIDS dementia complex by spectroscopic imaging. *Journal of Magnetic Resonance and Imaging*, 9, 10–18.

Narayana, P. A. (2005). Magnetic resonance spectroscopy in the monitoring of multiple sclerosis. *Journal of Neuroimaging*, 15, 46S–57S.

Narayana, P. A., Doyle, T. J., Lai, D., & Wolinsky, J. S. (1998). Serial proton magnetic resonance spectroscopic imaging, contrast-enhanced magnetic resonance imaging, and quantitative lesion volumetry in multiple sclerosis. *Annals of Neurology*, 43, 56–71.

Narayanan, S., De Stefano, N., Pouwels, P., Barkhof, F., Filippi, M., & Arnold, D. L. (2005). The effect of oral glatiramer acetate treatment on axonal integrity in multiple sclerosis: results from the multicentre CORAL MRS substudy. *Multiple Sclerosis*, 11(Suppl 1), 560.

Narayanan, S., Fu, L., Pioro, E., De Stefano, N., Collins, D. L., Francis, G. S., et al. (1997). Imaging of axonal damage in multiple sclerosis: spatial distribution of magnetic resonance imaging lesions. *Annals of Neurology*, 41, 385–391.

Nath, A., Schiess, N., Venkatesan, A., Rumbaugh, J., Sacktor, N., & McArthur, J. (2008). Evolution of HIV dementia with HIV infection. *International Review of Psychiatry*, 20, 25–31.

Offiah, C. E., & Turnbull, I. W. (2006). The imaging appearances of intracranial CNS infections in adult HIV and AIDS patients. *Clinical Radiology*, 61, 393–401.

Okuda, D. T., Mowry, E. M., Beheshtian, A., Waubant, E., Baranzini, S. E., Goodin, D. S., et al. (2009). Incidental MRI anomalies suggestive of multiple sclerosis: the radiologically isolated syndrome. *Neurology*, 72, 800–805.

Paul, R. H., Yiannoutsos, C. T., Miller, E. N., Chang, L., Marra, C. M., Schifitto, G., et al. (2007). Proton MRS and neuropsychological correlates in AIDS dementia complex: evidence of subcortical specificity. *Journal of Neuropsychiatry and Clinical Neuroscience, 19,* 283–292.

Peterson, J. W., Bo, L., Mork, S., Chang, A., & Trapp, B. D. (2001). Transected neurites, apoptotic neurons, and reduced inflammation in cortical multiple sclerosis lesions. *Annals of Neurology, 50,* 389–400.

Peterson, J. W., & Trapp, B. D. (2005). Neuropathobiology of multiple sclerosis. *Neurologic Clinics, 23,* 107–129, vi-vii.

Pike, G. B., De Stefano, N., Narayanan, S., Worsley, K. J., Pelletier, D., Francis, G. S., et al. (2000). Multiple sclerosis: magnetization transfer MR imaging of white matter before lesion appearance on T2-weighted images. *Radiology, 215,* 824–830.

Polman, C. H., Reingold, S. C., Banwell, B., Clanet, M., Cohen, J. A., Filippi, M., et al. (2011). Diagnostic criteria for multiple sclerosis: 2010 revisions to the McDonald criteria. *Annals of Neurology, 69,* 292–302.

Poptani, H., Gupta, R. K., Jain, V. K., Roy, R., & Pandey, R. (1995a). Cystic intracranial mass lesions: possible role of in vivo MR spectroscopy in its differential diagnosis. *Magnetic Resonance Imaging, 13,* 1019–1029.

Poptani, H., Gupta, R. K., Roy, R., Pandey, R., Jain, V. K., & Chhabra, D. K. (1995b). Characterization of intracranial mass lesions with in vivo proton MR spectroscopy. *American Journal of Neuroradiology, 16,* 1593–1603.

Poptani, H., Kaartinen, J., Gupta, R. K., Niemitz, M., Hiltunen, Y., & Kauppinen, R. A. (1999). Diagnostic assessment of brain tumours and non-neoplastic brain disorders in vivo using proton nuclear magnetic resonance spectroscopy and artificial neural networks. *Journal of Cancer Research and Clinical Oncology, 125,* 343–349.

Salvan, A. M., Confort-Gouny, S., Cozzone, P. J., & Vion-Dury, J. (1999). Atlas of brain proton magnetic resonance spectra. Part III: Viral infections. *Journal of Neuroradiology, 26,* 154–161.

Salvan, A. M., Vion-Dury, J., Confort-Gouny, S., Nicoli, F., Lamoureux, S., & Cozzone, P. J. (1997). Brain proton magnetic resonance spectroscopy in HIV-related encephalopathy: identification of evolving metabolic patterns in relation to dementia and therapy. *AIDS Research and Human Retroviruses, 13,* 1055–1066.

Sarchielli, P., Presciutti, O., Pelliccioli, G. P., Tarducci, R., Gobbi, G., Chiarini, P., et al. (1999). Absolute quantification of brain metabolites by proton magnetic resonance spectroscopy in normal-appearing white matter of multiple sclerosis patients. *Brain, 122* (Pt 3), 513–521.

Sarchielli, P., Presciutti, O., Tarducci, R., Gobbi, G., Alberti, A., Pelliccioli, G. P., et al. (2002). Localized (1)H magnetic resonance spectroscopy in mainly cortical gray matter of patients with multiple sclerosis. *Journal of Neurology, 249,* 902–910.

Schroth, G., Gawehn, J., Thron, A., Vallbracht, A., & Voigt, K. (1987). Early diagnosis of herpes simplex encephalitis by MRI. *Neurology, 37,* 179–183.

Sharma, R., Narayana, P. A., & Wolinsky, J. S. (2001). Grey matter abnormalities in multiple sclerosis: proton magnetic resonance spectroscopic imaging. *Multiple Sclerosis, 7,* 221–226.

Simone, I. L., Federico, F., Tortorella, C., Andreula, C. F., Zimatore, G. B., Giannini, P., et al. (1998). Localised 1 H-MR spectroscopy for metabolic characterisation of diffuse and focal brain lesions in patients infected with HIV. *Journal of Neurology Neurosurgery & Psychiatry, 64,* 516–523.

Srinivasan, R., Sailasuta, N., Hurd, R., Nelson, S., & Pelletier, D. (2005). Evidence of elevated glutamate in multiple sclerosis using magnetic resonance spectroscopy at 3 T. *Brain, 128,* 1016–1025.

Staffen, W., Zauner, H., Mair, A., Kutzelnigg, A., Kapeller, P., Stangl, H., et al. (2005). Magnetic resonance spectroscopy of memory and frontal brain region in early multiple sclerosis. *Journal of Neuropsychiatry and Clinical Neurosciences, 17,* 357–363.

Takanashi, J., Sugita, K., Ishii, M., Aoyagi, M., & Niimi, H. (1997). Longitudinal MR imaging and proton MR spectroscopy in herpes simplex encephalitis. *Journal of Neurological Sciences, 149,* 99–102.

Tarasow, E., Wiercinska-Drapalo, A., Kubas, B., Dzienis, W., Orzechowska-Bobkiewicz, A., Prokopowicz, D., et al. (2003). Cerebral MR spectroscopy in neurologically asymptomatic HIV-infected patients. *Acta Radiology, 44,* 206–212.

Tartaglia, M. C., Narayanan, S., De Stefano, N., Arnaoutelis, R., Antel, S. B., Francis, S. J., et al. (2002). Choline is increased in pre-lesional normal appearing white matter in multiple sclerosis. *Journal of Neurology, 249,* 1382–1390.

Tedeschi, G., Lundbom, N., Raman, R., Bonavita, S., Duyn, J. H., Alger, J. R., et al. (1997). Increased choline signal coinciding with malignant degeneration of cerebral gliomas: a serial proton magnetic resonance spectroscopy imaging study. *Journal of Neurosurgery, 87,* 516–524.

Tien, R. D., Felsberg, G. J., & Osumi, A. K. (1993). Herpesvirus infections of the CNS: MR findings. *American Journal of Roentgenology, 161,* 167–176.

Trapp, B. D., Peterson, J., Ransohoff, R. M., Rudick, R., Mork, S., & Bo, L. (1998). Axonal transection in the lesions of multiple sclerosis. *New England Journal of Medicine, 338,* 278–285.

Trotot, P. M., & Gray, F. (1997). Diagnostic imaging contribution in the early stages of HIV infection of the brain. *Neuroimaging Clinics of North America, 7,* 243–260.

van Waesberghe, J. H., van Walderveen, M. A., Castelijns, J. A., Scheltens, P., Lycklama a Nijeholt, G. J., Polman, C. H., et al. (1998). Patterns of lesion development in multiple sclerosis: longitudinal observations with T1-weighted spin-echo and magnetization transfer MR. *American Journal of Neuroradiology, 19,* 675–683.

von Einsiedel, R. W., Fife, T. D., Aksamit, A. J., Cornford, M. E., Secor, D. L., Tomiyasu, U., et al. (1993). Progressive multifocal leukoencephalopathy in AIDS: a clinicopathologic study and review of the literature. *Journal of Neurology, 240,* 391–406.

Wilkinson, I. D., Miller, R. F., Miszkiel, K. A., Paley, M. N., Hall-Craggs, M. A., Baldeweg, T., et al. (1997). Cerebral proton magnetic resonance spectroscopy in asymptomatic HIV infection. *AIDS, 11,* 289–295.

Wolinsky, J. S., Narayana, P. A., & Fenstermacher, M. J. (1990). Proton magnetic resonance spectroscopy in multiple sclerosis. *Neurology, 40,* 1764–1769.

Wylezinska, M., Cifelli, A., Jezzard, P., Palace, J., Alecci, M., & Matthews, P. M. (2003). Thalamic neurodegeneration in relapsing-remitting multiple sclerosis. *Neurology, 60,* 1949–1954.

Yiannoutsos, C. T., Ernst, T., Chang, L., Lee, P. L., Richards, T., Marra, C. M., et al. (2004). Regional patterns of brain metabolites in AIDS dementia complex. *Neuroimage, 23,* 928–935.

Yousry, T. A., Major, E. O., Ryschkewitsch, C., Fahle, G., Fischer, S., Hou, J., et al. (2006). Evaluation of patients treated with natalizumab for progressive multifocal leukoencephalopathy. *New England Journal of Medicine, 354,* 924–933.

Epilepsy

Jullie Pan and Hoby Hetherington

University of Pittsburgh Medical Center, Pittsburgh, PA, USA

INTRODUCTION

The strength of magnetic resonance spectroscopy (MRS) in the human brain has always been its ability to noninvasively evaluate the relatively high concentration (1–10 mM) compounds associated with brain metabolism. It is therefore not surprising that a neurological disorder such as epilepsy (i.e., spontaneous recurrent seizures), which displays highly aberrant metabolism, can be particularly well investigated by MRS. Notably however, the interest in the MR spectroscopic imaging (MRSI) of epilepsy is not solely based on the interesting metabolic pathophysiology of hyperexcitable networks but also due to the very clinical need to better identify the seizure-onset zone. As much clinical effort has shown, surgical resection of the seizure-onset zone can be a highly effective therapeutic avenue for seizure control (Wiebe et al., 2001; Engel et al., 2003; Erba et al., 2012). However, the challenge of identifying this brain area can be high, as many "localization-related epilepsy" patients can exhibit structural MR imaging (MRI) that is either negative or is ambiguous, i.e., there is an evident anomaly that may or may not localize to seizure onset.

In this chapter we review the various approaches that MR spectroscopic studies have taken for epilepsy, covering ^{31}P and ^{1}H MRS. As has been already discussed (in Chapters 1.1–1.3), single-voxel, multivoxel, and spectroscopic imaging methods are several avenues of spectroscopic study, with varying levels of complexity in acquisition and interpretation. In epilepsy, single-voxel spectroscopy is primarily of use where the region of seizure onset is already known. With well-positioned and adequately small voxel sizes to minimize dilutional effects from adjacent normal (gray and white) tissue, such studies can be informative. It is clear, however, that for many cases of epilepsy where the abnormalities may be both small and cryptic

(i.e., in an unknown location), spectroscopic imaging is a more informative approach. The challenges of spectroscopic imaging, however, are high, requiring excellent performance in both B_0 field homogeneity and B_1 amplitudes, components not commonly a problem for many types of structural imaging. However, for many advanced imaging systems, the performance of these components has been optimized through combinations of hardware and acquisition methods, and will be described in the studies below. Finally, alternative approaches to studying the metabolic state of the brain are available, in particular with intelligent use of ^{13}C-labeled substrates. The challenge of ^{13}C, however, remains its low sensitivity and consequent large voxel sizes (^{13}C is commonly acquired with voxel sizes greater than 50 cc). For epilepsy there would be required modeling with multiple compartments of unknown size, which can thereby make interpretation of the metabolic fluxes less definitive. Nonetheless, it is clear that additional work that can improve sensitivity of such measures are of great interest (see Chapters 4.2 and 4.3). For most of the studies described later in this chapter, higher (3, 4, and 7 T) magnetic fields have been used to garner the greatest sensitivity.

^{31}P STUDIES OF HIGH-ENERGY PHOSPHATES IN EPILEPSY

As is well known, ^{31}P spectroscopy allows the *in vivo* concentrations of phosphocreatine (PCr), adenosine triphosphate (ATP), and inorganic phosphate (Pi) to be imaged noninvasively and provides a direct evaluation of the bioenergetics state of the brain. In the brain, the creatine kinase equilibrium enables the use of PCr as a buffer for ATP such that when the demand for energy exceeds production, PCr is hydrolyzed to maintain ATP stores at constant levels. It is notable that the creatine

172

kinase system is not present in all tissues, and is absent in the kidney and liver, even though the metabolic demand of the kidney is very high (compared to brain, the oxygen consumption of kidney is more than twofold higher). In a teleological sense, the creatine kinase system appears to exist in tissues for which there is high variability in energetic demand (e.g., skeletal, cardiac muscle and brain), and likely physiologically makes use of PCr to temporally maintain constant levels of ATP.

Because of the reduced sensitivity of the ³¹P nucleus in comparison to the ¹H nucleus, lower concentration (1–4 mM), and spin multiplicity, ³¹P studies require greater data averaging to obtain sufficient signal-to-noise ratio (SNR) for interpretation. The large numbers of acquisitions required for SNR purposes also can be used to obtain spatial information simultaneously if phase-encoding is used. Given the absence of a large resonance requiring suppression (e.g., water for ¹H studies), which decreases the absolute requirement for homogeneity and the needed data averaging, strategies that map the entire brain simultaneously are advantageous. At higher fields, it may be thought that the increased linewidths (due to effect of chemical shift anisotropy vs. dipolar relaxation) could be counterproductive; however, the improved SNR has been shown to still result in major improvements (Bogner et al., 2011). At high field (>3 T), 3D SI sequences can generate 6–12 cc voxel resolutions with 40–50 min of acquisition (Hetherington et al., 2001). Although the sequence to acquire the data is elementary, the need for double-tuned radiofrequency (RF) coils (¹H and ³¹P nucleus) to provide both ³¹P images for metabolic information and ¹H images for anatomic interpretation (Vaughan et al., 1994) has even now limited its widespread use on clinical systems.

It should be stated that because of the variation in T_1 values between the high-energy phosphates, the ratios of high-energy phosphates can vary between different experimental conditions based on T_1, tip angle, and TR. This has been extensively discussed (Spencer & Fishbein, 2000; Bottomley et al., 2002) and occurs as a result of the chemical equilibria and magnetization transfer between different ³¹P pools of varying T_1 and the need (in brain spectroscopic studies) for signal averaging and phase encoding with some consequent degree of saturation. Thus for a given set of experimental conditions, the ratios cannot be readily compared to a different set of experimental conditions, and to calculate accurate values, some degree of modeling of the interacting high-energy phosphate pools is needed. Nonetheless, in spite of this, given that the expression of the chemical equilibria directly involves many of the measured ratios of the high-energy phosphates, consistently measured ratios of PCr/Pi and PCr/ATP have still found excellent utility and sensitivity.

In epilepsy ³¹P spectroscopy has been used by numerous groups to find impairments in bioenergetics, specifically decreases in PCr/ATP and PCr/Pi as a consistent finding for a variety of epilepsies, including Lennox–Gastaut syndrome, absence epilepsy, and in localization-related epilepsy (Hugg et al., 1992; Kuzniecky et al., 1992; Laxer et al., 1992; Garcia et al., 1994; Chu et al., 1998; Pan et al., 1999). In children with Lennox–Gastaut and absence epilepsy, nonfocal epilepsies, PCr/ATP was decreased in the cortical gray matter in comparison with that of control subjects (Pan et al., 1999). In patients with frontal lobe epilepsy, Garcia and colleagues (1994) reported elevations of Pi, consistent with a decrease in overall energy charge. Thus the finding of bioenergetic impairment in numerous epilepsy types may reflect a basic pathophysiologic process underlying seizures and seizure propagation.

Because of the numerous hypotheses that link the ketogenic diet (a well-established therapy for epilepsy) to metabolic and bioenergetics shifts (Devivo et al., 1978; Pan et al., 1999; Lutas & Yellen, 2013), we used ³¹P spectroscopic imaging to examine energetic changes induced by the diet in epilepsy patients. This study was performed at 4.1 T using a double-tuned ¹H-³¹P transverse electromagnetic volume coil with ³¹P pulse acquire spectroscopic imaging using a circularly sampled 16 × 16 × 16 matrix, with an effective spherical voxel size of ~11.5 cc (total duration ³¹P study 52 min). Although this study was limited in patient size (a total of seven patients), gray matter ratios of PCr/ATP and PCr/Pi were found, comparing measurements made before versus after initiation of the ketogenic diet: PCR/ATP 0.61 ± 0.08 to 0.69 ± 0.08 and PCr/Pi 2.45 ± 0.27 to 2.99 ± 0.44, before and after, respectively ($p < 0.025$ for both; Fig. 3.3.1). Selecting voxels from white matter did not show a substantial change in these parameters. While this is a small dataset, this showed that the improved seizure control and ketosis were found together with increases in PCr/ATP, raising the notion that in epilepsy, brain bioenergetics could be changed through dietary manipulation.

While many have considered epilepsy as a disorder characterized by aberrant electrical activity from a single location, much animal, clinical, and human research work has also shown that seizures display network properties, involving distorted networks of normal brain function. An obvious example of this has been the thalamus, commonly considered a central integration and regulator of normal whole brain activity. ¹⁸Fluoro-deoxyglucose-positron emission tomography (FDG-PET) studies have shown abnormalities in thalamic metabolism ipsilateral to temporal lobe epilepsy, as well as in linked subcortical nuclei (Benedek et al., 2004). In a similar vein, even with the comparatively large voxel sizes of whole-brain

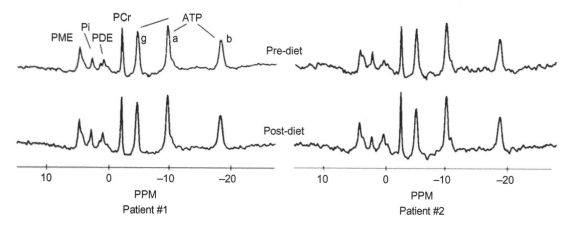

FIGURE 3.3.1   Pre- and post-diet ^{31}P spectroscopic imaging data from two epilepsy patients. The seizures of Patient #2 (right) improved with the diet while Patient #1 (left) did not substantially change. (From Pan et al., 1999, with permission.)

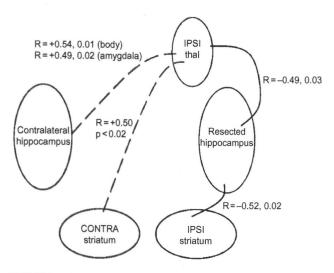

FIGURE 3.3.2   A diagram showing the correlations of the ipsilateral thalamus PCr/ATP with histology (total glial count) of the resected hippocampus and PCr/ATP from other loci. The solid lines represent histological-imaging relationships, the dotted lines are imaging relationships. IPSI, ipsilateral; CONTRA, contralateral.

^{31}P spectroscopic imaging ($\sim 12\,cc$), correlations of PCr/ATP from the ipsilateral thalamus, bilateral hippocampus, and basal ganglia show many significant correlations in temporal lobe epilepsy patients; these relationships are not present in controls, or in the "contralateral" direction (i.e., contralateral thalamus to hippocampi or basal ganglia). Furthermore, with histologic data from the tissue of resected patients, the PCr/ATP values in the ipsilateral thalamus also negatively correlate with glial numbers (but not with neuronal counts). This has been interpreted as a measure of propagated injury (rather than remaining function), within an asymmetric bioenergetic network in temporal lobe epilepsy with the greatest declines of PCr/ATP in the ipsilateral medial temporal lobe (see Fig. 3.3.2).

^{1}H SPECTROSCOPY IN EPILEPSY

What Can be Evaluated

With its greater sensitivity, ^{1}H spectroscopy has been used to a greater extent in the evaluation of epilepsy than ^{31}P. The most commonly studied ^{1}H spectroscopic compounds in MRSI has been N-acetyl-aspartate (NAA), creatine, myo-inositol, glutamate, and GABA. NAA is synthesized only in neuronal mitochondria (Patel & Clark, 1979; Urenjack et al., 1992) and is strongly correlated with oxidative metabolism (Goldstein, 1969; Heales et al., 1995; Bates, et al., 1996). As a result, many studies of a variety of brain disorders have found NAA to be an informative measure of neuronal function (Chapter 2.1). Creatine, as a key component of PCr to be highly useful as a normalization factor for many bioenergetic parameters, is consistent over a cross section of species and within a given tissue type, as discussed by Connett (1988; Chapter 2.2). While found in both neurons and astrocytes, the highest concentration of creatine is in the astrocytes and thus when considering an integrated unit of neuronal function, many groups have used the ratio of NAA/Cr as a normalized parameter. We characterize NAA/Cr as reflecting the bioenergetics of the neuronal/glial unit ("bGNU"), finding it to be very informative for identifying regions of energetic and neuronal dysfunction (Suhy et al., 2000; Muñoz-Maniega et al., 2008; Guevara et al., 2010).

The comparison between MRSI and FDG-PET is inevitable, and while these are clearly complementary measurements, it is worthwhile considering some of the pertinent differences and similarities. FDG-PET evaluates total glucose consumption, and has been long used to measure differences in glucose consumption in varying tissue types (FDG uptake in gray matter is approximately $3\times$ that of white matter,

Huisman et al., 2012) and with various states of activation. The amount of uptake reflects the amount of tissue present in the voxel of interest, and thus decreases in uptake can result from both decreased cerebral consumption and/or tissue atrophy (with potential for distortion of white and gray matter contributions). There is commonly variation in voxel size or point spread function with location in PET, but given improvements with human high-resolution research tomography (HRRT) cameras, the voxel resolution has improved to better than 2–3 mm in-plane resolution (Eggers et al., 2009). For application to epilepsy, the success rate of FDG-PET in identifying the region of seizure onset very much depends on the population studied with the best localization rates of ∼80–90% in temporal lobe epilepsy, although it is probably less successful in the nonlesional neocortical epilepsy patients (for review, see Spencer, 1996; Téllez-Zenteno et al., 2005; Spencer & Huh 2008). This lesser success rate reflects the challenge in neocortical epilepsy, with the region of seizure onset commonly much less well defined, with variations in propagation paths and volume of injury.

In MRSI, the use of the NAA/Cr ratio largely eliminates the sensitivity of the parameter to tissue volume due to minimal NAA and Cr in the cerebrospinal fluid (CSF); however there is sensitivity to tissue type (gray, white matter), with the majority of workers finding that NAA/Cr is smaller in gray than in white matter (reflecting primarily a higher creatine concentration in gray; Hetherington et al., 1996; Pouwels & Frahm, 1998; Schuff et al., 2001). With most sampling strategies, the sampling volume of MRSI is regionally constant, and for practicable time limits of study, are

typically 0.64–2 cc. Thus in epilepsy, where tissue atrophy can be variably gross or subtle, the ability of MRSI to detect dysfunction using the bGNU with tissue-type correction is potentially excellent as it does not require use of asymmetry indices and is relatively independent of tissue atrophy.

Medial Temporal Lobe Epilepsy

MRS work in patients with overtly identified cortical malformations has revealed that NAA changes were specific to the epileptogenic zone, and were "normal" in patients whose seizures were well controlled. Furthermore, in patients with ongoing seizures, the regions that were anatomically abnormal but nonepileptogenic also displayed normal NAA levels (Kuzniecky et al., 1997). As a result, many of the studies using MRS have shown the frequent occurrence of bilateral involvement in temporal lobe epilepsy (e.g., Fig. 3.3.3A), which has since also been reported by conventional and diffusion weighted imaging (Concha et al., 2005; Seidemberg et al., 2005; Araújo et al., 2006). Although the sensitivity to bilateral disease may be counterproductive, commonly the more severely injured temporal lobe is readily detected and many groups have used the NAA and bGNU to localize the seizure-onset zone in medial temporal lobe epilepsy (MTLE) with high sensitivity, 70–100% similar to FDG-PET (Cendes et al., 1994; Connelly et al.,1994; Hetherington et al., 1995). Our recent data (Hetherington et al., 2007; Pan et al., 2013) in temporal lobe epilepsy has demonstrated that the decrements in NAA are not just localized to the ipsilateral hippocampus, but consistent with existing PET and the

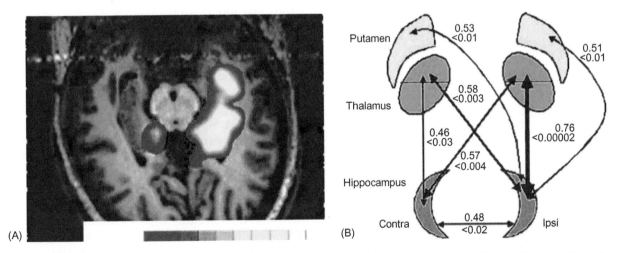

FIGURE 3.3.3 (A) MRSI statistical map showing the bilateral but dominant left hippocampal abnormalities in NAA/Cr. These data are corrected for tissue content variability and are independent of CSF and parenchymal tissue volume. The color bar indicates level of statistical significance, starting at $p < 0.05$ (red). (B) A limbic network of involved loci is seen in MTLE that heavily links the ipsilateral epileptogenic hippocampus with the ipsilateral anterior thalamus, and therein links with numerous other areas including contralateral limbic structures. For each pair of linked structures is shown its R value and significance.

previously mentioned ^{31}P studies are also found in a network of involved limbic and subcortical nuclei, as shown in Fig. 3.3.3A and B.

While it is not surprising that metabolic dysfunction follows from uncontrolled seizure activity, it has also been known that mild to moderate oxidative stress can also cause major abnormalities in GABA (and glutamate). Saransaari and Oja (1997) studied the mouse hippocampus with variable levels of peroxide stress to show increases in basal GABA release, ranging from 30% to >550%. These observations are of particular interest for epilepsy where GABA is thought to be a key component underlying the abnormal hyperexcitability. Given this and the known high energetic cost of neurotransmission and synaptic activity (Atwell & Laughlin, 2001; also Chapter 3.11), we anticipated that GABA neurotransmission and metabolic function might be correlated, certainly in the seizure-onset zone. This may be especially important given the recent *in vitro* work that has suggested GABA function may be either anticonvulsant or proconvulsant (Woo et al., 2002; Palma et al., 2006). This was evaluated in human epilepsy patients undergoing intracranial electroencephalography (EEG) and microdialysis analysis. Their microdialysis measurements of extracellular GABA (ecGABA) were compared to preoperative measures of the bGNU, or NAA/Cr. All data from this study were acquired from the hippocampus, including patients with either hippocampal epilepsy or non-hippocampal (neocortical) epilepsy. Fig. 3.3.4 shows the correlations from this study, finding very strong correlations between ecGABA and NAA/Cr. In the MTLE patients, ecGABA strongly negatively correlated with decreasing NAA/Cr, $R = -0.94$, $p < 0.001$ (Fig. 3.3.4) and implies that ecGABA and mitochondrial function are largely representing parallel processes. There are numerous neurochemical and neurophysiological injury studies that specifically link metabolic function with GABA. For example, Nguyen and Picklo (2002) suggested that injury-produced lipid peroxidation products inhibit the tricarboxylic acid (TCA) cycle enzyme succinic semialdehyde dehydrogenase (which metabolically degrades GABA). This would result in both decreased TCA cycle flow and decreased GABA clearance. Alternatively, electrophysiological data have suggested that in the context of injury and dysfunctional chloride transport, ecGABA can become excitatory (Woo et al., 2002) and can further propagate seizure-linked injury. While these data cannot specify which of several of these injurious processes may be ongoing in the seizure-onset zone, it is evident that the relationship of ecGABA with NAA/Cr within the ipsilateral hippocampus is clearly distinctive in comparison to ecGABA correlations in the non-MTLE group.

In the neocortical epilepsy patients and outside of the seizure-onset zone, the relationship between ecGABA and NAA/Cr, is also significant but positive with $R = +0.70$ $p < 0.015$. In these neocortical patients, the hippocampus studied was ipsilateral to the cortical seizure-onset region and thus may be a site of proximal propagation. Nonetheless, as it is not the seizure focus, these data remain conceptually similar to the results of Petroff et al. (2001), who found that well outside the seizure focus (studying the occipital lobe), patients with better seizure control have higher tissue GABA levels. Similar to the previous data, these correlational data do not permit the determination of the specific relationship between ecGABA and mitochondrial function. However, as these data were made in relatively healthier tissue, the physiological relationships that link these parameters are likely to be different in comparison to that seen in the seizure focus. For example, a potentially common source for increased ecGABA even in healthy brain has been suggested from the readily reversible GABA transporter GAT-1 (Richerson & Wu, 2003).

Thus comparing the *in vivo* human ecGABA and bGNU measure is consistent with rodent data showing relationships between metabolic injury with abnormal ecGABA concentrations, and probably neurotransmission as well. It is of note, however, that it is the hippocampal epilepsy patients (Fig. 3.3.4, filled circles) that show the increased ecGABA and is therefore consistent with the directionality of mitochondrial function causing elevated ecGABA as suggested by Saransaari & Oja (1997). The data from the non-hippocampal epilepsy patients may be more reflective of normal GABA and metabolic interdependence; it is clear that more work will be needed to better understand the poise of these relationships.

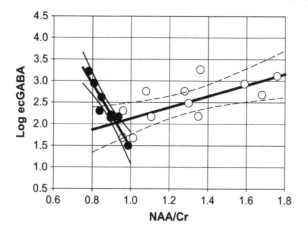

FIGURE 3.3.4　Interictal ecGABA measurements were measured by quantitative zero flow microdialysis, which estimates the true basal concentrations of extracellular fluid neurochemicals such as glutamate, glutamine, and GABA (Cavus et al., 2005). Closed circles from hippocampal epilepsy patients; open circles from non-hippocampal (neocortical) epilepsy patients.

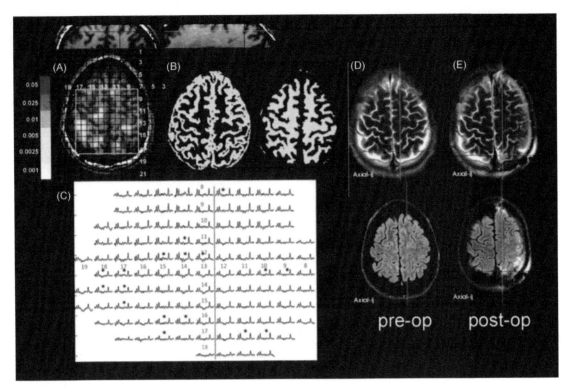

FIGURE 3.3.5 Data from a neocortical epilepsy patient, showing the (A) scout with statistical overlay, (B) segmentation data showing gray and white matter masks, (C) spectra, and (D, E) preoperative and postoperative clinical imaging showing the area of resection in the precuneus. There are multiple areas of NAA/Cr abnormality seen in both hemispheres.

Neocortical Epilepsy

While temporal lobe epilepsy, and, in particular, MTLE, is reasonably well defined from the perspective of anatomy and clinical seizure type, localization of extratemporal and neocortical epilepsies is commonly much more challenging. This arises in part from the limited size, relative clarity, and consistency of medial temporal lobe structures, enabling better identification of abnormalities. For neocortical epilepsy it is not surprising, given the large volume of neocortex that has potential for seizure onset (i.e., that which is either MRI negative, or MRI ambiguous), and the potential for variable propagation paths and variation between different subjects for volume of seizure onset, that this is a much more challenging problem. Nonetheless, given the success of surgery with accurate identification of seizure-onset zone is high (Spencer 1996; Siegel et al., 2001; Téllez-Zenteno et al., 2005; Jayakar et al., 2008), additional information that can help guide this process is desirable. As now routinely performed between neurosurgery and neurology, intracranial EEG monitoring is used to more accurately localize seizure onset; however, it is clear that positioning of electrodes is a critical step: if electrodes do not include an adequate sample of the seizure-onset zone, the likelihood for success for seizure localization is low. Our

group has hypothesized that the high sensitivity of the bGNU measure can help to better localize and understand neocortical epilepsy. The approach taken is to use high-resolution 7 T MRSI to study pertinent brain lobes as indicated from the available clinical information. The extent of overlap between the bGNU abnormality with surgical resection (none, partial, or complete) was compared with patient outcome (International League Against Epilepsy, ILAE, classification dichotomized to I–III and IV–VI). These studies, performed at 7 T for high SNR, made use of high degree and order B_0 shimming to accommodate large volumes of study as well as B_1 RF shimming to overcome known problems B_1 inhomogeneity and amplitude present at 7 T (Avdievich et al., 2009; Pan et al., 2012a).

Fig. 3.3.5 shows data from a patient with neocortical epilepsy with a history of childhood meningitis who had unilateral (left) intracranial EEG coverage based on semiology. The resulting resection surgery included the left precuneus, which did overlap with the bGNU abnormality. Postoperatively this patient did well initially for 3 months, but has had an ILAE class IV outcome. In a group of 25 patients, all of whom eventually underwent resective surgical treatment, we have assessed the coherence of the bGNU with resection region (i.e., did the region of resection overlap with metabolic abnormality or not) and eventual outcome.

TABLE 3.3.1   Concordance between bGNU Abnormality and Surgical Resection with ILAE Outcome

$N = 25$ patients ($p < 0.001$, $\chi^2 = 15.2$)	ILAE I–III	ILAE IV–VI
Complete concordance	A: 14	D: 0
Partial concordance	B: 2	E: 4
Discordant	C: 1	F: 4

While it is clear that this is a small patient group, a Fisher's exact 3×2 contingency statistical test found that the concordance between MRSI and surgical resection was significantly related to good outcome, $p < 0.001$ (see Table 3.3.1).

From an imaging perspective, it may be questioned as to how such studies may be optimally performed, in particular whether the 7 T ultrahigh field is requisite in comparison to the much more commonly available 3 T platform. In such studies that assess all types of localization-related epilepsy (neocortical and medial temporal), the needed volume resolution has not been optimized and thus with minimal *a priori* knowledge, there is a need for excellent spectral quality and spatial resolution. Toward these goals, ongoing developments at ultrahigh field MR are realizing the advantage of the anticipated field improvements in SNR (Tkác et al., 2009; Hale et al., 2010), which specifically in terms of field homogeneity and RF performance (Avdievich et al., 2009; Hetherington et al., 2010, Pan et al., 2012a) have made these high-resolution studies possible. Nonetheless it should be noted that while such technologic developments have been critical for 7 T work, they have immediate relevance for 3 T or 4 T, which is known to suffer from similar (but somewhat milder) problems, especially in lower brain regions (Maudsley et al., 2010a,b). In particular, the temporal lobe is a very commonly involved region in epilepsy, and more consistent success may be obtained by using separate acquisitions rather than 3D whole-brain studies at 3 T or 7 T.

Measurements of GABA and Glutamate

Other important resonances identified for epilepsy include glutamate, GABA, myo-inositol lactate, and glutamine. Glutamate and GABA, in particular, are important targets given their role in neurotransmission. However, as coupled resonances, these compounds generally require more care in detection and analysis, either via short-echo spectroscopy or through editing sequences. While short-echo spectroscopy is a relatively reliable approach, there are potential significant problems due to the variable macromolecule baseline that is present. Our group has targeted the

detection of coupled resonances using a J-refocused coherence transfer (double-echo) sequence that enables longer echo times, which minimizes the macromolecule baseline due to T_2 decay (Chapter 1.4) and yet retains excellent sensitivity to coupled resonances. Fig. 3.3.6 shows the performance of the coherence transfer sequence in comparison to a short-echo acquisition and shows the elevated glutamine resonance in an epilepsy patient being treated with valproic acid.

We have adapted the J-refocused approach to also edit for the C-4 3.0 ppm resonance of GABA (Pan et al., 2012b). This is based on initial suppression of the C-4 3.0 ppm resonance (and overlapping/adjacent resonances including creatine, choline, and macromolecules) via an inversion recovery sequence followed by a homonuclear polarization transfer sequence, resulting in transferred magnetization from the C-3 1.9 ppm GABA resonance to the C-4 3.0 ppm. This magnetization is, therefore, detected without the overlapping and adjacent resonances. The efficiency of this detection is $\sim 50\%$ and is performed in spectroscopic imaging mode as shown in Fig. 3.3.7. As tested in a small epilepsy group, this study found that the thalamic GABA/Cr in poorly controlled epilepsy patients ($n = 6$) was 0.054 ± 0.013 in comparison to controls ($n = 8$) at 0.071 ± 0.015.

Animal Models of Epileptogenesis

MRS has long been proposed to be useful for noninvasively evaluating the process of epileptogenesis (van Eijsden et al., 2004; Gomes et al., 2007). The more recent work of Filibian (2012) used a pilocarpine rat model to study the process of epileptogenesis, using short-echo Point RESolved Spectroscopy (PRESS) and 16 μl voxel sizes in the hippocampus. This report found progressive increases in myo-inositol and glutathione with decreases in NAA in the immediate days after status epilepticus, most likely characterizing microglial activation, edema, and neuronal injury (Fig. 3.3.8). In the chronic epileptic rat, similar findings were reported. This interesting study raises the question of what these changes may mean for epileptogenesis. The absence of changes in GABA and glutamate is notable, given the many rodent studies that have found pertinent changes in these neurotransmitter systems. In human studies, while the reliable detection of myo-inositol has been difficult, increases have been reported in the ipsilateral temporal lobe of MTLE patients (Woermann et al., 1999). It should be noted, however, that in general, short-echo spectroscopy faces problems with the macromolecule baseline, which can be substantial (Hofmann et al., 2001), and may vary depending on pathologic state (Hwang et al., 1996; Graham et al.,

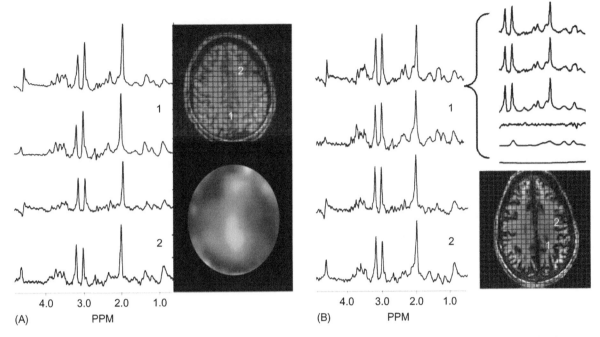

FIGURE 3.3.6 Spectroscopic imaging data from a healthy volunteer (A) and an epilepsy patient on valproic acid (b). Studies are acquired from similar planes for comparability. For both studies, two sets of spectra are shown, J-refocused (top) and short echo (bottom). In the healthy volunteer study, a magnitude glutamate image is shown. In the patient study (B), fitting of the J-refocused spectrum is shown (top to bottom): phased spectrum without baseline correction, spectrum with baseline correction, fitted spectrum, residual, macromolecule baseline, and overall baseline correction. These data were all acquired with a TE = 40 ms at 7 T, nominal voxel size 0.64. Note the generally lower NAA/Cr values and higher myo-inositol present in the epilepsy patient compared to the control.

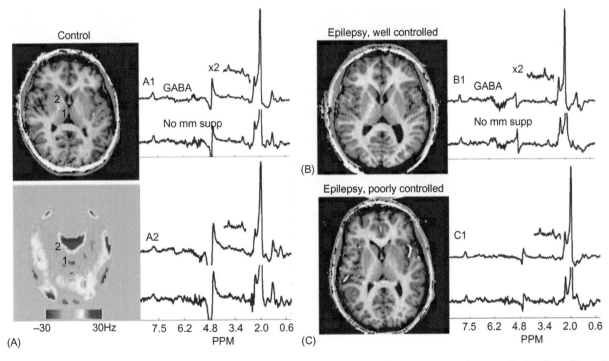

FIGURE 3.3.7 Data from a control (A) and two epilepsy patients (B, C). For each volunteer, scout and spectra (loci indicated) are shown. For the control, a B_0 map is also shown. At each locus indicated, the GABA (macromolecule suppressed) spectrum is shown with 2× magnification. The well-controlled epilepsy patient shows a much larger thalamic GABA resonance than compared with control or the poorly controlled patient. Data were acquired at TE = 40 ms, 16 × 16 encoding (nominal voxel size, 1.44 cc).

3. APPLICATIONS OF ¹H-MRS

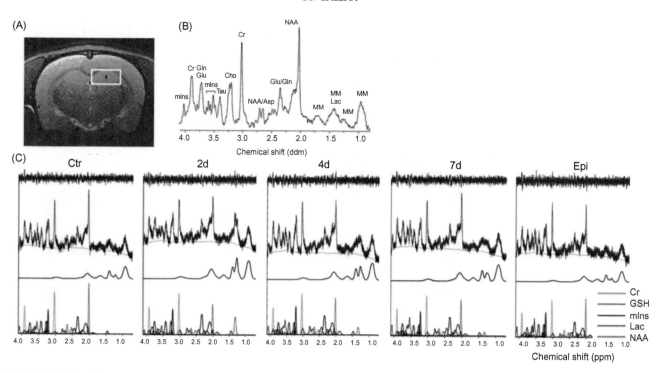

FIGURE 3.3.8 ¹H spectra (7 T 16 μl single-voxel TE 10 ms PRESS) from a pilocarpine rat model of epilepsy, showing progression of abnormalities. Fitted data from (C): spectrum, macromolecule, and fitted resonances (top noise line represents difference residual). (From Filibian et al., 2012.)

2001). With macromolecule components that directly underlie glutamate, GABA, and extend to overlap with glutamine, NAA etc., accurate ratios and concentrations of these compounds can be difficult. Nonetheless as animal model studies, such as that from Filibian et al. (2012), have identified changes in many of these compounds that link with epileptogenesis and seizure-related injury; these remain important targets for continuing MR studies for human epilepsy.

CONCLUSIONS

There are many bases for the metabolic contributions to seizures and epilepsy, in particular those resulting from the close physiological relationship between brain function and metabolism, the uncontrolled energetic demands that seizures place on the brain with consequent injury, and the abundant evidence showing disturbed neurotransmission that occurs under conditions of metabolic dysfunction. As a result, we believe that MRS and MRSI provide many critical tools that help to understand how the *in vivo* brain functions in epilepsy, both on a pathophysiologic and a clinical plane. With improved SNR at ultrahigh field combined with rapid encoding methods, we anticipate that the sensitive detection of key metabolites of NAA, creatine, glutamate, myo-inositol, GABA,

and other metabolically active compounds will enable a deeper understanding of epilepsy and how it can be better clinically managed.

References

Araújo, D., Santos, A. C., Velasco, T. R., Wichert-Ana, L., Terra-Bustamante, V. C., Alexandre, V., et al. (2006). Volumetric evidence of bilateral damage in unilateral mesial temporal lobe epilepsy. *Epilepsia, 47*, 1354–1359.

Atwell, D., & Laughlin, S. (2001). An energy budget for signaling in the gray matter of the brain. *Journal of Cerebral Blood Flow and Metabolism, 21*(10), 1133–1145.

Avdievich, N. I., Pan, J. W., Baehring, J. M., Spencer, D. D., & Hetherington, H. P. (2009). Short echo spectroscopic imaging of the human brain at 7 T using transceiver arrays. *Magnetic Resonance in Medicine, 62*, 17–25.

Bates, T. E., Strangward, M., Keelan, J., Davey, G. P., Munro, P. M., & Clark, J. B. (1996). Inhibition of N-acetylaspartate production: implications for 1 H MRS studies in vivo. *Neuroreport, 7*, 1397–1400.

Benedek, K., Juhász, C., Muzik, O., Chugani, D. C., & Chugani, H. T. (2004). Metabolic changes of subcortical structures in intractable focal epilepsy. *Epilepsia, 45*, 1100–1105.

Bogner, W., Chmelik, M., Andronesi, O. C., Sorensen, A. G., Trattnig, S., & Gruber, S. (2011). In vivo ³¹P spectroscopy by fully adiabatic extended image selected in vivo spectroscopy: a comparison between 3 T and 7 T. *Magnetic Resonance in Medicine, 66*(4), 923–930.

Bottomley, P. A., Ouwerkerk, R., Lee, R. F., & Weiss, R. G. (2002). Four angle saturation transfer method for measuring creatine kinase reactions rates in vivo. *Magnetic Resonance in Medicine, 47*, 850–863.

Cavus, I., Kasoff, W. S., Cassaday, M. P., Jacob, R., Gueorguieva, R., Sherwin, R. S., et al. (2005). Extracellular metabolites in the cortex and hippocampus of epileptic patients. *Annals of Neurology, 57*(2), 226–235.

Cendes, F., Andermann, F., Preul, M. C., & Arnold, D. L. (1994). Lateralization of temporal lobe epilepsy based on regional metabolic abnormalities in proton magnetic resonance spectroscopic images. *Annals of Neurology, 35*, 211–216.

Chu, W. J., Hetherington, H. P., Kuznicky, R. I., et al. (1998). Lateralization of human temporal lobe epilepsy by ^{31}P NMR spectroscopic imaging at 4.1 T. *Neurology, 51*, 472–479.

Concha, L., Beaulieu, C., & Gross, D. W. (2005). Bilateral limbic diffusion abnormalities in unilateral temporal lobe epilepsy. *Annals of Neurology, 57*, 188–196.

Connelly, A., Jackson, G. D., Duncan, J. S., King, M. D., & Gadian, D. G. (1994). Magnetic resonance spectroscopy in temporal lobe epilepsy. *Neurology, 44*, 1411–1417.

Connett, R. J. (1988). Analysis of metabolic control: new insights using scaled creatine kinase model. *American Journal of Physiology, 254*(6 Pt 2), R949–R959.

DeVivo, D. C., Leckie, M. P., Ferrendelli, J. S., & McDougal, D. B., Jr. (1978). Chronic ketosis and cerebral metabolism. *Annals of Neurology, 3*(4), 331–337.

Eggers, C., Hilker, R., Burghaus, L., Schumacher, B., & Heiss, W. D. (2009). High resolution positron emission tomography demonstrates basal ganglia dysfunction in early Parkinson's disease. *Journal of the Neurological Sciences, 276*(1-2), 27–30.

Engel, J., Jr, Wiebe, S., French, J., Sperling, M. R., Williamson, P. D., Spencer, D. D., et al. (2003). Practice parameters: temporal lobe and localized neocortical resections for epilepsy—report of the Quality Standards Subcommittee of the American Academy of Neurology, in association with the American Epilepsy Society and the American Association of Neurological Surgeons. *Neurology, 60*, 538–547.

Erba, G., Moja, L., Bevhi, E., Messina, P., & Pupillo, E. (2012). Barriers toward epilepsy surgery. A survey among practicing neurologists. *Epilepsia, 53*(1), 35–43.

Filibian, M., Frasca, A., Maggioni, D., Micotti, E., Vezzani, A., & Ravizza, T. (2012). In vivo imaging of glia activation using ^{1}H-magnetic resonance spectroscopy to detect putative biomarkers of tissue epileptogenicity. *Epilepsia, 53*(11), 1907–1916.

Garcia, P. A., Laxer, K. D., van der Grond, J., et al. (1994). Phosphorus magnetic resonance spectroscopic imaging in patients with frontal lobe epilepsy. *Annals of Neurology, 35*, 217–221.

Goldstein, F. B. (1969). The enzymatic synthesis of N-acetyl-aspartic acid by sub-cellular preparation of rat brain. *Journal of Biological Chemistry, 244*, 4257–4260.

Gomes, W. A., Lado, F. A., de Lanerolle, N. C., Takahashi, K., Pan, C., & Hetherington, H. P. (2007). Spectroscopic imaging of the pilocarpine model of human epilepsy suggests that early NAA reduction predicts epilepsy. *Magnetic Resonance in Medicine, 58*(2), 230–235.

Graham, G. D., Hwang, J. H., Rothman, D. L., & Prichard, J. W. (2001). Spectroscopic assessment of alterations in macromolecule and small-molecule metabolites in human brain after stroke. *Stroke, 32*(12), 2797–2802.

Guevara, C. A., Blain, C. R., Stahl, D., Lythgoe, D. J., Leigh, P. N., & Barker, G. J. (2010). Quantitative magnetic resonance spectroscopic imaging in Parkinson's disease, progressive supranuclear palsy and multiple system atrophy. *European Journal of Neurology, 17*(9), 1193–1202.

Hale, J. R., Brookes, M. J., Hall, E. L., Zumer, J. M., Stevenson, C. M., Francis, S. T., et al. (2010). Comparison of functional connectivity in default mode and sensorimotor networks at 3 and 7 T. *MAGMA, 23*(5-6), 339–349.

Heales, S. J. R., Davies, S. E. C., Bates, T. E., & Clark, J. B. (1995). Depletion of brain glutathione is accompanied by impaired mitochondrial function and decreased N-acetylaspartate concentration. *Neurochemical Research, 20*, 31–38.

Hetherington, H. P., Avdievich, N. I., Kuznetsov, A. M., & Pan, J. W. (2010). RF Shimming for spectroscopic localization in the human brain at 7 T. *Magnetic Resonance in Medicine, 63*(1), 9–19.

Hetherington, H. P., Kuznicky, R. I., Pan, J. W., Mason, G. F., Morawetz, R., Harris, C., et al. (1995). Proton nuclear magnetic resonance spectroscopic imaging of human temporal lobe epilepsy at 4.1 T. *Annals of Neurology, 38*, 396–404.

Hetherington, H. P., Kuznicky, R. I., Vives, K., Devinsky, O., Pacia, S., Luciano, D., et al. (2007). A subcortical network of dysfunction in TLE measured by MR spectroscopy. *Neurology, 69*, 2256–2265.

Hetherington, H. P., Pan, J. W., Mason, G. F., Adams, D., Vaughn, M. J., Twieg, D. B., et al. (1996). Quantitative ^{1}H spectroscopic imaging of human brain at 4.1 T using image segmentation. *Magnetic Resonance in Medicine, 36*(1), 21–29.

Hetherington, H. P., Spencer, D. D., Vaughan, J. T., et al. (2001). Quantitative ^{31}P spectroscopic imaging of human brain at 4 T: assessment of gray and white matter differences of phosphocreatine and ATP. *Magnetic Resonance in Medicine, 45*, 46–52.

Hofmann, L., Slotboom, J., Boesch, C., & Kreis, R. (2001). Characterization of the macromolecule baseline in localized ^{1}H MR spectra of human brain. *Magnetic Resonance in Medicine, 46*(5), 855–863.

Hugg, J. W., Laxer, K. D., Matson, G. B., et al. (1992). Lateralization of human focal epilepsy by ^{31}P magnetic resonance spectroscopic imaging. *Neurology, 42*, 2011–2018.

Huisman, M. C., van Golen, L. W., Hoetjes, N. J., Greuter, H. N., Schober, P., Ijzerman, R. G., et al. (2012). Cerebral blood flow and glucose metabolism in healthy volunteers measured using a high-resolution PET scanner. *EJNMMI Research, 2*(1), 63.

Hwang, J. H., Graham, G. D., Behar, K. L., Alger, J. R., Prichard, J. W., & Rothman, D. L. (1996). Short echo time proton magnetic resonance spectroscopic imaging of macromolecule and metabolite signal intensities in the human brain. *Magnetic Resonance in Medicine, 35*(5), 633–639.

Jayakar, P., Dunoyer, C., Dean, P., Ragheb, J., Resnick, T., Morrison, G., et al. (2008). Epilepsy surgery in patients with normal or nonfocal MRI scans: integrative strategies offer long-term seizure relief. *Epilepsia, 49*(5), 758–764.

Kuznicky, R., Elgavish, G. A., Hetherington, H. P., et al. (1992). In vivo ^{31}P nuclear magnetic resonance spectroscopy of human temporal lobe epilepsy. *Neurology, 42*, 1586–1590.

Kuznicky, R., Hetherington, H., Pan, J., Hugg, J., Palmer, C., Gilliam, F., et al. (1997). Proton spectroscopic imaging at 4.1 tesla in patients with malformations of cortical development and epilepsy. *Neurology, 48*, 1018–1024.

Laxer, K. D., Hubesch, B., Sappey-Marinier, D., et al. (1992). Increased pH and inorganic phosphate in temporal seizure foci demonstrated by ^{31}P MRS. *Epilepsia, 33*, 618–623.

Lutas, A., & Yellen, G. (2013). The ketogenic diet: metabolic influences on brain excitability and epilepsy. *Trends in Neuroscience, 36*(1), 32–40.

Maudsley, A. A., Domenig, C., Ramsay, R. E., & Bowen, B. C. (2010a). Application of volumetric MR spectroscopic imaging for localization of neocortical epilepsy. *Epilepsy Research, 88*(2-3), 127–138.

Maudsley, A. A., Domenig, C., & Sheriff, S. (2010b). Reproducibility of serial whole-brain MR spectroscopic imaging. *NMR in Biomedicine, 23*, 251–256.

Muñoz Maniega, S., Cvoro, V., Chappell, F. M., Armitage, P. A., Marshall, I., Bastin, M. E., et al. (2008). Changes in NAA and lactate following ischemic stroke: a serial MR spectroscopic imaging study. *Neurology, 71*(24), 1993–1999.

Nguyen, E., & Picklo, M. J., Sr. (2002). Inhibition of succinic semialdehyde dehydrogenase activity by alkenal products of lipid peroxidation. *Biochim Biophys Acta, 1637*(1), 107–112.

Palma, E., Amici, M., Sobrero, F., Spinelli, G., Di Angelantonio, S., Ragozzino, D., et al. (2006). Anomalous levels of Cl- transporters in the hippocampal subiculum from temporal lobe epilepsy patients make GABA excitatory. *Proceedings of the National Academy of Sciences USA, 103*(22), 8465–8468.

Pan, J. W., Bebin, E. M., Chu, W. J., & Hetherington, H. P. (1999). Ketosis and epilepsy: ^{31}P spectroscopic imaging at 4.1 T. *Epilepsia, 40*(6), 703–707.

Pan, J. W., Duckrow, R. B., Spencer, D., Avdievich, N., & Hetherington, H. P. (2013). Spectroscopic imaging of GABA in human brain at 7 T. *Magnetic Resonance in Medicine, 69*(2), 310–316.

Pan, J. W., Lo, K. M., & Hetherington, H. P. (2012a). Role of high degree and order B0 shimming for spectroscopic imaging at 7 T. *Magnetic Resonance in Medicine, 68*(4), 1007–1017.

Pan, J. W., Spencer, D. D., Kuzniecky, R., Duckrow, R. B., Hetherington, H., & Spencer, S. S. (2012b). Metabolic networks in epilepsy by MR spectroscopic imaging. *Acta Neurologica Scandinavica, 126*(6), 411–420.

Patel, T. B., & Clark, J. B. (1979). Synthesis of *N*-acetyl-L-aspartate by rat brain mitochondria and its involvement in mitochondrial/cytosolic carbon transport. *Biochemistry Journal, 184*, 539–546.

Petroff, O. A., Hyder, F., Rothman, D. L., & Mattson, R. H. (2001). Homocarnosine and seizure control in juvenile myoclonic epilepsy and complex partial seizures. *Neurology, 56*(6), 709–715.

Pouwels, P. J., & Frahm, J. (1998). Regional metabolite concentrations in human brain as determined by quantitative localized proton MRS. *Magnetic Resonance in Medicine, 39*(1), 53–60.

Richerson, G. B., & Wu, Y. (2003). Dynamic equilibrium of neurotransmitter transporters: not just for reuptake anymore. *Journal of Neurophysiology, 90*(3), 1363–1374.

Saransaari, P., & Oja, S. S. (1997). Enhanced GABA release in cell-damaging conditions in the adult and developing mouse hippocampus. *International Journal of Developmental Neuroscience, 15*(2), 163–174.

Schuff, N., Ezekiel, F., Gamst, A. C., Amend, D. L., Capizzano, A. A., Maudsley, A. A., et al. (2001). Region and tissue differences of metabolites in normally aged brain using multislice ^{1}H magnetic resonance spectroscopic imaging. *Magnetic Resonance in Medicine, 45*(5), 899–907.

Seidemberg, M., Kelly, K. G., Parrish, J., et al. (2005). Ipsilateral and contralateral MRI volumetric abnormalities in chronic unilateral temporal lobe epilepsy and their clinical correlates. *Epilepsia, 46*, 420–430.

Siegel, A. M., Jobst, B. C., Thadani, V. M., Rhodes, C. H., Lewis, P. J., Roberts, D. W., et al. (2001). Medically intractable, localization-related epilepsy with normal MRI: presurgical evaluation and surgical outcome in 43 patients. *Epilepsia, 42*(7), 883–888.

Spencer, R. G. S., & Fishbein, K. W. (2000). Measurement of spin-lattice relaxation times and concentrations in systems with chemical exchange using the one-pulse sequence: breakdown of the Ernst model for partial saturation in NMR spectroscopy. *Journal of Magnetic Resonance, 142*, 120–135.

Spencer, S., & Huh, L. (2008). Outcomes of epilepsy surgery in adults and children. *Lancet Neurology, 7*(6), 525–537.

Spencer, S. S. (1996). Long-term outcome after epilepsy surgery. *Epilepsia, 37*(9), 807–813.

Suhy, J., Rooney, W. D., Goodkin, D. E., Capizzano, A. A., Soher, B. J., Maudsley, A. A., et al. (2000). ^{1}H MRSI comparison of white matter and lesions in primary progressive and relapsing-remitting MS. *Multiple Sclerosis, 6*(3), 148–155.

Téllez-Zenteno, J. F., Dhar, R., & Wiebe, S. (2005). Long-term seizure outcomes following epilepsy surgery: a systematic review and meta-analysis. *Brain, 128*(Pt 5), 1188–1198.

Tkác, I., Oz, G., Adriany, G., Uğurbil, K., & Gruetter, R. (2009). In vivo ^{1}H NMR spectroscopy of the human brain at high magnetic fields: metabolite quantification at 4 T vs. 7 T. *Magnetic Resonance in Medicine, 62*(4), 868–879.

Urenjack, J., Williams, S. R., Gadian, D. G., & Noble, M. (1992). Specific expression of *N*-acetyl aspartate in neurons, oligodendrocyte type 2 astroyte progenitors and immature oligodendrocytes in vitro. *Journal of Neurochemistry, 59*, 55–61.

van Eijsden, P., Notenboom, R. G., Wu, O., de Graan, P. N., van Nieuwenhuizen, O., Nicolay, K., et al. (2004). In vivo ^{1}H magnetic resonance spectroscopy, T2-weighted and diffusion-weighted MRI during lithium-pilocarpine-induced status epilepticus in the rat. *Brain Research, 1030*(1), 11–18.

Vaughan, J., Hetherington, H. P., Harrison, J., et al. (1994). High frequency coils for clinical nuclear magnetic resonance imaging and spectroscopy. *Magnetic Resonance in Medicine, 32*(2), 206–218.

Wiebe, S., Blume, W. T., Girvin, J. P., & Eliasziw, M. (2001). A randomized controlled trial of surgery for temporal lobe epilepsy. *New England Journal of Medicine, 345*, 311–318.

Woermann, FG, McLean, MA, Bartlett, PA, Parker, GJ, Barker, GJ, & Duncan, JS. (1999). Short echo time single-voxel ^{1}H magnetic resonance spectroscopy in magnetic resonance imaging-negative temporal lobe epilepsy: different biochemical profile compared with hippocampal sclerosis. *Annals of Neurology, 45*(3), 369–376.

Woo, N., Lu, J., England, R., McClellan, R., Dufour, S., Mount, D., et al. (2002). Hyperexcitability and epilepsy associated with disruption of the mouse neuronal specific K-Cl cotransporter gene. *Hippocampus, 12*(2), 258–268.

3.4

Stroke and Cerebral Ischemia

Andrew Bivard[1], Peter Stanwell[2] and Mark Parsons[2]

[1]University of Melbourne, Melbourne Brain Centre, Melbourne, Australia [2]University of Newcastle,
New South Wales, Australia

INTRODUCTION

In developed countries, stroke is the second most common cause of death and the leading cause of adult disability (Senes, 2006). It has also been projected that as the proportion of elderly in the population increases over the next two decades, the total number of strokes per year worldwide may rise 60% (Rothwell, 2001). In Western countries, 85% of strokes are ischemic and 15% are hemorrhagic, with a higher proportion of hemorrhage in Asian countries.

ISCHEMIC STROKE

An ischemic stroke occurs when the blood supply in or to the brain is impaired, typically due to a blood clot. The cells that are solely supplied by the occluded blood vessel undergo necrosis within a few minutes, in an area termed the infarct core. Surrounding the infarct core is a larger area of brain that is hypoperfused but does not infarct rapidly due to an alternate source of blood flow from intact collateral vessels; it is termed the ischemic penumbra. Tissue within the penumbra can be saved from infarction if blood flow is restored promptly by unblocking the occluded vessel. This increases blood flow to the penumbral area above the perfusion threshold for imminent cellular death and prevents the tissue from infarcting. However, if the occlusion persists, the penumbra progressively dies as the collateral blood supply is either not sufficient to sustain the penumbra tissue for the long term or there is collateral vessel failure (Fig. 3.4.1). Rescuing the ischemic penumbra from infarction is the primary target of acute stroke therapies, such as thrombolysis and clot retrieval techniques (Vijay et al., 2010).

Survival of the penumbra can vary from patient to patient from <3–48 h. As a general rule, however, 90% of patients with supratentorial large artery occlusion (typically middle cerebral artery) have a clinically significant volume of penumbra tissue at 3 h after stroke onset (Furlan et al., 1999; Lees et al., 2010). By 6 h, only 75–80% of patients still have some penumbral tissue. Thus, ~25% of patients in the 3–6 h window are unlikely to benefit from thrombolysis if the standard clinical criteria are applied, almost certainly because a significant proportion of their penumbral tissue has been converted to infarct core. It has also been demonstrated that in the 3–6 h time window, that the size of the infarct core was the strongest predictor of outcome (Singer et al., 2008), regardless of the extent of residual penumbra. Further, the volume of the infarct core varies considerably from patient to patient despite similar times after stroke onset, likely due to large differences in the volume of collateral supply. The cerebral watershed areas, i.e., the areas between major vascular territories such as between the middle cerebral and anterior cerebral artery, are more susceptible to ischemic injury. Watershed areas receive blood supply from both of the nearby major arteries, therefore if one artery is blocked, there is a significant decline in blood supply, and the other nearby major artery does not provide enough blood supply to maintain tissue about the ischemic threshold. Additionally, posterior artery occlusions more often result in significant infarction due to the mild symptoms patients experience that delay treatment, and the small size of the vessel that limits the action of thrombolytic treatments.

During ischemia, there is a reduced supply of energy substrates such as glucose and oxygen. The neuronal injury cascade starts following failure of energy-dependent processes such as sodium pumps (Taoufik & Probert, 2008). Following hypoperfusion, cells resort to anaerobic glycolysis to compensate for the reduced energy supply, which results in an

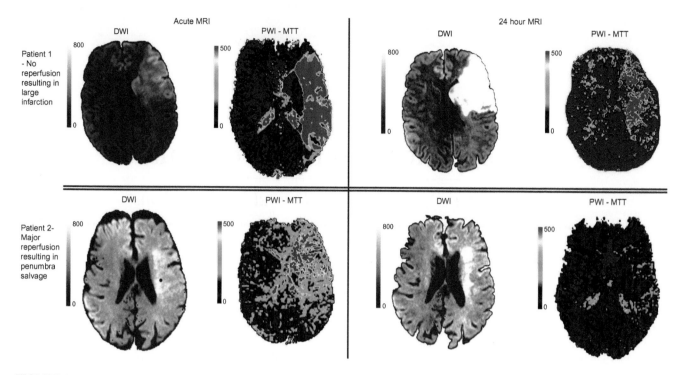

FIGURE 3.4.1   Acute and 24 h MRI of stroke patients showing the effect of reperfusion therapy. Patient 1 has a very large acute perfusion lesion on the PWI-MTT map, and a small acute infarct core on DWI. However, thrombolysis was not successful and the middle cerebral artery remained occluded resulting in a large area of infarction (increased DWI lesion volume) and persistent hypoperfusion on PWI-MTT. Patient 2 also had a middle cerebral artery occlusion on acute PWI-MTT maps and minimal acute infarction. After successful reperfusion therapy, the PWI-MTT map showed increased blood transit to the previously ischemic area with minimal infarction of follow-up DWI. These two patients had the same site of vessel occlusion but very different outcomes. This demonstrates the power of successful reperfusion therapy to treat acute ischemic stroke.

increase in lactic acid. Lactic acid byproducts are toxic at high concentrations and can disrupt tissue metabolism further or destroy cells (Back et al., 2004). The failure of sodium pumps also causes the excitotoxic release of glutamate due to the reversal of glutamate transporters, moving glutamate into the extracellular space. Excessive extracellular glutamate is highly detrimental to tissue and causes an influx of intracellular calcium that can lead to apoptosis or mitochondrial failure, leading to further energy depletion (see Chapter 2.4). Evidence is emerging that ischemic damage can continue to occur weeks after the acute event due to factors such as systemic hypotension, intracranial hypertension, or hyperglycemia (Merino & Warach, 2010), all of which affect the neuronal metabolism and may lead to further injury or impair recovery.

HEMORRHAGIC STROKE

Intracerebral hemorrhage (ICH) involves blood flowing through the blood–brain barrier into brain parenchyma and represents 15–20% of all strokes (Broderick et al., 2007) with a 50% mortality rate at day 30 (Broderick et al., 1993). African or Asian descent, hypertension, age, anticoagulant therapy, and amyloid angiopathy are significant risk factors for ICH (Hart et al., 2005). Factors associated with poor outcome include large hematoma volume (> 30 ml), posterior fossa and infratentorial location (Meretoja et al., 2012), older age, and admission mean arterial blood pressure > 130 mmHg (Fogelholm et al., 2005). Traumatic brain injury causes 15% of ICH while 85% of ICHs are spontaneous events caused by rupture of penetrating arteries and arterioles that may be damaged by hypertension (60%; Thrift et al., 1998) or amyloid angiopathy (30%; Qureshi et al., 2001).

MAGNETIC RESONANCE IMAGING IN STROKE

Acute stroke imaging can be used to confirm the diagnosis of stroke; identify the site of vessel occlusion, the extent of the perfusion deficit, and the age of the lesion; and define the tissue pathophysiology. Clinical evaluation is not an accurate predictor of these features and cannot differentiate stroke subtypes and imitators. Therefore, acute brain imaging is a mandatory requirement in the management of all strokes, or suspected stroke patients.

Magnetic resonance imaging (MRI) is the examination of choice for most neurological conditions, including stroke (Seenan et al., 2007; Annemans et al., 2010). The strengths of MRI are high soft tissue resolution, high sensitivity for tissue edema, and whole-brain coverage (with perfusion imaging). Unlike computed tomography (CT), MRI does not use ionizing radiation, and MRI has a much higher sensitivity for hemispheric and especially brainstem ischemia, particularly in a hyperacute situation (<12 h after onset) with diffusion-weighted imaging (DWI). However, there are some practical disadvantages of MRI; depending on number and length of imaging acquisition sequences, an MRI of a stroke patient can take up to 40 min, thus delaying the initiation of time-critical acute reperfusion therapy (intravenous thrombolysis or clot retrieval). For this reason, stroke centers that do perform acute stroke MRI prior to reperfusion therapy use the bare minimum of sequences to reduce treatment delays. Typically, these sequences include a T_1-weighted sequence, DWI, time of flight intracranial angiography, fluid attenuated inversion recovery, T_2^*w gradient echo sequence, and (depending on local expertise/preferences) dynamic susceptibility contrast perfusion-weighted imaging (DSC-PWI; Fig. 3.4.2).

The earliest morphological changes that are detectable are mostly due to edema with shortening of cortical sulci and distortions of the ventricular areas due to brain volume changes and retention of cerebral blood volume, both of which are best viewed with T_1 imaging. Changes on T_2 imaging are a result of the development of vasogenic edema, which develops after the acute stroke phase around 6−8 h after onset. Restricted diffusion is thought to occur within minutes of onset of ischemia due to cytotoxic edema (Kidwell et al., 2000; Bristow et al., 2008) or astrocyte swelling. Cytotoxic edema is a consequence of dysfunction of cellular metabolism (Bykowski et al., 2006) resulting in the failure of sodium and potassium pumps causing retention of sodium and water. This is an earlier pathophysiologic process than vasogenic edema, which occurs as a result of a breakdown of the blood—brain barrier, causing a build-up of intravascular proteins and fluid in the cerebral parenchymal extracellular space. T_2-weighted MRI is a conventional MR sequence that is able to detect vasogenic edema but not cytotoxic edema or astrocyte swelling, so like noncontrast CT, is often normal in the first 6 h after stroke onset. DWI is considered the "gold-standard" method to image the acute infarct core in clinical practice because it can measure cytotoxic edema in the acute phase of stroke (Chemmanam et al., 2010) and has been validated to be a measure of the acute infarct core. Currently, angiography and perfusion studies have shown very little dynamic changes after 15 min from occlusion, and as such perfusion imaging is used as a static marker of penumbra volume when a perfusion threshold is applied. The perfusion threshold

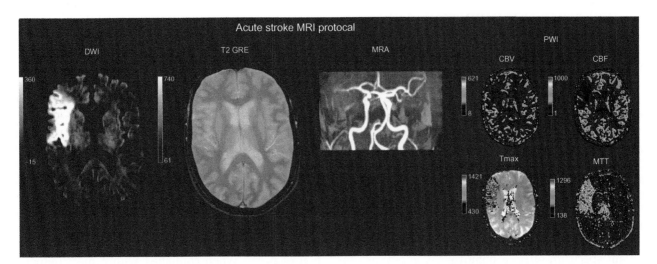

FIGURE 3.4.2 These maps are from the same acute ischemic stroke patient MRI, demonstrating the usefulness of multimodal MRI. The DWI map is used as the current gold standard for infarct core detection, represented by the hyperintense white region. Magnetic resonance angiography (MRA) is used to identify the site of vessel occlusion and measure the collateral circulation. This patient has a right middle cerebral artery occlusion with minimal collateral blood flow circumventing the site of vessel occlusion. Finally, the PWI map, which involves the injection of a contrast agent to quantify the cerebral blood flow (CBF) of the ischemic region, showed hypoperfusion in the middle cerebral artery region. PWI post processing results in four maps of cerebral blood volume (CBV), CBF, time to peak of the residual function (Tmax), and mean transit time (MTT, which is the ratio of CBF/CBV). The Tmax/MTT map shows very low flow in this DWI lesion area, indicating that there is minimal acute penumbra to be salvaged from reperfusion therapy.

does not change with time in the human clinical setting and is typically calculated as an increase of 2 s for contrast to reach tissue compared to the average contralateral hemisphere (Bivard & Parsons, 2012).

Another potential disadvantage of MR in acute stroke assessments is that 10–15% patients cannot have an MRI due to the presence of pacemakers or other metallic objects, claustrophobia, or an inability to lie still, which is more commonly seen in acute stroke patients compared to other patient groups due to cerebral irritability or acute cognitive deficits. Finally, immediate access to MRI in many hospitals worldwide is not available due to the expensive nature of installing and running an MRI, and because MRI is not often available at short notice due to high demand. Nonetheless, in an ideal world with immediate access to MRI, a streamlined protocol, and no patient contraindications, MRI is considered the gold-standard imaging for hyperacute stroke. In the subacute situation, where there is more time to screen for MRI compatibility and arrange access to the MRI scanner, there is no doubt that MRI is the superior imaging modality in terms of diagnosis, planning secondary prevention treatment, and predicting likely recovery. Predicting recovery/prognosis after stroke is predominantly where magnetic resonance spectroscopy (MRS) has been studied to date. Currently, because the role of MRS in acute stroke diagnosis and treatment selection in still evolving, most centers do not routinely perform MRS as part of hyperacute stroke MR protocols.

SPECTROSCOPY: PROTON MRS

In MRI the recorded signal intensity is the sum of the signals from all the hydrogen-containing molecules in a given volume (mostly fat and water); however, in localized proton spectroscopy of the brain the signal arising from water is much stronger ($\times 10^3$ more concentrated) then the cerebral metabolites of interest and therefore must be suppressed to allow for the detection of these low concentration neurochemicals of interest. The low concentration of metabolites of interest also ultimately leads to the low inherent signal-to-noise ratio (SNR) of the MRS experiment therefore demanding either comparatively large voxel size, long measurement time, or a trade-off between these two parameters. The resultant spectrum offers a noninvasive, *in vivo* assessment of brain neurochemistry with interpretation and analysis of such spectra based on the assessment of several key parameters including: (1) chemical shift, (2) metabolite signal intensity, and (3) spin–spin (J) coupling. Chemical shifts and J-couplings afford information regarding metabolite composition, while signal intensity affords information regarding metabolite

concentration. ^{1}H MRS is currently the most widely applied *in vivo* technique in stroke as it can be undertaken in a timely fashion (<5 min) using the same hardware as standard MRI. *In vivo* it records signals from *N*-acetylaspartate (NAA), choline-containing compounds (tCho), total creatine (Cr), myo-inositol (mI), lactate (Lac), lipids (Lip), and glutamine plus glutamate (Glx). These metabolites are present in the human brain at greater than millimolar (mM) concentrations and have spectra at known positions, which are expressed as parts per million (ppm; Fig. 3.4.3).

Single-voxel MRS is the most commonly used technique using Point RESolved Spectroscopy (PRESS) or STimulated Echo Acquisition Mode (STEAM) sequences. Clinically, MRS is readily available and is increasingly used due to short acquisition times (around 4–5 min for a single voxel) and the usefulness of information that MRS provides on the changes in concentration of metabolites post stroke (Ford et al., 1992; Gillard et al., 1996).

NAA

The largest metabolite signal in the normal adult brain, resonating at 2.02 ppm, is due to the acetyl moiety of NAA, with a smaller contribution from *N*-acetylaspartylglutamate or NAAG (see Chapter 2.1). NAA has been shown to be primarily localized to neurons, axons, and dendrites within the central nervous system. Moreover, studies of diseases known to involve neuronal or axonal loss have consistently shown NAA to be decreased. Accordingly, NAA is considered a neuronal marker with its concentration roughly equal in both white and gray matter (Tallan et al., 1956); however, the exact function of NAA is unknown.

The level of NAA detected using ^{1}H MRS was found to decrease dramatically after a stroke, and to continue to decline up to 1 week after stroke (Saunders et al., 1995). This therefore suggests that there is significant neuronal loss due to ischemia and that ischemic damage continues after the acute period. However, the continued decline of NAA may not necessarily reflect ongoing damage but might be the action of macrophages in clearing already dead cells. Moreover, low NAA is not specific for stroke as it can be seen in many other neurological disorders. Clinically, the concentration of NAA, when combined with a measurement of the acute infarct core (<6 h) on $T_{2}*w$ imaging, was a better predictor of patient outcome than either measure alone (Pereira et al., 1999). Therefore it appears that the concentration of NAA is clinically relevant to patient outcome and is a marker of the extent of ischemic damage. NAA and Lac are the only metabolites with an established clinical link in stroke.

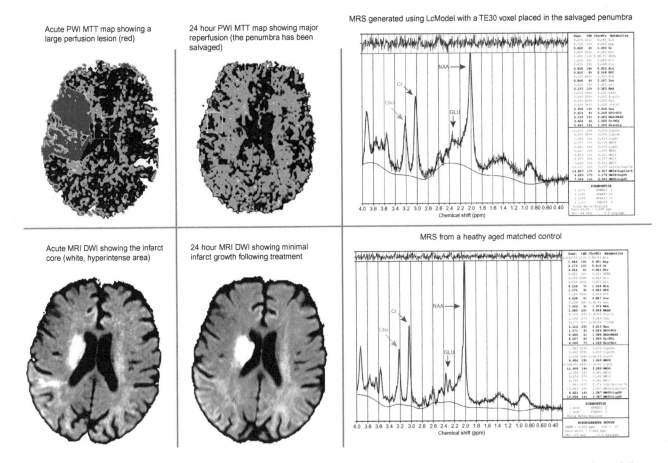

FIGURE 3.4.3 Spectroscopy of the reperfused penumbra. This patient had an acute ischemic stroke with an occlusion in the middle cerebral artery resulting in a small acute infarct core and large penumbra (seen as the mismatch between the acute DWI lesion and the PWI-MTT lesion). This patient was treated with thrombolysis that resulted in major reperfusion in the ischemic region and a large area of penumbra salvage (seen as minimal lesion growth between acute and 24 h DWI lesion volume, and normal 24 h PWI-MTT). On follow-up MRI, this patient also had an MRS single voxel placed in the reperfused penumbra. The MRS showed normal NAA, but major reductions in glutamate and Cr when compared to a control MRS. Metabolite concentrations are highlighted on the right (MRS processed by LCModel, and all other MRI processed on MiStar).

Cr

The total Cr signal resonates at 3.02 ppm and is a composite resonance consisting of Cr and phosphocreatine, compounds that are involved in energy metabolism through the Cr kinase reaction generating adenosine triphosphate (ATP; see Chapter 2.2). Cr concentration varies between glial cells and neurons, and the Cr concentration in white matter signal is lower than gray matter. There are also regional differences with supratentorial white and gray matter displaying lower levels of Cr than the cerebellum and insular cortex. Representing the energy buffer and phosphate transport system in neurons and glial cells, measurements of total Cr reflect the available metabolic energy in the brain. While Cr and phosphocreatine peaks can be separated using high strength scanners (>3 T) (Provencher, 1993), such measurements are best undertaken with ^{31}P MRS (Chu et al., 1998). Total Cr as measured using ^1H MRS has been found to continue to decline for up to 10 days post stroke (Saunders et al., 1995). This may be due to a change in cell population (reflected by a decrease in NAA) resulting in altered metabolic energy availability and use. However, the decline in Cr may also be a delay in clearing cellular fragments from infarcted tissue. Gray matter contains a larger total Cr signal from MRS than white matter (Hetherington et al., 1996), suggesting that changes in the total Cr level may represent preferential damage to gray matter. However, glial cells are also known to contain a higher level of Cr than neurons (Urenjak et al., 1993), and as such changes in total Cr may reflect glial proliferation in response to injury or preferential damage to glial cells.

Around 6 weeks after a stroke, it has been shown that the ratio of NAA/Cr is increased around the stroke lesion, likely due to a loss of NAA signal, which then returns to near normal at 1 year post stroke (Mountz, 2007). The correction of the NAA/Cr ratio may be due to an increase in NAA that reestablishes the NAA/Cr ratio or a reduction in Cr, as a result of a reduced cell population that requires less phosphate stored by Cr. The implications of these metabolite changes are unknown, but show that the brain is metabolically reorganizing for a very long time post stroke. Biologically, changes in metabolite concentrations could be due to delayed ischemia, delayed clearance by macrophages, or changes in demand for metabolites due to neural plasticity.

Choline

The signal from choline-containing compounds resonates at 3.21 ppm and arises from the trimethylamine groups of glycerophosphocholine (GPC), phosphocholine (PC), and free choline, which are measured together as total choline concentration (tCho; see Chapter 2.3). These compounds are known to be involved in cell membrane synthesis and degradation, and are perceived as a marker of cell membrane integrity. In a healthy, intact brain, choline reflects the levels of GPC and PC, which are involved in membrane synthesis and degradation (Miller, 1991), with increases of tCho in stroke thought to reflect gliosis or damage to myelin, and decreases of tCho as a result of edema, necrosis, and cell loss. Changes in the choline peak have been noted post stroke; however, the implications and direction of these changes are unknown and inconsistent (Gideon et al., 1992; Graham et al., 1993). One year post stroke, it has been shown that there is an increase in the Cr/Cho ratio in the hemisphere contralateral to the stroke lesion as well as an increase in cerebral blood flow (Mountz, 2007), which may be due to plasticity and reorganization.

Theoretically, demyelination (such as in multiple sclerosis) results in an increase in choline-containing metabolites. However, if there is significant tissue damage, as in stroke, demyelination monitoring by measuring tCho may not directly reflect cell membrane damage or integrity. Therefore tCho changes should be measured with other metabolites such as NAA to understand if cellular membranes are damaged, or if the cell itself is dead.

Lac

The signal from Lac is observed as a doublet (1.33 ppm). Healthy tissues do not have sufficient Lac concentration for *in vivo* detection by proton MRS, although it may be detectable in cerebrospinal fluid (CSF) due to higher concentrations or longer T_2 relaxation values in CSF than brain. However, Lac can be detected as a product of anaerobic glycolysis when the brain is starved of oxygen. Additionally, interruption of the Krebs cycle by mitochondrial damage and absence or inhibition of pyruvate dehydrogenase can also result in a detectable Lac signal (see Chapter 2.5).

During a stroke there is severe hypoperfusion resulting in a shutdown of the ATP-driven sodium pumps. This results in an increase in anaerobic metabolism due to a reduction in blood-delivered oxygen, which in turn results in an increase in anaerobic byproducts such as Lac. The increase in Lac has been shown to persist for months in the peri-infarct stroke lesion (Graham et al., 1993), and Lac has been found outside of the stroke-affected perfusion lesion (Saunders, 1995), even in the contralateral hemisphere (Gillard et al., 1996). This shows that the effects of ischemia extend far beyond the perfusion lesion, and mean that even oligemic hypoperfusion (hypoperfusion that does not cause infarction) results disruption of ATP synthesis.

Myo-inositol

Myo-inositol (mI) generates four groups of resonances; a doublet-of-doublets centered at 3.52 ppm and a triplet at 3.61 ppm each corresponding to two protons. *myo*-Inositol is a carbohydrate and structural foundation for secondary messengers in eukaryotic cells and various inositol phosphates. Observations of MRS applied to stroke have reported no consistent increase or decrease in mI.

Glutamate and Glutamine

Glutamine is a precursor and storage form of glutamate and is located within astrocytes, while glutamate is the major excitatory neurotransmitter in the human brain, as well as, a component of intermediary energy metabolism. The sum of glutamate plus glutamine (Glx) produces a characteristic spectral pattern between 2.12 and 2.35 ppm, as well as at 3.74 and 3.75 ppm.

The link between elevated glutamate, the N-methyl-D-aspartate (NMDA) receptor, and the etiology of stroke is firmly established (Brott & Bogousslavsky, 2000). In humans following stroke there is a large and persistent release of glutamate into the intracellular space during the first few minutes of stroke (Bullock et al., 1995). This release of glutamate is not limited to just the ischemic area and can affect regions distal to the infarction. Also, high levels of glutamate have also been measured in plasma and CSF in patients with acute ischemic stroke (Dávalos et al., 1997).

Excitotoxicity is thought to be the primary cause of cellular dysfunction after acute stroke treatment with thrombolytics. A decrease in the ATP levels of astrocytes cause glutamate efflux due to a reversal of the ionic gradients that drive transporter function (Hazell, 2007). Although under normal conditions astrocytes remove neuronally released glutamate via active transport and conversion to glutamine (see Chapter 3.11). Under ischemic conditions dysregulation of this process may lead to impaired glutamate uptake and elevated levels (Rossi et al., 2007). Astrocyte swelling due to excessive K^+ spatial buffering or glutamate uptake can result in depolarization of cells, leading to release of glutamate via transporter reversal. These processes lead to increased extracellular glutamate concentration and excitotoxic-mediated cell dysfunction.

MRS IN THE PENUMBRA AND INFARCT CORE

Previous MRS studies have struggled to separate the processes taking place in the infarct core and penumbra (see Fig. 3.4.4). Animal experiments have shown that the excitotoxic release of glutamate occurs extremely rapidly after ischemic onset, and is rarely present at 6–24 h after ischemic stroke. Additionally, the concentration of glutamate is not significantly different at the border zone between the infarct core and penumbra, making glutamate a poor marker of either infarct core or penumbra in the acute setting. If energy metabolism is impaired in the penumbra, it would be expected that there would be a decrease in the concentration of glutamate due to its role in mitochondrial energy production. Moreover, if there were disruption in glutamate metabolism, there would be a difference in the concentration of glutamate and glutamine compared to healthy individuals. However, due to technical constraints, measurements of both glutamate and glutamine have not been done in human ischemic stroke patients.

Lac has been consistently reported to be the metabolite of choice to separate core and penumbra, with the infarct core undergoing a more rapid increase in the level of Lac than the penumbra due to a greater degree of hypoperfusion resulting in a more rapid onset of anaerobic metabolism in the core versus penumbra. Moreover, the concentration of Lac in the infarct core can be equal to that of NAA, while in the penumbra it may rise to 2 mM, therefore, while there is a rise of Lac in both the infarct core and penumbra, there is still a significant difference in the concentration between the two tissue pathophysiologies. Following reperfusion, the Lac levels dramatically reduce in the penumbra compared to ischemic conditions. Low levels of Lac observed in reperfused human tissue indicate that the tissue is still viable, whereas persistent high Lac likely reflects chronic hypoperfusion and lack of tissue viability and impending infarction at later time windows (>6 h).

Changes in brain metabolic concentrations, as detected by ^1H MRS, are observed beyond the volume of the penumbra and infarct core. The effect of stroke has been seen in the hippocampus in patients with a large middle cerebral artery occlusion (Tang et al., 2011). A decreased NAA/Cr ratio seen in the hippocampus post stroke is similar but not as severe as that seen in Alzheimer's disease, suggesting significant tissue damage leading to future memory impairment.

SPECTRAL EDITING

The spectra for glutamate, GABA, and glutamine overlap considerably, making quantification difficult. Spectral editing methods, such as TE averaging and MEGA-PRESS that target a specific metabolite, are available to investigate these metabolites (Mescher et al., 1998). A frequency-selective editing technique (MEGA) combined with the point-resolved spectroscopy sequence (PRESS) method (MEGA-PRESS) allows the detection of the outer two peaks of the GABA triplet at 3.0 ppm, while editing out signal due to Cr and sacrificing the central peak of the triplet. GABA consists of six coupled proton spins, and their chemical shifts are as follows: H2 and H2' = 3.01 ppm, H3 and H3' = 1.89 ppm, and H4 and H4" = 2.28 ppm. One of the most accurate ways to measure GABA is using MEGA-PRESS, using the J-coupling between the GABA-H2 resonance at 3.01 ppm and GABA-H3 resonance at 1.89 ppm to reveal the GABA resonance with the following parameters: echo time (TE) = 68 ms, repetition time (TR) = 3000 ms, 96 averages, 2048 acquisition points. Two subsequent editing acquisitions are made, each with scan-to-scan switching of the editing frequency between 1.9 and 7.5 ppm. Furthermore, raw MEGA-PRESS data can be analyzed as a standard single-voxel spectroscopy (SVS) TE = 68 sequence. The SVS spectra can then be used to measure other metabolites such as NAA and Lac and glutamine. This approach has been validated and published in multiple disorders, with the exception of stroke. Despite the availability of these techniques, no studies have been reported in ischemic stroke.

DIASCHISIS

Diaschisis has been defined as a loss of function within a region distant to the site of the lesion and results from deafferentation of neurons as a result of

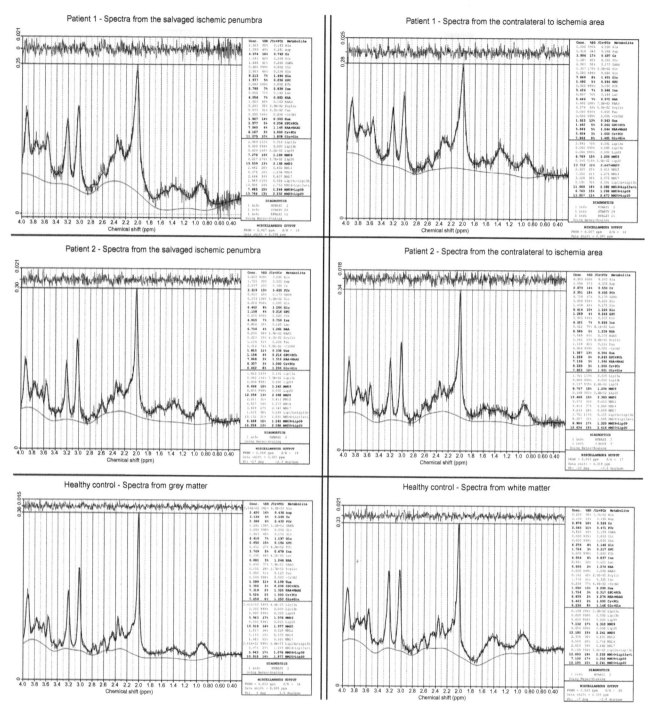

FIGURE 3.4.4   This figure demonstrates the MRS single-voxel results from two patients with major reperfusion resulting in penumbra salvage. Voxels were placed in the penumbra (first column) and contralateral to ischemic stroke region (second column) to demonstrate a variety of different results as well as compare to two control voxels taken from one participant (bottom row). The stroke MRS voxels show a range of NAA and glutamate reduction, but a consistent decrease in Cr when compared to the contralateral and control voxels. Metabolite concentrations are highlighted on the right (MRS processed by LCModel).

axon damage caused by stroke. This results in reduced metabolic activity in the regions affected by the loss of neuronal input, and can be observed with MRS as changes in NAA and Cr. MRS studies of stroke survivors have shown a decrease in NAA distal to stroke regions, indicating neuronal loss, but not caused by the acute ischemic injury. Therefore, it is hypothesized that neurons whose inputs have been damaged by stroke are removed from tissue as they are no longer functioning normally due to their severed input (Chu et al.,

2002). Regions of diaschisis show a decreased Cr/NAA ratio and decreased rCBF on perfusion imaging, which may be a result of reduced neuronal activity, leading to a reduced need for Cr storage. Patients with normal Cr/NAA ratios 48 h after ischemia were more likely to recover from diaschisis (Mountz et al., 2003), indicating that neuronal activity can be restored in areas with preserved Cr levels and normal NAA, making the Cr/NAA ratio a marker of tissue fate.

STROKE AND DEPRESSION

The damage caused by an ischemic stroke does not stop after the acute period (24 h). The incidence of post-stroke depression is around 20% in stroke survivors. When considering post-stroke depression it is important to remember that the cause and biological reasoning behind depression is poorly understood. Studies of depression suggest affect regulation involving the frontal lobe may be dysregulated in a wide range of depressive disorders that may cause or result in frontal lobe structural changes (Soares & Mann, 1997), glucose metabolism abnormalities (Kimbrell et al., 2002), and altered patterns of functional MRI activations (Beauregard et al., 1998). ^{1}H MRS studies suggest that glutamate levels in the frontal lobe are increased in patients that develop depression within 10 days of ischemic stroke (Glodzik-Sobanska et al., 2006). The notion of glutamate deregulation during depression has been relevant for some time (Yuksel & Ongur, 2010), and confirmed with the near instant clinical resolution of symptoms with the administration of the NMDA antagonist ketamine, confirming the role of a glutamatergic mechanism in major depression (Berman et al., 2000; Zarate et al., 2006). However, whether the increase in glutamate is caused by the ischemic process itself or is actually secondary to depression is uncertain. One study of 31 ischemic stroke patients using ^{1}H MRS showed that patients with depression in the immediate post-stroke phase had significantly higher Glx/Cr ratios in the contralesional hemisphere than nondepressive patients. However, these metabolite changes were not persistent at 4 months post stroke (Glodzik-Sobanska et al., 2006). This suggests that stroke may cause changes in the glutamatergic transmission that can provoke depression. It is very difficult to identify if these glutamate changes were indeed due to a depression mechanism or the excitotoxic processes taking place post stroke.

Stroke can also result in a patient showing apathy, defined as a flattened affect, lack of interest, and diminished motivation, which is not as severe as in depression (Okada et al., 1997). Apathy prevents patients from engaging in rehabilitation and leads to poor physical and mental improvements post stroke. The prefrontal cortex as well as the nucleus accumbens, ventral pallidum, ventral tegmental area, and limbic system have all been implicated in apathy (Marin, 1996). A ^{1}H MRS in stroke study assessed apathy in 31 ischemic stroke survivors and showed patients with apathy had lower NAA/Cr ratios in the right frontal lobe than non-apathetic patients (Glodzik-Sobanska et al., 2006).

Another study found that in patients with post-stroke depression there was a significant difference in the ratios of NAA/Cr and Cho/Cr in the bilateral hippocampus and thalami (Huang et al., 2010). Following treatment with an antidepressant (paroxetine), the NAA/Cr ratio increased and the Cho/Cr ratio decreased in both the left and right hippocampi. While the effectiveness of antidepressants in stroke survivors remains unproven, these results show that in patients that respond to antidepression medication there is a neurobiological change in metabolites (Ende et al., 2000; Pears et al., 2005).

SPECTROSCOPY IN THE RECOVERING BRAIN

After the initial insult, the primary mechanism with which patients overcome the disabling affect of a stroke is thought to be through cortical reorganization, termed plasticity. ^{1}H MRS holds much promise for the assessment of plasticity through measurement of NAA, Cr, and Glu as the brain recovers from a stroke and a patient regains functional abilities. One study in hemorrhagic stroke showed that in the ipsilateral hemisphere, the NAA/Cr ratio was decreased, indicating neuronal loss. After 1 month, patients with poor outcome demonstrated a reduction of NAA/Cr over the bilateral frontal lobes, while patients with a good clinical outcome showed NAA increases (Kobayashi et al., 2001). Another longitudinal study in ischemic stroke with 27 participants showed a significant increase in the ratio of NAA/Cr in the contralateral to ischemic stroke hemisphere, suggesting plasticity. Increased NAA/Cr ratio was significantly related to better functional ability after stroke. Increases in NAA concentrations are likely due to increases in brain tissue density post stroke while increase in Cr represent an increase or normalization of energy storage in the tissue. Decreases in metabolite concentration are difficult to explain because we cannot know if they are due to the clearance of dead cells, or a reduction in the demand for local metabolites caused by a stroke. Human plasticity post stroke is currently poorly understood, yet is the underlying premise of rehabilitation therapy. Spectroscopy likely has the strongest

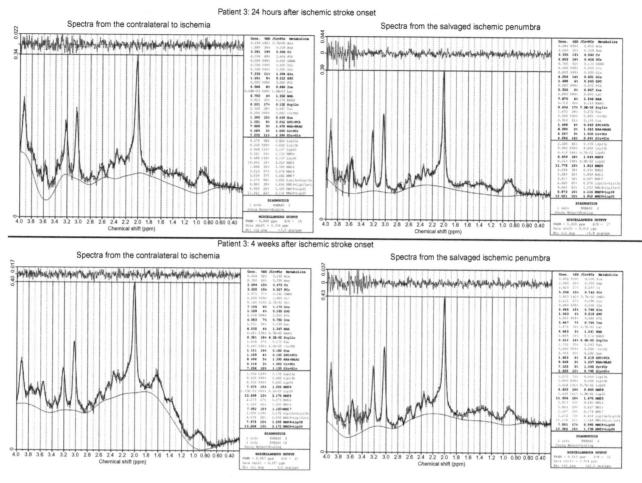

FIGURE 3.4.5 A follow-up MRS study showing changes in MRS results between 24 h after ischemic stroke and 1 month. This single patient had an MRS single voxel placed in the salvaged ischemic penumbra and contralateral to ischemic stroke. These data show that there was an increase in total Cr (6.157–7.125), glutamate (4.256–5.665), and NAA (7.675–8.843) in the salvaged penumbra. However, in the contralateral area, there was a large increase in NAA (6.755–8.235). These changes in metabolites likely reflect clearance of dead cells and restoration of energy stores and plasticity in the contralateral hemisphere. Metabolite concentrations are highlighted on the right (MRS processed by LCModel).

use in stroke rehabilitation studies that seek to enhance neuroplasticity, as we can directly monitor the changes in brain metabolites and monitor the effect of an intervention (see Fig. 3.4.5).

PROBLEMS WITH MRS ACQUISITION IN STROKE

Spectroscopy of the infarct core and in areas where there is hemorrhage suffer from an inability to achieve adequate localized shimming that results in a low inherent SNR, with broad resonances that are difficult to interpret. For the infarct core, the clinical importance of spectroscopy data from the core is questionable, as the tissue is dead and beyond salvage. Last, it is important to also set an appropriate TE when trying to acquire the concentration of a specific metabolite.

For example, when investigating the concentration of glutamate, a low TE of below 40 ms is the most appropriate to avoid spectra overlap with other metabolites and maximize the glutamate signal.

In spectra recorded at short echo times, broad signals originating from macromolecules with short T_2 relaxation time can be detected that underlie metabolite resonances and perturb the spectral baseline. The assignment of these macromolecules includes contributions from cytosolic proteins and Lips. Although these signals are normally fairly small, pathologic processes such as necrosis or apoptosis can cause substantial increases to occur. Substantial elevation of signals that resonate at 0.9 and 1.3 ppm are most likely due to the methylene and methyl groups of mobile saturated Lips that accumulate as a result of cell membrane degradation. However, a single-subject autopsy study with MRS suggested that the narrow 0.9 and 1.3 ppm resonances are due to macrophage infiltration that contains mobile Lip droplets (Petroff et al., 1992). The evidence of macromolecule signals relating to macrophages requires further investigation, but should the link be strengthened, there is a great deal that the previously ignored macromolecule signals can teach us about the time course of cellular processes post stroke in humans and animals.

Long-term studies of spectroscopy monitoring changes in metabolites are difficult to interpret due to the difficulty of placing a voxel on the exact same location for all repeat scans. However, increases in NAA and Cr after a stroke are consistently seen in the literature and are most likely due to plasticity. Measuring a decrease in a metabolite concentration in stroke patients is very difficult, because we do not know why a metabolite is reduced in concentration, whether it is due to cellular degradation, reduced local energy demand resulting in reduced energy storage, or random error in our acquisition. For this reason, MRS studies should be combined with other imaging modalities such as perfusion or DWI in order to confirm or explain a result. Additionally, combining MRS studies of patients with stroke, dementia, and/or epilepsy may lead to common findings and translation of treatments from one patient pool to another.

Multivoxel MRS has a significant role to play in stroke research, but not in clinical decision making (Dani et al., 2012). Acute stroke imaging with multivoxel MRS was shown to not significantly improve the quality of treatment decision making, despite clear results regarding NAA loss in infracted areas. This was mainly because the commonly used DWI acquisition is the gold standard for infarct core identification and takes less time to acquire than MRS. Therefore using MRS and DWI adds limited information to a clinician, despite the volume of the infarct core being the best predictor of outcome and treatment response. Additionally, a major weakness of multivoxel MRS is that it cannot accurately detect as many metabolites as single-voxel MRS. The benefit of multivoxel sequences is that they can measure metabolite changes across tissue. Therefore multivoxel MRS is a prime tool for research into the progression of plasticity during the stroke recovery period, and is especially useful when combined with other whole-brain techniques such as arterial spin labeling perfusion imaging (ASL) and measure of white matter tracts from diffusion tensor imaging (DTI). Such multimodal scanning studies can identify the effect of NAA loss post stroke by measuring the changes in NAA with MRS, the thinning of white matter tracts with DTI and the relationship with these changes and perfusion imaging on ASL, the infarct core volume on DWI, and overall brain volumes from volumetric MRI sequences. Such studies

will be able to identify if white matter is preferentially lost compared to gray matter by comparing tract loss (DTI) with gray matter volume reduction and NAA decline. These types of studies pose great potential for post-stroke treatments, as they may identify a particular group who always has a more rapid recovery. By identifying such positive rehabilitation groups, it may be possible to develop medications that can promote positive rehabilitation in nonresponders.

MRS is the only technique available that can characterize what is occurring to the metabolite and tissue structure of the brain during acute, subacute, and chronic ischemic stroke. However, technical limitations and the requirement of expert staff limit the clinical utility of MRS. MRS experimentation ideally requires a high field strength (3 T or greater), which is not always available, as well as staff who are familiar and confident with the placement of voxels. Voxel placement also requires technicians who are extremely familiar with neuro-anatomy and stroke topography. There is also significant variation in metabolites across brain regions, gender, and age. Therefore exact and reliable quantification for study purposes requires careful participant selection. Overall MRS is unlikely to be used routinely clinically in ischemic stroke; however, MRS may be used for studies in ischemic stroke that aim to investigate interventions aimed at improving stroke recovery.

References

Annemans, L., Wittrup-Jensen, K., & Bueno, H. (2010). A review of international pharmacoeconomic models assessing the use of aspirin in primary prevention. *Journal of Medical Economics*, 13(3), 418–427.

Back, T., Hemmen, T., & Schüler, O. G. (2004). Lesion evolution in cerebral ischemia. *Journal of Neurology*, 251(4), 388–397.

Beauregard, M., Leroux, J. M., Bergman, S., Arzoumanian, Y., Beaudoin, G., & Bourgouin, P. (1998). The functional neuroanatomy of major depression: an fMRI study using an emotional activation paradigm. *Neuroreport*, 9, 3253–3258.

Berman, R. M., Cappiello, A., Anand, A., Oren, D. A., Heninger, G. R., Charney, D. S., et al. (2000). Antidepressant effects of ketamine in depressed patients. *Biological Psychiatry*, 47, 351–354.

Bivard, A., & Parsons, M. (2012). ASPECTaSaurus (a dinosaur)? *International Journal of Stroke*, 7(7), 564.

Bristow, M. S., Poulin, B. W., & Simon, J. E. (2008). Identifying lesion growth with MR imaging in acute ischemic stroke. Journal of Magnetic Resonance Imaging, *2008 Oct, 28*(4), 837–846.

Broderick, J., Connolly, S., Feldmann, E., Hanley, D., Kase, C., Krieger, D., et al. (2007). Guidelines for the management of spontaneous intracerebral hemorrhage in adults: 2007 update: a guideline from the American Heart Association/American Stroke Association Stroke Council, High Blood Pressure Research Council, and the Quality of Care and Outcomes in Research Interdisciplinary Working group. *Stroke, 38*, 2001–2023.

Broderick, J. P., Brott, T. G., Duldner, J. E., Tomsick, T., & Huster, G. (1993). Volume of intracerebral hemorrhage. A powerful and easy-to-use predictor of 30-day mortality. *Stroke, 24*, 987–993.

Brott, T., & Bogousslavsky, J. (2000). Drug therapy: treatment of acute ischemic stroke. *New England Journal of Medicine, 343*, 710–722.

Bullock, R., Zauner, A., Woodward, J., & Young, H. F. (1995). Massive persistent release of excitatory amino acids following human occlusive stroke. *Stroke, 26*, 2187–2189.

Bykowski, J., Schellinger, P. D., & Warach, S. (2006). Diffusion and perfusion MRI. In R. R. Edelman, J. R. Hesselink, & M. B. Zatkin (Eds.), *Clinical magnetic resonance imaging* (3rd ed., pp. 1538–1570). Philadelphia: Saunders-Elsevier.

Chemmanam, T., Campbell, B. C., Christensen, S., & Nagakane, Y. (2010). Desmond PM, Bladin CF, Parsons MW, Levi CR, Barber PA, Donnan GA, Davis SM (2010). Ischemic diffusion lesion reversal is uncommon and rarely alters perfusion-diffusion mismatch. *Neurology, 75*(12), 1040–1047 Sep 21.

Chu, W., Mason, G., Pan, J., Hetherington, H., & Liu, H. (2002). Regional cerebral blood flow and magnetic resonance spectroscopic imaging findings in diaschisis from stroke. *Stroke, 33*, 1243–1248.

Chu, W. J., Hetherington, H. P., Kuzniecky, R. I., Simor, T., Mason, G. F., & Elgavish, G. A. (1998). Lateralization of human temporal lobe epilepsy by 31P NMR spectroscopic imaging at 4.1 T. *Neurology, 51*, 472–479.

Dani, K. A., An, L., Henning, E. C., Shen, J., & Warach, S. (2012). Multivoxel MR spectroscopy in acute ischemic stroke: comparison to the stroke protocol MRI. *Stroke, 43*(11), 2962–2967 Nov.

Dávalos, D., Castillo, J., Serena, J., & Noya, M. (1997). Duration of glutamate release after acute ischemic stroke. *Stroke, 28*, 708–710.

Ende, G., Braus, D. F., Walter, S., Weber-Fahr, W., & Henn, F. A. (2000). The hippocampus in patients treated with electroconvulsive therapy: a proton magnetic resonance spectroscopic imaging study. *Archives of General Psychiatry, 57*, 937–943.

Fogelholm, R., Murros, K., Rissanen, A., & Avikainen, S. (2005). Long term survival after primary intracerebral haemorrhage: a retrospective population based study. *Journal of Neurology, Neurosurgery, & Psychiatry, 76*, 1534–1538.

Ford, C. C., Griffey, R. H., Matwiyoff, N. A., & Rosenberg, G. A. (1992). Multivoxel ^{1}H MRS of stroke. *Neurology, 42*(7), 1408–1412 1992 Jul.

Furlan, A., Higashida, R., Wechsler, L., Gent, M., Rowley, H., Kase, C., et al. (1999). Intra-arterial prourokinase for acute ischemic stroke: The PROACT II Study: a randomized controlled trial. *JAMA, 282*(21), 2003–2011.

Gideon, P., Henriksen, O., Sperling, B., Christiansen, P., Olsen, T. S., Jørgensen, H. S., et al. (1992). Early time course of N-acetylaspartate, creatine and phosphocreatine, and compounds containing choline in the brain after acute stroke. A proton magnetic resonance spectroscopy study. *Stroke, 23*, 1566–1572.

Gillard, J. H., Barker, P. B., van Zijl, P. C., Bryan, R. N., & Oppenheimer, S. M. (1996). Proton MR spectroscopy in acute middle cerebral artery stroke. *American Journal of Neuroradiology, 17*(5), 873–886 1996 May.

Glodzik-Sobanska, L., Slowik, A., Kieltyka, A., Kozub, J., Sobiecka, B., Urbanik, A., et al. (2006). Single voxel proton magnetic resonance spectroscopy in post-stroke depression. *Psychiatry Research: Neuroimaging, 148*, 111–120.

Graham, G. D., Blamire, A. M., Rothman, D. L., Brass, L. M., Fayad, P. B., Petroff, O. A., et al. (1993). Early temporal variation of cerebral metabolites after human stroke. A proton magnetic resonance spectroscopy study. *Stroke, 24*, 1891–1896.

Hart, R. G., Tonarelli, S. B., & Pearce, L. A. (2005). Avoiding central nervous system bleeding during antithrombotic therapy: recent data and ideas. *Stroke, 36*, 1588–1593.

Hazell, A. S. (2007). Excitotoxic mechanisms in stroke: an update of concepts and treatment strategies. *Neurochemistry International, 50*, 941–953 2007.

Hetherington, H. P., Pan, J. W., Mason, G. F., Adams, D., Vaughn, M. J., Twieg, D. B., et al. (1996). Quantitative ^{1}H spectroscopic imaging of human brain at 4.1 T using image segmentation. *Magnetic Resonance in Medicine, 36*, 21–29 1996.

Huang, Y., Chen, W., Li, Y., Wu, X., Shi, X., & Geng, D. (2010). Effects of antidepressant treatment on N-acetyl aspartate and choline levels in the hippocampus and thalami of post-stroke depression patients: a study using ^{1}H magnetic resonance spectroscopy. *Neuroimaging, 182*, 48–52.

Kimbrell, T. A., Ketter, T. A., George, M. S., Little, J. T., Benson, B. E., Willis, M. W., et al. (2002). Post. Regional cerebral glucose utilization in patients with a range of severities of unipolar depression. *Biological Psychiatry, 51*, 237–252 2002.

Kidwell, C. S., Saver, J. L., & Mattiello, J. (2000). Thrombolytic reversal of acute human cerebral ischemic injury shown by diffusion/perfusion magnetic resonance imaging. *Annals of Neurology, 47*, 462–469 2000.

Kobayashi, M., Takayama, H., Suga, S., & Mihara, B. (2001). Longitudinal changes of metabolites in frontal lobes after hemorrhagic stroke of basal ganglia: a proton magnetic resonance spectroscopy study. *Stroke, 32*, 2237–2245 2001.

Lees, K. R., Bluhmki, E., & von Kummer, R. (2010). Time to treatment with intravenous alteplase and outcome in stroke: an updated pooled analysis of ECASS, ATLANTIS, NINDS, and EPITHET trials. *Lancet, 375*(9727), 1695–1703.

Marin, R. S. (1996). Apathy: concept, syndrome, neural mechanisms, and treatment. *Seminars in Clinical Neuropsychiatry, 1*, 304–314.

Meretoja, A., Strbian, D., Putaala, J., Curtze, S., Haapaniemi, E., Mustanoja, S., et al. (2012). SMASH-U: A proposal for etiologic classification of intracerebral hemorrhage. *Stroke, 43*, 2592–2597 2012.

Merino, J. G., & Warach, S. (2010). Imaging of acute stroke. *Nature Reviews Neurology, 6*(10), 560–571 2010 Oct.

Mescher, M., Merkle, H., Kirsch, J., Garwood, M., & Gruetter, R. (1998). Simultaneous *in vivo* spectral editing and water suppression. *NMR in Biomedicine, 11*, 266–272 1998.

Miller, B. L. (1991). A review of chemical issues in 1H NMR spectroscopy: N-acetyl-L-aspartate, creatine and choline. *NMR in Biomedicine, 4*, 47–52 1991.

Mountz, J. M. (2007). Nuclear medicine in the rehabilitative treatment evaluation in stroke recovery. role of diaschisis resolution and cerebral reorganization. *Eura Medicophysica, 43*, 221–239 2007.

Mountz, J. M., Lui, H. G., & Deutch, G. (2003). Neuroimaging in cerebrovascular disorders: measurement of cerebral physiology after stroke and assessment of stroke recovery. *Seminars in Nuclear Medicine, 33*(1), 56–76 2003 Jan.

Okada, K., Kobayashi, S., Yamagata, S., Takahashi, K., & Yamaguchi, S. (1997). Poststroke apathy and regional cerebral blood flow. *Stroke, 28*, 2437–2441.

Pears, M. R., Cooper, J. D., Mitchison, R. J., Mortishi re-Smith, R. J., Pearce, D. A., & Griffin, J. L. (2005). High resolution 1 H NMR-based metabolomics indicates a neurotransmitter cycling deficit in cerebral tissue from a mouse model of Batten disease. *Journal of Biological Chemistry, 280*, 42508–42514.

Petroff, O. A. C., Graham, G. D., Blamire, A. M., Al-Rayess, M., Rothman, D. L., Fayad, P. B., et al. (1992). Spectroscopic imaging of stroke in man: Histopathology correlates of spectral changes. *Neurology, 42*, 1349–1354.

Pereira, A. C., Saunders, D. E., Doyle, V. L., Bland, J. M., Howe, F. A., Griffiths, J. R., et al. (1999). Measurement of initial N-acetyl aspartate concentration by magnetic resonance spectroscopy and initial infarct volume by MRI predicts outcome in patients with middle cerebral artery territory infarction. *Stroke, 30*, 1577–1582 1999.

Provencher, S. W. (1993). Estimation of metabolite concentrations from localized *in vivo* proton NMR spectra. *Magnetic Resonance in Medicine, 30*, 672–679.

Qureshi, A. I., Tuhrim, S., Broderick, J. P., Batjer, H. H., Hondo, H., & Hanley, D. F. (2001). Spontaneous intracerebral hemorrhage. *New England Journal of Medicine, 344*, 1450–1460.

Rossi, D. J., Brady, J. D., & Mohr, C. (2007). Astrocyte metabolism and signaling during brain ischemia. *Nature Neuroscience, 10*, 1377–1386.

Rothwell, P. M. (2001). The high cost of not funding stroke research: a comparison with heart disease and cancer. *Lancet, 357*(9268), 1612–1616 2001 May 19

Saunders, D. E., Howe, F. A., van den Boogaart, A., McLean, M. A., Griffiths, J. R., & Brown, M. M. (1995). Continuing ischemic damage after acute middle cerebral artery infarction in humans demonstrated by short-echo proton spectroscopy. *Stroke, 26*, 1007–1013.

Seenan, P., Long, M., & Langhorne, P. (2007). Stroke units in their natural habitat: systematic review of observational studies. *Stroke, 38*(6), 1886–1892.

Senes, S. (2006). How we Manage Stroke In Australia. AIHW Cat No CVD 31. Canberra: Australian Institute of Health and Welfare.

Singer, O. C., Humpich, M. C., Fiehler, J., Albers, G. W., Lansberg, M. G., Kastrup, A., et al. (2008). MR Stroke Study Group Investigators. Risk for symptomatic intracerebral hemorrhage after thrombolysis assessed by DWI MRI. *Annals of Neurology, 63*, 52–60.

Soares, J. C., & Mann, J. J. (1997). The anatomy of mood disorders-review of structural neuroimaging studies. *Biological Psychiatry, 41*, 86–106.

Tallan, H. H., Moore, S., & Stein, W. H. (1956). N-acetyl-L-aspartic acid in brain. *Journal of Biological Chemistry, 219*, 257–264.

Tang, X., Wang, C., Xia, L., Zhu, W., Zhao, L., & Zhu, W. (2011). Volumetric MRI and ^{1}H MRS study of hippocampus in unilateral MCAO patients: Relationship between hippocampal secondary damage and cognitive disorder following stroke. *European Journal of Radiology* 24 2011 Sep

Taoufik, E., & Probert, L. (2008). Ischemic neuronal damage. *Current Pharmaceutical Design, 14*(33), 3565–3573.

Thrift, A. G., McNeil, J. J., Forbes, A., & Donnan, G. A. (1998). Three important subgroups of hypertensive persons at greater risk of intracerebral hemorrhage. *Melbourne Risk Factor Study Group. Hypertension, 31*, 1223–1229.

Urenjak, J., Williams, S. R., Gadian, D. G., & Noble, M. (1993). Proton nuclear magnetic resonance spectroscopy unambiguously identifies different neural cell types. *Journal of Neuroscience, 13*, 981–989.

Yuksel, C., & Ongur, D. (2010). Magnetic resonance spectroscopy studies of glutamate-related abnormalities in mood disorders. *Biological Psychiatry, 68*, 785–794.

Zarate, C. A., Singh, J. B., Carlson, P. J., Brutsche, N. E., Ameli, R., & Luckenbaugh, D. A. (2006). A randomized trial of an N-methyl-D-aspartate antagonist in treatment-resistant major depression. *Archives of General Psychiatry, 63*, 856–864.

Use of MRS in Inborn Errors of Metabolism: Canavan's Disease and MRS in Differential Diagnosis

Kim M. Cecil

Cincinnati Children's Hospital Medical Center, Departments of Radiology, Pediatrics, and Environmental Health, University of Cincinnati College of Medicine, OH, USA

INTRODUCTION

Magnetic resonance spectroscopy (MRS) provides a powerful tool in deriving or confirming a diagnosis of an inborn error of metabolism. Levels of key metabolites such as lactate, *N*-acetylaspartate (NAA), creatine (Cr), cholines (Cho) and myo-inositol (mI) can suggest metabolic dysfunction and support findings of acidosis, neuroaxonal loss, hypomyelination, demyelination, and gliosis. The temporal course of a disease and the ongoing developmental maturation in children influence not only the clinical and imaging presentations, but also the spectroscopic findings. Metabolic changes within the earliest stages of a disease will often differ significantly from those observed in the later stages. Early assessment in a disease process provides important information for narrowing a differential diagnosis and often offering prognostic features. Later assessment of disease course can offer the ability to monitor disease progression and may measure treatment response. Brain development, particularly myelination, may also be proceeding at a normal or near normal pace in lesser affected regions. Interpretation of metabolite changes requires consideration of the evolving developmental changes to the spectroscopy profile occurring in the background in addition to pathologic changes.

Unfortunately, the literature provides only a limited number of case reports and patient series employing MRS in the diagnosis and monitoring of inborn errors of metabolism since these disorders are relatively rare and tend to present during childhood.

Identifying a child with a metabolic disease can be complex. There are several screening procedures for select metabolic diseases in the newborn. Upon ruling out birth-related injury, the sickest newborns hospitalized can be screened for a variety of metabolic disorders. Unfortunately, some infants with metabolic diseases are misclassified under the "cerebral palsy" category and the progressive nature of metabolic disease is not recognized until later childhood. For children with a normal postnatal period, the identification of metabolic disease in early childhood (6 months to 4 years) first occurs by the pediatrician when the child is not meeting developmental milestones. Referral to a pediatric neurologist usually results in an MR imaging (MRI) study ordered for those children with suspicion of metabolic disease. An unknown subset of the children with an MRI order will also have MRS performed. For many patients, MRS is only ordered late in the disease course after several nonspecific laboratory and imaging studies have been performed. Only a few conditions, such as Canavan's disease, and Cr deficiency syndromes, have an MRS profile that is disease specific. The next "MRS-positive" group of findings (elevated lactate, elevated lipids, reduced NAA, abnormal Cho, elevated mI) support imaging diagnoses, but are usually not specific for a given class of disorders or an individual disease. Taken with the inherent limitations of MRS, which include the learning curve for acquisition and interpretation, including the ability to only primarily detect cellular events (neuronal dysfunction, lactic acidemia, abnormal myelination, gliosis, etc.), relatively low signal-to-noise ratio (SNR), and in the United States, limited reimbursement for the expense of the procedure, reports of MRS findings in these disorders are few with many obtained from dedicated research studies of known patients with a given disorder. The goal of this chapter is to provide the reader with a survey of inborn errors in metabolism with the presentation, metabolic, pathologic, MRI, and MRS features described with illustrative images. Given the space constraints, genetic features of selected diseases are included in Table 3.5.1.

TABLE 3.5.1

Disease or disorder	Gene name; abbreviation (locus)	Phenotype MIM	Inheritance mode	Primary grouping	Primary defect
Neonatal ALD	*PTS1* and *Peroxin* genes	202370	Autosomal-recessive	Peroxisomal	Deficiency in oxidizing VLCFAs
X-linked ALD	ATP-binding cassette, subfamily *D* (*ALD*), member 1, *ABCD1* (Xq28)	300100	X-linked	Peroxisomal	Inability to oxidize VLCFAs into shorter chain fatty acids
Alexander's disease	Glial fibrillary acidic protein (GFAP); (17q21.31)	203450	Autosomal-dominant	Leukodystrophy	Presence of Rosenthal fibers, GFAPs in astrocytes
Canavan's disease	ASPA (17p13.2)	271900	Autosomal-recessive	Leukodystrophy	Enzyme deficiency, ASPA deficiency, inability to metabolize NAA into aspartate and acetate
Childhood ataxia with diffuse CNS hypomyelination	*EIF2B1-5* (12q24.31, 14q24.3, 1p34.1, 2p23.3, 3q27)	603896	Autosomal-recessive	Leukodystrophy	Gene defect in eukaryotic translation initiation factor (mRNA translated into proteins)
Cr deficiency: Cr transporter defect	*SLC6A8* (Xq28)	300036	X-linked	Miscellaneous	Cr transport compromised to the brain
Cr deficiency: AGAT deficiency	*AGAT* (15q21.1)	602360	Autosomal-recessive	Miscellaneous	Cr synthesis compromised
Cr deficiency: GAMT deficiency	*GAMT* (19p13.3)	601240	Autosomal-recessive	Miscellaneous	Creatine synthesis compromised
Galactosemia	*GALT* (9p13.3)	230400	Autosomal-recessive	Miscellaneous	Defect encoding galactose-1-phosphate uridyltransferase
Globoid cell leukodystrophy (Krabbe disease)	Galactocerebrosidase; *GALC* (14q31.3)	245200	Autosomal-recessive	Lysosomal	Enzyme deficiency-galactocerebroside β-galactosidase deficiency
Glutaric aciduria	Type I: glutaryl-CoA-dehydrogenase; (19p13.2)	231670	Autosomal-recessive	Organic or amino acid	Enzyme deficiency altering metabolism of lysine, hydroxylysine, and tryptophan
Glutaric aciduria	Type II: multiple acyl-CoA dehydrogenase genes; (19q13.41, 15q24.2-q24.3, 4q32.1)	231680	Autosomal-recessive	Organic or amino acid	Disorder of fatty acid, amino acid, and Cho metabolism
L-Hydroxyglutaric aciduria	*L2HGDH* (14q21.3)	236792	Autosomal-recessive	Organic or amino acid	Defect in oxidizing L2HG
LBSL	*DARS2* (1q25.1)	611105	Autosomal-recessive	Leukodystrophy	Defect in the gene encoding mitochondrial aspartyl-tRNA synthetase
MSUD	Mutations in the catalytic subunit genes of the branched chain α-keto acid dehydrogenase	248600	Autosomal-recessive	Organic or amino acid	Defect in the genes of the branched chain α-keto acid dehydrogenase blocking oxidative decarboxylation

(Continued)

3. APPLICATIONS OF ¹H-MRS

TABLE 3.5.1   (Continued)

Disease or disorder	Gene name; abbreviation (locus)	Phenotype MIM	Inheritance mode	Primary grouping	Primary defect
	complex; (19q13.2, 7q31.1, 6q14.1, 1p21.2)				
MLD	*Arylsulfatase A; ASA/ARSA* (22q13.33)	250100	Autosomal-recessive	Lysosomal	Decreased arylsulfatase A, ARSA activity
NCL	*CLN3* (16p11.2)	204200	Autosomal-recessive	Lysosomal	Defects involve lysosomal function
NPC	*NPC 1* (18q11.2)	257220	Autosomal-recessive	Lysosomal	Defective cholesterol esterification due to a deficiency of sphingomyelinase
NKH	Multiple genes (*GCSH* 16q23.2, *GLDC* 9p24.1, *AMT* 3p21.31)	605899	Autosomal-recessive	Amino aciduria	Defective mitochondrial enzyme involved in glycine cleavage
IRD	*PEX 1* 7q21.2, *PXMP3* 8q21.11, *PEX26* 22q11.21	266510	Autosomal-recessive	Peroxisomal	Phytanic acid oxidase deficiency
Vacuolating MLC (with subcortical cysts)	*MLC1* (22q13.33)	604004	Autosomal-recessive	Leukodystrophy	Uncertain
ZS	Several genes involved in peroxisome biogenesis	214100	Autosomal-recessive	Peroxisomal	Decreased dihydroxyacetone phosphate acyltransferase activity

PRIMARY LEUKODYSTROPHIES

The word leukodystrophy describes conditions that are both *genetically determined* and *progressive*. Leukodystrophies arise as a result of a gene defect that manages production or metabolism of exclusively one component of myelin, which causes imperfect growth and development or maintenance of myelin sheaths. While these conditions may eventually involve and alter gray matter, the primary features impact the white matter.

Canavan's Disease

Canavan's disease usually presents in the first 3–6 months of life with macrocephaly, poorly controlled head movement, lack of motor development, and feeding problems. Left untreated, life expectancy is between 3 and 10 years. It occurs when there is a deficiency of the enzyme aspartocylase, a cytosolic enzyme found in oligodendrocytes (Madhavarao et al., 2004). Aspartoacylase (ASPA) hydrolyzes NAA to acetate and aspartic acid (see Chapter 2.1). With this enzymatic defect, NAA accumulates in the brain, accompanied by vacuolization in the lower layers of the cerebral cortex and subcortical white matter with intramyelinic swelling and myelin loss. (Moffett et al., 2006). Histologic examination has demonstrated that the disease originates in a peripheral location within the brain, involving the U-fibers of the subcortical white matter of the cerebral hemispheres, and reflecting dysfunctional ASPA activity within regions of greatest myelination occurring in brain development. Later, the disease progresses and encompasses the deep white matter structures of both cerebral hemispheres, and eventually it extends to the cerebellum and spinal cord. The involvement of the U-fibers of the white matter is diffuse, with evidence of vacuoles within the subcortical white matter and extending into the adjacent cortex.

Fig. 3.5.1 illustrates typical imaging and spectroscopy findings associated with Canavan's disease. Proton MRS performed within cerebral white matter demonstrates significant elevation of the resonance positioned at 2.0 parts per million (ppm), representing NAA. (Toft et al., 1993; Engelbrecht et al., 1995; Wittsack et al., 1996; Aydinli et al., 1998; Bluml et al., 2001; Gordon et al., 2001; Moreno et al., 2001; Krawczyk & Gradowska, 2003) A dramatic elevation of the NAA concentration, which can be represented as NAA/Cr or any NAA/metabolite ratio, will appear in patients with Canavan's disease. The NAA elevation is pronounced on MRS acquisitions, regardless of echo time. In the course of clinical MRS examinations in patients without the Canavan's features, one may encounter what appears as a slight increase in the NAA to Cr ratio. These are usually due to

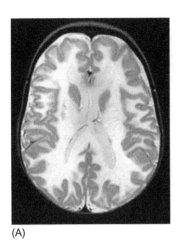
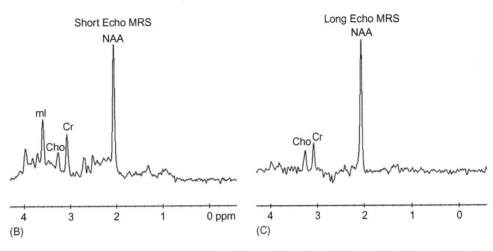

FIGURE 3.5.1 Twelve-month-old female diagnosed with Canavan's disease. (A) Axial T$_2$-weighted image displays hyperintense signal throughout the white matter. (B) Short-echo (35 ms) and (C) long-echo (288 ms) MR spectra show dramatic elevation of NAA.

developmental effects, depending upon the reference point (e.g., normative curves for metabolite ratios, comparison to prior studies) and technical factors. Major elevations of NAA/Cr are distinctive; minor elevations are not characteristic and should not be confused with Canavan's disease. Urine and plasma NAA levels can support the diagnosis for Canavan's disease in accordance with described imaging and clinical findings.

Megalencephalic Leukoencephalopathy with Subcortical Cysts

Megalencephalic leukoencephalopathy with subcortical cysts (MLC) presents within the first year of life with macrocrania and macrocephaly (van der Knaap et al., 1995). Initially, normal mental and motor development occurs with almost all patients having epilepsy at an early age, which is usually controlled by medication. There is a gradual onset of ataxia, spasticity, and extrapyramidal findings. Mild mental deterioration occurs late in the disease and is much milder than the motor symptoms. Severity of the disease varies with some patients able to walk into their forties, while others lose their independence after only a few years.

MRI demonstrates widespread signal abnormalities throughout the white matter, with relative sparing of deep structures (Leegwater et al., 2002). Diffusely abnormal and swollen white matter of the cerebral hemispheres and the presence of subcortical cysts in the anterior temporal region are strongly suggestive of MLC. Cysts are typically identified in the subcortical temporal lobes, and less frequently in the frontal, parietal, or occipital lobes (see Fig. 3.5.2).

Spectroscopic analyses of affected white matter in patients with MLC revealed marked reduction of NAA, Cr, and Cho with normal values for mI, consistent with axonal loss and astrocytic proliferation. (Brockmann et al., 2003c; van der Voorn et al., 2006). This distinct profile can be easily distinguished from Canavan's disease.

Alexander's Disease

The most commonly encountered presentation of Alexander's disease is the infantile form, presenting in the first 2 years of life. The onset of symptoms appears at birth, with delay in development, hypotonia, seizures, and progressive macrocephaly. Children with the infantile form of disease rarely survive to the second decade. The juvenile form presents after 4 years of age with speech and swallowing difficulties, ataxia, and spasticity. Progression is slower, with a more prolonged survival. Adult-onset disease has a more variable clinical and imaging presentation, and is occasionally diagnosed incidentally at autopsy. Alexander's disease begins by involving the periventricular white matter, typically involving the frontal lobes, and then extends into the parietotemporal and finally, the occipital regions. Eventually, there is involvement of the cerebellar white matter and spinal cord.

MRI findings for the infantile form demonstrate macrocephaly with hyperintensity on T$_2$-weighted images involving the white matter areas, beginning in the frontal areas with progression posteriorly to involve other parts of the cerebral hemispheres. Van der Knaap et al. (2001) identified five characteristics of Alexander's disease on MRI that can be applied to suspected cases in order to make a presumptive diagnosis. These characteristics include extensive cerebral white matter changes with frontal predominance, a periventricular rim with high signal on T$_1$-weighted images and low

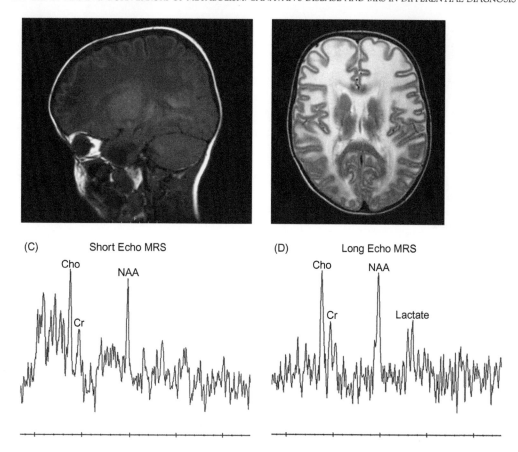

FIGURE 3.5.2   Four-year-old male with MLC with subcortical cysts. (A) Sagittal T_1-weighted and (B) axial T_2-weighted images reveal diffuse white matter signal abnormalities (hypointense T_1 and hyperintense T_2), decreased sulcation pattern, and thinning of cortical gray matter, with temporal and frontal cysts. (C) Short-echo (35 ms) and (D) long-echo (288 ms) MR spectra acquired from left frontal white matter show significant reduction of all metabolites as evidenced with the low SNR level within the spectrum.

signal on T_2-weighted images, brainstem signal abnormalities, signal abnormalities with swelling or volume loss in the basal ganglia and thalami, and contrast enhancement of one or more of the following structures: optic chiasm, fornix, ventricular lining, periventricular rim of tissue, white matter of the frontal lobes, basal ganglia, thalamus, dentate nucleus, or brainstem structures. Although many of these abnormalities may be seen in other leukodystrophies, the association of four or more appears to be relatively specific for Alexander's disease. The extent and pattern of contrast enhancement and the distinctive periventricular rim of abnormal signal are not commonly encountered in other leukodystrophies. However, recent reports document patients with significant numbers of Rosenthal fibers upon pathological examination confirming Alexander's disease, yet demonstrate unusual and atypical imaging features and often discrepant with a relatively benign clinical course (van der Knaap et al., 2005, 2006b; Dinopoulos et al., 2006).

Brockmann et al. (2003a) employed proton MRS to identify metabolic abnormalities in four patients genetically confirmed with infantile Alexander's disease. Elevated concentrations of mI with normal or increased Cho compounds in gray and white matter, basal ganglia, and cerebellum suggest astrocytosis and demyelination. Neuroaxonal degeneration, as reflected by a reduction of NAA, was found in cerebral and cerebellar white matter. The accumulation of lactate in affected white matter supports the presence of infiltrating macrophages. Recently, a linear discriminant analysis approach for disease classification in juvenile Alexander's disease was published (van der Voorn et al., 2006). This study suggested that spectral features might play a stronger role in determining the nature of Alexander's disease. The lactate elevations found on proton MRS could arise from non-oxidative glycolysis due to the metabolic disruption of disordered astrocytes. As the Rosenthal fibers accumulate, the astrocytes demonstrate hyperplasia and hypertrophy and produce mI elevations. Fig. 3.5.3 provides an example of imaging and spectroscopy findings associated with Alexander's disease.

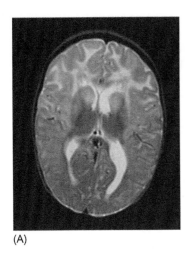
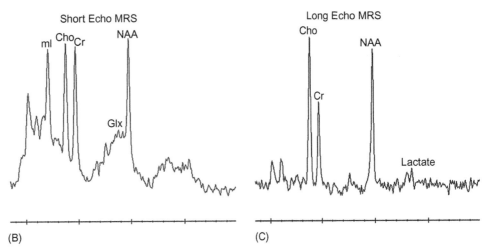

FIGURE 3.5.3   Eight-month-old female with Alexander's disease. (A) Axial T₂-weighted image features hyperintense signal in the frontal white matter. (B) Short-echo (35 ms) and (C) long-echo (288 ms) MR spectra acquired from left frontal white matter demonstrate reduced NAA/Cr, with elevations of Cho/Cr and mI/Cr accompanied by a small lactate peak visible in (C) at 1.3 ppm.

Childhood Ataxia with Central Nervous System Hypomyelination or Leukoencephalopathy with Vanishing White Matter

Childhood ataxia with central nervous system (CNS) hypomyelination (CACH) is a prevalent inherited leukodystrophy with more than 250 patients recognized (Bugiani et al., 2010). The age at onset inversely correlates with disease severity. Stresses, such as acute fright, febrile infections, and minor head trauma can induce onset of symptoms with rapid and major neurologic deterioration. In childhood onset, CACH can present in such crisis periods with hypotonia, epilepsy, vomiting, irritability accompanied by impaired consciousness spanning from somnolence to coma, and in some patients, death. Outside of these periods, the disease can present with cerebellar ataxia, and less frequently, spasticity and optic atrophy with preservation of cognition. While the disease is eventually fatal, the course is slowly progressive outside of episodes of major neurological deterioration. The adolescent and adult forms of the disease have milder but more protracted clinical courses with less prominent episodes of major deterioration. The clinical symptoms in adults feature seizures, complicated migraine, and psychiatric features. CACH is now regarded as an axonopathy rather than a hypomyelination or demyelination process (van der Knaap et al., 2006a).

Although the genes responsible are housekeeping genes, CACH is primarily a brain disorder, with glial vulnerability a key feature. The neuropathological findings consist of severe, cystic white matter degeneration with only small amounts of myelin breakdown products (Van Haren et al., 2004; Pronk et al., 2006). Foamy oligodendrocytes, dysmorphic astrocytes and oligodendrocytes, oligodendrocytosis, and apoptotic losses of oligodendrocytes are present. The oligodendrocytes undergo apoptosis in response to major neurologic crises with only a subset of oligodendrocytes remaining functional.

The clinical and MRI findings in the classic childhood form were specific to enable recognition of this disease as a distinct entity, with subsequent genetic characterization (van der Knaap et al., 1997). Clinical diagnosis of the childhood form can be narrowed with recognition of MRI features. CACH appears on imaging as a diffuse cerebral hemispheric leukoencephalopathy, with abnormal white matter progressing over time indicating rarefaction and cystic degeneration. Abnormal white matter demonstrates hyperintense signal on fluid-attenuated inversion recovery (FLAIR), proton density, and T₂-weighted imaging sequences. FLAIR, proton density, and T₁-weighted imaging reveal a radiating, stripe-like pattern with remaining tissue strands. This feature corresponds with widened blood vessels with reactive astrocytes. The U-fibers can be affected; however, the fornix, optic tracts, anterior commissure, the internal capsules, and the outer part of the corpus callosum appear to be less affected. The cortical gray matter, basal ganglia, and brainstem nuclei appear normal (van der Knaap et al., 1997, 2006a; Bugiani et al., 2010). There has been no evidence of contrast enhancement with CACH as the disease lacks inflammatory changes. The correlation between the MRI findings and the detection of the mutations in eIF2B1-5 genes is very high, but the genotype-phenotype correlation is poor due to wide variations in the phenotype.

The pathological course demonstrates different features upon proton MRS. A normal spectral profile is preserved early in the disease; however, upon rarefaction and cystic degeneration of the white matter, a dramatic decrease occurs for NAA, Cr, Cho, and lipids in white matter. In the advanced stages, there is a virtual absence of all parenchymal metabolites with only the presence of cerebrospinal fluid (CSF) metabolites, primarily lactate and glucose (Hanefeld et al., 1993; Schiffmann et al., 1994; Tedeschi et al., 1995; van der Knaap et al., 1997, 1998, 2006a; Dreha-Kulaczewski et al., 2008).

Leukoencephalopathy with Brainstem and Spinal Cord Involvement and Elevated White Matter Lactate

For many with leukoencephalopathy with brainstem and spinal cord involvement and elevated white matter lactate (LBSL), initial child development is normal, with the deterioration of motor skills beginning in childhood, adolescence or for some, not until adulthood. In some patient reports, independent walking begins late and demonstrates instability from the start. The pattern of involvement includes a slowly progressive cerebellar ataxia, spasticity, and dorsal column dysfunction with more involvement of the legs than the arms. Most patients have normal cognitive function; however, some may develop learning problems and experience mild cognitive decline, with reports of treatable epilepsy for some patients.

Since the clinical features resemble a spinocerebellar ataxia, imaging findings can help distinguish LBSL from other entities (van der Knaap et al., 2003). The MRI pattern is quite distinct as the progressive white matter abnormalities, spotty or confluent, spread from the periventricular region outward with sparing of the subcortical U-fibers. The corpus callosum is affected with posterior preference. The pyramidal tracts are affected over their entire length from the posterior limb of the internal capsule and brainstem into the lateral corticospinal tracts of the spinal cord. The sensory tracts are involved from the dorsal columns in the spinal cord to the medial lemniscus throughout the brainstem up to the level of the thalamus and the corona radiata above the level of the thalamus. The cerebellar involvement progresses over time to the point of significant volume loss. These patterns suggest that defects in mitochondrial translation related to DARS2 mutation are responsible for dysfunction of long tract-associated glia (Labauge et al., 2011).

Proton MRS studies of affected white matter may demonstrate a highly significant lactate elevation for patients. For one patient, the elevated lactate within regions of signal abnormality has been monitored for several years (Fig. 3.5.4). However, lactate elevation is not a requirement for diagnosis as several case reports describe adult patients without lactate elevation in affected white matter (Petzold et al., 2006; Labauge et al., 2007). Cho and mI elevations with diminished NAA concentrations are also featured within regions of signal abnormality (van der Knaap et al., 2003; Linnankivi et al., 2004; Serkov et al., 2004; Tavora et al., 2007; Uluc et al., 2008). In regions without signal abnormalities on imaging, the spectra are within normal levels.

LYSOSOMAL STORAGE DISEASES

Many neurodegenerative diseases are characterized by the accumulation of non-degradable molecules in cells or at extracellular sites in the brain. The lysosomes are intracellular organelles responsible for degrading lipids, proteins, and complex carbohydrates. For many lysosomal storage disorders the genetic mutation resulting in the absence or partial deficiency of an enzyme or protein is known and functionally understood. Generally, the substrate for the defective enzyme builds up to produce intralysosomal storage. While the diseases are complex, mechanical disruption of the cell due to the storage of non-degradable material leads to cellular dysfunction. Usually, the pathology primarily involves neuronal dysfunction rather than loss, with the exception of differential loss of Purkinje cells, which characterizes several storage diseases, including Niemann—Pick disease type C (NPC) and the massive cell loss that occurs in neuronal ceroid lipofuscinoses (NCL). Unknown is whether the storage material affects cellular function only when it begins to accumulate in extralysosomal sites or if problems in cell homeostasis are triggered while the material is still confined to the lysosome. Lysosomal disorders are typically inherited as autosomal recessive traits, usually afflict infants and young children, involve brain pathology, and are untreatable. The collective frequency of lysosomal storage diseases is estimated to be approximately 1 in 8000 live births, with some occurring at high frequency in select populations. The common biochemical hallmark of these diseases is the storage of macromolecules in the lysosome.

Globoid Cell Leukodystrophy (Krabbe Disease)

Globoid cell leukodystrophy (GLD) arises from a deficiency in the enzyme, β-galactocerebrosidase, leading to the accumulation of cerebroside and galactosylsphingosine within the lysosome and inducing apoptosis in the oligodendrocyte cell lines. Also known as Krabbe disease, it is seen predominantly in

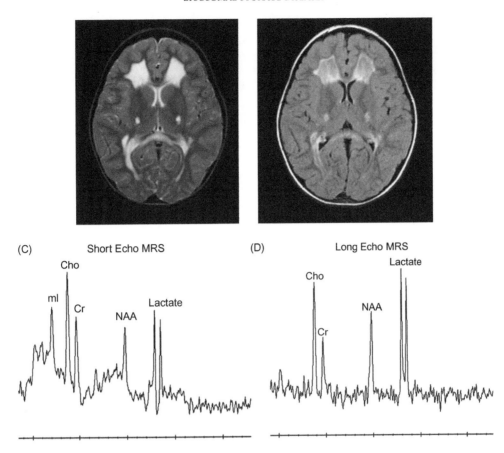

FIGURE 3.5.4 Four-year-old female with LBSL. (A) Axial T_2 and (B) axial FLAIR images feature significant signal abnormalities in the central white matter, the corpus callosum, and the posterior aspects of the posterior limbs of the internal capsule. (C) Short-echo (35 ms) and (D) long-echo (288 ms) MR spectra sampling within the left posterior parietal white matter demonstrate significant reduction of NAA and elevation of Cho with dramatically large lactate resonances.

young children with the most common form, infantile, presenting with irritability between 3 and 6 months after birth. The disease progresses with symptoms mimicking encephalitis with motor deterioration, difficulties in feeding, and atypical seizures. At the end stage of the disease, the child exists in a vegetative state with decerebrate posturing.

The disease predominantly involves the white matter of the cerebral hemispheres, cerebellum, and spinal cord. Pathologic changes include a marked toxic reduction in the number of oligodendrocytes. Multinucleated globoid-appearing cells, as well as reactive macrophages with cerebroside, are scattered throughout the white matter and around blood vessels (Kumar et al., 2005). Hypomyelination may be extensive leading eventually to gliosis and scarring in the white matter. Gray matter involvement in the basal ganglia region can be found accompanied by punctate calcification.

Delayed myelination may be the first feature observed on MRI in infants. The imaging appearance demonstrates one of two patterns. Patchy hyperintense periventricular signal on T_2-weighted imaging, consistent with hypomyelination, may eventually evolve into a more diffuse pattern in the white matter, often with involvement of the thalami. A second pattern is patchy low signal on T_2-weighted images representing a paramagnetic effect arising from calcium deposition. Early changes include abnormal signal in the thalami, cerebellum, caudate heads, and brainstem that may precede the changes in the white matter of the centrum semiovale. Symmetric enlargement of the optic nerves is presumed to reflect accumulation of proteolipid in globoid cells. Changes within the cerebellar white matter have also been reported, with hyperintensity noted on T_2-weighted images. The findings within the spinal cord are visualized as atrophic changes. Diffuse volume loss and periventricular white matter abnormalities predominate in the latter stages of this disease.

Reduced NAA with elevated Cho and mI have been reported. Diminished NAA is expected with neuroaxonal loss, but spectroscopy has also revealed disturbances in glial cell metabolism associated with hypomyelination. Brockmann (2003b) found different

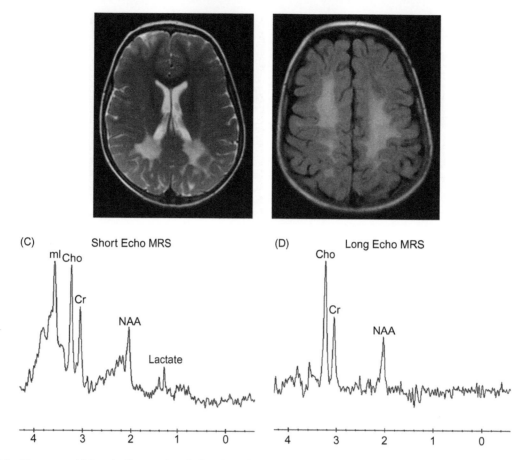

FIGURE 3.5.5   Four-year-old female diagnosed with GLD (Krabbe disease). (A) Axial T$_2$-weighted image shows hyperintense signal in the parietal white matter. (B) Axial FLAIR image shows significant signal abnormalities in the central white matter. (C) Short-echo (35 ms) and (D) long-echo (288 ms) MR spectra acquired from right parietal white matter show reduced NAA/Cr, with elevations of Cho/Cr and mI/Cr with a small lactate peak visible in (C) at 1.3 ppm.

metabolic profiles dependent upon the presentation (infantile, juvenile, and adult onset) consistent with recognized histopathologic features. For infantile presentation of Krabbe, pronounced Cho and mI elevations in affected white matter reflected astrocytosis, demyelination, and glial proliferation with reductions in NAA representing neuroaxonal loss. For juvenile-onset patients, the white matter MRS reflected metabolic changes consistent with neuroaxonal loss and astrocytosis, analogous to the infantile form with lesser NAA reduction. In an adult-onset patient, white matter spectroscopy approximated normal metabolic concentrations (see Fig. 3.5.5).

Metachromatic Leukodystrophy

Metachromatic leukodystrophy (MLD) arises from a deficiency in the enzyme arylsulfatase A, which cleaves the sulfate from sulfate-containing lipids, resulting in the accumulation of cerebroside sulfate within the lysosome. There are four presentations of metachromatic leukodystrophy: congenital, late infantile, juvenile, and

adult. The most common form, late infantile, presents from around 14 months to 4 years of age. The early presentation begins with an unsteady gait that eventually progresses to severe ataxia and flaccid paralysis, dysarthria, mental retardation, and decerebrate posturing.

Histologic analysis of affected white matter demonstrates a complete loss of myelin with evidence of axonal degeneration. Metachromatic granules are reported within engorged lysosomes in white matter, neurons, and on peripheral nerve biopsies. Oligodendrocytes are reduced in number, and areas of demyelination predominate throughout the deep white matter region. Macrophages with vacuolated cytoplasm containing crystalloid sulfatide structures are scattered in the white matter (Kumar et al., 2005). Early sparing of the subcortical arcuate white matter fibers (U-fibers) occurs until late in the disease process. An inflammatory response is typically absent, which accounts for the lack of contrast enhancement in this disorder, but eventually, myelinated white matter is replaced by astrogliosis and scarring. On T$_2$-weighted imaging, there is marked hyperintensity of the white matter

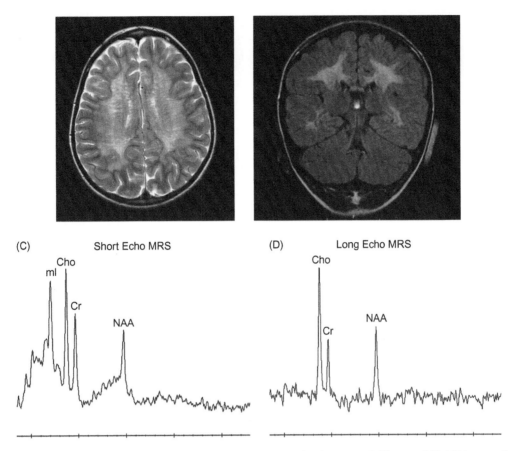

FIGURE 3.5.6 Seven-year-old male diagnosed with MLD. (A) Axial T_2-weighted image and (B) coronal FLAIR images show hyperintense signal in periventricular white matter with sparing of subcortical U-fibers. (C) Short-echo (35 ms) and (D) long-echo (288 ms) MR spectra acquired from left posterior parietal white matter feature reduced NAA and Cr and elevated Cho and from the short-echo MRS, an elevated mI level.

fiber tracts involving the cerebral hemispheres extending to the cerebellum, brainstem, and spinal cord. The findings are initially focal and patchy, but later develop into a diffuse, hyperintense T_2 signal of the centrum semiovale. On T_1-weighted imaging, the white matter fibers may be isointense with or hypointense to gray matter. Over time, a diffuse volume loss of all regions emerges with marked compensatory enlargement of the ventricles and extra-axial fluid spaces. At this end stage, differentiation of this condition from diffuse hypoxic/ischemic injury or other late-stage neurodegenerative/metabolic diseases is difficult from imaging findings alone.

Proton MRS investigations of patients with MLD have demonstrated reduced NAA as expected from axonal degeneration and neuroaxonal loss. Disturbances in glial cell metabolism indicated by elevated mI and Cho may reflect the loss of myelin. In one study, Kruse (1993) found that in contrast to other leukodystrophies, late infantile and juvenile MLD patients demonstrate two- to threefold increases in brain mI. This elevation may reflect a specific aspect of

the pathophysiology of demyelination associated with MLD. Van der Voorn et al. (2006) supports this finding, with highly significant elevations of mI and Cho as useful for classification of demyelinating disorders (see Fig. 3.5.6).

NCL

NCL, a common neurodegenerative syndrome with an incidence estimated between 2 and 4 per 100,000 newborns, is a disorder or group of disorders characterized by striking volume loss of brain parenchyma. Clinical manifestations include seizures and abnormal eye movements, with subsequent vision loss, dementia, hypotonia, and speech and motor deficits. At pathology, these disorders are characterized by distinctive granular inclusions in neuronal lysosomes, referred to as granular osmiophilic deposits. Imaging findings lag behind the clinical presentation in all subtypes, with the exception of the infantile form of NCL, and feature progressive cerebral and cerebellar volume

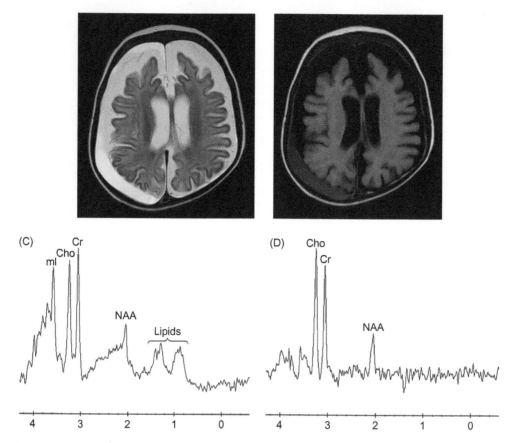

FIGURE 3.5.7   Nine-month-old male followed for a neuropathic form of osteopetrosis who presented with MRI and MRS findings consistent with NCL. (A) Axial T$_2$-weighted image reveals hyperintense signal from CSF-associated supratentorial volume loss. (B) Axial FLAIR image illustrating volume loss and subdural collection. (C) Short-echo (35 ms) and (D) intermediate-echo (144 ms) MR spectra acquired from right parietal lobe demonstrate reduced NAA, with elevations of lipids and mI/Cr.

loss. Later disease stages are characterized by development of a band of hyperintense signal in the periventricular white matter on T$_2$-weighted images. Proton MRS has shown progressive decreases in NAA and relative increases in mI in NCL. An example from a 9-month-old patient with NCL is demonstrated in Fig. 3.5.7.

Confort-Gouny et al. (1993) reported MRS findings from the basal ganglia of a 4-year-old patient with infantile NCL displaying an unusual increase of mI and taurine levels with a reduction of NAA. The patient demonstrated extensive cerebral atrophy. Brockmann et al. (1996) described a series of five patients with NCL using proton MRS. Juvenile NCL demonstrated normal metabolite levels, while infantile NCL was characterized by a complete loss of NAA, marked reductions of Cr and Cho, and increases of mI and lactate in both gray and white matter. Reduced NAA and elevated lactate were also detected in gray and white matter of late-infantile NCL; however, not only mI, but also Cr and Cho were increased in white matter. Seitz et al. (1998) sampled parietal lobe white matter in three patients with late-infantile NCL and

compared the findings with healthy control participants. Again, reduced NAA with elevated mI levels relative to Cr were reported. Vanhanen et al. (2004) examined eight infantile patients with MRI, MRS acquired in the thalamus and parietal-occipital white matter, and perfusion single-photon emission computed tomography. Using clinical features, Vanhanen et al. (2004) described the disease presentations as ranging from preclinical (stage 0) to late stage (stage 4). While not specific for infantile NCL, MRS indicated cerebral abnormalities before symptoms, structural changes, or blood flow changes appeared in the patients. Patients between 3 and 5 months of age, classified as stage 0 with normal developmental milestones, demonstrated reduced NAA and elevated Cho levels to Cr. By 17 months, classified as stage 2 where onset of microcephaly and muscular hypotonia presents, decreased NAA and Cho were accompanied by increased mI in the thalamus and parietal white matter. By stage 4 with rapid developmental deterioration and neurological symptoms, NAA and Cho levels declined significantly with lipids, lactate, and mI increased. Reduction of NAA in the thalamus and white matter possibly reflected neuroaxonal damage or changes in the function of the remaining cells. As Cho mainly represents structural components of the cell membrane, especially myelin sheaths in white matter, an increase of Cho and Cho/Cr reflected demyelination. High Cho and increasing mI indicated progression of demyelination with glial proliferation. Increased levels of mI, lipids, and lactate also indicated gliosis, cell loss, and abnormal anaerobic metabolism of the macrophages, and possibly, atrophic thalamic astrocytes filled with abnormal storage material (Vanhanen et al., 2004). At stage 4, the spectrum also featured lipid signals, which could serve as markers of myelin breakdown product. The complete absence of NAA, minimally detectable Cho and Cr, and relatively high mI and lipids indicated almost complete neuroaxonal loss, ongoing demyelination, and gliosis.

NPC

NPC is an autosomal-recessive, neurovisceral, lysosomal lipid storage disorder that results from defective cholesterol esterification and is associated with impaired intracellular lipid trafficking leading to accumulation of cholesterol and glycosphingolipids in the brain, the liver, the spleen, and the lung. NPC has a very heterogeneous clinical presentation from a neonatal rapidly fatal disorder to an adult-onset chronic neurodegenerative disease. The initial presentation is visceral, with systemic signs of cholestatic jaundice in the neonatal period. Presentation during infancy or childhood can feature isolated splenomegaly or hepatosplenomegaly. In the early infantile, late infantile, and juvenile period, a wide range of nonspecific and progressive neurologic symptoms varies according to the age at onset. The first neurological symptoms may include delay in developmental motor milestones (early infantile period), falls, clumsiness, cataplexy, and academic difficulties (late infantile and juvenile period). Seizures, dysarthria, dysphagia, ataxia, and psychiatric disturbances can occur within the disease course. The most characteristic sign is vertical supranuclear gaze palsy. The prognosis generally correlates with the age at onset of the neurological manifestations, with better prognosis at later onset. NPC is currently described as a cellular cholesterol trafficking defect, but in the brain, the prominently stored lipids are gangliosides.

Tedeschi et al. (1998) evaluated 10 patients with NPC using proton spectroscopic imaging (MRSI) and compared the findings with those obtained from 15 healthy controls. NAA/Cr levels were decreased in the frontal and parietal cortices, centrum semiovale, and caudate nucleus. Cho/Cr levels were increased in the frontal cortex and centrum semiovale. Strong correlations were found between clinical staging scale scores and MRSI abnormalities.

Cholesterol-lowering agents effectively decrease hepatic lipids in NPC patients. Sylvain et al. (1994) described the effects of such agents on neurologic features using proton MRS in a 9-month-old boy with progressive hepatosplenomegaly and neurodevelopmental delay. MRS acquired within a supraventricular volume of central white and gray matter revealed an abnormally elevated lipid signal. The patient treatment included cholesterol-lowering agents (i.e., cholestyramine, lovastatin). Repeat standardized neurodevelopmental assessments using Peabody and Griffith scales at 13 and 19 months were normal. MRS no longer detected the previously observed abnormal lipid resonance.

Miglustat (N-butyl-deoxynojirimycin), an inhibitor of glycosphingolipid synthesis, is approved to treat patients in the United States and Europe, but questions remain regarding its efficacy. Galanaud et al. (2009) acquired proton MRS in three locations (centrum semiovale, basal ganglia, and cerebellum) for three adults with NPC treated with Miglustat for 24 months. All patients reported mild clinical improvement or stabilization. With multiple time points assessed, the abnormally elevated Cho/Cr levels within the parietal white matter (centrum semiovale) were observed in all three patients to decrease over time. Although preliminary, Miglustat demonstrated beneficial effects on brain dysfunction in NPC.

PEROXISOMAL DISORDERS PRODUCING LEUKODYSTROPHIES

Peroxisomes are organelles within a cell that hold enzymes responsible for critical cellular processes, including biosynthesis of membrane phospholipids (plasmalogens), cholesterol, and bile acids, conversion of amino acids into glucose, oxidation of fatty acids, reduction of hydrogen peroxide by catalases, and prevention of excess oxalate synthesis.

Four different disorders make up the genetically heterogeneous peroxisomal biogenesis disorders group: Zellweger syndrome (ZS), infantile Refsum's disease (IRD), neonatal adrenoleukodystrophy (NALD), and rhizomelic chondrodysplasia punctata. X-linked adrenoleukodystrophy (ALD) is the prototypical peroxisomal disorder in which the morphology of the organelle is found to be normal on electron microscopy, but a single enzyme defect leads to the accumulation of very long chain fatty acids (VLCAs) and progressive CNS deterioration in the form of a chronic progressive encephalopathy.

ZS

ZS is an autosomal recessive disease characterized by defective peroxisomal functions. Infants are symptomatic early, with hypotonia, seizures, large liver size, and limb and facial anomalies that are easily recognizable at birth. There is a diffuse lack of myelination throughout the white matter combined with cortical dysplasia. The gyri are broad, with shallow intervening sulci found mainly in the anterior frontal and temporal lobes but also over the convexities in the perirolandic area. Variants of ZS have also been described that do not follow the typical prototype, but demonstrate many common features to ZS. Clinical overlap may occur with other conditions including NALD, IRD, and hyperpipecolic acidemia. The difference among ZS, NALD, and IRD is one of severity. ZS is the most severe, with death occurring in the first year of life, whereas survival for NALD is limited to childhood, and patients with IRD can survive into adulthood.

MRS performed in older patients with ZS and IRD finds similar features with dramatic lipid and choline elevations, minor mI elevations, and reduced NAA levels for sampled white matter (Fig. 3.5.8). ZS presents with cortical dysplasia and neuronal heterotopia on imaging. Proton MRS illustrates the neuropathologic aspects of ZS, which include neuronal degeneration, abnormal myelination, and compromised liver function. Bruhn et al. (1992) reported MRS of infants ($N = 4$) with impaired peroxisomal function classified as variants of ZS revealed a marked decrease of NAA in white and gray matter, thalamus, and cerebellum with two patients also demonstrating an increase of cerebral glutamine and a decrease of the cytosolic mI in gray matter and striatum reflecting impaired hepatic function. Two subjects in the Bruhn study exhibited a notable elevation of mobile lipids and/or cholesterol in white matter.

NALD

NALD is characterized by the presence of multiple recognizable enzyme deficiencies with grossly normal, but reduced numbers of peroxisomes. Specific conditions include pipecolic and phytanic acidemia and a deficiency of plasmalogen synthetase. This condition also presents with hypotonia in the first months of life, but without many of the facial features of ZS. Cortical abnormalities in the form of a dysplasia can be found in this condition as well with hypomyelination in cerebral white matter. An example of proton MRS in NALD is shown in Fig. 3.5.9.

X-Linked ALD

For X-linked ALD, the morphology of the organelle is found to be normal on electron microscopy; however, a single enzyme defect, acyl-CoA synthetase, and a failure of the incorporation into cholesterol esters for myelin synthesis results in the accumulation of VLCFAs and progressive CNS deterioration in the form of a chronic progressive encephalopathy. The "classic" form of ALD is an X-linked disorder (Xq28) with a clinical onset between the ages of 5–7 years, which includes behavioral problems, followed by a rapidly progressive decline in neurologic function, and death within the ensuing 5–8 year period. Clinical symptoms may begin with subtle alterations in neurocognitive function, but eventually progress to severe

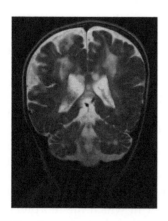
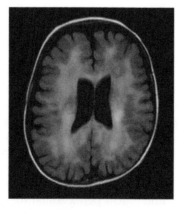
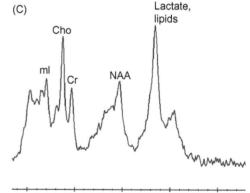

FIGURE 3.5.8 Three-year-old male diagnosed with ZS. (A) Coronal T_2 image and (B) axial FLAIR show diffuse periventricular white matter hyperintensities. (C) Short-echo (35 ms) MR spectrum shows elevated lactate and lipids, as well as increased choline, with a reduction of NAA.

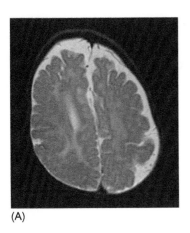
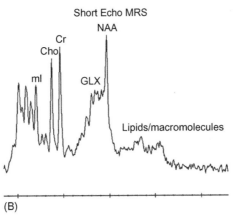
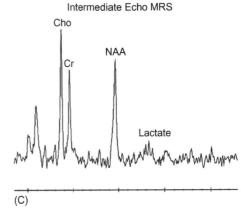

FIGURE 3.5.9 Twelve-month-old male diagnosed with neonatal ALD. (A) Axial T_2-weighted image reveals diffuse white matter signal abnormalities. (B) Short-echo MR spectrum shows elevated Glx and macromolecules. (C) Intermediate-echo (144 ms) MR spectrum demonstrates the reduced NAA and slight elevation of Cho and lactate.

spasticity and visual deficits, ultimately leading to a vegetative state and death.

X-linked ALD demonstrates a loss of myelin with relative preservation of the subcortical U-fibers along with lymphocytic inflammation and gliosis (Kumar et al., 2005). It has been described with a typical appearance on MRI with predominately posterior involvement that over time progresses from posterior to anterior into the frontal lobes, and from the deep white matter to the peripheral subcortical white matter. The involvement appears symmetrical in a butterfly distribution across the splenium of the corpus callosum, surrounded on its periphery by an enhancing zone. Three zones are readily distinguished on MRI: an inner zone of astrogliosis and scarring that appears hypointense on T_1-weighted imaging and hyperintense on T_2-weighted sequences, an intermediate zone of active inflammation that appears isointense on T_1-weighted images and isointense or hypointense on T_2-weighted imaging, and an outer zone of active demyelination that appears minimally hypointense on T_1-weighted images and hyperintense on T_2-weighted imaging. Rarely, involvement can be entirely anterior in a butterfly distribution; however, unilateral and asymmetrical involvement has also been described. Following a bone marrow transplant, the disappearance of gadolinium contrast enhancement within the intermediate zone of inflammation is observed on MRI. The progression of disease from posterior to anterior and from deep white matter to the periphery of the brain may be slower compared to its previous course; however, hyperintense signal changes are not significantly reversed (Fig. 3.5.10).

X-linked ALD patients evaluated with proton MRS demonstrate abnormal spectra within regions of abnormal imaging signal as well as normal-appearing white matter (NAWM). The spectral profile for NAWM of neurologically asymptomatic patients is characterized by slightly elevated concentrations of Cho compounds, with an increase of Cho and mI reflecting the onset of demyelination. Markedly elevated concentrations of Cho, mI, and glutamine in affected white matter suggest active demyelination and glial proliferation. A simultaneous reduction of the concentrations of NAA and glutamate is consistent with neuronal loss and injury. Elevated lactate is consistent with inflammation and/or macrophage infiltration. The more severe metabolic disturbances in ALD correspond to progressive demyelination, neuroaxonal loss, and gliosis leading to clinical deterioration and eventually death. The detection of MRS abnormalities before the onset of neurological symptoms may help in the selection of patients for bone marrow transplantation and stem cell transplant. Stabilization and partial reversal of metabolic abnormalities is demonstrated in some patients after therapies. The spectral profiles can be used to monitor disease evolution and the effects of therapies.

AMINO ACIDURIA

Non-ketotic hyperglycinemia (NKH), also referred to as glycine encephalopathy, is an autosomal recessive disorder of glycine metabolism. The defective glycine cleavage enzyme yields elevated concentrations of glycine in plasma, urine, CSF, and CNS, instead of the normal conversion to serine. Confirmation with an enzyme assay of liver tissue or mutational analysis can be definitive for diagnosis.

The toxic effects of glycine accumulation rapidly become clinically apparent, with the majority of patients presenting in the neonatal period. Approximately 85%

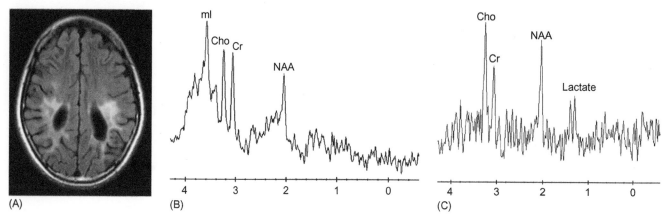

FIGURE 3.5.10   Fifteen-year-old diagnosed with X-linked ALD, approximately 6 months post bone marrow transplant. (A) Axial FLAIR image shows diffuse signal hyperintensities in the parietal white matter. (B) The short-echo (35 ms) spectrum displays decreased NAA and elevated mI. (C) The long-echo (288 ms) spectrum shows decreased NAA and elevated lactate; however, the low SNR reflects contribution of CSF from the adjacent lateral ventricle. The patient imaging was stable, with no abnormal contrast enhancement or abnormal diffusion signal, for at least 1 year on follow-up studies.

of NKH patients have the severe neonatal form of the disorder. Patients can present with hiccups, poor feeding, lethargy, severe hypotonia, and early infantile seizures with myoclonic jerks associated with burst-suppression pattern on electroencephalography. Most will have repeated episodes of severe and prolonged apnea that can lead to death. Surviving infants usually have profound intellectual disabilities and intractable seizures. Some patients can present with atypical, milder forms of the disorder if residual enzyme activity remains present.

The glycine cleavage enzyme maintains extracellular glycine concentrations as glycine serves as an excitation modulator of *N*-methyl-D-aspartate (NMDA) receptors in the brain. The excessive activation of these receptors produces neuronal and axonal injury. NMDA receptors also play an important role in neurogenesis. Thus, the excess glycine concentration can potentially impair neurogenesis and produce cellular neurotoxicity. Patients are treated with sodium benzoate to reduce glycine levels in the blood and CSF, and with dextromethorphan to counteract the neurostimulatory effect of high glycine levels on NMDA receptors. Unfortunately, these pharmacological therapies often fail suggesting that irreversible glycine-induced brain damage occurs *in utero*.

Imaging features support the notion of fetal injury with abnormalities demonstrated on neonatal MRI, which generally include thinning or agenesis of the corpus callosum with hypomyelination. Pathology in NKH is characterized by vacuolation, astrocytosis, and demyelination, also called vacuolating myelinopathy. Because these changes only occur in myelinated white matter, in the neonate they are restricted to the dorsal limbs of the internal capsule, dorsal brainstem,

pyramidal tracts in the coronal radiata, and lateral thalamus. Significant volume loss is also appreciated with enlarged ventricles and prominent sulci. Fig. 3.5.11 illustrates the MRI and MRS findings in a patient with a neonatal NKH presentation.

Heindel et al. (1993) first employed proton MRS to describe the findings from two children diagnosed with NKH. In a 2-month-old female, the signal of the inhibitory neurotransmitter glycine was present with equal signal intensity and prominence in the parieto-occipital white matter and in the basal ganglia region. In a 10-day-old female with follow-up studies performed within the first 4 months of life, a reduction of glycine in brain tissue corresponded more reliably with clinical findings than the stable values in plasma and cerebrospinal fluid. Gabis et al. (2001) monitored the course of treatment with sodium benzoate and dextromethorphan in a male child at 10 and 13 months of age. Over that period, a small increase in glycine coupled with a dramatic elevation of the composite glutamate and glutamine (Glx) was observed. These findings were correlated with glycine and glutamine levels monitored in the blood. Choi et al. (2001) evaluated a patient with neonatal presentation of NKH at 6, 12, and 17 days of life before expiration at 20 days. Proton MRS supported initial diagnosis with the prominent glycine resonance, reflected improvement at 12 days with reduced glycine, and indicated distress with the appearance of a lactate resonance at 17 days. These three studies described elevated glycine in terms of a ratio to brain Cr. Huisman et al. (2002) employed a quantitative proton MRS approach that allowed for the determination of elevated glycine concentrations in the basal ganglia, cerebellar, parieto-occipital, and frontal white matter for a male at 7 days of life. Results were

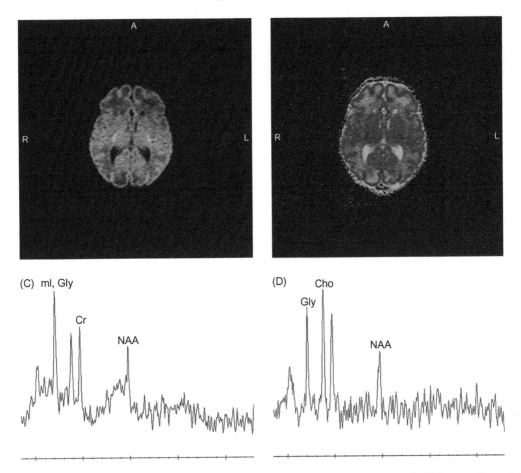

FIGURE 3.5.11 Neonate diagnosed with NKH. (A) Axial DWI. (B) ADC image. (C) Short-echo MRS. (D) Intermediate-echo (144 ms) MRS. The short-echo spectrum reveals a composite mI and glycine resonance at 3.5 ppm. The intermediate-echo spectrum features the elevated signal at 3.5, which arises from glycine.

in agreement with findings obtained at day 9 upon autopsy conducted 12 h postmortem. Other metabolite concentrations were within normal limits for the site. This contrasts an *in vitro* study of the blood, CSF, and *in vivo* brain from patients with NKH. Viola et al. (2002) reported elevated Cr levels in addition to elevations of glycine for blood, fluids, and brain. Increased lactate, pyruvate, alanine, proline, and sulfur amino acids were also observed in the blood and CSF. These elevations were thought to represent the consequence of glycine disposal via several metabolic pathways. With longitudinal monitoring of two patients, the *in vivo* elevation of creatine was noted by comparing the individual metabolite area with the total area of all measured metabolites. Comparing two patients with *in vivo* MRS acquired, a low NAA/glycine level was found in the fatal case suggesting it may represent a prognostic marker for poorer outcomes. For these two patients, vigabatrin was part of a medication regimen to control seizures. However, Tekgul et al. (2006) reported vigabatrin-associated deterioration in two infants with NKH.

ORGANIC ACIDURIAS

Glutaric Acidurias

Glutaric aciduria type 1 (GA-I), an inborn error of lysine, hydroxylysine, and tryptophan metabolism, usually presents between birth and 18 months of life with acute striatal degeneration with neurologic dysfunction characterized by encephalopathy and subtle neurologic signs in infancy (irritability or hypotonia), to dystonia, choreoathetosis, loss of milestones, and seizures. The diagnosis of GA-I is confirmed with the presence of increased urinary glutaric acid and 3-hydroxyglutaric acid. The disorder features a deficiency or absence of glutaryl-CoA dehydrogenase in cultured fibroblasts. Hoffman et al. (1996) found that 20−30% of patients had "chronic" subdural effusions and hematomas identified on neuroimaging studies. The presence of subdural effusions on imaging in GA-I can mimic abusive head trauma; however, appropriate biochemical and imaging can normally be used to distinguish the two entities. Another prominent clinical

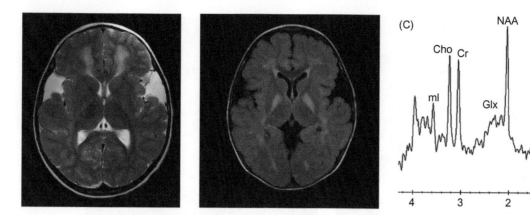

FIGURE 3.5.12   Twenty-two-month-old male diagnosed with GA-I. (A) Axial T$_2$-weighted and (B) axial FLAIR images demonstrate abnormal, symmetric signal within the globus pallidus and white matter. There is also symmetric, bilateral widening of the Sylvian fissures. (C) Short-echo MRS sampled from the basal ganglia illustrates elevated Cho levels.

feature of infants and children with GA-I is macrocephaly, but not megalencephaly. Hoffman et al. (1996) found that 70% of the patients with GA-I studied had either macrocephaly or increasing head circumference past the 97th percentile. Common features on neuroimaging include widened or enlarged Sylvian fissures, increased spaces anterior to the frontotemporal lobes but no evidence of frontotemporal atrophy. Enlargement of the Sylvian fissure has been correlated with severity of the enzyme deficiency. Basal ganglia and white matter signal abnormalities have also been noted (see Fig. 3.5.12).

Early case reports employing proton and phosphorus MRS in GA-I were discrepant in their findings. Several reported cases with no spectral abnormalities. However, the absence of rigorous quantification and appropriate control groups or the examinations conducted during stable periods could explain the discrepancy with later case reports and series. Kurul et al. (2004) described findings in a 19-month-old male with GA-I. Short-echo MRS of right frontal white matter and right lentiform nuclei revealed decreased NAA/Cr levels, slightly increased Cho/Cr levels, and increased mI/Cr levels, compared with the age-matched control patients. Oguz et al. (2005) reported widespread restricted diffusion in the white matter and increased diffusion in bilateral putamen in an 11-month-old male diagnosed with GA-I. The MRS showed decreased NAA/Cr levels found on MRSI performed with an intermediate echo time compared with a sex- and age-matched control with no significant change in Cho/Cr levels. Elevated lactate levels were noted in affected basal ganglia and in normal-appearing regions of brain parenchyma. Sijens et al. (2006) employed an MRSI approach in two patients with GA-I and reported reductions in the white matter NAA signal, in the more severe case

accompanied by a loss of glutamate and the appearance of lactate signals. In the largest case series to date, Pérez-Dueñas (2009) examined symptomatic pediatric patients and asymptomatic siblings with GA-I with proton MRS. For the symptomatic patients, the MRI and MRS was performed between 3 and 8 days after the onset of acute encephalopathic crisis. For the encephalopathic patients, isotropic diffusion images showed high signal changes with corresponding low apparent diffusion coefficient (ADC) values within the putamen, caudate nuclei, and globus pallidus, and for one patient, the cerebral peduncles including the substantia nigra. The imaging for the asymptomatic siblings appeared normal. MRS showed decreased NAA/Cr levels at the basal ganglia in encephalopathic patients when compared to a group of sex- and age-matched controls.

Glutaric aciduria type II (GA-II), also known as multiple acyl-CoA dehydrogenase deficiency, is a mitochondrial electron transport chain disorder that impairs electron transfer flavoprotein or electron transfer flavoprotein-ubiquinone oxidoreductase (at coenzyme Q). The brain involvement is often revealed with abnormal T$_2$ prolongation within the basal ganglia, periventricular white matter, and the splenium of the corpus callosum. Firat et al. (2006) examined a 12-year-old female patient with GA-II and compared her results with data obtained from four healthy age- and sex-matched volunteers. During clinical exacerbation, frontal lobe Cho/Cr level was greater than the levels reported for the comparison participants. The NAA/Cr level was lower than normal limits. After successful riboflavin treatment and dietary restriction for proteins, the NAA/Cr level normalized; however, the Cho/Cr level remained below the normal range, suggesting riboflavin-responsive multiple acyl-CoA dehydrogenase deficiency. An elevated Cho/Cr ratio and decreased NAA/Cr ratio appeared consistent with a demyelinating process in the active phase of GA-II. MRS aided in monitoring the progress of the disease and the efficacy of treatment by demonstrating changes in NAA/Cr and Cho/Cr levels.

L-Hydroxyglutaric Aciduria

Elevated levels of L-2-hydroxyglutaric acid (L2HG) in urine, CSF, and to a lesser extent, plasma, are found in patients with the disorder. Most patients experience a slowly progressive clinical course. The most common presenting signs include developmental delay, hypotonia, epilepsy, hypotonia, spasticity, extrapyramidal symptoms, behavioral problems, and cerebellar ataxia.

Accumulation of L2HG is toxic to the human brain, producing an appearance similar to a leukoencephalopathy and increasing the susceptibility of a patient to develop tumors. The MRI pattern of signal abnormalities of the subcortical cerebral white matter, putamen, caudate nucleus, globus pallidus, and dentate nucleus has been described (D'Incerti et al., 1998; Seijo-Martinez et al., 2005; Topcu et al., 2005; Steenweg et al., 2009). Hanefeld et al. (1994) described the spectroscopic findings in L2HG with a case report of a 16-year-old female. Using quantitative short-echo proton MRS, the study found a 50% decrease of NAA, a 75% increase of mI, and a 40% decrease of Cho in white matter relative to age-matched controls. MRS findings upon follow-up 2 years later demonstrated further declines in NAA and increases in mI. Sener (2003) reported the detection of a singlet resonance at 2.50 ppm, suspected to represent L2HG, in a 10-month-old male with urinary levels of L2HG greater than 80 times normal. Aydin et al. (2003) reported a multiplet within the region of 2.1 and 2.5 ppm, for two male siblings (ages 10 and 12 years), which potentially could represent L2HG, coupled by the commonly observed Glx resonances.

Maple Syrup Urine Disease

Maple syrup urine disease (MSUD) is a rare autosomal recessive disorder caused by defective oxidative decarboxylation of the branched-chain amino acids valine, isoleucine, and leucine. The accumulation of metabolites in the urine leads to the characteristic odor resembling maple syrup. While cerebral imaging may initially be unremarkable, diffuse cerebral edema develops in the deep cerebellar white matter, posterior limb of the internal capsule, perirolandic white matter, dorsal brainstem, and pons. Imaging studies have shown reversible brain edema during acute metabolic decompensation.

Proton MRS of the brain appears to be useful for examining patients suffering from MSUD in different metabolic states. Felber et al. (1993) demonstrated the appearance of a previously unassigned resonance in a 3-year-old male with MSUD. This peak disappeared with normalization of branched-chain amino acids and oxoacids in the plasma and CSF. *In vitro* spectroscopy of these acids at 1.5 T confirmed the chemical shift position of the acid methyl components. The duration of lactate elevation correlated with the presence of brain edema and coma. Heindel et al. (1995) replicated the finding of accumulation of branched-chain amino acids and their corresponding 2-oxo acids in the brain of a 9-year-old girl suffering from classical MSUD. During acute metabolic decompensation, the compounds appeared as a resonance located at 0.9 ppm. The brain tissue concentration of these acids could be estimated as 0.9 mmol/L. Six patients with MSUD were evaluated by Jan et al. (2003) during acute presentation with metabolic decompensation. Follow-up examinations were performed after clinical and metabolic recovery. Diffusion weighted imaging (DWI) revealed marked diffusion restriction compatible with cytotoxic or intramyelinic sheath edema in the brainstem, basal ganglia, thalami, cerebellar and periventricular white matter, and the cerebral cortex. Long-echo MRS acquired in four of the six patients revealed the abnormal branched-chain amino acids and branched-chain α-keto acids peak at 0.9 ppm as well as elevated lactate on proton MRS. The changes were reversed with treatment without evidence of volume loss or persistent tissue damage. The presence of cytotoxic or intramyelinic edema as evidenced by restricted water diffusion on DWI, with the presence of lactate on spectroscopy, appear worrisome for irreversible injury; however, in the context of metabolic decompensation in MSUD, it appears that changes in cell osmolarity and metabolism can reverse completely after metabolic correction. An example of MRI and MRS findings in an infant diagnosed with MSUD is shown in Fig. 3.5.13.

Urea Cycle Defects

The urea cycle is responsible for the clearance of nitrogen, a waste product arising from protein metabolism. Normally nitrogen, accumulated in the form of ammonia, is removed from the blood and converted to urea. Urea is subsequently transferred into the urine and excreted. Five catalytic enzymes, a cofactor, and at least two transport proteins comprise the urea cycle. This cycle is also responsible for endogenous synthesis of arginine.

Severe deficiency or the complete absence of an enzyme or cofactor activity results in the accumulation

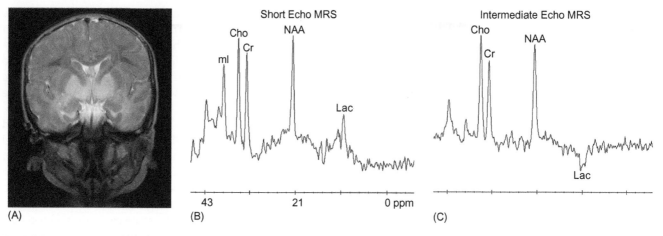

FIGURE 3.5.13   Infant diagnosed with MSUD. (A) Coronal T_2-weighted image. (B) Short-echo MRS. (C) Intermediate-echo (144 ms) MRS. On short-echo MRS, there is a composite of branched chain amino acids (0.9 ppm) with lactate (1.35 ppm). The lactate resonance becomes inverted on intermediate-echo MRS.

of ammonia and other precursor metabolites within the first days of life. Initially, infants with a urea cycle disorder are born without disease symptoms. However, a rapid deterioration occurs with acute onset of cerebral edema, lethargy, seizures, neurologic posturing, hyper- or hypoventilation, coma, and potentially death. In persons with partial enzyme deficiencies, a milder form can manifest later in life with less severe hyperammonemia and subtle symptoms (psychiatric symptoms such as hyperactive, self-injurious behaviors, and autistic features; vomiting, learning disorders, stroke-like episodes, etc.). Hyperammonemia can be exacerbated by illness or stress. Treatment regimes for patients with urea cycle defects include many approaches (dialysis, low protein-dietary restrictions, IV administration of glucose, arginine chloride, and nitrogen scavengers) for reducing ammonia concentrations and minimizing neurologic damage.

The acute and subacute imaging appearances of these disorders mimic hypoxic-ischemic encephalopathy with edema. The insular cortex, perirolandic cortex, basal ganglia, especially the globi pallidi and putamina, demonstrate swelling and abnormal signals with T_1 and T_2 prolongation. The subcortical white matter, including the U-fibers, is also involved. With prolonged durations of hyperammonemia, cortical volume loss and cystic changes are also appreciated.

Connelly et al. (1993) first reported an elevation of glutamine with reduction of NAA, Cr, and Cho levels found upon long-echo proton MRS examinations within the white matter of two female infants with partial ornithine transcarboxylase (OTC) defects hospitalized with encephalopathy associated with hyperammonemia. Kreis et al. (1992) reported elevated glutamine in patients with chronic hepatic encephalopathy. Ross et al. (1992) reported reduced mI levels in a 14-year-old male patient with partial OTC effectively treated with oral benzoate. Takanashi et al. (2002) later expanded the findings in OTC with a study of six patients with late onset OTC using a short-echo MRS approach. Upon comparison with age-matched controls, Glx levels within the centrum semiovale were increased in four patients, proportionally to clinical stage of the disease; Cho levels were reduced in the two patients with more severe disease; mI levels were reduced in five of six patients to undetectable levels for five symptomatic patients. NAA and Cr levels were normal for all four patients. This suggested a spectroscopic pattern of disease involvement with mI depletion and glutamine accumulation, followed by Cho depletion.

Kojic et al. (2005) described a 16-year-old female patient with well-controlled carbamoyl phosphate synthetase I (CPSI) who presented with hyperammonemia, which was corrected over 2 days. Despite maintenance of near normal ammonia levels, the patient suffered further neurologic deterioration. After being comatose for 5 days, short-echo proton MRS was acquired within the occipital gray and parietal white matter. The resonances within alpha (3.65–3.8 ppm), beta and gamma (2.02–2.5 ppm) regions corresponding to Glx levels were elevated, especially in gray matter. After 5 weeks and therapeutic efforts to reduce glutamine levels, the patient emerged from the coma. Five months after presentation, when the patient demonstrated an essentially complete recovery, a repeat MRS study indicated a decrease of Glx levels, but without normalization of the levels. Fig. 3.5.14 illustrates another patient with CPSI with MRI and MRS features.

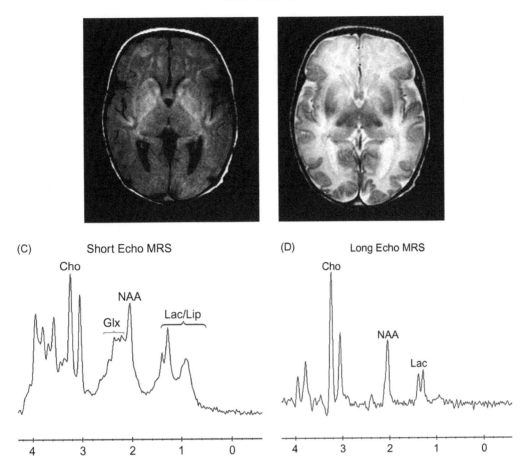

FIGURE 3.5.14   10-day-old female diagnosed with CPSI. (A) Axial proton density and (B) T_2-weighted images demonstrate hyperintense signal and swelling within the cortex and deep gray matter. (C) Short-echo and (D) long-echo MRS acquired from the basal ganglia. The short-echo MRS shows elevated glutamine, lactate, and lipids with reduced NAA. The long-echo MRS reveals the lactate elevation and NAA declines.

Miscellaneous Metabolic Disorders

Galactosemia

Galactosemia arises from mutations in the *GALT* gene that alter the galactose-1-phosphate uridylyltransferase protein responsible for proper metabolism of carbohydrates, specifically galactose. Due to the failure of the primary galactose metabolic pathway, an alternative enzyme activates such that aldose reductase catalyzes the conversion of galactose to galactitol. Excretion of abnormal quantities of galactitol in the urine is characteristic of galactosemia. Diagnosis of GALT enzyme activity is necessary to differentiate classic galactosemia (<5% controls) from Duarte variant galactosemia (5–25% control values). Infants with classic galactosemia have no GALT enzyme activity and cannot oxidize galactose to CO_2. Within days of ingesting breast milk or lactose-containing formulas, affected infants develop life-threatening complications including poor feeding, hypoglycemia, jaundice, hepatocellular damage, failure to thrive, bleeding diathesis,

and hyperammonemia. During the first 3–10 days of life, if a lactose–galactose-restricted diet is initiated, the symptoms resolve quickly and prognosis is good for prevention of liver failure, *Escherichia coli* sepsis, neonatal death, and intellectual disability. If treatment is delayed, complications such as intellectual disability, speech abnormalities, ocular cataracts, growth retardation, and primary ovarian failure in females can occur (Elsas, 2010).

Berry et al. (2001) first reported detection of galactitol with *in vivo* proton MRS acquired in the basal ganglia and occipital cortex of a 10-day-old infant patient with galactosemia. At 1.5 T, galactitol resonates with two resonance peaks located at 3.67 and 3.74 ppm. NAA, Cho, and mI/Cr levels were reduced in both regions upon comparison with metabolite levels from age-matched healthy control participants. In a subsequent study of 12 patients diagnosed with galactosemia, Wang et al. (2001) demonstrated that a correlation existed between the MRS-detected galactitol/Cr level acquired within the basal ganglia and the urine galactitol levels for the four neonates. For eight patients (ages 1.3–47 years) who had been on galactose-restricted diets since the neonatal period, cerebral galactitol was undetectable by proton MRS for six of the patients, with a small elevation observed for the remaining two. This suggested that in order to detect galactitol on *in vivo* brain proton MRS examination, high galactitol levels are requisite in the patient's urine. Galactosemic patients, who have been following a restricted diet for several years and maintain controlled levels of galactitol in the urine, do not demonstrate galactitol in the brain by *in vivo* MRS. Otaduy et al. (2006) further confirmed this with proton MRS revealing a doublet at 3.7 ppm indicating elevated galactitol in an undiagnosed 6-month-old female. *In vitro* proton MRS of the patient's urine confirmed the elevations of galactose and galactitol. Follow-up MRS performed at 2 years was within normal limits without galactitol as the patient was treated with a restricted lactose-free diet. These findings explain the early negative MRS findings in controlled patients described by Moller et al. (1995).

Inborn Errors of Cr Metabolism: Cerebral Cr Deficiency Syndromes

Cr (α-methyl-guanidinoacetic acid) plays an important role in energy metabolism. Creatine kinase is an essential enzyme to catalyze phosphorylation of Cr to provide a high-energy phosphate buffer system. In humans, Cr is synthesized in the liver, kidney, and pancreas where it is taken up via a sodium- and chloride-dependent Cr transporter (SLC6A8 protein) and ultimately transported via the blood to the muscles, heart, and nervous system, which are rich in creatine kinase.

Cr deficiency syndromes arise from one of three distinct defects, two involving Cr biosynthesis and one involving Cr transport. On proton MRS within the brain, all three disorders demonstrate a severely diminished or completely absent signal at 3.0 ppm for the composite resonance of Cr and phosphocreatine. Some degree of discrimination between synthesis and transporter defects could potentially be afforded from the MRS determination of Cr levels within skeletal muscle. Cr levels in the muscle of some patients with Cr biosynthesis defects are low. However, evidence suggests additional Cr transport mechanisms exist allowing passage of dietary sources of Cr (foods rich in Cr, creatine monohydrate supplements) into the muscle. Cr levels were described within normal limits for muscle in one patient with a transporter defect (deGrauw et al., 2003; Pyne-Geithman et al., 2004). However, the urine and plasma measurement of guanidinoacetic acid (GAA), Cr, and the excreted form creatinine are the most cost-efficient approaches for

narrowing the diagnostic differential. The next tier of testing includes molecular genetic testing; however, it too, can be inconclusive. Finally, enzyme activity and Cr uptake can discriminate among the three disorders. Diagnosis remains important as patients with synthesis defects can benefit from dietary Cr supplementation.

Cr Synthesis Defect: Arginine:Glycine Amidinotransferase Deficiency

Arginine:glycine amidinotransferase (AGAT) deficiency has been described in only seven individuals internationally (Item et al., 2001; Battini et al., 2002; Johnston et al., 2005; Edvardson et al., 2010). This autosomal recessive disorder can present with mild to moderate intellectual disability, psychomotor delay, language delay, failure to thrive, and autistic-like behavioral features. Patients with AGAT deficiency appear to respond favorably to creatine monohydrate dietary supplementation with dramatic improvement in neurological abnormalities (Mercimek-Mahmutoglu & Stockler-Ipsiroglu, 1993).

Cr Synthesis Defect: Guanidinoacetate Methyltransferase Deficiency

Guanidinoacetate methyltransferase (GAMT) deficiency was the first creatine deficiency syndrome recognized and now reportedly affects about 40 individuals worldwide (Mercimek-Mahmutoglu & Stockler-Ipsiroglu, 1993; Stockler et al., 1994). This autosomal recessive disorder can present with variable clinical features that include mental retardation, language and developmental delay, muscular hypotonia, weakness, extrapyramidal signs, epilepsy, autistic, and in some, hyperactivity and self-aggressive behavior (Mercimek-Mahmutoglu & Stockler-Ipsiroglu, 1993). In many patients, but not all with GAMT deficiency, abnormal hyperintense T_2 signal appears within the globus pallidus, which is thought to reflect neuronal injury from GAA accumulation. If early treatment is implemented, especially in the neonatal period, patients with GAMT defects demonstrate a positive response to creatine monohydrate dietary supplementation (Fig. 3.5.15). A dietary restriction of arginine in combination with ornithine supplementation reduces the accumulation of GAA by competitive inhibition of AGAT activity. In older patients, the prolonged accumulation of neurotoxic GAA limits the neurological benefits of Cr supplementation (Schulze et al., 1998, 2001, 2006; Leuzzi et al., 2000; Ensenauer et al., 2004; Mercimek-Mahmutoglu et al., 2006).

Cr Transporter Defect: SLC6A8 Deficiency

The discovery of the X-linked Cr transporter defect started with the observation of the absence of Cr upon proton MRS acquired within the basal ganglia and

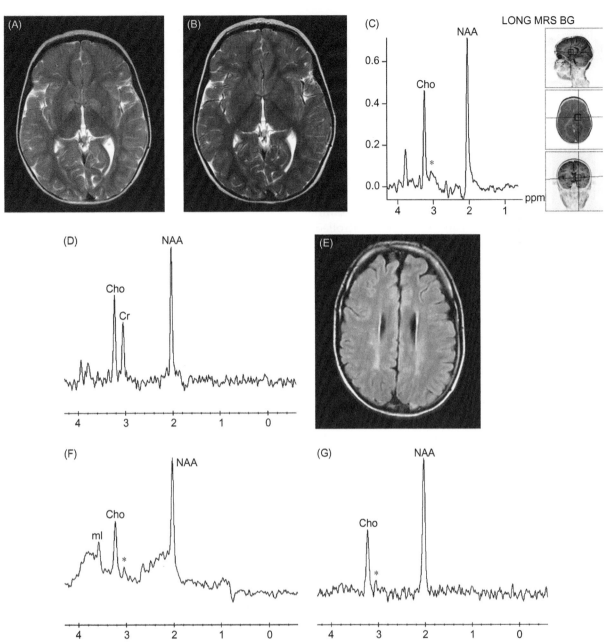

FIGURE 3.5.15 Two patients with distinct Cr deficiency syndromes. The first patient (images A–D) has a Cr synthesis defect known as GAMT deficiency. (A) Axial T_2-weighted imaging demonstrates signal abnormality within the globus pallidus due to the accumulation of guanidinoacetate. (B) Axial T_2 acquired after Cr supplementation demonstrates resolution of signal abnormality. (C) Long-echo MRS acquired presupplementation at 3 T with absent Cr peak (noted by the asterisk). (D) Long-echo MRS indicating an increase in Cr levels, acquired at 1.5 T following dietary supplementation. Cr transporter deficiency: (E) axial FLAIR image obtained at 15 years of age with posterior white matter signal abnormalities and (F) short-echo and (G) long-echo MRS acquired from the left frontal white matter demonstrates the absence of creatine signal at 3.0 (noted by the asterisk) and 3.9 ppm.

frontal lobes of a 6-year-old male evaluated for language delay and a head circumference at the 95th percentile (Cecil et al., 2001). Imaging was unremarkable (Fig. 3.5.15). Metabolic testing revealed elevated serum and urine Cr levels with normal substrates and products involved in Cr synthesis and excretion (glycine, ornithine, GAA. and creatine). Upon exclusion of a

synthesis defect, speculation about a novel mutation in the human Cr transporter gene, *SLC6A8*, located on Xq28 grew. Fibroblast from the 6-year-old male confirmed a hemizygous nonsense mutation (R514X; Salomons et al., 2001). The maternal female relatives were heterozygous for the mutation. The nonsense mutation most likely results in an unstable and/or inappropriately folded protein that is completely inactive, thereby inhibiting transport of Cr. Reports indicate that over 150 patients have been diagnosed with this disorder. It is now estimated that an incidence of Cr transporter deficiency ranges from 0.25 to 3.5%, making its diagnosis frequency second only to fragile X syndrome in X-linked mental retardation syndromes (Rosenberg et al., 2004, 2006; Newmeyer et al., 2005; Almeida et al., 2006; Clark et al., 2006; Lion-Francois et al., 2006; Arias et al., 2007; Betsalel et al., 2008; Puusepp et al., 2009; Edvardson et al., 2010). There is variability in the clinical presentation; however, common features include speech delay, intellectual disabilities and epilepsy. Epilepsy can usually be controlled with medication. Some patients with Cr transporter deficiency, especially older ones, demonstrate volume loss on MRI. Currently, there is no definitive therapy that can allow passage of Cr across the blood–brain barrier to restore brain Cr for patients with Cr transporter deficiency. Chilosi et al. (2008) reported neurological improvement in two patients with Cr transporter deficiency treated with arginine supplementation to promote cerebral Cr synthesis. However, this finding was not replicated in four patients supplemented with arginine (Fons et al., 2008). Recently, the development and successful treatment of brain-specific knockout mouse for Cr transporter deficiency syndrome has been reported (Kurosawa et al., 2012).

CONCLUSIONS

Most inborn errors of metabolism require integration of clinical symptoms, family histories, laboratory (metabolic and molecular) test results, MRI, and MRS interpretation to formulate disease diagnosis. Understanding the role that MRS can provide will facilitate patient care and ultimately improve our collective knowledge of pediatric brain disorders.

References

Almeida, L. S., Rosenberg, E. H., Martinez-Munoz, C., Verhoeven, N. M., Vilarinho, L., Jakobs, C., et al. (2006). Overexpression of GAMT restores GAMT activity in primary GAMT-deficient fibroblasts. *Molecular Genetics and Metabolism, 89*(4), 392–394.

Arias, A., Corbella, M., Fons, C., Sempere, A., Garcia-Villoria, J., Ormazabal, A., et al. (2007). Creatine transporter deficiency: prevalence among patients with mental retardation and pitfalls in metabolite screening. *Clinical Biochemistry, 40*(16-17), 1328–1331.

Aydin, K., Ozmen, M., Tatli, B., & Sencer, S. (2003). Single-voxel MR spectroscopy and diffusion-weighted MRI in two patients with l-2-hydroxyglutaric aciduria. *Pediatric Radiology, 33*(12), 872–876.

Aydinli, N., Caliskan, M., Calay, M., & Ozmen, M. (1998). Use of localized proton nuclear magnetic resonance spectroscopy in Canavan's disease. *Turkish Journal of Pediatrics, 40*(4), 549–557.

Battini, R., Leuzzi, V., Carducci, C., Tosetti, M., Bianchi, M. C., Item, C. B., et al. (2002). Creatine depletion in a new case with AGAT deficiency: clinical and genetic study in a large pedigree. *Molecular Genetics and Metabolism, 77*(4), 326–331.

Berry, G. T., Hunter, J. V., Wang, Z., Dreha, S., Mazur, A., Brooks, D. G., et al. (2001). *In vivo* evidence of brain galactitol accumulation in an infant with galactosemia and encephalopathy. *Journal of Pediatrics, 138*(2), 260–262.

Betsalel, O. T., van de Kamp, J. M., Martinez-Munoz, C., Rosenberg, E. H., de Brouwer, A. P., Pouwels, P. J., et al. (2008). Detection of low-level somatic and germline mosaicism by denaturing high-performance liquid chromatography in a EURO-MRX family with SLC6A8 deficiency. *Neurogenetics, 9*(3), 183–190.

Bluml, S., Moreno, A., Hwang, J. H., & Ross, B. D. (2001). 1-^{13}C glucose magnetic resonance spectroscopy of pediatric and adult brain disorders. *NMR in Biomedicine, 14*(1), 19–32.

Brockmann, K., Dechent, P., Meins, M., Haupt, M., Sperner, J., Stephani, U., et al. (2003a). Cerebral proton magnetic resonance spectroscopy in infantile Alexander disease. *Journal of Neurology, 250*(3), 300–306.

Brockmann, K., Dechent, P., Wilken, B., Rusch, O., Frahm, J., & Hanefeld, F. (2003b). Proton MRS profile of cerebral metabolic abnormalities in Krabbe disease. *Neurology, 60*(5), 819–825.

Brockmann, K., Finsterbusch, J., Terwey, B., Frahm, J., & Hanefeld, F. (2003c). Megalencephalic leukoencephalopathy with subcortical cysts in an adult: quantitative proton MR spectroscopy and diffusion tensor MRI. *Neuroradiology, 45*(3), 137–142.

Brockmann, K., Pouwels, P. J., Christen, H. J., Frahm, J., & Hanefeld, F. (1996). Localized proton magnetic resonance spectroscopy of cerebral metabolic disturbances in children with neuronal ceroid lipofuscinosis. *Neuropediatrics, 27*(5), 242–248.

Bugiani, M., Boor, I., Powers, J. M., Scheper, G. C., & van der Knaap, M. S. (2010). Leukoencephalopathy with vanishing white matter: a review. *Journal of Neuropathology and Experimental Neurology, 69*(10), 987–996.

Cecil, K. M., Salomons, G. S., Ball, W. S., Jr., Wong, B., Chuck, G., Verhoeven, N. M., et al. (2001). Irreversible brain creatine deficiency with elevated serum and urine creatine: a creatine transporter defect? *Annals of Neurology, 49*(3), 401–404.

Chilosi, A., Leuzzi, V., Battini, R., Tosetti, M., Ferretti, G., Comparini, A., et al. Treatment with L-arginine improves neuropsychological disorders in a child with creatine transporter defect. *Neurocase, 14* (2):151–161.

Choi, C. G., Lee, H. K., & Yoon, J. H. (2001). Localized proton MR spectroscopic detection of nonketotic hyperglycinemia in an infant. *Korean Journal of Radiology, 2*(4), 239–242.

Clark, A. J., Rosenberg, E. H., Almeida, L. S., Wood, T. C., Jakobs, C., Stevenson, R. E., et al. (2006). X-linked creatine transporter (SLC6A8) mutations in about 1% of males with mental retardation of unknown etiology. *Human Genetics, 119*(6), 604–610.

Confort-Gouny, S., Chabrol, B., Vion-Dury, J., Mancini, J., & Cozzone, P. J. (1993). MRI and localized proton MRS in early infantile form of neuronal ceroid-lipofuscinosis. *Pediatric Neurology, 9*(1), 57–60.

Connelly, A., Cross, J. H., Gadian, D. G., Hunter, J. V., Kirkham, F. J., & Leonard, J. V. (1993). Magnetic resonance spectroscopy shows increased brain glutamine in ornithine carbamoyl transferase deficiency. *Pediatric Research, 33*(1), 77–81.

D'Incerti, L., Farina, L., Moroni, I., Uziel, G., & Savoiardo, M. (1998). L-2-Hydroxyglutaric aciduria: MRI in seven cases. *Neuroradiology, 40*(11), 727–733.

deGrauw, T. J., Cecil, K. M., Byars, A. W., Salomons, G. S., Ball, W. S., & Jakobs, C. (2003). The clinical syndrome of creatine transporter deficiency. *Molecular and Cellular Biochemistry, 244*(1-2), 45–48.

Dinopoulos, A., Gorospe, J. R., Egelhoff, J. C., Cecil, K. M., Nicolaidou, P., Morehart, P., et al. (2006). Discrepancy between neuroimaging findings and clinical phenotype in Alexander disease. *American Journal of Neuroradiology, 27*(10), 2088–2092.

Dreha-Kulaczewski, S. F., Dechent, P., Finsterbusch, J., Brockmann, K., Gartner, J., Frahm, J., et al. (2008). Early reduction of total N-acetyl-aspartate-compounds in patients with classical vanishing white matter disease. A long-term follow-up MRS study. *Pediatric Research, 63*(4), 444–449.

Edvardson, S., Korman, S. H., Livne, A., Shaag, A., Saada, A., Nalbandian, R., et al. (2010). l-arginine:glycine amidinotransferase (AGAT) deficiency: clinical presentation and response to treatment in two patients with a novel mutation. *Molecular Genetics and Metabolism, 101*(2-3), 228–232.

Elsas, Louis J. Galactosemia. In R. A. Pagon, T. C. Bird C.R. Dolan (Eds.), *GeneReviews [Internet].* Accessed 26.10.10.

Engelbrecht, V., Rassek, M., Gartner, J., Kahn, T., & Modder, U. (1995). Magnetic resonance tomography and localized proton spectroscopy in 2 siblings with Canavan's disease. *Rofo, 163*(3), 238–244.

Ensenauer, R., Thiel, T., Schwab, K. O., Tacke, U., Stockler-Ipsiroglu, S., Schulze, A., et al. (2004). Guanidinoacetate methyltransferase deficiency: differences of creatine uptake in human brain and muscle. *Molecular Genetics and Metabolism, 82*(3), 208–213.

Felber, S. R., Sperl, W., Chemelli, A., Murr, C., & Wendel, U. (1993). Maple syrup urine disease: metabolic decompensation monitored by proton magnetic resonance imaging and spectroscopy. *Annals of Neurology, 33*(4), 396–401.

Firat, A. K., Karakas, H. M., & Yakinci, C. (2006). Magnetic resonance spectroscopic characteristics of glutaric aciduria type II. *Developmental Medicine and Child Neurology, 48*(10), 847–850.

Fons, C., Sempere, A., Arias, A., Lopez-Sala, A., Poo, P., Pineda, M., et al. (2008). Arginine supplementation in four patients with X-linked creatine transporter defect. *Journal of Inherited Metabolic Diseases, 31*(6), 724–728.

Gabis, L., Parton, P., Roche, P., Lenn, N., Tudorica, A., & Huang, W. (2001). In vivo ^{1}H magnetic resonance spectroscopic measurement of brain glycine levels in nonketotic hyperglycinemia. *Journal of Neuroimaging, 11*(2), 209–211.

Galanaud, D., Tourbah, A., Lehericy, S., Leveque, N., Heron, B., Billette de Villemeur, T., et al. (2009). 24 month-treatment with miglustat of three patients with Niemann-Pick disease type C: follow up using brain spectroscopy. *Molecular Genetics and Metabolism, 96*(2), 55–58.

Gordon, N. (2001). Canavan disease: a review of recent developments. *European Journal of Paediatric Neurology, 5*(2), 65–69.

Hanefeld, F., Holzbach, U., Kruse, B., Wilichowski, E., Christen, H. J., & Frahm, J. (1993). Diffuse white matter disease in three children: an encephalopathy with unique features on magnetic resonance imaging and proton magnetic resonance spectroscopy. *Neuropediatrics, 24*(5), 244–248.

Hanefeld, F., Kruse, B., Bruhn, H., & Frahm, J. (1994). In vivo proton magnetic resonance spectroscopy of the brain in a patient with L-2-hydroxyglutaric acidemia. *Pediatric Research, 35*(5), 614–616.

Heindel, W., Kugel, H., & Roth, B. (1993). Noninvasive detection of increased glycine content by proton MR spectroscopy in the brains of two infants with nonketotic hyperglycinemia. *American Journal of Neuroradiology, 14*(3), 629–635.

Heindel, W., Kugel, H., Wendel, U., Roth, B., & Benz-Bohm, G. (1995). Proton magnetic resonance spectroscopy reflects metabolic decompensation in maple syrup urine disease. *Pediatric Radiology, 25*(4), 296–299.

Hoffmann, G. F., Athanassopoulos, S., Burlina, A. B., Duran, M., de Klerk, J. B., Lehnert, W., et al. (1996). Clinical course, early diagnosis, treatment, and prevention of disease in glutaryl-CoA dehydrogenase deficiency. *Neuropediatrics, 27*(3), 115–123.

Huisman, T. A., Thiel, T., Steinmann, B., Zeilinger, G., & Martin, E. (2002). Proton magnetic resonance spectroscopy of the brain of a neonate with nonketotic hyperglycinemia: in vivo-in vitro (ex vivo) correlation. *European Radiology, 12*(4), 858–861.

Item, C. B., Stockler-Ipsiroglu, S., Stromberger, C., Muhl, A., Alessandri, M. G., Bianchi, M. C., et al. (2001). Arginine:glycine amidinotransferase deficiency: the third inborn error of creatine metabolism in humans. *American Journal of Human Genetics, 69*(5), 1127–1133.

Jan, W., Zimmerman, R. A., Wang, Z. J., Berry, G. T., Kaplan, P. B., & Kaye, E. M. (2003). MR diffusion imaging and MR spectroscopy of maple syrup urine disease during acute metabolic decompensation. *Neuroradiology, 45*(6), 393–399.

Johnston, K., Plawner, L., Cooper, L., Salomons, G. S., Verhoeven, N. M., Jakobs, C., et al. (2005). *The second family with AGAT deficiency (creatine biosynthesis defect): diagnosis, treatment and first prenatal diagnosis.* Paper presented at the American Society of Human Genetics, Salt Lake City, Utah.

Kojic, J., Robertson, P. L., Quint, D. J., Martin, D. M., Pang, Y., & Sundgren, P. C. (2005). Brain glutamine by MRS in a patient with urea cycle disorder and coma. *Pediatric Neurology, 32*(2), 143–146.

Krawczyk, H., & Gradowska, W. (2003). Characterisation of the ^{1}H and ^{13}C NMR spectra of N-acetylaspartylglutamate and its detection in urine from patients with Canavan disease. *Journal of Pharmaceutical and Biomedical Analysis, 31*(3), 455–463.

Kreis, R., Ross, B. D., Farrow, N. A., & Ackerman, Z. (1992). Metabolic disorders of the brain in chronic hepatic encephalopathy detected with ^{1}H MR spectroscopy. *Radiology, 182*(1), 19–27.

Kruse, B., Hanefeld, F., Christen, H. J., Bruhn, H., Michaelis, T., Hanicke, W., et al. (1993). Alterations of brain metabolites in metachromatic leukodystrophy as detected by localized proton magnetic resonance spectroscopy in vivo. *Journal of Neurology, 241* (2), 68–74.

Kumar, V., Abbas, A. K., & Fausto, N. (2005). *Robbins and Cotran Pathologic Basis of Disease* (7th ed.). Philadelphia: Elsevier Saunders.

Kurosawa, Y., Degrauw, T. J., Lindquist, D. M., Blanco, V. M., Pyne-Geithman, G. J., Daikoku, T., et al. (2012). Cyclocreatine treatment improves cognition in mice with creatine transporter deficiency. *Journal of Clinical Investigation, 122*(8), 2837–2846.

Kurul, S., Cakmakci, H., & Dirik, E. (2004). Glutaric aciduria type 1: proton magnetic resonance spectroscopy findings. *Pediatric Neurology, 31*(3), 228–231.

Labauge, P., Dorboz, I., Eymard-Pierre, E., Dereeper, O., & Boespflug-Tanguy, O. (2011). Clinically asymptomatic adult patient with extensive LBSL MRI pattern and DARS2 mutations. *Journal of Neurology, 258*(2), 335–337.

Labauge, P., Roullet, E., Boespflug-Tanguy, O., Nicoli, F., Le Fur, Y., Cozzone, P. J., et al. (2007). Familial, adult onset form of leukoencephalopathy with brain stem and spinal cord involvement: inconstant high brain lactate and very slow disease progression. *European Neurology, 58*(1), 59–61.

Leegwater, P. A., Boor, P. K., Yuan, B. Q., van der Steen, J., Visser, A., Konst, A. A., et al. (2002). Identification of novel mutations in MLC1 responsible for megalencephalic leukoencephalopathy with subcortical cysts. *Human Genetics, 110*(3), 279–283.

Leuzzi, V., Bianchi, M. C., Tosetti, M., Carducci, C., Cerquiglini, C. A., Cioni, G., et al. (2000). Brain creatine depletion: guanidinoacetate methyltransferase deficiency (improving with creatine supplementation). *Neurology, 55*(9), 1407–1409.

Linnankivi, T., Lundbom, N., Autti, T., Hakkinen, A. M., Koillinen, H., Kuusi, T., et al. (2004). Five new cases of a recently described leukoencephalopathy with high brain lactate. *Neurology, 63*(4), 688–692.

Lion-Francois, L., Cheillan, D., Pitelet, G., Acquaviva-Bourdain, C., Bussy, G., Cotton, F., et al. (2006). High frequency of creatine deficiency syndromes in patients with unexplained mental retardation. *Neurology, 67*(9), 1713–1714.

Madhavarao, C. N., Moffett, J. R., Moore, R. A., Viola, R. E., Namboodiri, M. A., & Jacobowitz, D. M. (2004). Immunohistochemical localization of aspartoacylase in the rat central nervous system. *Journal of Comparative Neurology, 472*(3), 318–329.

Mercimek-Mahmutoglu, S., Stockler-Ipsiroglu, S. (1993). Creatine Deficiency Syndromes. In R. A. Pagon, T. C. Bird, C.R. Dolan (Eds.), *GeneReviews [Internet].* Jan. 15, 2009 ed.

Mercimek-Mahmutoglu, S., Stoeckler-Ipsiroglu, S., Adami, A., Appleton, R., Araujo, H. C., Duran, M., et al. (2006). GAMT deficiency: features, treatment, and outcome in an inborn error of creatine synthesis. *Neurology, 67*(3), 480–484.

Moffett, John R., Tieman, Suzannah, B., Weinberger, Daniel, R., Coyle, Joseph, T., & Namboodiri, Aryan, M. A. (2006). *N-acetylaspartate: A Unique Neuronal Molecule in the Central Nervous System (Advnaces in Experimental Medicine and Biology.* New York: Springer.

Moller, H. E., Ullrich, K., Vermathen, P., Schuierer, G., & Koch, H. G. (1995). In vivo study of brain metabolism in galactosemia by ^{1}H and ^{31}P magnetic resonance spectroscopy. *European Journal of Pediatrics, 154*(7 Suppl 2), S8–S13.

Moreno, A., Ross, B. D., & Bluml, S. (2001). Direct determination of the *N*-acetyl-L-aspartate synthesis rate in the human brain by ^{13}C MRS and [1-^{13}C]glucose infusion. *Journal of Neurochemistry, 77*(1), 347–350.

Newmeyer, A., Cecil, K. M., Schapiro, M., Clark, J. F., & Degrauw, T. J. (2005). Incidence of brain creatine transporter deficiency in males with developmental delay referred for brain magnetic resonance imaging. *Journal of Developmental and Behavioral Pediatrics, 26*(4), 276–282.

Oguz, K. K., Ozturk, A., & Cila, A. (2005). Diffusion-weighted MR imaging and MR spectroscopy in glutaric aciduria type 1. *Neuroradiology, 47*(3), 229–234.

Otaduy, M. C., Leite, C. C., Lacerda, M. T., Costa, M. O., Arita, F., Prado, E., et al. (2006). Proton MR spectroscopy and imaging of a galactosemic patient before and after dietary treatment. *American Jouranl of Neuroradiology, 27*(1), 204–207.

Pérez-Dueñas, B., De La Osa, A., Capdevila, A., Navarro-Sastre, A., Leist, A., Ribes, A., et al. (2009). Brain injury in glutaric aciduria type I: the value of functional techniques in magnetic resonance imaging. *European Journal of Paediatric Neurology, 13*(6), 534–540.

Petzold, G. C., Bohner, G., Klingebiel, R., Amberger, N., van der Knaap, M. S., & Zschenderlein, R. (2006). Adult onset leucoencephalopathy with brain stem and spinal cord involvement and normal lactate. *Joural of Neurology, Neurosurgergy and Psychiatry, 77*(7), 889–891.

Pronk, J. C., van Kollenburg, B., Scheper, G. C., & van der Knaap, M. S. (2006). Vanishing white matter disease: a review with focus on its genetics. *Mental Retardation and Developmental Disabilities Research Review, 12*(2), 123–128.

Puusepp, H., Kall, K., Salomons, G. S., Talvik, I., Mannamaa, M., Rein, R., et al. (2009). The screening of SLC6A8 deficiency among Estonian families with X-linked mental retardation. *Journal of inherited metabolic disease.*

Pyne-Geithman, G. J., deGrauw, T. J., Cecil, K. M., Chuck, G., Lyons, M. A., Ishida, Y., et al. (2004). Presence of normal creatine in the muscle of a patient with a mutation in the creatine transporter: a case study. *Molecular and Cellular Biochemistry, 262*(1-2), 35–39.

Rosenberg, E. H., Almeida, L. S., Kleefstra, T., deGrauw, R. S., Yntema, H. G., Bahi, N., et al. (2004). High prevalence of SLC6A8 deficiency in X-linked mental retardation. *American Journal of Human Genetics, 75*(1), 97–105.

Rosenberg, E. H., Munoz, C. M., Degrauw, T. J., Jakobs, C., & Salomons, G. S. (2006). Overexpression of wild-type creatine transporter (SLC6A8) restores creatine uptake in primary SLC6A8-deficient fibroblasts. *Journal of Inherited Metabolic Disease, 29*(2-3), 345–346.

Ross, B., Kreis, R., & Ernst, T. (1992). Clinical tools for the 90s: magnetic resonance spectroscopy and metabolite imaging. *European Journal of Radiology, 14*(2), 128–140.

Salomons, G. S., van Dooren, S. J., Verhoeven, N. M., Cecil, K. M., Ball, W. S., Degrauw, T. J., et al. (2001). X-linked creatine-transporter gene (SLC6A8) defect: a new creatine-deficiency syndrome. *American Journal of Human Genetics, 68*(6), 1497–1500.

Schiffmann, R., Moller, J. R., Trapp, B. D., Shih, H. H., Farrer, R. G., Katz, D. A., et al. (1994). Childhood ataxia with diffuse central nervous system hypomyelination. *Annals of Neurology, 35*(3), 331–340.

Schulze, A., Ebinger, F., Rating, D., & Mayatepek, E. (2001). Improving treatment of guanidinoacetate methyltransferase deficiency: reduction of guanidinoacetic acid in body fluids by arginine restriction and ornithine supplementation. *Molecular Genetics and Metabolism, 74*(4), 413–419.

Schulze, A., Hoffmann, G. F., Bachert, P., Kirsch, S., Salomons, G. S., Verhoeven, N. M., et al. (2006). Presymptomatic treatment of neonatal guanidinoacetate methyltransferase deficiency. *Neurology, 67*(4), 719–721.

Schulze, A., Mayatepek, E., Bachert, P., Marescau, B., De Deyn, P. P., & Rating, D. (1998). Therapeutic trial of arginine restriction in creatine deficiency syndrome. *European Journal of Pediatrics, 157*(7), 606–607.

Seijo-Martinez, M., Navarro, C., Castro del Rio, M., Vila, O., Puig, M., Ribes, A., et al. (2005). L-2-hydroxyglutaric aciduria: clinical, neuroimaging, and neuropathological findings. *Archives of Neurology, 62*(4), 666–670.

Seitz, D., Grodd, W., Schwab, A., Seeger, U., Klose, U., & Nagele, T. (1998). MR imaging and localized proton MR spectroscopy in late infantile neuronal ceroid lipofuscinosis. *American Journal of Neuroradiology, 19*(7), 1373–1377.

Sener, R. N. (2003). L-2 hydroxyglutaric aciduria: proton magnetic resonance spectroscopy and diffusion magnetic resonance imaging findings. *Journal of Computer Assisted Tomography, 27*(1), 38–43.

Serkov, S. V., Pronin, I. N., Bykova, O. V., Maslova, O. I., Arutyunov, N. V., Muravina, T. I., et al. (2004). Five patients with a recently described novel leukoencephalopathy with brainstem and spinal cord involvement and elevated lactate. *Neuropediatrics, 35*(1), 1–5.

Sijens, P. E., Smit, G. P., Meiners, L. C., Oudkerk, M., & van Sprronsen, F. J. (2006). Cerebral ^{1}H MR spectroscopy revealing white matter NAA decreases in glutaric aciduria type I. *Molecular Genetics and Metabolism, 88*(3), 285–289.

Steenweg, M. E., Salomons, G. S., Yapici, Z., Uziel, G., Scalais, E., Zafeiriou, D. I., et al. (2009). L-2-Hydroxyglutaric aciduria: pattern of MR imaging abnormalities in 56 patients. *Radiology, 251*(3), 856–865.

Stockler, S., Holzbach, U., Hanefeld, F., Marquardt, I., Helms, G., Requart, M., et al. (1994). Creatine deficiency in the brain: a new, treatable inborn error of metabolism. *Pediatric Research, 36*(3), 409–413.

Sylvain, M., Arnold, D. L., Scriver, C. R., Schreiber, R., & Shevell, M. I. (1994). Magnetic resonance spectroscopy in Niemann-Pick disease type C: correlation with diagnosis and clinical response to cholestyramine and lovastatin. *Pediatric Neurology, 10*(3), 228–232.

Takanashi, J., Kurihara, A., Tomita, M., Kanazawa, M., Yamamoto, S., Morita, F., et al. (2002). Distinctly abnormal brain metabolism in late-onset ornithine transcarbamylase deficiency. *Neurology, 59*(2), 210—214.

Tavora, D. G., Nakayama, M., Gama, R. L., Alvim, T. C., Portugal, D., & Comerlato, E. A. (2007). Leukoencephalopathy with brainstem and spinal cord involvement and high brain lactate: report of three Brazilian patients. *Arquivos Neuro-Psiquiatria, 65*(2B), 506—511.

Tedeschi, G., Bonavita, S., Barton, N. W., Betolino, A., Frank, J. A., Patronas, N. J., et al. (1998). Proton magnetic resonance spectroscopic imaging in the clinical evaluation of patients with Niemann-Pick type C disease. *Journal of Neurology, Neurosurgery, and Psychiatry, 65*(1), 72—79.

Tedeschi, G., Schiffmann, R., Barton, N. W., Shih, H. H., Gospe, S. M., Jr., Brady, R. O., et al. (1995). Proton magnetic resonance spectroscopic imaging in childhood ataxia with diffuse central nervous system hypomyelination. *Neurology, 45*(8), 1526—1532.

Tekgul, H., Serdaroglu, G., Karapinar, B., Polat, M., Yurtsever, S., Tosun, A., et al. (2006). Vigabatrin caused rapidly progressive deterioration in two cases with early myoclonic encephalopathy associated with nonketotic hyperglycinemia. *Journal of Child Neurology, 21*(1), 82—84.

Toft, P. B., Geiss-Holtorff, R., Rolland, M. O., Pryds, O., Muller-Forell, W., Christensen, E., et al. (1993). Magnetic resonance imaging in juvenile Canavan disease. *European Journal of Pediatrics, 152*(9), 750—753.

Topcu, M., Aydin, O. F., Yalcinkaya, C., Haliloglu, G., Aysun, S., Anlar, B., et al. (2005). L-2-hydroxyglutaric aciduria: a report of 29 patients. *Turkish Journal of Pediatrics, 47*(1), 1—7.

Uluc, K., Baskan, O., Yildirim, K. A., Ozsahin, S., Koseoglu, M., Isak, B., et al. (2008). Leukoencephalopathy with brain stem and spinal cord involvement and high lactate: a genetically proven case with distinct MRI findings. *Jouranl of the Neurological Sciences, 273*(1-2), 118—122.

van der Knaap, M. S., Barth, P. G., Gabreels, F. J., Franzoni, E., Begeer, J. H., Stroink, H., et al. (1997). A new leukoencephalopathy with vanishing white matter. *Neurology, 48*(4), 845—855.

van der Knaap, M. S., Barth, P. G., Stroink, H., van Nieuwenhuizen, O., Arts, W. F., Hoogenraad, F., et al. (1995). Leukoencephalopathy with swelling and a discrepantly mild clinical course in eight children. *Annals of Neurology, 37*(3), 324—334.

van der Knaap, M. S., Kamphorst, W., Barth, P. G., Kraaijeveld, C. L., Gut, E., & Valk, J. (1998). Phenotypic variation in leukoencephalopathy with vanishing white matter. *Neurology, 51*(2), 540—547.

van der Knaap, M. S., Naidu, S., Breiter, S. N., Blaser, S., Stroink, H., Springer, S., et al. (2001). Alexander disease: diagnosis with MR imaging. *American Journal of Neuroradiology, 22*(3), 541—552.

van der Knaap, M. S., Pronk, J. C., & Scheper, G. C. (2006a). Vanishing white matter disease. *Lancet Neurology, 5*(5), 413—423.

van der Knaap, M. S., Ramesh, V., Schiffmann, R., Blaser, S., Kyllerman, M., Gholkar, A., et al. (2006b). Alexander disease: ventricular garlands and abnormalities of the medulla and spinal cord. *Neurology, 66*(4), 494—498.

van der Knaap, M. S., Salomons, G. S., Li, R., Franzoni, E., Gutierrez-Solana, L. G., Smit, L. M., et al. (2005). Unusual variants of Alexander's disease. *Annals of Neurology, 57*(3), 327—338.

van der Knaap, M. S., van der Voorn, P., Barkhof, F., Van Coster, R., Krageloh-Mann, I., Feigenbaum, A., et al. (2003). A new leukoencephalopathy with brainstem and spinal cord involvement and high lactate. *Annals of Neurology, 53*(2), 252—258.

van der Voorn, J. P., Pouwels, P. J., Hart, A. A., Serrarens, J., Willemsen, M. A., Kremer, H. P., et al. (2006). Childhood white matter disorders: quantitative MR imaging and spectroscopy. *Radiology, 241*(2), 510—517.

Van Haren, K., van der Voorn, J. P., Peterson, D. R., van der Knaap, M. S., & Powers, J. M. (2004). The life and death of oligodendrocytes in vanishing white matter disease. *Journal of Neuropathology and Experimental Neurology, 63*(6), 618—630.

Vanhanen, S. L., Puranen, J., Autti, T., Raininko, R., Liewendahl, K., Nikkinen, P., et al. (2004). Neuroradiological findings (MRS, MRI, SPECT) in infantile neuronal ceroid-lipofuscinosis (infantile CLN1) at different stages of the disease. *Neuropediatrics, 35*(1), 27—35.

Viola, A., Chabrol, B., Nicoli, F., Confort-Gouny, S., Viout, P., & Cozzone, P. J. (2002). Magnetic resonance spectroscopy study of glycine pathways in nonketotic hyperglycinemia. *Pediatric Research, 52*(2), 292—300.

Wang, Z. J., Berry, G. T., Dreha, S. F., Zhao, H., Segal, S., & Zimmerman, R. A. (2001). Proton magnetic resonance spectroscopy of brain metabolites in galactosemia. *Annals of Neurology, 50*(2), 266—269.

Wittsack, H. J., Kugel, H., Roth, B., & Heindel, W. (1996). Quantitative measurements with localized 1H MR spectroscopy in children with Canavan's disease. *Journal of Magnetic Resonance Imaging, 6*(6), 889—893.

MRS of Psychiatric Disorders

Matthew Taylor

Department of Psychosis Studies, Institute of Psychiatry, London, UK

INTRODUCTION

Magnetic Resonance Spectroscopy (MRS) has a growing relevance to the study of psychiatric conditions. Proton MRS in particular is being applied to the study of a wide range of disorders, impacting our understanding of pathophysiology and vulnerability to illness. Emerging evidence suggests that in the future, MRS could even gain a clinical role to supplement conventional clinical assessment.

Although psychiatric illnesses can have profound effects on mental function, reflecting striking alterations in underlying brain function, gross brain structure typically appears normal. Structural brain imaging does reveal average differences between unwell populations and healthy controls. One of the first described and most striking anatomical findings is lateral ventricular enlargement in schizophrenia (Lawrie & Abukmeil, 1998; Wright et al., 2000). However, these effects are not necessarily disorder specific; for example, meta-analysis reveals that lateral ventricular enlargement is also evident, albeit at lesser magnitude, in bipolar disorder (Kempton et al., 2008) and unipolar depression (Kempton et al., 2011). These structural abnormalities are also typically too subtle to be evident at an individual level. This is in keeping with a growing awareness that psychiatric disorders more commonly reflect disruptions in function of extended networks of brain structures rather than of the effects of focal lesions (Bassett & Bullmore, 2009; Price & Drevets, 2012). Following this distributed model of psychiatric illness, MRS studies to date have generally focused on anatomical regions of interest believed to play a functional role in the illness rather than any overt lesions.

MRS studies have revealed some consistent neurochemical abnormalities present during episodes of mental illness. Emerging evidence indicates that some of these abnormalities persist after clinical recovery, and may even be present prior to the onset of illness, suggesting a possible role as markers of vulnerability or resilience to disease. Here we will review the use of MRS so far in improving our understanding of psychiatric conditions. MRS findings inform our understanding of a wide range of psychiatric disorders as diverse as autistic spectrum disorders (Chugani, 2012) and dementia (Griffith et al., 2009). For reasons of space here a particular focus is made on findings in affective and psychotic illnesses as examples of the utility of this approach.

FINDINGS DURING EPISODES OF ILLNESS

Initial studies using MRS in psychiatric illness understandably tended to focus on the study of the brain during episodes of illness. Psychiatric illness can involve profound abnormalities in cognition and emotion, so it is perhaps not surprising that a number of abnormalities across a range of disorders have been demonstrated using MRS.

Psychosis

Schizophrenia is the archetypal psychotic illness, and can be associated with a diverse range of symptoms including delusional beliefs, hallucinations, disorganization of thoughts and negative symptoms such as lack of motivation or speech, and even movement abnormalities (van Os & Kapur, 2009). Schizophrenia is associated with gray matter reductions across several brain regions including frontal and temporal lobes and thalamus (Shepherd et al., 2012). A number of MRS studies have compared levels of the neuronal

222

marker, *N*-acetylaspartate (NAA), in patients with schizophrenia and control populations. Recent meta-analysis of data from almost one hundred separate studies demonstrated that reductions in NAA levels are found in frontal lobe, temporal lobe, and thalamus in both first episode and chronic schizophrenia (Brugger et al., 2011). The effect size of this reduction is greater than 0.3. The reduced neuronal integrity or dysfunction suggested by this effect may be secondary to abnormalities in glutamatergic function, given the close relationship between NAA and glutamate neurotransmission (Reynolds & Harte, 2007).

There has been increasing interest in using MRS to measure glutamate directly in psychotic illnesses. There is growing evidence from a range of directions indicating that schizophrenia may be associated with disturbances in glutamatergic function (Coyle, 2006). For example, it appears that a number of putative risk genes for schizophrenia appear to converge on the glutamatergic synapse (Harrison & Weinberger, 2005). Further, a number of environmental risk factors for the development of psychosis, such as stress, cannabis use, and maternal infection, can all result in glutamatergic dysfunction (Egerton et al., 2012b).

MRS studies in schizophrenia have often investigated medial frontal cortex, including anterior cingulate cortex (ACC). In a recent meta-analysis of data from 28 studies including over 600 patients with schizophrenia and a similar number of controls, medial frontal cortical glutamate was decreased and glutamine was increased in patients with schizophrenia compared with healthy individuals (Marsman et al., 2011). Interestingly, both glutamate and glutamine levels in the frontal region appear to decrease progressively with age in patients with schizophrenia. This parallels the available data from structural brain imaging, which also point to progressive structural brain abnormalities affecting both gray and white matter (Olabi et al., 2011). Whether such apparently progressive changes reflect the intrinsic pathophysiology of the disorder, or are secondary to other factors such as medication or lifestyle choices, remains unclear (Zipursky et al., 2012).

Emerging data from people treated for a first psychotic episode points to a link between these glutamatergic findings and treatment response. It was recently reported that in a group of first-episode patients, those responding well to antipsychotic treatment differed in their post-treatment MRS glutamate levels from those who remained symptomatic (Egerton et al., 2012a). ACC glutamate levels were higher in those remaining symptomatic after initial treatment, and higher levels were also linked to lower general functioning. At least one study (http://www.optimisetrial.eu/) is currently underway to assess whether such MRS markers differ at baseline sufficiently to act as predictors of response to treatment. An alternative explanation could be that effective antipsychotic treatment acts to lower glutamate levels, since in one recent study elevated levels of total Glx (composed mainly of glutamate and glutamine) and GABA were observed in unmedicated patients but not in an otherwise similar group receiving treatment, consistent with a normalization of levels by antipsychotic medication (Kegeles et al., 2012).

New treatments following the glutamatergic hypothesis are in development with several compounds targeting various aspects of glutamatergic transmission; clinical trials have yielded some encouraging results (Egerton & Stone, 2012). It may be that novel glutamatergic agents will allow a greater number of individuals to achieve a good symptomatic recovery from psychosis in the future.

Mood Disorders

Mood disorders are another area where glutamatergic dysfunction is increasingly implicated, and there is also interest in the potential of glutamatergic agents to provide new therapeutic approaches (Zarate et al., 2010; Sanacora et al., 2012). In mood disorders, a clinical distinction is drawn between bipolar disorder, sometimes known as manic depression, where both abnormal episodes of depressed mood and also episodes of abnormally elevated mood (hypomania or mania) are experienced, and recurrent depressive disorder, or unipolar depression, where only depressive episodes are experienced. Bipolar disorder and unipolar depression differ in a number of respects including optimal treatment.

Depressive episodes are characterized by a range of symptoms and not simply low mood and lack of enjoyment, but commonly also disturbances of sleep and appetite and cognitive distortions with guilt and hopelessness commonly encountered. Depression is clinically similar in both bipolar and unipolar disorder, although on average some features are more commonly encountered in one or the other disorder (Mitchell et al., 2008).

MRS studies during episodes of depression have often been performed, with glutamatergic measures commonly expressed as total Glx, rather than individually resolved glutamate and glutamine estimates. One of the earliest reports was of a decrease in ACC levels of Glx in a predominantly unipolar depressed group compared to controls (Auer et al., 2000). This finding of reduced Glx in unipolar depression has been well replicated since, and found to be present even in the absence of medication (Hasler et al., 2007). In contrast, with depression associated with bipolar disorder the opposite effect, elevated Glx, tends to be observed (Yüksel & Öngür, 2010).

This pattern of contrasting reduced Glx in unipolar versus elevated Glx in bipolar disorder is clearest in medial frontal cortex, and appears to be region specific. For example, in unipolar depression glutamate in occipital cortex is increased rather than decreased (Sanacora et al., 2004). MRS measures of the major inhibitory neurotransmitter, GABA, are technically more challenging, and thus less widely reported. On available evidence it appears that GABA levels are reduced during episodes of depression in both prefrontal (Hasler et al., 2007) and occipital cortex (Sanacora et al., 2004). The functional effects of the contrasting glutamatergic abnormalities in frontal and occipital cortex remain unclear. One intriguing hypothesis, emerging from a synthesis of animal and human data, suggests these glutamatergic findings may reflect more widespread differences in resting state activity between ventral and dorsal midline structures in unipolar depression (Alcaro et al., 2010).

Manic episodes can appear clinically as the antithesis of depression, with elated or irritable mood, increased energy, decreased need for sleep, and positive rather than negative cognitive distortions, for example, grandiose or unrealistically optimistic plans or beliefs in one's own abilities. Interestingly, during episodes of mania an elevation in the ratio of glutamate to glutamine in both anterior cingulate and parieto-occipital cortex is observed (Öngür et al., 2008). This increased glutamate/glutamine ratio is thought to indicate increased glutamatergic function. Interestingly in schizophrenia a trend toward a similar elevation in glutamate/glutamine ratios in frontal cortex is also seen (Marsman et al., 2011). This similarity of MRS finding between mania and psychosis echoes growing evidence of overlap between bipolar disorder and schizophrenia from the genetic level (Owen et al., 2007) through to clinical presentation (Goldberg et al., 2009).

were better understood it might improve our ability to delay or prevent onset and relapse in psychiatric disorders.

Mood Disorders

One of the notable features of mood disorders is that they do tend generally to be episodic, i.e., full clinical remission is often achieved between episodes of illness, whether spontaneously or following treatment. Although people may be fully recovered and asymptomatic after a previous episode of depression, they do remain at substantially elevated risk of future episodes (Müller et al., 1999). In recent years a growing body of evidence has revealed persistent neurobiological abnormalities in people clinically recovered from mood disorders, investigated by a range of techniques including MRS (Bhagwagar & Cowen, 2008).

In people with a history of depressive episodes who are now asymptomatic, and also medication free to reduce possible confounding neurobiological effects of treatment, a replicated finding is that the decreased glutamate in ACC notable during episodes of illness appears to normalize (Hasler et al., 2005; Taylor et al., 2009). In contrast, with parieto-occipital cortex there appears to be a persistent elevation after clinical recovery, alongside a persistent reduction in GABA (Bhagwagar et al., 2007). This evidence points to a dissociation of glutamatergic MRS effects in depression, with some representing state effects of depressed mood, and others as potential markers of vulnerability or after effects (akin to "scarring") of previous episodes.

In bipolar disorder, it appears that glutamatergic findings tend to persist after clinical recovery, so Glx elevations are observed in currently euthymic people with bipolar disorder in both occipital cortex (Bhagwagar et al., 2007) and ACC (Soeiro-de-Souza, et al., 2013).

ABNORMALITIES AFTER CLINICAL RECOVERY

While biological features of episodes of psychiatric illness are certainly of interest, they are not the only question to which MRS has contributed answers in recent years. Just as the study of cardiovascular disease is not restricted to the nature of myocardial infarction, instead incorporating and benefitting from the study of factors such as hypertension or cholesterol levels that affect risk, so there is growing interest in understanding the processes that underlie vulnerability and resilience to psychiatric illness. If these factors

ABNORMALITIES IN HIGH-RISK GROUPS

If these glutamatergic changes represent vulnerability markers, rather than some after effect of illness or its treatment, one might expect to see them present before onset of illness. The practicalities of neuroimaging limit the extent to which population studies can be performed, but one general approach is to perform a comparison of higher and lower risk groups for the disorder in question, expecting the vulnerability marker to be more evident in the higher risk group. Where possible of course, it is ideal to recruit a cohort of participants and follow-up over time to link imaging findings to clinical onset of illness.

Psychosis

For psychosis, a recent breakthrough in research and clinical practice has been the development of clinical criteria to identify a high-risk or prodromal state. The so-called at risk mental state (ARMS) has been defined during which people are at a substantially higher risk of progressing to develop psychosis, although such progression is far from inevitable. When the ARMS criteria were initially developed, it was found that among symptomatic individuals with either a family history of psychotic disorder, schizotypal personality disorder, subthreshold psychotic symptoms, or brief transient psychotic symptoms, 41% developed a psychotic disorder within 12 months of follow-up (Yung et al., 2003). This clinical definition has become widely employed at centers internationally, and a recent meta-analysis of 27 studies, with data from a total of 2502 patients, found that rates of transition to a psychotic episode from the ARMS high-risk state were 18% after 6 months of follow-up, 22% after 1 year, 29% after 2 years, and 36% after 3 years (Fusar-Poli et al., 2012). Given that lifetime risk of psychosis in the general population is on the order of 1%, it can be seen that this ARMS cohort is indeed at substantially increased risk of transition.

MRS studies are contributing substantially to our understanding of the at-risk state for psychosis and transition to psychosis. As noted earlier, established psychosis is associated with frontal lobe abnormalities in both NAA and glutamate and glutamine. Meta-analysis of MRS studies indicates that the decreased levels of NAA in frontal lobe in psychosis are present during the first psychotic episode, but are not apparent in that region during the high-risk stage preceding its onset (Brugger et al., 2011). In light of these data, it is intriguing to speculate that some intervention that maintained NAA might have a role in avoiding onset of psychosis. In support of this hypothesis, there is some initial clinical data suggesting that antidepressant medication use might reduce onset of psychosis in high-risk populations (Fusar-Poli et al., 2007), and initial data suggesting that in some groups they may also act to increase frontal NAA levels (Taylor et al., 2012), consistent with recent neurotrophic theories of antidepressant action (Schmidt & Duman, 2007).

A different pattern is observed with the use of glutamate MRS in the ARMS group. It appears that glutamate MRS abnormalities may well predate onset of psychosis, and also correlate with other measures where early abnormalities are seen such as imaging of dopaminergic function and brain structure. It appears that ARMS subjects have significantly lower levels of glutamate than control subjects in the thalamus (Stone et al., 2009). This thalamic glutamate level correlates with gray matter volume in the medial temporal cortex and insula (Stone et al., 2009). In a recent study, 16 individuals with ARMS mental state and 12 control subjects had measures both of MRS glutamate and a positron emission tomography (PET) measure of striatal dopamine function. In the ARMS population, a significant negative relationship between hippocampal glutamate levels and striatal dopamine function was observed (Stone et al., 2010). This glutamate—dopamine interaction may have clinical significance, since even in this small study there was a trend for the interaction between hippocampal glutamate and 18 F-DOPA uptake to predict later transition to psychosis (Stone et al., 2010).

Mood Disorders

In mood disorders, prodromal clinical populations are not similarly defined at present in clinical practice, although there are developing definitions for bipolar disorder that may become more widely adopted in due course (Bechdolf et al., 2010). For unipolar depression, one established high-risk group are the children of parents with a history of mood disorder. Such individuals are at significantly increased risk of depression themselves. By young adulthood it appears that around 40% of children of parents with a history of a clinical mood disorder will have experienced a personal episode of depression (Beardslee et al., 1998). In a recent study we found that participants with a parental history of depression had significantly higher levels of glutamate than controls in parieto-occipital cortex (Taylor et al., 2011a). This suggests that the glutamatergic abnormalities in this brain region, also observed during and between episodes of depression, may indeed represent a trait vulnerability marker for depression.

One limitation of these cross-sectional studies is that it is unclear whether a putative vulnerability factor represents a static and immutable personal characteristic, like eye color, or if it is a more dynamic measure of a vulnerability mechanism, like blood pressure, which might be more suggestive of a potential for future modification. For these glutamatergic abnormalities in depression, a key question is therefore whether the MRS picture changes within an individual when their depression risk is modified. Clearly, stable factors such as parental history are not suitable to answer this question. However, there is a natural experiment provided by a treatment for liver disease that incidentally increases the risk of depression in those receiving it.

Interferon-α (IFN-α) is a naturally occurring cytokine that forms part of the immune response, particularly to fight viral infection. Treatment with IFN-α can become necessary in a number of illnesses, one of which is chronic infection with hepatitis C virus. Unfortunately, IFN-α for the treatment of hepatitis C is associated with a significant incidence of depressive symptoms, with up to 40% of patients developing major depression over 3 months of IFN-α therapy (Hauser et al., 2002; Raison et al., 2005). This emergent depression can cause substantial problems and may necessitate early termination of therapy leaving persistent viral infection. Unsurprisingly, there has been growing interest in better understanding this clinical problem, to allow prediction or prevention of the depression side effect. Sadly, to date, attempts to use antidepressants to prevent its occurrence have lacked convincing effectiveness (Diez-Quevedo et al., 2011).

Interestingly this IFN-associated depression ties in with growing interest in the possible role of inflammatory mechanisms in the pathophysiology of mood disorders more generally (Raison et al., 2006). For example, across several studies it appears that depressed patients on average have elevated plasma levels of pro-inflammatory mediators such as tumor necrosis factor and interleukin-6 (Dowlati et al., 2010).

Recently we studied MRS effects of treatment with IFN-α over 4–6 weeks. This allowed us to compare within the same individual MRS measures in both a lower risk baseline state and a higher risk state during treatment, but before the onset of any major depressive episode. Preliminary analysis indicates that IFN leads to an elevation in ACC MRS Glx (Taylor et al., 2011b). The mechanism of this effect of an immune intervention on central glutamate function is unclear although possibilities include effects mediated via altered tryptophan metabolism (Miller et al., 2009) or an impairment of the ability of astrocytes to take up synaptic glutamate (Tavares et al., 2002).

It is interesting to note that an elevated ACC Glx is more similar to the characteristic spectroscopic findings described earlier for bipolar disorder rather than unipolar depression. In keeping with this, clinical data do indicate that manic symptoms may emerge during IFN treatment (Constant et al., 2005) and pretreatment reports of subsyndromal manic symptoms predict higher rates of psychiatric complications during IFN treatment (Lim et al., 2010). This may suggest a rationale to test established treatments for bipolar disorder in the prevention of psychiatric side effects of IFN-α treatment.

CLINICAL ROLE

As noted previously, the examples of mood disorders and psychotic illness provide evidence of the way MRS has contributed to our understanding of these disease processes, both during episodes of illness and in vulnerability before or between episodes. Looking to the future it is possible to conceive of possible clinical roles, for example, using MRS in addition to conventional clinical assessment to refine definitions of high-risk prodromal states for psychosis or bipolar disorder. Clearly, longitudinal studies will be necessary to test such hypothetical approaches.

One promising avenue for study would be to test the use of MRS to differentiate bipolar depression from unipolar. Bipolar disorder is commonly mistaken for unipolar depression; indeed this is unavoidable with current diagnostic frameworks given that depressive episodes may predate any hypomanic or manic episodes. Unfortunately, it is known that those who go on to be diagnosed with bipolar disorder have often had a poor course of illness and apparent treatment resistance when treated as unipolar (Goodwin, 2012; Li et al., 2012). Given the qualitatively different MRS Glx findings in ACC during unipolar and bipolar depression described earlier, this may be an area where MRS could contribute constructively by prospectively identifying those with a neurobiological pattern most like bipolar disorder.

CONCLUSIONS

MRS plays an increasingly important role in improving our understanding of psychiatric illnesses. Well-replicated findings demonstrate neurochemical abnormalities in normal-appearing brain tissue both during episodes of psychiatric illness and as possible vulnerability markers. Studies in high-risk and prodromal populations demonstrate findings that predate the onset of illness. Future studies will investigate whether such MRS findings can usefully complement clinical assessment and allow for more appropriate and directed treatment.

References

Alcaro, A., Panksepp, J., Witczak, J., Hayes, D. J., & Northoff, G. (2010). Is subcortical-cortical midline activity in depression mediated by glutamate and GABA? A cross-species translational approach. *Neuroscience and Biobehavioral Reviews, 34*(4), 592–605.

Auer, D. P., Pütz, B., Kraft, E., Lipinski, B., Schill, J., & Holsboer, F. (2000). Reduced glutamate in the anterior cingulate cortex in depression: an in vivo proton magnetic resonance spectroscopy study. *Biological Psychiatry, 47*(4), 305–313.

Bassett, D. S., & Bullmore, E. T. (2009). Human brain networks in health and disease. *Current Opinion in Neurology, 22*(4), 340–347.

Beardslee, W. R., Versage, E. M., & Gladstone, T. R. (1998). Children of affectively ill parents: a review of the past 10 years. *Journal of the American Academy of Child and Adolescent Psychiatry, 37*(11), 1134–1141.

Bechdolf, A., Nelson, B., Cotton, S. M., Chanen, A., Thompson, A., Kettle, J., et al. (2010). A preliminary evaluation of the validity of at-risk criteria for bipolar disorders in help-seeking adolescents and young adults. *Journal of Affective Disorders, 127*(1-3), 316–320.

Bhagwagar, Z., & Cowen, P. J. (2008). 'It's not over when it's over': persistent neurobiological abnormalities in recovered depressed patients. *Psychological Medicine, 38*(3), 307–313.

Bhagwagar, Z., Wylezinska, M., Jezzard, P., Evans, J., Ashworth, F., Sule, A., et al. (2007). Reduction in occipital cortex gamma-aminobutyric acid concentrations in medication-free recovered unipolar depressed and bipolar subjects. *Biological Psychiatry, 61* (6), 806–812.

Brugger, S., Davis, J. M., Leucht, S., & Stone, J. M. (2011). Proton magnetic resonance spectroscopy and illness stage in schizophrenia–a systematic review and meta-analysis. *Biological Psychiatry, 69*(5), 495–503.

Chugani, D. C. (2012). Neuroimaging and neurochemistry of autism. *Pediatric Clinics of North America, 59*(1), 63–73.

Constant, A., Castera, L., Dantzer, R., Couzigou, P., de Ledinghen, V., Demotes-Mainard, J., et al. (2005). Mood alterations during interferon-alfa therapy in patients with chronic hepatitis C: evidence for an overlap between manic/hypomanic and depressive symptoms. *Journal of Clinical Psychiatry, 66*(8), 1050–1057.

Coyle, J. T. (2006). Glutamate and schizophrenia: beyond the dopamine hypothesis. *Cellular and Molecular Neurobiology, 26*(4-6), 365–384.

Diez-Quevedo, C., Masnou, H., Planas, R., Castellví, P., Giménez, D., Morillas, R. M., et al. (2011). Prophylactic treatment with escitalopram of pegylated interferon alfa-2a-induced depression in hepatitis C: a 12-week, randomized, double-blind, placebo-controlled trial. *Journal of Clinical Psychiatry, 72*(4), 522–528.

Dowlati, Y., Herrmann, N., Swardfager, W., Liu, H., Sham, L., Reim, E. K., et al. (2010). A meta-analysis of cytokines in major depression. *Biological Psychiatry, 67*(5), 446–457.

Egerton, A., Brugger, S., Raffin, M., Barker, G. J., Lythgoe, D. J., McGuire, P. K., et al. (2012a). Anterior cingulate glutamate levels related to clinical status following treatment in first-episode schizophrenia. *Neuropsychopharmacology, 37*(11), 2515–2521.

Egerton, A., Fusar-Poli, P., & Stone, J. M. (2012b). Glutamate and psychosis risk. *Current Pharmaceutical Design, 18*(4), 466–478.

Egerton, A., & Stone, J. M. (2012). The glutamate hypothesis of schizophrenia: neuroimaging and drug development. *Current Pharmaceutical Biotechnology, 13*(8), 1500–1512.

Fusar-Poli, P., Bonoldi, I., Yung, A. R., Borgwardt, S., Kempton, M. J., Valmaggia, L., et al. (2012). Predicting psychosis: meta-analysis of transition outcomes in individuals at high clinical risk. *Archives of General Psychiatry, 69*(3), 220–229.

Fusar-Poli, P., Valmaggia, L., & McGuire, P. (2007). Can antidepressants prevent psychosis? *Lancet, 370*(9601), 1746–1748.

Goldberg, D. P., Andrews, G., & Hobbs, M. J. (2009). Where should bipolar disorder appear in the meta-structure? *Psychological Medicine, 39*(12), 2071–2081.

Goodwin, G. M. (2012). Bipolar depression and treatment with antidepressants. *British Journal of Psychiatry, 200*(1), 5–6.

Griffith, H. R., Stewart, C. C., & den Hollander, J. A. (2009). Proton magnetic resonance spectroscopy in dementias and mild cognitive impairment. *International Review of Neurobiology, 84*, 105–131.

Harrison, P. J., & Weinberger, D. R. (2005). Schizophrenia genes, gene expression, and neuropathology: on the matter of their convergence. *Molecular Psychiatry, 10*(1), 40–68.

Hasler, G., Neumeister, A., van der Veen, J. W., Tumonis, T., Bain, E. E., Shen, J., et al. (2005). Normal prefrontal gamma-aminobutyric acid levels in remitted depressed subjects determined by proton magnetic resonance spectroscopy. *Biological Psychiatry, 58*(12), 969–973.

Hasler, G., van der Veen, J. W., Tumonis, T., Meyers, N., Shen, J., & Drevets, W. C. (2007). Reduced prefrontal glutamate/glutamine and gamma-aminobutyric acid levels in major depression determined using proton magnetic resonance spectroscopy. *Archives of General Psychiatry, 64*(2), 193–200.

Hauser, P., Khosla, J., Aurora, H., Laurin, J., Kling, M. A., Hill, J., et al. (2002). A prospective study of the incidence and open-label treatment of interferon-induced major depressive disorder in patients with hepatitis C. *Molecular Psychiatry, 7*(9), 942–947.

Kegeles, L. S., Mao, X., Stanford, A. D., Girgis, R., Ojeil, N., Xu, X., et al. (2012). Elevated prefrontal cortex γ-aminobutyric acid and glutamate-glutamine levels in schizophrenia measured in vivo with proton magnetic resonance spectroscopy. *Archives of General Psychiatry, 69*(5), 449–459.

Kempton, M. J., Geddes, J. R., Ettinger, U., Williams, S. C. R., & Grasby, P. M. (2008). Meta-analysis, database, and meta-regression of 98 structural imaging studies in bipolar disorder. *Archives of General Psychiatry, 65*(9), 1017–1032.

Kempton, M. J., Salvador, Z., Munafo, M. R., Geddes, J. R., Simmons, A., Frangou, S., et al. (2011). Structural Neuroimaging Studies in Major Depressive Disorder: Meta-analysis and Comparison With Bipolar Disorder. *Archives of General Psychiatry, 68*(7), 675–690.

Lawrie, S. M., & Abukmeil, S. S. (1998). Brain abnormality in schizophrenia. A systematic and quantitative review of volumetric magnetic resonance imaging studies. *British Journal of Psychiatry, 172*, 110–120.

Li, C. -T., Bai, Y. -M., Huang, Y. -L., Chen, Y. -S., Chen, T. -J., Cheng, J. -Y., et al. (2012). Association between antidepressant resistance in unipolar depression and subsequent bipolar disorder: cohort study. *British Journal of Psychiatry, 200*(1), 45–51.

Lim, C., Olson, J., Zaman, A., Phelps, J., & Ingram, K. D. (2010). Prevalence and impact of manic traits in depressed patients initiating interferon therapy for chronic hepatitis C infection. *Journal of Clinical Gastroenterology, 44*(7), e141–146.

Miller, A. H., Maletic, V., & Raison, C. L. (2009). Inflammation and its discontents: the role of cytokines in the pathophysiology of major depression. *Biological Psychiatry, 65*(9), 732–741.

Mitchell, P. B., Goodwin, G. M., Johnson, G. F., & Hirschfeld, R. M. A. (2008). Diagnostic guidelines for bipolar depression: a probabilistic approach. *Bipolar Disorders, 10*(1 Pt 2), 144–152.

Olabi, B., Ellison-Wright, I., McIntosh, A. M., Wood, S. J., Bullmore, E., & Lawrie, S. M. (2011). Are there progressive brain changes in schizophrenia? A meta-analysis of structural magnetic resonance imaging studies. *Biological Psychiatry, 70*(1), 88–96.

Ongür, D., Jensen, J. E., Prescot, A. P., Stork, C., Lundy, M., Cohen, B. M., et al. (2008). Abnormal glutamatergic neurotransmission and neuronal-glial interactions in acute mania. *Biological Psychiatry, 64*(8), 718–726.

Owen, M. J., Craddock, N., & Jablensky, A. (2007). The genetic deconstruction of psychosis. *Schizophrenia Bulletin, 33*(4), 905–911.

Price, J. L., & Drevets, W. C. (2012). Neural circuits underlying the pathophysiology of mood disorders. *Trends in Cognitive Sciences, 16*(1), 61–71.

Raison, C. L., Borisov, A. S., Broadwell, S. D., Capuron, L., Woolwine, B. J., Jacobson, I. M., et al. (2005). Depression during pegylated interferon-alpha plus ribavirin therapy: prevalence and prediction. *Journal of Clinical Psychiatry, 66*(1), 41–48.

Raison, C. L., Capuron, L., & Miller, A. H. (2006). Cytokines sing the blues: inflammation and the pathogenesis of depression. *Trends in Immunology, 27*(1), 24–31.

Reynolds, G. P., & Harte, M. K. (2007). The neuronal pathology of schizophrenia: molecules and mechanisms. *Biochemical Society Transactions, 35*(2), 433.

Sanacora, G., Gueorguieva, R., Epperson, C. N., Wu, Y. -T., Appel, M., Rothman, D. L., et al. (2004). Subtype-specific alterations of gamma-aminobutyric acid and glutamate in patients with major depression. *Archives of General Psychiatry, 61*(7), 705–713.

Sanacora, G., Treccani, G., & Popoli, M. (2012). Towards a glutamate hypothesis of depression: an emerging frontier of neuropsychopharmacology for mood disorders. *Neuropharmacology, 62*(1), 63–77.

Schmidt, H. D., & Duman, R. S. (2007). The role of neurotrophic factors in adult hippocampal neurogenesis, antidepressant treatments and animal models of depressive-like behavior. *Behavioural Pharmacology, 18*(5-6), 391–418.

Shepherd, A. M., Laurens, K. R., Matheson, S. L., Carr, V. J., & Green, M. J. (2012). Systematic meta-review and quality assessment of the structural brain alterations in schizophrenia. *Neuroscience and Biobehavioral Reviews, 36*(4), 1342–1356.

Soeiro-de-Souza, M. G., Salvadore, G., Moreno, R. A., Otaduy, M. C. G., Chaim, K. T., Gattaz, W. F., et al. (2013). Bcl-2 rs956572 polymorphism is associated with increased anterior cingulate cortical glutamate in euthymic bipolar i disorder. *Neuropsychopharmacology, 38*(3), 468–475.

Stone, J. M., Day, F., Tsagaraki, H., Valli, I., McLean, M. A., Lythgoe, D. J., et al. (2009). Glutamate dysfunction in people with prodromal symptoms of psychosis: relationship to gray matter volume. *Biological Psychiatry, 66*(6), 533–539.

Stone, J. M., Howes, O. D., Egerton, A., Kambeitz, J., Allen, P., Lythgoe, D. J., et al. (2010). Altered relationship between hippocampal glutamate levels and striatal dopamine function in subjects at ultra high risk of psychosis. *Biological Psychiatry, 68*(7), 599–602.

Tavares, R. G., Tasca, C. I., Santos, C. E. S., Alves, L. B., Porciúncula, L. O., Emanuelli, T., et al. (2002). Quinolinic acid stimulates synaptosomal glutamate release and inhibits glutamate uptake into astrocytes. *Neurochemistry International, 40*(7), 621–627.

Taylor, M. J., Godlewska, B. R., Norbury, R., Selvaraj, S., Near, J., & Cowen, P. J. (2012). Early increase in marker of neuronal integrity with antidepressant treatment of major depression: 1H-magnetic resonance spectroscopy of N-acetyl-aspartate. *International Journal of Neuropsychopharmacology, 15*(10), 1541–1546. .

Taylor, M. J., Mannie, Z. N., Norbury, R., Near, J., & Cowen, P. J. (2011a). Elevated cortical glutamate in young people at increased familial risk of depression. *International Journal of Neuropsychopharmacology, 14*(2), 255–259.

Taylor, M. J., Near, J., & Cowen, P. J. (2011b). Neurochemical changes in an immunologically-induced high risk state for mood disorder: interferon-alpha treatment of chronic hepatitis C viral infection. *Journal of Psychopharmacology, 25*(S8), A13.

Taylor, M. J., Selvaraj, S., Norbury, R., Jezzard, P., & Cowen, P. J. (2009). Normal glutamate but elevated myo-inositol in anterior cingulate cortex in recovered depressed patients. *Journal of Affective Disorders, 119*(1-3), 186–189.

van Os, J., & Kapur, S. (2009). Schizophrenia. *Lancet, 374*(9690), 635–645.

Wright, I. C., Rabe-Hesketh, S., Woodruff, P. W., David, A. S., Murray, R. M., & Bullmore, E. T. (2000). Meta-analysis of regional brain volumes in schizophrenia. *American Journal of Psychiatry, 157*(1), 16–25.

Yung, A. R., Phillips, L. J., Yuen, H. P., Francey, S. M., McFarlane, C. A., Hallgren, M., et al. (2003). Psychosis prediction: 12-month follow up of a high-risk ("prodromal") group. *Schizophrenia Research, 60*(1), 21–32.

Yüksel, C., & Öngür, D. (2010). Magnetic resonance spectroscopy studies of glutamate-related abnormalities in mood disorders. *Biological Psychiatry, 68*(9), 785–794.

Zarate, C., Jr Machado-Vieira, R., Henter, I., Ibrahim, L., Diazgranados, N., & Salvadore, G. (2010). Glutamatergic modulators: the future of treating mood disorders? *Harvard Review of Psychiatry, 18*(5), 293–303.

Zipursky, R. B., Reilly, T. J., & Murray, R. M. (2012). The myth of schizophrenia as a progressive brain disease. *Schizophrenia Bulletin.* [Epub ahead of print]

Preclinical and Clinical Applications of ^{1}H MRS in the Spinal Cord

Amber Michelle Hill[1,2] *and Olga Ciccarelli*[1,3]

[1]Department of Brain Repair and Rehabilitation and [2]Department of Neuroinflammation, University College London Institute of Neurology, London, UK [3]National Institute for Health Research University College London Hospitals Biomedical Research Centre, London, UK

INTRODUCTION

Proton magnetic resonance spectroscopy (^{1}H MRS) is a noninvasive technique for quantifying, characterizing, and monitoring metabolic biomarkers involved in neurological disease pathology. Due to technical challenges, it has developed less quickly in spinal cord research than in brain research. However, spinal cord ^{1}H MRS is a cutting-edge technique that is increasingly becoming a useful tool that has important clinical applications.

This chapter will provide an overview of the importance of spinal cord ^{1}H MRS in preclinical and clinical research, then briefly review its methodological challenges and limitations. The applications of spinal cord ^{1}H MRS in neurological disorders, such as multiple sclerosis (MS), spinal cord injury (SCI), tumor, and amyotrophic lateral sclerosis (ALS), will also be reviewed. In this chapter, these disorders are used as disease "models" to illustrate the successful use of spinal cord ^{1}H MRS in preclinical and clinical research. Finally, we will discuss the future potential of spinal cord ^{1}H MRS and its promising applications.

IMPORTANCE OF ^{1}H MRS ADVANCES

Methodological challenges of ^{1}H MRS in the spinal cord have increased the importance of optimizing ^{1}H MRS techniques and protocols. Developments in high field scanner technology have improved the feasibility of examining smaller areas of interest and obtaining a good signal within the spinal cord. In particular, high field scanners allow for optimized spectral resolution, providing better distinction between metabolic peaks in spectra and the ability to quantify metabolites more precisely. This has allowed researchers to have access to a more detailed analysis of metabolic function in animals and humans than previously possible, thereby making it easier to reliably quantify metabolites and gradually increasing the value of spinal cord ^{1}H MRS studies for animal studies and clinical research.

Preclinical Developments

Preclinical spinal cord ^{1}H MRS is important in order to understand the mechanisms underlying pathological changes that cannot be directly tested in humans. Preclinical ^{1}H MRS methodology can be used to (1) track changes before and after the onset of neurological symptoms resulting from pathological changes, (2) monitor the time course of neurological illness noninvasively and prior to postmortem histology methods, and (3) provide biomarkers sensitive enough to detect clinical changes and responsiveness to treatments. These advantages allow researchers to precisely examine metabolites in animal models to determine their role in the pathogenesis of neurological diseases.

Correspondingly, improvements in experimental methodology are necessary to optimize preclinical ^{1}H MRS spectra and improve outcomes. Advancements have the potential to lead developments in clinical uses of ^{1}H MRS techniques. Preclinical researchers have developed several protocols to reliably quantify

229

the following metabolites: total *N*-acetylaspartate (NAA), total creatine (Cr), total choline (Cho), *myo*-inositol (mI), and glutamate (Glu) in the spinal cord of healthy rats and mice (Tachrount, et al., 2012).[1] Feasibility studies in the spinal cord demonstrated the viability of acquiring high-quality MR spectra from healthy rat spinal cord using implanted radiofrequency (RF) coils; these RF coils were implanted to optimize the signal and increase sensitivity in the small diameter of the spinal cord (Bilgen et al., 2001; Silver et al., 2001). The disadvantage of this invasive methodology is that it could result in strong magnetic field distortion, with subsequent distortions in the spinal cord homogeneity. Additionally, the procedure may also increase complications for animals that are ill from induced disease (Bilgen et al., 2001; Silver et al., 2001). Conversely, the feasibility of (optimized) high-resolution ¹H MRS in the spinal cord of mice and rats was demonstrated; this technique is noninvasive, and therefore could be applied safely for transgenic mouse models and other animal models to monitor and better understand pathology, such as neurodegeneration and neuroinflammation (Bilgen et al., 2001; Silver et al., 2001; Tachrount et al., 2012).

An important consideration concerning preclinical developments is that they allow the investigators to combine ¹H MRS with other structural and functional measures, which might be most useful in obtaining a complete view of spinal cord plasticity and neuroregeneration. Additionally, *in vivo* measurements obtained in preclinical studies can be complemented by histological examination in experiments that would not be feasible in humans.

Clinical Developments

Optimized imaging parameters for spinal cord ¹H MRS (Marliani et al., 2007; Table 3.7.1) and the use of statistical modeling of structural measures and NAA levels (Ciccarelli et al., 2010a) have been useful to detect metabolic abnormalities in the spinal cord of patients with neurological conditions, such as MS. ¹H MRS studies in the brain have often described correlations between the metabolite concentrations (mainly NAA, but also mI) and neurological disability, suggesting that these metabolites reflect pathological processes. These processes are likely to play a role in determining clinical disability and, therefore, should also be investigated in the spinal cord, which is a major factor that leads to clinical impairment in neurological conditions.

If optimized protocols are used, then ¹H MRS in the spinal cord allows the quantification of the major metabolites, including NAA, Cho, Cr, and mI, with acceptable confidence. Recent technical developments have made it possible to quantify more metabolites in the spinal cord, such as glutamate and glutamine, which are often studied in the brain, but have previously been very difficult to estimate in the spinal cord (Solanky et al., 2013). Forthcoming clinical studies are ongoing to explore the correlations between these new metabolites and clinical disability.

A goal of clinical research is to develop and validate spinal cord markers for testing the efficacy of novel treatment and monitoring patients' responses. Despite the fact that ¹H MRS has a greater pathologic specificity for axonal integrity and other pathological processes as compared to conventional MRI, it has been only rarely used in phase III clinical trials. This is mainly due to the technical difficulties related to the protocol implementation and standardization of data acquisition, position, and size of the volume of interest (VOI), postprocessing, and quantification procedures between centers. Recommendations for the application of MRS to clinical trials have been reported (De Stefano et al., 2007). For example, only a few clinical trials in patients with MS have included ¹H MRS in their MR protocols to assess the efficacy of new medications in MS (Sajja et al., 2008). These studies have performed a homogeneous acquisition procedure of single-voxel MRS and a centralized analysis of the MRS data. Future developments of spinal cord ¹H MRS have the potential to facilitate the use of this technique in clinical trials.

METHODOLOGICAL CHALLENGES AND CONSIDERATIONS

General ¹H MRS Considerations

¹H MRS has not been widely applied in the spinal cord due to technical challenges posed by its small diameter, magnetic field inhomogeneities, and physiological motion. Experimental designs have largely been limited to the cervical spinal cord in humans and lumbar region in animals, as these are spinal regions with larger cross-sectional areas close enough to the coil when lying flat to obtain a good signal-to-noise ratio (SNR) and have less magnetic field distortion due to its size. Although the optimization of sequences is

---

[1]The metabolites are generally measured with Cramér—Rao lower bounds estimated error of metabolite quantification, where metabolites with similar and strongly correlated overlapping resonances are quantified in terms of "total" concentration under the following constraints: tNAA = NAA + NAAG concentrations, tCr = PCr + Cr concentrations, and tCho = PCho + GPC concentrations.

TABLE 3.7.1   Summary of Clinical and Preclinical ^{1}H MRS Optimization Protocols in the Spinal Cord

Species	Reference	Region	Field strength	Sequence	RF coil	Acquisition time (ms)	Water suppression	VOI	Averages
Human	Marliani et al. (2007)	C2–C3	3 T	PRESS	Phased array spine coil	TE: 35TR: 2000	CHESS	$7 \times 9 \times 35$ mm (0.4 mL)	400
Mouse	Tachrount et al. (2012)	C3	11.75 T	PRESS	Volume coil	TE: 10TR: 4000	VAPOR	$2 \times 1.8 \times 1.1$ mm^3 (4 µL)	256
Rat	Balla et al. (2007)	L1	17.6 T	PRESS	Transmit—receive surface coil	TE: 60TR: 3000	VAPOR	$2 \times 2 \times 2$ to $2 \times 2 \times 4$ mm^3(8—16 µl)	512

PRESS, Point RESolved Spectroscopy; CHESS, CHEmical Shift Selective; VAPOR, Variable Pulse power and Optimized Relaxation.

commonly achieved by a physics team, several considerations and precautions for ^{1}H MRS experimental designs and analysis should be considered by preclinical and clinical researchers. This section provides a brief overview of common challenges that affect experimental methodology and outcomes.

Region of Interest

There are many challenges to consider when deciding on the region of interest (ROI) and voxel placement within the spinal cord, which include the position of the coil. The SNR is reduced compared with brain MRS due to the small volume of the spinal cord. Additionally, a sufficient SNR is more challenging to obtain in the spinal cord than in the brain due to magnetic susceptibility at tissue/air/bone interface and physiological cycles, such as respiration and cardiac motion, which can cause distortions and motion artifacts (Fig. 3.7.1) (Hock et al., 2012a; Tachrount et al., 2012). As a result, a precise quantification of metabolic concentrations may not be easily achievable. The SNR needs to be optimized to ensure high spectral quality; this will increase the opportunity for higher sensitivity and signal (Barker et al., 2010; Hock et al., 2012b). Other elements, such as the coil positioning, the location of the voxel, the size of the voxel, and a reduction of motion disturbance around the area of interest, need to be taken into account when designing an experiment. The use of either transmitter/receiving (surface) coil or multichannel-phased array coils is recommended for brain MRS. In preclinical studies of spinal cord rat MRS the former is commonly used (see Table 3.7.1). The latter provides a higher SNR, but metabolite quantification may be more challenging (Natt et al., 2005). In humans, surface coil, neck coil, or a combination of coils (for example, we often use at 3 T at the posterior half of a 12-channel head coil, the posterior part of a neck array coil, and the upper elements of a spine array coil) is used for spinal cord MRS.

From a methodological point of view, the spinal cord spectroscopic voxel includes both the white and gray matter. Novel acquisition techniques at 3 T, such as the fat-suppressed 3D slab-selective fast field echo sequence, have been used to demonstrate that the segmentation of white matter and gray matter in the human spinal cord is feasible (Yiannakas et al., 2012). Combining this sequence with single-voxel MRS has shown that the spectroscopic volume takes up most of the cross-sectional area of the spinal cord and incorporates both gray matter and white matter. Additionally, if there are lesions in the spinal cord, it is likely that the voxel will encompass the lesional tissue and its surrounding regions. This implies that the observed metabolic concentrations always represent an "averaged" concentration over spinal cord tissues.

Protocol Influences on the Analysis of Spectra

^{1}H MRS is the most sensitive *in vivo* spectroscopy technique because of the nuclear magnetic resonance characteristics of protons[2] in comparison to other nuclei that could be utilized in MRS. However, this advantage also has the disadvantage that extensive water-suppression techniques are necessary to remove large water signals and strengthen the magnetic field homogeneity, so that smaller chemical shifts of metabolite signals can be detected (Fig. 3.7.1). Shimming can be especially challenging in the spinal cords of animal models, such as rats or mice, and can be time-consuming. Timing should be taken into account when designing the experiment, particularly when dealing with sick animals and with neurological patients who cannot tolerate being scanned for a long time. Therefore, obtaining good water suppression and

---

[2]This is because the proton has the highest gyromagnetic ratio of nonradioactive nuclei and a high abundance. The gyromagnetic ratio is the ratio of its intrinsic magnetic dipole moment to its spin angular momentum.

shimming is particularly important to achieve good spectra, where metabolic peaks are easily distinguished from noise. Table 3.7.1 gives an example of the recommended protocols for spinal cord ¹H MRS in the human.

Animal Protocols

The diameter of the spinal cord of the animals, such as mice and rats, is even smaller than that of the humans (2–3 mm compared to ∼10 mm), and this has a significant impact on the time it takes to optimize parameters and acquire good spectra while the animal is stable under anesthesia.

Animal Preparation and Handling

Physiological measures and prescan preparation are essential for *in vivo* animal research. Animals must be anesthetized and stabilized under anesthesia. The amount of anesthesia along with the amount of saline intraperitoneally injected to keep the animal hydrated for the duration of the experiment is determined by the size of the animal. An optimized flow rate[3] and isoflurane concentrations[4] should be within range for the species of the animal examined and delivered through a nose cone (with a holder for the teeth). Temperature should be regulated by heating the gradient cooling system and monitored using a temperature probe; a warming pad might be necessary for a larger bore hole. Additionally, monitors for respiration, heart rate, and ideally blood oxidation levels should also be used to ensure the animal is stable while in the scanner. Each of these parameters will make a significant difference in the stabilization of the animal and thereby affect results.

Scanning Considerations

Researchers should also consider the challenges of scanning in the design of their experiment, particularly with regard to prepreparation and timing. The preparation of the animal for the scanner may require a minimum of 30–45 min for rodents and an hour or more for larger animals, such as piglets. The preparation time also largely depends on the number of physiological measures being monitored. All items secured to the animal, such as oxygenation sensors, should not reduce circulation, and the magnet should have a suitable animal bed and mask for long-term anesthetic delivery. If the bed, mask, or coil cords are not properly secured, the magnet may cause small vibra-

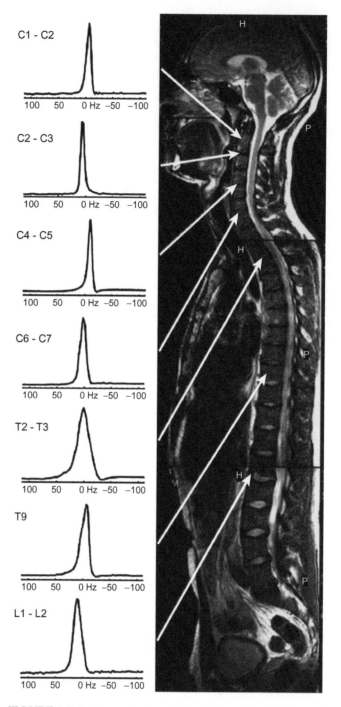

FIGURE 3.7.1 Demonstration of the challenges in obtaining optimized water suppression, or shim quality, at the lower levels of the spinal cord, thereby limiting current ¹H MRS methodology in clinical studies to the cervical levels of the spinal cord. This shows that sufficient shim convergence could not be reached in the thoracic (aside from the T9 region) and lumbar levels of spinal cord due to homogeneity problems of cerebral spinal fluid flow pattern and movement artifacts. (From Henning et al., 2008, with permission.)

---

[3]Approximately 250–300 mL/min for small rodents.

[4]Approximately 1.5–2% for small rodents.

tions that produce slight movements in the animal's position, separate from the animal's respiration. These vibrations may produce distorted peaks visible in combination with the respiratory readings, leading to an inability to determine whether the animal is stable and not distressed in the scanner.

To reduce motion artifacts, the respiration signal is taken using a pressure sensor within an air-filled balloon under the abdomen of the animal[5] and the acquisitions are gated to synchronize with the animals breathing motions. Likewise, if the mask is not suitable (i.e., a specific mask for the corresponding species of animal), the animal is at risk of waking up while in the scanner and jeopardizing the data already acquired. If the respiration shifts abruptly, an MRI scan can be used to check the positioning of the animal and assess the need to further optimize or re-start the experiment. Stable respiration and respiratory gating (i.e., a setting to acquire data between the peaks of respiration) should be in place before running any sequences.

Region of Interest

At the start of experimentation, anatomical images are usually acquired to ensure that the position of the ROI is at the isocenter of the coil where the sensitivity is optimal. Sometimes it is necessary to adjust the animal's position until a suitable position within the isocenter of the coil is established. This can be made easier by marking ruler measurements on the animal bed. Larger voxel sizes (increasing sensitivity) and longer acquisition times (allowing for more averages) will translate into better results (see Table 3.7.1 for more details). The L3–L5 region of the spinal cord is the widest area of the spinal cord, and thus this is the region that allows the largest spectroscopic voxel. It is also a region of the rodent spinal cord that is closest to the coil, thus increasing sensitivity for optimal results. However, the L1 region of the rodent spinal cord is commonly used also, as it is also close to the coil, a good size, and easy to locate with the ribs as its reference point.

PRECLINICAL AND CLINICAL ¹H MRS APPLICATIONS IN THE SPINAL CORD

Neurological diseases, particularly those affecting the spinal cord, cause metabolic and microstructural changes in the neuronal environment that may cause acute symptoms and/or chronic disability. ¹H MRS may provide *in vivo* information on the extent of pathological involvement that is not quantifiable using conventional imaging methods. In general, ¹H MRS in clinical studies can be used to (1) investigate correlations between metabolite concentrations and clinical disability, (2) identify predictors of clinical outcome, (3) improve accuracy of diagnosis, and (4) monitor patients' responses to treatment and test the efficacy if medications are used. This section will focus on the application of ¹H MRS in the spinal cord of patients with MS, SCI, tumors, and ALS, as "models" to demonstrate the various uses of ¹H MRS preclinically and clinically.

MS

MS (see also Chapter 3.2) is a chronic inflammatory demyelinating and immune-mediated disease of the central nervous system (CNS). Most people are diagnosed between the ages of 20–40 and develop symptoms that result in physical and cognitive disability. Conventional MR imaging (MRI) is currently used in patients with MS to facilitate the diagnosis of the disease and monitor the response to treatment. The applications of advanced MRI techniques, including ¹H MRS, to patients with MS have contributed to understanding the biological mechanisms responsible for the initiation of MS and its accumulation of disability during the secondary progressive phase of the disease. Additionally, experimental animal studies have greatly improved our current knowledge of these mechanisms and contributed to the development of new therapies.

Preclinical Applications in Models of MS

The autoimmune-mediated CNS inflammation, demyelination, and axonal damage that the experimental autoimmune encephalomyelitis (EAE) model produces, makes it one of the most widely used models of MS. EAE can be induced using active or passive methods, but despite versatile induction methods and range of pathology, it is still under debate as to whether or not it is the best model for MS (Nelson et al., 2004; Sriram & Steiner, 2005). Despite the challenges of modeling MS pathology, preclinical MR techniques have enabled greater understanding of disease pathology. Both laboratory methods, such as immunohistochemistry and imaging techniques, have dramatically improved the ability to more accurately associate live *in vivo* findings with *in vitro* and postmortem biological measures (Brochet et al., 2006; Budde et al., 2009; Abourbeh et al., 2012; Badawi et al., 2012; MacKenzie-Graham et al., 2012).

Prior to ¹H MRS developments, conventional EAE and other animal studies have required histological examination of tissue, which is limited by a terminal

---

[5]Rapid Biomedical (Rimpar, Germany) or SA Instruments (Stony Brook, New York).

experiment, and fixed-time point investigation of the tissue. Immunohistochemical evaluation is limited by its reliance on fixation techniques as well as monoclonal and polyclonal antibodies that may not be reliable, or fully representative of, the biological component being explored. *In vivo* ^{1}H MRS allows serial evaluation over multiple time points, which can now be *supported* with histological examination of the tissue, rather than fully reliant on the fixed-time point evaluations.

There has only been one feasibility study ($n = 8$) that employed ^{1}H MRS *in vivo* in the spinal cord of EAE animals (250–300 g, 7–10 weeks of age, voxel positioned at T13/L1) (Zelaya et al., 1996). This study observed changes in NAA, Cho, and resonances caused by macromolecules, which are characteristic of EAE and studies in MS patients (Zelaya et al., 1996). These observations suggest that ^{1}H MRS *in vivo* is sensitive to detect changes that are associated with inflammation and demyelination in EAE (Zelaya et al., 1996). This has demonstrated the potential to answer questions regarding the pathogenesis of MS that cannot be otherwise obtained in human studies.

Clinical Applications in Patients with MS

Studies in MS using ^{1}H MRS in the spinal cord have used different MR scanners at different magnetic field strengths and different patient groups, making the comparison between studies very challenging (Table 3.7.2). Nevertheless, studies published have been concordant in demonstrating a reduction in NAA concentration in patients with MS compared to healthy controls; the reduction has varied between 21 and 39% (Table 3.7.2 and Fig. 3.7.2; Blamire et al., 2007; Ciccarelli et al., 2007; Marliani et al., 2010). NAA is synthesized in neurons and present in very high concentrations in the CNS (Benarroch, 2008). Therefore, reduced NAA concentrations in the spinal cord of MS patients compared to controls indicates axonal loss and/or metabolic dysfunction, both in the lesions and in the tissue outside the lesions (or normal-appearing

white matter; Kendi et al., 2004; Blamire et al., 2007; Moffett et al., 2007; Henning et al., 2008; Ciccarelli et al., 2010a; Marliani et al., 2010; Hock et al., 2012a).

Correlations between lower spinal cord levels of NAA and higher disability, as assessed by cerebellar functional score (Blamire et al., 2007) and 9-hole peg test (Ciccarelli et al., 2007), suggest that this metabolite reflects pathological processes that may play a role in determining a patient's disability. However, significant correlations between NAA and disability, as measured by the Expanded Disability Status Scale (EDSS), which is a scale commonly used to quantify disability in MS, are often not seen (Ciccarelli et al., 2007; Marliani et al., 2010).

Mechanisms of spinal cord repair and their relative contribution to clinical recovery were measured in patients with MS after cervical cord relapse, using spinal cord ^{1}H MRS and volumetric imaging (Ciccarelli et al., 2010a). Results indicated that patients who showed a higher increase in NAA after one month were those who presented the greater clinical improvement. Longer disease duration at study entry predicted a worse clinical recovery (Ciccarelli et al., 2010a). Since the partial recovery in NAA levels after the relapse was concurrent with a decline in cord cross-sectional area, we suggested that the increase in NAA concentration may be driven by increased axonal mitochondrial metabolism (Ciccarelli et al., 2010a).

In a subsequent study we proposed that the indirect estimation of mitochondrial metabolism *in vivo* could be estimated by statistically modeling the NAA concentration, estimated in the spinal cord, in combination with other spinal cord MRI techniques, such as diffusion tensor imaging (DTI) and atrophy (Ciccarelli et al., 2010b). These studies are in agreement with previous brain studies that suggested decreases in NAA concentrations reflect a reduction in mitochondrial metabolism in addition to a reduced axonal number (Davie et al., 1994; De Stefano et al., 1995; Mader et al., 2000). In fact, preclinical ^{1}H MRS *in vitro*

TABLE 3.7.2   Summary of the Methods and Results of Clinical ^{1}H MRS Studies in Patients with MS

Reference	Field strength	Spinal cord level	Type of MS	EDSS	Tissue included in the voxel	Reduced NAA in patients vs. control
Kendi et al. (2004)	1.5 T	C3–C7	NR	NR	NAWM	Yes, but no information provided
Blamire et al. (2007)	2 T	C3	4 RRMS, 7 SPMS	4.5	NR	32%
Ciccarelli et al. (2007)	1.5 T	C1–C3	13 RRMS, 1 SPMS	4	Acute lesion	39%
Marliani et al. (2010)	3 T	C2–C3	15 RRMS	NR	Chronic lesion	21% (NAA/Cho)

NR, not reported; Cho, choline-containing compounds; NAWM, normal-appearing white matter; RRMS, relapsing-remitting MS; SPMS, secondary progressive MS.

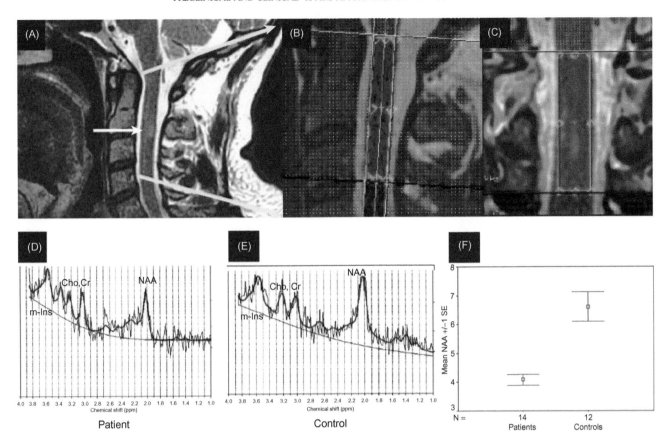

FIGURE 3.7.2   Spinal cord spectroscopy in humans. (A–C) Sagittal T_2-weighted image of the spinal cord of a patient that shows a posterior lesion at C2–C3 (white arrow; A). Location of a spectroscopic VOI between C1 and C3 on the sagittal (B) and coronal (C) images. (D) Spectrum of a MS patient. (E) Spectrum of a healthy subject. Graph indicating the difference in NAA concentrations between patients with an acute lesion in the spectroscopic voxel at the onset of an acute relapse and healthy subjects. (From Ciccarelli et al., 2007, with permission.)

studies of mitochondrial respiratory chain inhibitors of complexes I, II, IV, and V showed irreversible mitochondrial NAA production, which was thought to reflect impaired mitochondrial energy production, rather than neuronal cell loss (Bates et al., 1996). Interestingly, a study carried out in patients with MS reported no correlation between NAA and spinal cord atrophy (Blamire et al., 2007), which is considered to reflect neurodegeneration, suggesting that the two measures may be complementary in detected *in vivo* pathological processes.

Other metabolites can be measured with ^{1}H MRS, such as Cho, Cr, and mI, but these have not been found to be consistently (and significantly) different in patients with MS when compared to healthy controls (Blamire et al., 2007; Ciccarelli et al., 2007; Marliani et al., 2010). In particular, mI, which is a marker of glial activation and proliferation (see Chapter 2.5), has been found to increase, although nonsignificantly, in patients when compared to controls (between 8 and 15%; Blamire et al., 2007; Ciccarelli et al., 2007; Marliani et al., 2010). We found a correlation between

higher mI in the acute spinal cord lesions and greater disability, which warrants further investigation (Ciccarelli et al., 2007).

SCI

Traumatic SCI is characterized by a loss of sensorimotor functions, which adversely affects organ tissue causing cellular death, demyelination, and axonal degeneration. Primary injury to sensorimotor pathways in SCI is followed by an extended period of secondary injury, which ultimately causes progressive tissue degeneration. The pathology of SCI plays a central role in modulating motor and pain transmission. The use of ^{1}H MRS permits the ability to record the time course of the pathology and monitoring the effects of neuroprotective developments in SCI.

Preclinical Uses of ^{1}H MRS in SCI

Several studies on SCI have been investigated preclinically. Qian et al. (2010) monitored longitudinal changes in tissue degeneration in SCI using ¹H MRS and immunohistochemical examination in three sections of the spinal cord of rats. SCI was induced by a laminectomy and damage at the level of T6–T8 vertebra; significant decreases in NAA and Cr were found in all three spinal cord segments affected from 2 to 8 weeks postinjury (Qian et al., 2010). In contrast, Cho levels significantly increased in all segments of SCI rats at 2 weeks postinjury, then all but the most rostral region (T6) recovered to baseline by 8 weeks. Immunohistochemical examination in this study was advantageous in regard to confirming the following: (1) neuronal cell death in the gray matter, (2) axonal degeneration in the white matter, and (3) astrocytic activity, which is suggested by the various shifts in metabolic concentrations. However, histology is limited by fixed-point methodology rather than the ability to confirm these changes *in vivo* and at the various time points of the study.

Tachrount et al. (2011) followed the previous study with similar methodology using a combination of MRS, DTI for longitudinal structural measures, and immunohistochemical examination. The researchers demonstrated a marked reduction in NAA in mice with injured spinal cords, as well as changes in Glu, Cr, Cho, and mI 5 days postinjury, followed by a slow and progressive increase. Cr, a marker of cellular density, recovered to pre-injury levels within 2 weeks of post injections and then continued to increase. NAA reached full recovery level 4 weeks postinjury. The concentration of mI, a marker of glial activation and proliferation, had an abrupt increase above the pre-injection baseline, then leveled back down to recovery levels after 5 weeks. The most rapid recovery was seen in Cho, a marker of cell membrane metabolism, recovering within a few days. These results suggest

significant plasticity may have lead to a full recovery in axonal integrity following SCI. The spike in mI is likely to be related to the glial immune response resulting from the initial injury, but may also mediate some of the recovery, as it is the last to return to baseline. The sequence of events may also be an early indicator of the mechanism underlying biochemical changes leading to recovery. However, an assessment of whether or not these changes indicate functional recovery would need to be assessed in behavioral measures outside of the scanner.

In a follow-up SCI study at C3 and C4, Callot et al. (2012), used a multimodal approach including MRS, diffusion and perfusion, and histological analyses in order to characterize the metabolic post-traumatic events in correlation with structural, vascular measures (Fig. 3.7.3). Widespread lesions from rostral to caudal and lateral white matter and gray matter changes were seen. After SCI, mice suffered from forelimb paralysis with force-decrease over time. In the acute phase (1 day postinjury), the primary MR features were fiber disruption, ischemia, and axonal and neuronal loss. In the early postinjury phase (i.e., between days 3 and 5 postinjury), changes in the apparent diffusion coefficient were observed and a rapid increase in spinal cord blood flow (SCBF) values. This was attributed to angiogenesis, which was thought to be in response to an energy demand for tissue regeneration. After 7 days postinjury, extended perfusion overreached the basal level and mI concentrations increased as well as diffusion in the gray matter, suggesting gliosis. Mice presented sustained abnormalities in metabolic, structural, and vascular parameters revealing an incomplete recovery that was confirmed by histology (Callot et al., 2012). Using this multimodal approach, combining MRS with other MRI

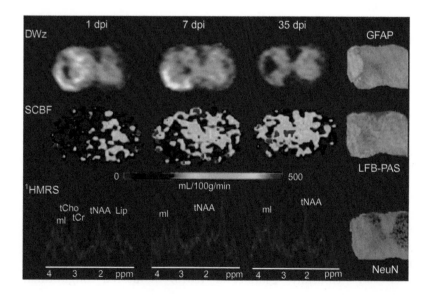

FIGURE 3.7.3 Diffusion weighted imaging (DW₂), SCBF, and spectroscopy (¹H MRS) at 1 day postinjury (1 dpi), 7 dpi, and 35 dpi. Immunohistochemistry with labeling of astrocyte activity using glial fibrillary acidic protein (GFAP), myelin shown by luxol fast blue labeling (LFB-PAS), and neurons shown by neuron-specific nuclear protein (NeuN) labeling. (From Callot et al., 2012, with permission.)

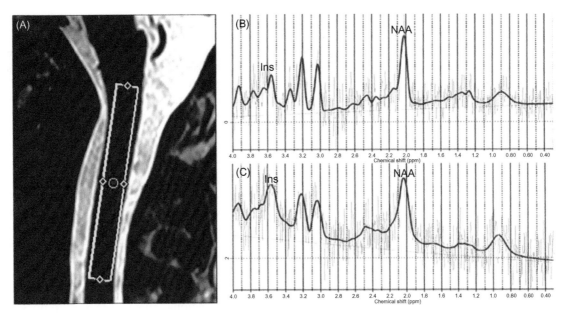

FIGURE 3.7.4 (A) Sagittal T_2-weighted image of a healthy control showing the spectroscopic voxel between C1 and C3 (in yellow) on the T_2-weighted sagittal image of one control. (B) Spectrum derived from voxel in (A) that shows reduced levels of mI with respect to total Cr levels (m-Ins/Cr = 1.37 [%SD = 11]) in comparison with a spectrum obtained in a patient (m-Ins/Cr = 2.11 [%SD = 10]) (C). (From Kachramanoglou et al., 2013, with permission.)

techniques, the researchers were able to further characterize the time course of pathology of post-traumatic events following moderate and severe SCI. Furthermore, this approach helps to improve postprocessing results and define the most relevant markers of post-traumatic disease and disease progression.

Clinical Analysis of SCI using ¹H MRS

Recent developments and advances in imaging acquisition and the increased use of high field scanners have made it possible to apply MRS to the spinal cord of patients with SCI. Clinical applications of spinal cord MRS have been scarce and limited to a few studies that were carried out in patients with brachial plexus injury, chronic whiplash, and cervical spondylotic myelopathy. These studies have demonstrated that MRS of the spinal cord provides information on the underlying mechanisms of the disease by reflecting pathological changes that are not detectable with conventional MRI techniques.

BRACHIAL PLEXUS INJURY

The avulsion of all the dorsal and ventral roots from C5 to T1 (brachial plexus) leads to a completely paralyzed and anesthetic arm, with associated neuropathic pain. It is effectively a CNS injury and often described as "longitudinal spinal cord injury." The re-implantation of the avulsed ventral roots back in the spinal cord may provide some improvement in the motor function. Kachramanoglou and colleagues (2013) studied 10 patients with brachial plexus

avulsion who underwent re-implantation of C5 to T1 ventral roots on average 5.5 years earlier. All patients and a group of healthy subjects underwent single-voxel MRS at 3 T; the voxel was positioned from C1 to C3. Patients showed significantly higher levels of mI normalized to Cras compared with healthy subjects (Fig. 3.7.4; Kachramanoglou et al., 2013). This finding suggests that reactive gliosis, perhaps in response to the Wallerian degeneration of avulsed fibers, may occur in the spinal cord above the site of injury, as demonstrated in animal model of root avulsion (Koliatsos et al., 1994). Interestingly, greater mI/Cr values were associated with worse function of the affected arm, as assessed by the Disability for Arm, Shoulder, and Hand (DASH) scale (Kachramanoglou et al., 2013), suggesting that these values reflect pathological processes that are clinically relevant.

CHRONIC WHIPLASH

Elliott et al. (2012) recently studied a case series of five patients with chronic whiplash (>6 months postinjury) and seven healthy controls. All subjects underwent single-voxel MRS at 3 T and the voxel was located from the top of C1 to the upper part of C3. Patients showed reduced levels of NAA with respect to Cr when compared with healthy controls (Elliott et al., 2012), suggesting underlying axonal degeneration and/or metabolic dysfunction, which may be secondary to the damage of the peripheral structures, which, in turn, causes an abnormal afferent input.

CERVICAL MYELOPATHY

A similar reduction in the NAA/Cr ratio has been detected in the spinal cord of patients with cervical myelopathy (Holly et al., 2009). Cervical myelopathy is caused by degenerative changes in the disc and the facet joints that lead to a narrowing of the spinal cord, which is often visible on conventional MRI. Conventional MRI can also demonstrate a T_2-weighted, hyperintense lesion in the spinal cord at the level of the canal narrowing. It is caused rarely by tumor. Holly and colleagues (2009) studied 21 patients with chronic cervical myelopathy and 13 healthy controls. Thirteen out of 21 patients had T_2-weighted, hyperintense signal abnormalities in the spinal cord. The authors used a 1.5 T scanner and a neck coil; the voxels were positioned at the C2 level of the spinal cord, which was above the region of spinal cord compression in all cases. Patients showed reduced NAA when compared with controls (Holly et al., 2009), suggesting neuroaxonal injury. One-third of the patients showed a lactate peak (Holly et al., 2009), which is a marker of increased anaerobic glycolysis, and which was absent in the control group. This peak was more frequent in patients showing a T_2 lesion in the spinal cord, suggesting that the spinal cord is undergoing ischemic changes under the effect of the spinal cord compression (see Fig. 3.7.5).

Other Neurological Conditions

We will now briefly describe the results of clinical studies carried out in patients with tumor and ALS; preclinical studies of these conditions have not been yet published.

Tumor

A tumor (or neoplasm; see Chapter 3.1 for MRS of tumors within the brain) of the CNS is characterized by a large mass lesion. Tumors are complex and under the conditions of conventional MR techniques, may closely resemble lesions seen in other neurological diseases (Hock et al., 2012). ^{1}H MRS may be of diagnostic value for spinal cord tumors because it gives in vivo information on the underlying pathological processes.

Kim et al. (2004) utilized ^{1}H MRS in spinal cord tumors of varying mass lesion, to examine metabolic changes between tumors and other neurological diseases. Using a 1.5 T MRI scanner, the group examined 14 patients with tumor compared to other mass lesions including non-multiple sclerosis myelitis, disc herniation, dermoid cyst, and tuberculosis. They reported the general observation, although without associated quantifications, that Cho was present only in spinal tumors, whereas other metabolic changes were similar to those of CNS tumors (Kim et al., 2004). This preliminary observation warrants follow-up studies as it suggests a potential for in vivo ^{1}H MRS to distinguish spinal cord tumors from the other CNS lesions tested in this study.

Using a higher field scanner (3 T), Dydak et al. (2005) reported increases in lactate and mI and lower NAA, visually shown in ^{1}H MRS spectra, of one patient with a primary spinal cord tumor compared to healthy controls. They examined various tumor regions of the cervical spinal cord including the pons, medulla oblongata, C1/C2, and C3/C4. Spectra from the spinal cord tumors were reported to be similar to spectra from brain tumors; however, upper cord region presented a different challenge of shimming than lower regions. This is due to inhomogeneities and differences in susceptibility of connective tissue and vertebral processes. Similarly, Henning et al. (2008) reported quantified decreases in NAA, Cr, Cho, and mI and increases in lactate and glutamine/glutamate in two patients with intramedullary spinal cord tumors. The observations were in two separate regions (C4–C5 in one patient and T9 in the other).[6] These results demonstrate that ^{1}H MRS methodology is sensitive enough to monitor metabolic changes in spinal cord tumors and despite challenges in some tissue ROIs, it may be a useful diagnostic criterion to differentiate these types of tumors from other types of diseases.

Hock et al. (2012) reported 3 patients with neoplastic lesions in the spinal cord compared to 13 healthy volunteers and 13 patients with MS. Spectra showed strongly reduced NAA/Cr, increased Cho/Cr, and strongly increased mI/Cr in addition to lipids and lactate compared to metabolite over Cr ratios measured in healthy controls. A unique feature of this study is that it shows a differentiation between low-grade neoplasia and demyelination—a distinction that might ultimately prevent a patient from biopsies or unnecessary surgeries. This study further supports the sensitivity and use of ^{1}H MRS in the differential diagnosis of varying types of spinal cord tumors and neuropathologies, despite limitations of SNR.

ALS

ALS is a rapidly progressive and fatal neurodegenerative disease, initially described in 1865 by Charcot (1865). ALS is characterized by selective degeneration of the upper and lower motor neurons, causing severe

---

[6]Sufficient shimming at the T9 level was accomplished at 12 Hz (full-width at half-maximum of the water peak).

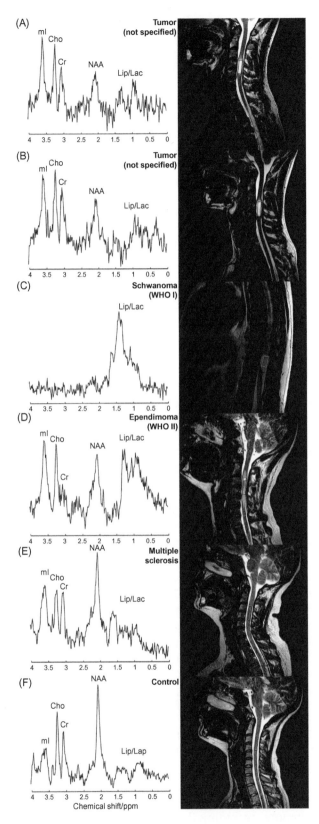

FIGURE 3.7.5 A demonstration of changes in metabolic concentrations according to neurological condition. (A–D) Spectra of patients with tumors, (C) Schwannoma, and (D) ependymoma in the spinal cord. (E) Spectra of a patient with MS. (F) spectra of a healthy control. (From Hock et al., 2012, with permission.)

muscle weakness and wasting. The axonal loss and ultimate loss of motor neurons results in a cascade of progressive paralysis affecting the skeletal musculature leaving the sufferer unable to walk and eventually unable to swallow or breathe. The cause of ALS is unknown and more than 90% of cases are sporadic (Hideyama & Kwak, 2011).

In familial cases of ALS, several genes have been implicated in the illness including a mutation in the Cu/Zn superoxide dismutase (SOD1) gene (Rosen et al., 1993; Jackson et al., 1997; Hideyama & Kwak, 2011), FUS/TLS (Kwiatkowski et al., 2009; Vance et al., 2009), and TARDBP (TDP-43; Kabashi et al., 2008; Sreedharan et al., 2008; Van Deerlin et al., 2008; Yokoseki et al., 2008). However, similar to other neurological disease studies, conventional methods such as the use of histological methods at a fixed-time point could be used to investigate the pathology of disease in the mouse model of familial ALS. Figure 3.7.6 shows collapsed myelin where axons have degenerated in the lumbar spinal cord below the ventral horn of mutant SOD1 transgenic mouse model of ALS shown by toll blue staining.

Spinal cord ^{1}H MRS has been recently applied to study ALS in patients (Pineda-Alonso et al., 2009; Carew et al., 2011a). Carew et al. (2011a) showed reduced NAA/Cr and NAA/mI in 14 ALS patients as compared to 16 controls (by 40 and 38%, respectively). The reduction in NAA/mI and NAA/Cho was found to be associated with clinical parameters, indicating that ^{1}H MRS may be a beneficial tool to assess pathological progression (Carew et al., 2011a).

A follow-up study by the same group examined the hypothesis that the onset of neurodegeneration might precede neurological symptoms appearing in early adulthood (Carew et al., 2011b). The group examined ^{1}H MRS on the cervical spinal cords of 24 presymptomatic SOD1-positive volunteers, 29 healthy controls, and 23 ALS patients. The study reported reduced ratios of NAA/Cr and NAA/mI in the SOD1-positive subjects (by 39.7 and 18%, respectively) and patients with ALS (41.2 and 24%, respectively) when compared to controls. The study also reported that mI/Cr was reduced in SOD1-positive subjects when compared to controls (by 10.3%); however, no difference was found between ALS patients and controls. NAA/Cho was also reduced in patients with ALS compared to controls (by 24%), but not in presymptomatic SOD1-positive volunteers. This study suggests that the ratios of metabolic concentrations are important in predicting signs of ALS prior to the onset of symptoms. These findings support the role of ^{1}H MRS in the spinal cord as a valuable tool to detect neurometabolic changes early in the course of disease.

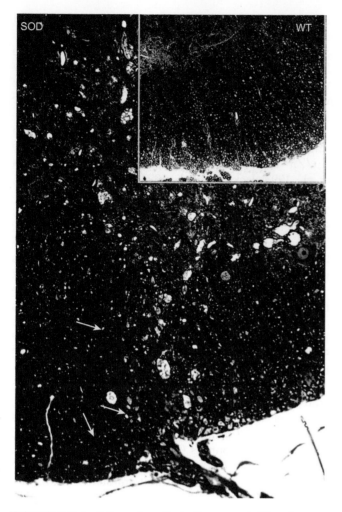

FIGURE 3.7.6 Collapsed myelin (yellow arrows), filling the space where axons have degenerated in L3 of the mutant SOD animal model of familial ALS compared to a wild-type (WT) control, as shown by Toll Blue staining. (Unpublished image courtesy of Amber Michelle Hill.)

FUTURE POTENTIAL OF ¹H MRS IN THE SPINAL CORD

At present, ¹H MRS studies are limited by small cohort sizes and technical limitations. These limitations have inevitably reduced our ability to monitor pathological changes throughout the entire spinal cord using live *in vivo* methodology. However, despite the challenges of ¹H MRS, published studies have shown the potential of ¹H MRS within the spinal cord of patients with neurological illnesses and animal models. Larger, prospective longitudinal studies are now needed to corroborate the findings to date and assess how long-term outcomes relate to changes in MRS metabolite concentrations at the time of acute injury.

Additionally, improvements in the technical aspects of ¹H MRS will provide reduced scanning time, increased spectral quality, and more accurate postprocessing. Optimization of ¹H MRS methodology will also allow for novel protocols in lower regions of the spinal cord, such as the lumbar and thoracic regions in human studies, which are at present not possible because these regions are too far from the surface coils for optimal sensitivity and movement distortions are too severe. As ultrahigh field scanners (7 T) increase in prevalence, they may enable the expansion of ¹H MRS techniques to other regions of the spinal cord, providing a more complete view of pathology in the CNS. Advances in magnetic resonance technology will improve the diagnosis, monitoring, and development of therapeutic drugs for neurological illnesses and perhaps empower targeted treatments for individual patients.

A key question that needs to be answered is whether MRS of the spinal cord provides biomarkers that are sensitive to clinical change and responsive to treatments. An important goal of clinical research that will provide more insight into the detection of biomarkers via a combination of MRS with structural and functional MR techniques is to obtain a complete view of spinal cord plasticity. More ¹H MRS research in the spinal cord and optimized protocols will improve our understanding of biomarkers and underlying mechanisms involved in the pathogenesis of various neurological diseases. These advanced insights into the pathogenesis of neurological diseases may be provided by the *in vivo* quantification of such metabolites in the future.

CONCLUSIONS

¹H MRS in the spinal cord is a valuable tool for the evaluation of biochemical changes and the diagnosis of several neurological conditions. ¹H MRS provides a noninvasive way to obtain additional information on the microenvironment within the spinal cord. The information on biochemical conditions in the spinal cord provided by ¹H MRS, also complemented by conventional MR techniques, provides more accurate diagnosis and monitoring of the pathogenesis of various neurological illnesses.

Spinal cord ¹H MRS allows the *in vivo* quantification of metabolites, which reflects specific pathological processes. Therefore, it provides insights into the underlying pathophysiological processes that are not detectable with conventional MR techniques. Technical limitations, including the small size of the cord, motion artifacts, and image distortions from the magnetic susceptibility at tissue/bone/air interface, have limited the use of ¹H MRS in preclinical and clinical settings. However, recent developments in imaging acquisition and postprocessing, as well as the increased availability of high-field scanners, have enabled the application of ^{1}H MRS in the spinal cord for clinical and preclinical investigation. Applications of ^{1}H MRS in the spinal cord may eventually become a standard for diagnostic criteria, differential diagnosis, and monitoring of therapeutic methodologies for individuals with spinal cord pathology.

References

Abourbeh, G., Thézé, B., Maroy, R., Dubois, A., Brulon, V., Fontyn, Y., et al. (2012). Imaging microglial/macrophage activation in spinal cords of experimental autoimmune encephalomyelitis rats by positron emission tomography using the mitochondrial 18 kDa translocator protein radioligand [^{18}F]DPA-714. *Journal of Neuroscience, 32*(17), 5728–5736.

Badawi, A. H., Kiptoo, P., Wang, W., Choi, I., Lee, P., Vines, C. M., et al. (2012). Suppression of EAE and prevention of blood-brain barrier breakdown after vaccination with novel bifunctional peptide inhibitor. *Neuropharmacology, 62*, 1874–1881.

Barker, P. B., Bizzi, A., Stefano, N., Gullapalli, R., & Lin, D. M. D. (2010). *Clinical MR Spectroscopy: Techniques and Applications.* Cambridge, UK: Cambridge University Press.

Bates, T. E., Strangward, M., Keelan, J., Davey, G. P., Munro, P. M. G., & Clark, J. B. (1996). Inhibition of N-acetylaspartate production: implications for 1H MRS studies *in vivo. Neuroreport, 7*, 1397–1400.

Benarroch, E. E. (2008). N-Acetylaspartate and N-acetylaspartylglutamate: neurobiology and clinical significance. *Neurology, 70*, 1353.

Bilgen, M., Elshaficy, I., & Narayana, P. A. (2001). *In vivo* magnetic resonance microscopy of rat spinal cord at 7 T using implantable RF coils. *Magnetic Resonance in Medicine, 46*, 1216–1222.

Blamire, A. M., Cader, S., Lee, M., Palace, & Matthews, P. M. (2007). Axonal damage in the spinal cord of multiple sclerosis patients detected by magnetic resonance spectroscopy. *Magnetic Resonance Spectroscopy, 58*, 880–885.

Brochet, B., Deloire, M. S. A., Touil, T., Anne, O., Caillé, J. M., Dousset, V., et al. (2006). Early macrophage MRI of inflammatory lesions predicts lesion severity and disease development in relapsing EAE. *Neuroimage, 32*, 266–274.

Budde, M. D., Xie, M., Cross, A. H., & Song, S. (2009). Axial diffusivity is the primary correlate of axonal injury in the experimental autoimmune encephalomyelitis spinal cord: a quantitative pixel-wise analysis. *Journal of Neuroscience, 29*(9), 2805–2813.

Callot, V., Tachrount, M., Laurin, J., Mauès de Paula, A., Marqueste, T., Decherchi, P., et al. (2012). Multimodal spinal cord MRI for temporal characterization of posttraumatic vascular, metabolic and structural events in a mouse model of spinal cord injury. *Proceedings of the International Society of Magnetic Resonance Medicine, 20*, 616.

Carew, J. D., Nair, G., Anderson, P. M., Wuu, J., Gronka, S., Hu, X., et al. (2011a). Presymptomatic spinal cord neurometabolic findings in *SOD1*-positive people at risk for ALS. *Neurology, 77*, 1370–1375.

Carew, J. D., Nair, G., Pineda-Alonso, N., Usher, S., Hu, X., & Benatar, M. (2011b). Magnetic resonance spectroscopy of the cervical cord in amyotrophic lateral sclerosis. *Amyotrophic Lateral Sclerosis, 12*, 185–191.

Charcot, J. M. (1865). Sclérose des cordons latéraux de la moelleépiniere chez une femme hystérique, atteinte de contracture permanente des quantremembres. *Bulletins et Memoires de la Societe Medicale des Hopitaux de Paris, 2*, 24–35 Second series.

Ciccarelli, O., Altmann, D. R., McLean, M. A., Wheeler-Kingshot, C. A., Wimpey, K., Miller, D. H., et al. (2010a). Spinal cord repair in MS: does mitochondrial metabolism play a role? *Neurology, 74*(9), 721–727.

Ciccarelli, O., Toosy Ahmed, T., De Stefano, N., Wheeler-Kingshott, C. A. M., Miller, D. H., & Thompson, A. J. (2010b). Assessing neuronal metabolism *in vivo* by modelling imaging measures. *Journal of Neuroscience, 30*(45), 15030–15033.

Ciccarelli, O., Wheeler-Kingshott, C. A., McLean, M. A., Cercignani, M., Wimpey, K., Miller, D. H., et al. (2007). Spinal cord spectroscopy and diffusion-based tactography to assess acute disability in multiple sclerosis. *Brain, 130*, 2220–2231.

Davie, C. A., Hawkins, C. P., Barker, G. J., Brennan, A., Tofts, P. S., Miller, D. H., et al. (1994). Serial proton magnetic resonance spectroscopy in acute multiple sclerosis lesions. *Brain, 117*(pt 1), 49–58.

De Stefano, N., Filippi., M., Miller, D., Pouwels, P. J., Rovira, A., Gass, A., et al. (2007). Guidelines for using proton MR spectroscopy in multicenter clinical MS studies. *Neurology, 69*(20), 1942–1952.

De Stefano, N., Matthews, P. M., & Arnold, D. L. (1995). Reversible decreases in N-acetylaspartate after acute brain injury. *Magnetic Resonance in Medicine, 34*, 721–727.

Dydak U., Kollias, S., Schär, M., Meier, D., & Boesiger, P. (2005).MR spectroscopy in different regions of the spinal cord and in spinal cord tumors. In: *Proceedings of the Annual Meeting of the International Society of Magnetic Resonance in Medicine, Miami Beach, Florida*, pp. 813.

Elliott, J. M., Pedler, A. R., Cowin, G., Sterling, M., & McMahon, K. (2012). Spinal cord metabolism and muscle water diffusion in whiplash. *Spinal Cord, 50*(6), 474–476.

Henning, A., Schar, M, Kollias, S. S., Boesiger, P., & Dydak, U. (2008). Quantitative magnetic resonance spectroscopy in the entire human cervical spinal cord and beyond at 3 T. *Magnetic Resonance in Medicine, 59*(6), 1250–1258.

Hideyama, T., & Kwak, S. (2011). When does ALS start? ADAR2-GluA2 hypothesis for the etiology of sporadic ALS. *Frontiers in Molecular Neuroscience, 4*, 33.

Hock, A., Fuchs, A., Boesiger, P, et al. (2012a). Spinal cord MRS spectroscopy in neoplastic lesions. In: *Proceedings of the Annual Meeting of the International Society of Magnetic Resonance in Medicine, Victoria, Australia*.

Hock, A., Henning, A., Boesiger, P., & Kollias, S. S. (2012b). ^{1}H-MR spectroscopy in the human spinal cord. *American Journal of Neuroradiology*, [Epub ahead of print].

Holly, L. T., Freitas, B., McArthur, D. L., & Salamon, N. (2009). Proton magnetic resonance spectroscopy to evaluate spinal cord axonal injury in cervical spondyloticmyelopathy. *Journal of Neurosurgery Spine, 10*(3), 194–200.

Jackson, M., Al-Chalabi, A., Enayat, Z. E., Chioza, B., Leigh, P. N., & Morrison, K. E. (1997). Copper/zinc superoxide dismutase 1 and sporadic amyotrophic lateral sclerosis: analysis of 155 cases and identification of a novel insertion mutation. *Annals of Neurology, 42*, 803–807.

Kabashi, E., Valmanis, P. N., Dion, P., Spiegelman, D., McConkey, B. J., Velde, V. C., et al. (2008). TARDBP mutations in individuals with sporadic and familial amyotrophic lateral sclerosis. *Nature Genetics, 40*, 572–574.

Kachramanoglou, C., De Vita, E., Thomas, D. L., Wheeler-Kingshott, C. A., Balteau, E., Carlstedt, T., et al. (2013). Metabolic changes in the spinal cord after brachial plexus root re-implantation. *Neurorehabilitation and Neural Repair, 27*(2), 118–124.

Kendi, A. T. K., Tan, F. U., Kendi, M., Huvaj, S., & Tellioğlu, S. (2004). MR spectroscopy of cervical spinal cord in patients with multiple sclerosis. *Neuroradiology, 46*, 764–769.

Kim, Y. G, Choi, G. H., Kim, D. H., Kim, Y. D., Kang, Y. K., & Kim, J. K. (2004). *In vivo* proton magnetic resonance spectroscopy of human spinal mass lesions. *Journal of Spinal Disorders and Technology, 17*(5), 405–411.

Koliatsos, V. E., Price, W. L., Pardo, C. A., & Price, D. L. (1994). Ventral root avulsion: an experimental model of death of adult motor neurons. *Journal of Comparative Neurology, 342*(1), 35–44.

Kwiatkowski, T. J., Jr., Bosco, D. A., Leclerc, A. L., Tamrazian, E., Vanderburg, C. R., Russ, C., et al. (2009). Mutations in the FUS/TLS gene on chromosome 16 cause familial amyotrophic lateral sclerosis. *Science, 323*, 1205–1208.

MacKenzie-Graham, A., Rinek, G. A., Avedisian, A, Gold, S. M., Frew, A. J., Aguilar, C., et al. (2012). Cortical atrophy in experimental autoimmune encephalomyelitis: *In vivo* imaging. *Neuroimage, 60*, 95–106.

Mader, I., Roser, W., Kappos, I., Hagberg, G., Seelig, J., Radue, E. W., et al. (2000). Serial proton MR spectroscopy of contrast-enhancing multiple sclerosis plaques: absolute metabolic values over 2 years during a clinical pharmacological study. *American Journal of Neuroradiology, 21*, 1220–1227.

Marliani, A. F., Clementi, V., Albini-Riccioli, L., Agati, R., Carpenzano, M., Salvi, F., et al. (2010). Quantitative cervical spinal cord 3 T proton MR spectroscopy in multiple sclerosis. *American Journal of Neuroradiology, 31*, 180–184.

Marliani, A. F., Clementi, V., Albini-Riccioli, L., Agati, R., & Leonardi, M. (2007). Quantitative proton magnetic resonance spectroscopy of the human cervical spinal cord at 3 tesla. *Magnetic Resonance in Medicine, 57*, 160–163.

Moffett, J. R., Ross, B., Arun, P., & Madhavarao, C. N. (2007). N-Acetylaspartate in the CNS: from neurodiagnostics to neurobiology. *Progress in Neurobiology, 81*, 89–131.

Natt, O., Bezkorovaynyy, V., Michaelis, T., & Frahm, J. (2005). Use of phased array coils for a determination of absolute metabolite concentrations. *Magnetic Resonance in Medicine, 53*, 3–8.

Nelson, A. L. A., Bieber, A. J., & Rodriguez, M. (2004). Contrasting murine models of MS. *International MS Journal, 11*, 95–99.

Pineda-Alonso, N., Benatar, M., Hu, X., & Carew, J. (2009). Proton magnetic resonance spectroscopy (1H-MRS) on the spinal cord in amyotrophic lateral sclerosis (ALS) at 3 T. *Proceedings of the Annual Meeting of the International Society of Magnetic Resonance in Medicine, 17*, 3325 Honolulu, Hawaii.

Qian, J., Herrera, J. J., & Narayana, P. A. (2010). Neuronal and axonal degeneration in experimental spinal cord injury: in vivo proton magnetic resonance spectroscopy and histology. *Journal of Neurotrauma, 27*, 599–610.

Rosen, D. R., Siddique, T., Patterson, D., Figlewicz, D. A., Sapp, P., Hentati, A., et al. (1993). Mutations in Cu/Zn superoxide dismutase gene are associated with familial amyotrophic lateral sclerosis. *Nature, 362*, 59–62.

Sajja, B. R., Narayana, P. A., Wolinsky, J. S., Ahn, C. W., & PROMiSe Trial MRSI Group (2008). Longitudinal magnetic resonance spectroscopic imaging of primary progressive multiple sclerosis patients treated with glatiramer acetate: multicenter study. *Multiple Sclerosis, 14*(1), 73–80.

Silver, X., Ni, W. X., Mercer, E. V., Beck, B. L., Bossart, E. L., Inglis, B., et al. (2001). *In vivo* ¹H magnetic resonance imaging and spectroscopy of the rat spinal cord using an inductively-coupled chronically implanted RF coil. *Magnetic Resonance in Medicine, 46*, 1216–1222.

Solanky, B. S., Abdel-Aziz, K., Yiannakas, M. C., Berry, A. M., Ciccarelli, O., & Wheeler-Kingshott, C. A. (2013). *In vivo* magnetic resonance spectroscopy detection of combined glutamate-glutamine in a healthy upper cervical cord at 3 T. *NMR in Biomedicine, 23*(3), 357–366.

Sreedharan, J., Blair, I. P., Tripathi, V. B., Hu, X., Vance, C., Rogelj, B., et al. (2008). TDP-43 mutations in familial and sporadic amyotrophic lateral sclerosis. *Science, 319*, 1668–1672.

Sriram, S., & Steiner, I. (2005). Experimental allergic encephalomyelitis: a misleading model of MS. *Annals of Neurology, 58*(6), 939–945.

Tachrount, M., Duhamel, G., Laurin, J., Marqueste, T., Maues de Paula, A., Decherchi, P., et al. (2012). *In vivo* short TE localized ¹H MR Spectroscopy of mouse cervical spinal cord at very high magnetic field (11.75 T). *Magnetic Resonance in Medicine, 68* (6), 1–7.

Tachrount, M., Duhamel, G., Maues de Paula, A., Laurin, J., Marqueste, T., Decherchi, P., et al. (2011). Medullar and thalamic metabolic alterations following spinal cord injury (SCI): a preliminary mice study, combining early and longitudinal follow-ups using high-spatial resolved MRS and DTI at high field. *Annual meeting of ISMRM, 401*.

Van Deerlin, V. M., Leverenz, J. B., Bekris, L. M., Bird, T. D., Yuan, W., Elman, L. B., et al. (2008). TARDBP mutations in amyotrophic lateral sclerosis with TDP-43 neuropathology: a genetic and histopathological analysis. *Lancet Neurology, 7*, 409–416.

Yiannakas, M. C., Kearney, H., Samson, R. S., Chard, D. T., Ciccarelli, O., Miller, D. H., et al. (2012). Feasibility of grey matter and white matter segmentation of the upper cervical cord in vivo: A pilot study with application to magnetisation transfer measurements. *Neuroimage, 63*(3), 1054–1059.

Yokoseki, A., Shiga, A., Tan, C. F., Tagawa, A., Kaneko, H., Koyama, A., et al. (2008). TDP-43 mutation in familial amyotrophic lateral sclerosis. *Annals of Neurology, 63*, 538–542.

Zelaya, F. O., Chalk, J. B., Mullins, P., Brereton, I. M., & Doddrell, D. M. (1996). Localized ¹H NMR spectroscopy of rat spinal cord in vivo. *Magnetic Resonance in Medicine, 35*, 443–448.

Interindividual Differences in Behavior and Plasticity

Velicia Bachtiar and Charlotte J. Stagg

Oxford Centre for Functional MRI of the Brain (FMRIB), Nuffield Department of Clinical Neurosciences, University of Oxford, UK

INTRODUCTION

Considerable differences exist between individuals both in the way the brain functions normally and how it recovers from injury. Plasticity can be defined as the reorganization of brain connectivity through experience, and animal studies have shown that modulation of intracortical inhibitory circuits is necessary for plasticity induction to occur. There is significant interest among both the clinical and neuroscience communities in investigating the role of inhibitory processes in normal brain function and in how this can help us understand pathophysiology in disease. Since the pioneering work of Rothman and colleagues (Rothman et al., 1993), it is now possible to measure the main inhibitory neurotransmitter γ-amino butyric acid (GABA) in humans using magnetic resonance spectroscopy (MRS). The ability to measure GABAergic inhibition *in vivo* has sparked interest in investigating interindividual differences in the role of GABA in behavior and the effects on GABA concentrations following plasticity-induction paradigms. This chapter will summarize what has been learned about interindividual differences in behavior from MRS studies and explore its potential use in the future.

SUMMARY OF GABA METABOLISM

Within GABAergic neurons, GABA is primarily produced from glutamate via the enzyme glutamic acid decarboxylase (GAD) and is metabolized to succinic acid semialdehyde in the astrocytes by GABA transaminase (GABA-T; Petroff & Rothman, 1998). Two molecular forms of GAD (65 and 67 kDa) exist and these are thought to regulate the two major pools of GABA: the cytoplasmic pool found throughout the neuron and the vesicular pool found in their presynaptic boutons (Martin & Barke, 1998). Cytoplasmic GABA is primarily produced by the tonically active GAD67 and is found almost evenly distributed throughout the neuron. It is thought to be the rate-limiting step in GABA production (Chattopadhyaya et al., 2007) and has an activity-dependent role in GABA synthesis such that decreased network activity leads to decreased expression of GAD67, which in turn leads to lower GABA levels (Lau & Murthy, 2012). Vesicular GABA on the other hand, is found in high concentrations within the presynaptic boutons and is regulated by the phasically active GAD65, playing a key role in inhibitory synaptic neurotransmission (Martin & Rimvall, 1993). For a more detailed account on the biochemistry of GABA synthesis, see Chapter 2.5.

Evidence suggests that extracellular GABA is related to intracellular GABA (Petroff & Rothman, 1998). The level of GABA present in synaptic terminals and in the extracellular fluid depends on the metabolic cycle between neurons and glia. Nerve-terminal GABA is synthesized from glutamate, and enters the extracellular fluid by neurotransmitter release from where it is either recycled back into the nerve terminal or taken up by astrocytes (Petroff, 2002).

Two main subtypes of receptors mediate the synaptic effects of GABA within the cortex: fast-acting ionotropic $GABA_A$ receptors that gate chloride ions and slow-acting $GABA_B$ metabotropic receptors that activate potassium channels (Schousboe et al., 2007). GABA also acts at nonsynaptic $GABA_A$ receptors, producing the so-called "GABAergic tone" (Martin & Rimvall, 1993).

243

DATA FROM ANIMAL MODELS OF PLASTICITY INDUCTION

Plasticity occurs in the neocortex via a multitude of mechanisms over a wide range of timescales, from the relatively rapid strengthening of existing synaptic connections and unmasking of latent synapses (synaptic plasticity), to longer term mechanisms such as the formation of new synapses, and new neuronal structures. This chapter will concentrate on one of the earliest plasticity mechanisms, synaptic plasticity, and, in particular, on long-term potentiation (LTP)-like synaptic changes, which are dependent on the modulation of both glutamatergic and GABAergic signaling (Bear & Malenka, 1994). In the motor cortex, reduction of local inhibition is a necessary first step in the induction of LTP-like plasticity in primary motor cortex (M1) horizontal fiber pathways (Jacobs & Donoghue, 1991), and is thought to be responsible for the remodeling of motor representations in M1 (Hess & Donoghue, 1994). Animal studies have shown that preventing this GABAergic decrease results in an inability to induce LTP-like plasticity within the cortex (Castro-Alamancos et al., 1995), whereas reducing GABA inhibition facilitates LTP-like plasticity induction (Trepel & Racine, 2000).

QUANTIFYING GABA IN HUMANS IN VIVO

The role of GABA is well established in the induction of LTP-like processes underpinning neuroplastic mechanisms in animal models. In humans, it has been less straightforward to investigate the role of GABA in these processes in vivo. However, recent technological and methodological advances in neuroimaging and in noninvasive brain stimulation have lead to new insights into the mechanisms that underlie neuroplastic processes in humans.

MRS

GABA was first detected in vivo in the rat brain using ^{1}H nuclear magnetic resonance (NMR) spectroscopy (Rothman et al., 1984). MRS is the commonly used term for in vivo application of ^{1}H NMR using MR imaging (MRI) and allows for the accurate quantification of endogenous metabolites within a localized region (or voxel) of tissue. As described in detail in Chapter 1.1, the MRS signal is derived from differences in the molecular structure of metabolites with chemically specific frequencies. If the MRS signal is plotted as a function of frequency, individual peaks can be identified in the spectrum, which represent signal intensity from different metabolites. The chemical shift is most commonly reported in units of parts per million (ppm) of the proton frequency, a measure independent of the scanner field strength. For example, N-acetylaspartate (NAA), a marker of neuronal mitochondrial function found in high concentrations in the brain and often utilized as a reference peak, is shown to give a signal at 2.0 ppm regardless of the scanner used.

In humans, quantifying GABA in vivo has been less straightforward than some other neurochemicals due to its low concentrations in the brain and the overlap between its resonances and those of other molecules found in higher concentration such as creatine, glutamate, and glutamine. Since the pioneering work of Rothman and colleagues (1993), we can now accurately quantify GABA in the human brain. The MEscher–GArwood-Point RESolved Spectroscopy (MEGA-PRESS) method is currently the most widely applied, which allows for simultaneous 3D voxel localization, water suppression, and editing for accurate quantification of GABA (Mescher et al., 1998). The GABA concentration is often reported relative to a standard reference metabolite, most commonly NAA or creatine, which are both found at relatively high concentrations in the brain. Unlike referencing to water or reporting absolute concentrations of GABA, referencing to standard metabolites acquired in the same spectra has the added benefit of controlling for any nonspecific changes in neuronal density, for example, caused by edema. However, internal referencing to these metabolites can be problematic in clinical studies as these levels can vary with disease states and drug interventions (Ongur et al., 2009).

Another disadvantage of MRS GABA-edited methods is their reliance upon the subtraction of signals to remove strong overlapping frequencies from the spectrum in order to reveal GABA (Puts & Edden, 2012). Any experimental noise in the form of instrumental factors or subject movement can result in subtraction artifacts, which can then obscure the edited GABA signal (Waddell et al., 2007). Furthermore, some macromolecules, which primarily contain proteins (Behar et al., 1994) have a resonance at 3.0 ppm that is coupled to a resonance at 1.7 ppm near the GABA peak. Thus at lower field strengths the edited "GABA" peak may include a contribution from those macromolecules that need to be considered in quantification.

It is possible that many of these limitations can be improved with increasing magnetic field strength above 3 T (Tkac & Gruetter, 2005), which allows for increased signal-to-noise ratio (SNR), far less contamination of the spectrum and thus, improved editing of macromolecular contributions (Henry et al., 2001).

The number of sites with the more powerful 7 T magnets is currently limited, although such magnets are likely to be used more widely for better quantification of GABA in the future.

Transcranial Magnetic Stimulation

Another method for assessing GABAergic activity in humans is via transcranial magnetic stimulation (TMS). TMS is a noninvasive neurostimulation technique that induces a flow of current in the brain via the principles of electromagnetic induction (Hallett, 2000). A magnetic field is generated via a brief current flowing through a figure-of-eight coil of wire placed on the scalp, which in turn induces an electric current in the underlying brain tissue (Fig. 3.8.1). When TMS is applied to the primary motor cortex it can elicit a peripheral response and its effects can be measured via the study of electromyographic (EMG) recordings of affected muscles. TMS is typically targeted to the

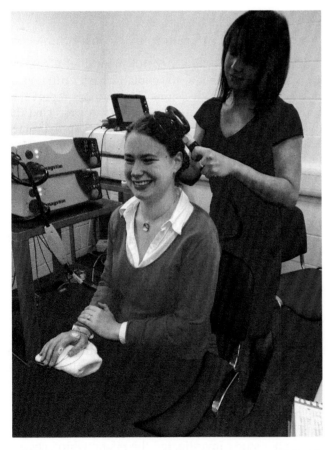

FIGURE 3.8.1 A typical experimental setup using TMS. The figure-of-eight coil is placed on the scalp, which in turn induces an electric current in the underlying brain tissue. A peripheral response is measured by EMG recordings from the target muscle on the hand and the MEP recorded within the target muscle using electrodes. This figure is reproduced in color in the color plate section.

primary motor cortex by finding the "motor hotspot," the scalp position at which the lowest intensity TMS pulse evokes a just noticeable response, or a motor evoked potential (MEP) within the targeted muscle. The intensity of stimulation is then calibrated for an individual subject by modulating the intensity of the stimulation to elicit an MEP of a predefined size. The intensity of the TMS pulse that elicits an MEP of $>50\,\mu V$ in 5 of 10 pulses is known as the resting motor threshold and gives an index of the ease with which signals can pass from M1 to the muscles.

Within the primary motor cortex, GABAergic activity can be measured using paired-pulse TMS approaches, which involve giving two magnetic stimuli delivered in close sequence to the same cortical region through a single stimulation coil. An interstimulus interval (ISI) of 2–4 ms results in short-interval intracortical inhibition (SICI) and is thought to reflect $GABA_A$-mediated inhibition (Kujirai et al., 1993). The first (conditioning) stimulus is set at a subthreshold intensity that is low enough to stimulate the smaller cortical interneurons but not the pyramidal neurons. This then modulates the effects of the second (test) suprathreshold stimulus, giving a smaller magnitude of response due to the influence of GABAergic interneurons. Increasing the ISI to 50–200 ms with a suprathreshold conditioning stimulus results in long-interval intracortical inhibition (LICI) and is thought to reflect $GABA_B$ activity (Valls-Sole et al., 1992).

It is also possible to induce inhibition of the pyramidal neurons using an SICI protocol with an interstimulus of 1 ms. It is less clear exactly what this inhibition reflects, but it is known to be a GABAergic phenomenon with a distinct mechanism from the 2–4 ms ISI SICI and has been postulated to reflect extrasynaptic GABAergic tone (Stagg et al., 2011d).

Another TMS protocol used to investigate inhibitory phenomena is to measure the cortical silent period (CSP). The CSP is the period of "silence" observed as the absence of activity from the muscle of interest in EMG after an MEP caused by the TMS pulse. The CSP is measured by applying a TMS pulse during tonic contraction of a target muscle. The recovery of the EMG signal is thought to depend on the recovery of motor cortical excitability from GABAergic inhibition following the TMS pulse (Fuhr et al., 1991). It is likely that this inhibition is $GABA_B$ dependent, although it does not appear to reflect identical circuits as LICI (Wassermann et al., 2008).

Although TMS is a powerful tool for investigating inhibitory cortical circuits, the TMS protocols mentioned are not entirely specific. For example, studies have shown that SICI and LICI interact with each other and it still remains unclear whether the same population of neurons mediates both these measures (for review, see Reis et al., 2008). CSP measures have high intrinsic variability and are dependent on various experimental factors such as coil positioning and TMS strength (Orth & Rothwell, 2004). Furthermore, it is possible that each behavioral state studied with TMS could condition fundamentally different cortical interactions (Allen et al., 2007), and care should be taken when making generalizing conclusions on the role of inhibitory and excitatory processes beyond the behaviors specifically tested.

The relationship between MRS-assessed GABA and TMS-assessed GABA is currently unclear. This is likely due to the lack of specificity of both TMS protocols (for review, see Sandrini et al., 2011) and MRS methods (Stagg et al., 2011b). The spatial scale over which the two techniques are sensitive to GABAergic activity differs greatly. MRS requires a relatively large voxel volume, commonly $2 \times 2 \times 2$ cm or greater to obtain enough SNR for accurate quantification of GABA. It is not precisely clear over what spatial scale TMS is sensitive. This makes direct comparisons between the two methods problematic (Stagg et al., 2011d). Studies that have compared the two techniques suggest that MRS-GABA does not solely reflect either $GABA_A$ or $GABA_B$ activity alone or in combination (Stagg et al., 2011d), but appears to be most sensitive to extrasynaptic GABA tone. It is important to note, however, that there is a close relationship between intracellular and extracellular GABA concentrations (see Chapter 2.5).

However, although this relationship has been demonstrated between TMS and MRS measures at baseline it should not be inferred that decreases in GABA concentration seen with plasticity induction protocols are due solely to decreases in extrasynaptic GABAergic tone, but are likely to reflect changes in both synaptic activity and extrasynaptic activity.

CHAPTER OUTLINE

Despite the methodological considerations (as discussed in the MRS section and in Chapter 2.5), MRS is still a powerful tool to investigate the role of GABA in the human cortex *in vivo*. Although traditionally it has been used within a clinical context (Laxer, 1997), MRS is increasingly used in cognitive neuroscience to study the healthy human brain. Over the past decade MRS studies have flourished, and can be grouped loosely into four types of studies: those investigating interindividual differences in GABA concentration in healthy subjects, those investigating differences in GABA levels within clinical populations, those investigating changes in GABA with a behavioral intervention, and correlational studies using multi-modality imaging.

INTERINDIVIDUAL DIFFERENCES IN GABA CAN BE RELATED TO BEHAVIOR

Studies looking at interindividual differences in humans have traditionally focused on higher level cognitive functions at the level of personality and intelligence. Interindividual differences in data of more basic functions such as motor control are often treated as a source of noise and studies typically focus on the change in mean response associated with an experimental manipulation (Kanai & Rees, 2011). However, this averaging process precludes the use of potentially meaningful information on natural variations in behavior and ignores individual differences. Recent studies using MRS have shown that, in addition to relationships between GABA levels and higher level cognitive functions, there are also significant differences in the neural basis of more basic cognitive functions, such as sensorimotor behavior. Higher GABA levels have been related both to better and worse performance across a range of tasks and brain regions.

Interindividual Differences in Healthy Subjects

Sumner and colleagues (2010) quantified GABA in the frontal eye fields to explain basic differences in individual action decisions. The authors report that individual differences in baseline GABA predicted the ability to rapidly resolve competitive action decisions, here measured in the form of saccades to visual targets presented with distractors, such that people with higher GABA levels were less influenced by the presence of distractors.

Similarly, differences in baseline GABA concentration in the supplementary motor area (SMA) between subjects predicted their ability to suppress subliminal motor activations evoked by visual priming (Boy et al., 2010). The SMA is a region previously associated with automatic motor control and the authors demonstrate that subjects with naturally higher levels of inhibition within the SMA were more likely to have less suppression of the initial subliminal motor activation evoked by early visual priming than those with lower GABA levels. Given the SMA functions as part of a network with other regions, the direction of these findings imply that the SMA is involved upstream in the production of suppression rather than the site of inhibition.

Another study investigated the relationship between GABA levels within a sensorimotor voxel and performance of a tactile discrimination task. The authors demonstrated a significant relationship, such that subjects with higher levels of GABA were better at performing the task (Puts et al., 2011).

However, with less complex behaviors, particularly those involving the primary motor and visual regions, there is an inverse relationship between GABA levels and behavior. For example, Stagg et al. (2011a) demonstrated that subjects with higher baseline GABA levels had slower reaction times and also smaller motor task-related blood oxygen level-dependent (BOLD) signal change in response to a visually cued motor task. This relationship was observed only in the primary motor cortex and not in a control voxel placed on the visual cortex, suggesting a specific regional and task-relevant relationship. Similar findings are also shown with measurements from the primary visual cortex (Muthukumaraswamy et al., 2009). Baseline GABA concentration in the visual cortex was both inversely correlated with the magnitude of the BOLD response induced by a simple visual gating stimulus (Fig. 3.8.2B) and positively correlated with the gamma oscillation frequency as measured by magnetoencephalography (MEG; Fig. 3.8.2A), suggesting that functional neuroimaging metrics are dependent on the excitation and inhibition balance in an individual's cortex, here measured by resting GABA levels.

In all these studies, GABA differences were found in the voxel of interest related to the task, but not in a control voxel located in regions unrelated to the task. This highlights the regional specificity of baseline levels of GABA. Thus, in interpreting MRS studies it is important to remember that the GABA levels are measured from an *a priori* defined area of interest. The measurements cannot be used to infer global relationships; rather, they reflect regionally specific correlations. This places extra importance on a strong *a priori* hypothesis for targeting specific brain regions in the experimental design. Studies measuring GABA from a less defined area are likely to be more difficult to interpret.

Mechanisms Underlying Interindividual Differences

It is still unclear why natural differences in baseline GABA concentration occur, and what factors determine their regional specificity. Physiologically, these differences could reflect natural variation in the density of GABA interneurons in a given area, the number of synapses per neuron, or the concentration of GABA per synapse. Methodological limitations currently prevent the direct pinpointing of the cellular mechanisms involved, but it is likely that a combination of all these factors leads to the degree of variability in GABA levels between subjects. Despite this, a study investigating *in vivo* intracerebral GABA using ^{1}H MRS has shown good intrasubject and intersubject reproducibility (Bogner et al., 2010), suggesting that MRS has good potential to be used in clinical and scientific settings to detect even small alterations in brain GABA.

GABA CHANGES IN CLINICAL POPULATIONS

The understanding of natural differences in inhibition in normal brain function can give important insights into the pathophysiology of disorders where GABA-mediated inhibition has been implicated. Abnormalities in GABA concentrations have been

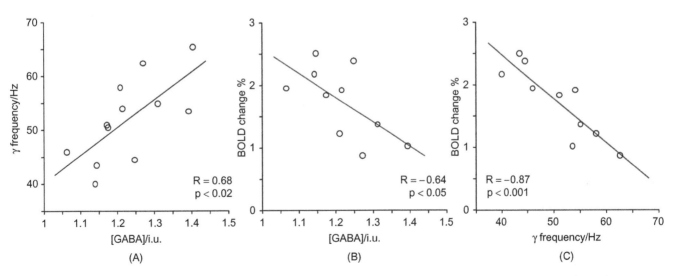

FIGURE 3.8.2 Baseline GABA and MEG gamma oscillations. Correlation plots with best-fit regression lines showing for each participant the relationship between (A) peak gamma oscillation frequency and GABA concentration, (B) BOLD response magnitude and GABA concentration, and (C) BOLD response magnitude versus peak gamma oscillation frequency. (From Muthukumaraswamy et al., 2009)

reported in a wide range of neurological and psychiatric disorders including schizophrenia and epilepsy. For example, it has been shown that reduced GABA levels are found in the basal ganglia of early stage schizophrenic patients (Goto et al., 2009), whereas increased GABA levels were found in the prefrontal cortex of drug-naive patients with schizophrenia (Choe et al., 1994). With regards to epilepsy there is great interest in the role of GABA in understanding the pathophysiology of seizures and in terms of its use as drug treatments. Low cortical GABA is reported in untreated epileptics who frequently have seizures and drugs such as vigabatrin can elevate brain GABA (for review, see Petroff et al., 2002). For an extensive review on the role of GABA in schizophrenia and epilepsy, see Chapters 3.6 and 3.3, respectively.

Within neurodevelopmental syndromes such as the autism spectrum disorders (ASDs), there is accumulating evidence that points toward a dysfunction in GABAergic inhibitory signaling as being responsible for the behavioral symptoms observed. These findings are primarily from genetic and postmortem gene-expression data (for review, see Coghlan et al., 2012) and *in vivo* human evidence is currently limited. One MRS study reported reduced GABA levels in the frontal lobe of patients with autism (Harada et al., 2011) but not in the basal ganglia. However, as most subjects were sedated before the scan, the interpretations of the results are difficult. Other studies have used TMS to examine intracortical inhibition in ASD, but have shown confounding results, with two studies showing reduced inhibition only in some subgroups of patients (Enticott et al., 2010; Oberman et al., 2010), and one large study reporting no significant differences in intracortical inhibition between ASD adults and controls (Enticott et al., 2012). The use of MRS in the future to reconcile findings from genetic and epigenetic data will be crucial in understanding the pathophysiology of ASD and the role of GABA in its development.

Abnormalities in GABA processing have also been demonstrated in dystonia, a neurological diagnosis characterized by sustained muscle contractions leading to repetitive movements or abnormal posturing. Patients have been shown to have decreased GABA levels within the affected M1 compared with controls (Levy & Hallett, 2002). In addition, patients do not show the characteristic decrease in SICI seen in healthy controls during movement preparation (Stinear & Byblow, 2004). It may be, however, that in this context the decreased GABA seen with MRS reflects a decrease in surround inhibition—a phenomenon where the cortical representations immediately surrounding a muscle preparing to move show increased inhibition—which would go some way toward explaining why the

spread of activity occurs from one muscle to another in dystonia (Beck et al., 2008, 2009a,b).

Evidently, abnormalities in brain metabolites are characteristic of a variety of neuropsychiatric disorders (Maddock & Buonocore, 2012). There is compelling evidence to suggest that deficits in the GABA system are closely involved in the pathophysiology of various disorders. However, the specific mechanisms are currently unclear and results are made more difficult to interpret with the range of medication that these patients take often from a young age. Future investigations should focus on characterizing the pattern of region-specific GABA to behavioral differences in healthy individuals to untangle the wide range of evidence on disorders with GABAergic abnormalities.

GABAERGIC CHANGES IN PLASTICITY INDUCTION

Despite the established role of GABA in cortical plasticity, studies investigating the changes in GABA

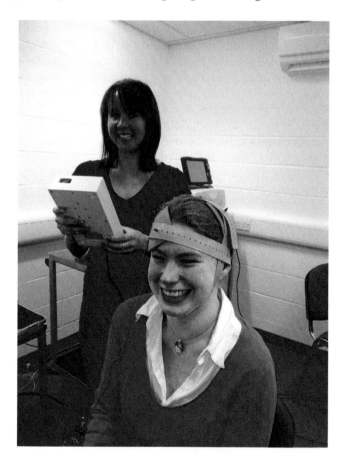

FIGURE 3.8.3 A typical experimental setup using tDCS. A DC stimulator delivers a current up to 2 mA to the brain via two electrodes. One electrode is placed above the area of interest, in this case M1, and the reference electrode is placed over the contralateral supra-orbital ridge. This figure is reproduced in color in the color plate section.

after behavioral interventions are still limited. Looking at changes in GABA during motor learning, decreased GABA levels were observed in the sensorimotor cortex during motor sequence learning but not during random movement or when subjects were at rest (Floyer-Lea et al., 2006). Similarly, temporary deafferentation of the hand with an ischemic nerve block, an intervention known to decrease GABA levels, has been shown to facilitate practice-dependent plasticity in the motor cortex (Ziemann et al., 2001).

In addition to endogenous modulation of plasticity within M1 via motor learning or acute deafferentation, a few studies have examined the response of the primary motor cortex to exogenous plasticity-induction paradigms using transcranial stimulation approaches. Stagg and colleagues (2009) investigated the effects of continuous theta burst stimulation (TBS) on GABA levels within the motor cortex. TBS is a TMS protocol whereby a burst of three supra-threshold TMS pulses are given at 50 Hz, with an interburst interval of 200 ms. If applied continuously for 40 s (a total of 600 pulses), TBS has been shown to decrease cortical excitability and induce long-term depression (LTD)-like plasticity (Huang et al., 2005).

In line with the finding that continuous TBS induces cortical inhibition, increased GABA levels were reported within M1 following continuous TBS stimulation (Stagg et al., 2009).

Studies have also investigated the effects of transcranial direct current stimulation (tDCS) on the GABAergic system (Stagg et al., 2009, 2011). tDCS is a noninvasive neuromodulatory technique that involves passing a small electric current (1–2 mA) through the brain for up to 20 min via two large (5 × 7 cm) electrodes placed on the scalp, the active electrode over the cortical region of interest (the primary motor cortex in the studies discussed here) and the reference over the contralateral supra-orbital ridge (Fig. 3.8.3). The effects of tDCS are dependent on the direction of current—anodal stimulation, where the current passes from the active electrode over M1 to the reference electrode over the contralateral supra-orbital ridge increases cortical excitability and is thought to induce LTP-like plasticity, whereas cathodal stimulation, where the current direction is reversed, decreases cortical excitability and leads to LTD-like effects (Nitsche & Paulus, 2000).

Anodal tDCS, which is facilitatory, leads to a significant decrease in GABA levels within M1 (Stagg et al.,

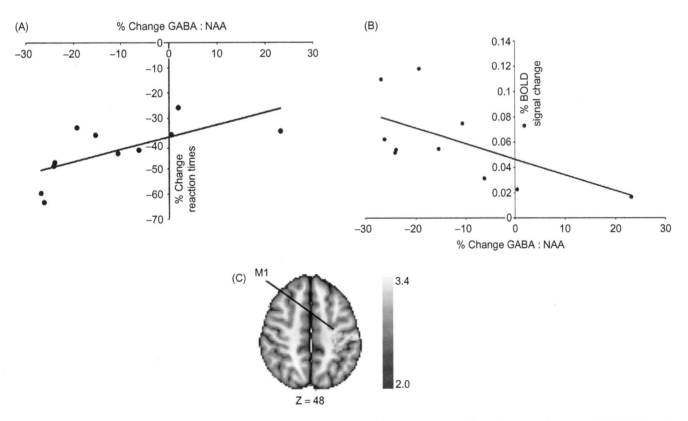

FIGURE 3.8.4 Changes in GABA with anodal tDCS modulation. (A) Significant positive correlation between change in GABA:NAA ratio due to anodal tDCS and change in reaction times due to learning ($r = 0.645$, $p = 0.03$). (B) One cluster in left primary motor cortex showed a negative correlation between learning-related change in fMRI activity and change in GABA:NAA ratios due to anodal tDCS. (C) Negative correlation between change in GABA:NAA ratios due to anodal tDCS and the learning-related change in fMRI activity in the left M1 region of interest (arbitrary units; $r = 20.59$, $p = 0.05$, uncorrected). (From Stagg et al., 2011a.) Part C is reproduced in color in the color plate section.

2009). In addition, it has been demonstrated that the degree of tDCS-induced GABA decrease is related to the degree of learning in a motor task performed on a separate day, such that subjects with the greatest drop in anodal tDCS-induced GABA also had the greatest drop in their reaction times during a motor task (Stagg et al., 2011a; Fig. 3.8.4A). Thus, subjects who were better learners were also the most responsive to anodal stimulation. The study also demonstrated that the degree of GABA decrease within M1 in response to anodal tDCS further correlated with the learning-related changes in functional MRI (fMRI) activity (Fig. 3.8.4B) specifically within the hand region of the primary motor cortex (Fig. 3.8.4C). These findings are consistent with the hypothesis from the animal literature that the induction of LTP-like plasticity is dependent on GABA modulation, and suggest that learning processes and GABA modulation are closely linked in humans, and further, that this relationship is specific to the region where learning is thought to occur.

However, it is important to note that the studies reported here by their nature measure correlations between GABA and behavioral interventions but do not infer causality. It is still unclear whether decreases in GABA are necessary for plasticity induction to occur in humans, or whether it is simply a closely linked phenomenon.

Clinical Implications for Exogenous GABA Modulation

The previously presented evidence that anodal tDCS can decrease GABA levels within the stimulated cortex and that this decrease is related to the degree of plasticity, raise the possibility that enhancement of the brain environment to promote plasticity could be a potential target for therapeutic interventions following damage to the human cortex. For example, there is increasing evidence of the beneficial effects of anodal tDCS applied to the ipsilesional M1 as an adjunct therapy in stroke rehabilitation (Stagg et al., 2011c; Butler et al., 2013). However, relatively little is known about the physiological mechanisms underlying the effects of tDCS after stroke and whether these beneficial effects are mediated via GABA modulation. Better understanding of changes in brain metabolites during transcranial stimulation in clinical populations is essential to evaluate the clinical applicability of these techniques and to optimize their use in a clinical setting. It is hoped that further investigation may eventually lead to individually tailored rehabilitation programs as a part of post-stroke care to reduce long-term disability. The use of MRS will help answer many of these questions.

RELATIONSHIP TO MRS-ASSESSED GABA AND INFORMATION DERIVED FROM OTHER IMAGING MODALITIES

A number of studies have investigated the relationship between MRS-derived measures of GABA and a number of other imaging modalities. Multimodal imaging has the potential to combine the strengths of different imaging methods to probe different aspects of how the GABAergic system functions within the brain.

GABA Levels and the BOLD Response

The molecular behavior of inhibitory and excitatory processes is relatively well understood in animal models. However, much less is known about the role of these processes in explaining variations in fMRI and other imaging measures. Recent multimodal imaging work has shown that baseline GABA concentrations are inversely correlated to the BOLD fMRI signal in the visual cortex (Muthukumaraswamy et al., 2009), and are directly correlated with negative task-BOLD responses in the anterior cingulate cortex (Northoff et al., 2007).

In addition to the commonly used BOLD fMRI contrast, other emerging hemodynamic contrasts such as arterial spin labeling (ASL) and vascular-space-occupancy (VASO) also show signal variations that have been linked to baseline GABA levels (Donahue et al., 2010). Similar to the BOLD signal (Fig. 3.8.5a), total cerebral blood volume to V1 as assessed by VASO measures (Fig.18.5b) are inversely related to baseline V1 GABA levels. ASL, which gives a measure of cerebral perfusion, shows a more complex trend and has a positive relationship with GABA levels in the primary visual cortex (V1; Fig. 3.8.5c). Taken together, these findings suggest that interindividual variability in hemodynamic MRI responses is at least partially related to variations in cortical inhibition. The exact nature of this relationship, and, in particular, the complex nature of the relationship between GABA levels and the BOLD response needs to be fully explored.

GABA Levels and Local Oscillatory Activity

In addition to the BOLD fMRI signal, baseline GABA levels also contribute to the variability seen in gamma oscillation frequencies as measured by MEG. Higher GABA concentrations in the primary visual cortex are correlated with both smaller BOLD response amplitudes (Fig. 3.8.2A) and higher gamma oscillation frequency (Fig. 3.8.2B) in the primary visual cortex, and an inverse relationship exists between BOLD response amplitudes and gamma

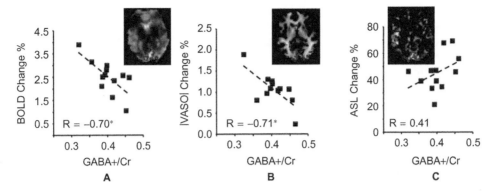

FIGURE 3.8.5   Baseline GABA and hemodynamic measures. Correlation plots between hemodynamic measures and baseline GABA in visual cortex. (A) BOLD mean signal change, (B) magnitude VASO mean signal change, (C) ASL mean signal change. (From Donahue et al., 2010.) This figure is reproduced in color in the color plate section.

oscillation frequency (Fig. 3.8.2C; Muthukumaraswamy et al., 2009). A similar relationship exists between baseline GABA concentration and motor cortex gamma oscillations (Gaetz et al., 2011). This has important implications as it confirms data from animal studies suggesting a causal link between GABA concentration and gamma-frequency oscillations in the brain, and is of relevance for the study of diseases where abnormalities in both GABA and naturally occurring oscillatory rhythms have been demonstrated. For example, it is hypothesized that impairment of GABA-mediated inhibition in schizophrenia can lead to a reduction in synchronized network oscillations, and that this might be causally linked to at least some of the symptoms observed in patients (Gonzalez-Burgos & Lewis, 2008).

CONCLUSIONS AND OUTSTANDING QUESTIONS

Harnessing the strengths of combined MRS, MEG, and fMRI studies is a powerful approach to understanding brain function, because it allows measurements of metabolites, neuronal currents, and hemodynamic activity *in vivo* without the need for contrast agents or neuroactive compounds. It not only gives a unique insight into the normal functioning of the brain, but also allows for comparisons to be made before and after behavioral intervention.

Furthermore, by using techniques such as TMS and tDCS we can probe the responsiveness of the GABA system. Combining this with different imaging modalities has meant that we can begin to answer important questions on the role of inhibitory processes in normal brain function and how this can help us understand pathophysiology in disease. Abnormalities in GABAergic inhibition have been linked to the pathophysiology of several important clinical conditions such as schizophrenia (Lewis et al., 2005), epilepsy (Petroff et al., 2002), depression (Luscher et al., 2010), and autism (Tannan et al., 2008). Understanding the basic mechanisms of normal brain function will have significant implications on the interpretation of these clinical disorders.

The past decade has seen great progress in the understanding of interindividual differences in behavior and plasticity. With advancements in neuroimaging and brain stimulation techniques we can now gain a clearer understanding of the importance of regional patterns of metabolites and its relevance to interindividual differences in behavior. However, a number of questions still remain to be answered before the full utility of GABA MRS can be exploited.

Of particular importance in future investigations is to determine what exactly the MRS-assessed GABA measure reflects. For example, are the natural variances seen among healthy individuals in resting GABA concentration a reflection of the density of GABA within a given area, the number of synapses per neuron, or does it reflect the concentration of GABA per synapse? Furthermore, by what mechanism is GABA decreased in LTP-like plasticity? And how will more powerful magnets increase our understanding of these relationships?

The use of MRS approaches is still in its infancy for applications in neuroscience and many important questions remain to be answered. Using well-defined experimental designs, the combination of multimodal imaging and stimulation techniques will help uncover some of these questions. However, despite these unanswered questions MRS is increasingly recognized as a robust and powerful tool for the *in vivo* investigations of metabolites in the human brain. It is evident that MRS is sensitive to biologically relevant GABAergic activity within a localized region of tissue. Dynamic changes in GABA concentration induced by noninvasive brain stimulation have important similarities with cortical changes underlying plasticity induction during learning of a motor task. Although it is still unclear exactly what is being measured with MRS on a cellular level and its relationship to neuronal activity, accumulating evidence suggests that it is a promising tool in investigating neurophysiological changes in humans.

References

Allen, E. A., Pasley, B. N., Duong, T., & Freeman, R. D. (2007). Transcranial magnetic stimulation elicits coupled neural and hemodynamic consequences. *Science, 317*(5846), 1918–1921.

Bear, M. F., & Malenka, R. C. (1994). Synaptic plasticity: LTP and LTD. *Current Opinion in Neurobiology, 4*(3), 389–399.

Beck, S., Richardson, S. P., Shamim, E. A., Dang, N., Schubert, M., & Hallett, M. (2008). Short intracortical and surround inhibition are selectively reduced during movement initiation in focal hand dystonia. *J Neurosci, 28*, 10363–10369.

Beck, S., Schubert, M., Richardson, S. P., & Hallett, M. (2009a). Surround inhibition depends on the force exerted and is abnormal in focal hand dystonia. *J Appl Physiol, 107*, 1513–1518.

Beck, S., Shamim, E. A., Richardson, S. P., Schubert, M., & Hallett, M. (2009b). Inter-hemispheric inhibition is impaired in mirror dystonia. *Eur J Neurosci, 29*, 1634–1640.

Behar, K. L., Rothman, D. L., Spencer, D. D., & Petroff, O. A. (1994). Analysis of macromolecule resonances in 1H NMR spectra of human brain. *Magnetic Resonance in Medicine, 32*(3), 294–302.

Bogner, W., Gruber, S., Doelken, M., Stadlbauer, A., Ganslandt, O., & Boettcher, U. (2010). In vivo quantification of intracerebral GABA by single-voxel ^{1}H-MRS-How reproducible are the results? etc. *European Journal of Radiology, 73*(3), 526–531

Boy, F., Evans, C. J., Edden, R. A., Singh, K. D., Husain, M., & Sumner, P. (2010). Individual differences in subconscious motor control predicted by GABA concentration in SMA. *Current Biology, 20*(19), 1779–1785.

Butler, A. J., Shuster, M., O'Hara, E., Hurley, K., Middlebrooks, D., & Guilkey, K. (2013). A meta-analysis of the efficacy of anodal transcranial direct current stimulation for upper limb motor recovery in stroke survivors. *Journal of Hand Therapy, 26*(2), 162–170 quiz 171.

Castro-Alamancos, M. A., Donoghue, J. P., & Connors, B. W. (1995). Different forms of synaptic plasticity in somatosensory and motor areas of the neocortex. *Journa of Neuroscience, 15*(7 Pt 2), 5324–5333.

Chattopadhyaya, B., Di Cristo, G., Wu, C. Z., Knott, G., Kuhlman, S., Fu, Y., et al. (2007). GAD67-mediated GABA synthesis and signaling regulate inhibitory synaptic innervation in the visual cortex. *Neuron, 54*(6), 889–903.

Choe, B. Y., Kim, K. T., Suh, T. S., Lee, C., Paik, I. H., Bahk, Y. W., et al. (1994). 1H magnetic resonance spectroscopy characterization of neuronal dysfunction in drug-naive, chronic schizophrenia. *Academy of Radiology, 1*(3), 211–216.

Coghlan, S., Horder, J., Inkster, B., Mendez, M. A., Murphy, D. G., & Nutt, D. J. (2012). GABA system dysfunction in autism and related disorders: From synapse to symptoms. *Neuroscience and Biobehavioral Reviews, 36*(9), 2044–2055.

Donahue, M. J., Near, J., Blicher, J. U., & Jezzard, P. (2010). Baseline GABA concentration and fMRI response. *Neuroimage, 53*(2), 392–398.

Enticott, P. G., Rinehart, N. J., Tonge, B. J., Bradshaw, J. L., & Fitzgerald, P. B. (2010). A preliminary transcranial magnetic stimulation study of cortical inhibition and excitability in high-functioning autism and Asperger disorder. *Developmental Medicine & Child Neurology, 52*(8), e179–e183.

Enticott, P. G., Kennedy, H. A., Rinehart, N. J., Tonge, B. J., Bradshaw, J. L., & Fitzgerald, P. B. (2012). GABAergic activity in autism spectrum disorders: an investigation of cortical inhibition via transcranial magnetic stimulation. *Neuropharmacology, 68*, 202–209.

Floyer-Lea, A., Wylezinska, M., Kincses, T., & Matthews, P. M. (2006). Rapid modulation of GABA concentration in human sensorimotor cortex during motor learning. *Journal of Neurophysiology, 95*(3), 1639–1644.

Fuhr, P., Agostino, R., & Hallett, M. (1991). Spinal motor neuron excitability during the silent period after cortical stimulation. *Electroencephalography and Clinical Neurophysiology, 81*(4), 257–262.

Gaetz, W., Edgar, J. C., Wang, D. J., & Roberts, T. P. (2011). Relating MEG measured motor cortical oscillations to resting gamma-aminobutyric acid (GABA) concentration. *Neuroimage, 55*(2), 616–621.

Gonzalez-Burgos, G., & Lewis, D. A. (2008). GABA neurons and the mechanisms of network oscillations: implications for understanding cortical dysfunction in schizophrenia. *Schizophrenia Bulletin, 34*(5), 944–961.

Goto, N., Yoshimura, R., Moriya, J., Kakeda, S., Ueda, N., Ikenouchi-Sugita, A., et al. (2009). Reduction of brain gamma-aminobutyric acid (GABA) concentrations in early-stage schizophrenia patients: 3 T Proton MRS study. *Schizophrenia Research, 112*(1–3), 192–193.

Hallett, M. (2000). Transcranial magnetic stimulation and the human brain. *Nature, 406*, 6792.

Harada, M., Taki, M. M., Nose, A., Kubo, H., Mori, K., Nishitani, H., et al. (2011). Non-invasive evaluation of the GABAergic/glutamatergic system in autistic patients observed by MEGA-editing proton MR spectroscopy using a clinical 3 tesla instrument. *Journal of Autism and Devevelomental Disorders, 41*(4), 447–454.

Henry, P. G., Dautry, C., Hantraye, P., & Bloch, G. (2001). Brain GABA editing without macromolecule contamination. *Magnetic Resonance in Medicine, 45*(3), 517–520.

Hess, G., & Donoghue, J. P. (1994). Long-term potentiation of horizontal connections provides a mechanism to reorganize cortical motor maps. *Journal of Neurophysiology, 71*(6), 2543–2547.

Huang, Y. Z., Edwards, M. J., Rounis, E., Bhatia, K. P., & Rothwell, J. C. (2005). Theta burst stimulation of the human motor cortex. *Neuron, 45*(2), 201–206.

Jacobs, K. M., & Donoghue, J. P. (1991). Reshaping the cortical motor map by unmasking latent intracortical connections. *Science, 251*(4996), 944–947.

Kanai, R., & Rees, G. (2011). The structural basis of inter-individual differences in human behaviour and cognition. *Nature Reviews Neuroscience, 12*(4), 231–242.

Kujirai, T., Caramia, M. D., Rothwell, J. C., Day, B. L., Thompson, P. D., Ferbert, A., et al. (1993). Corticocortical inhibition in human motor cortex. *Journal of Physiology, 471*, 501–519.

Lau, C. G., & Murthy, V. N. (2012). Activity-dependent regulation of inhibition via GAD67. *Journal of Neuroscience, 32*(25), 8521–8531.

Laxer, K. D. (1997). Clinical applications of magnetic resonance spectroscopy. *Epilepsia, 38*(Suppl. 4), S13–S17.

Levy, L. M., & Hallett, M. (2002). Impaired brain GABA in focal dystonia. *Annals of Neurology, 51*(1), 93–101.

Lewis, D. A., Hashimoto, T., & Volk, D. W. (2005). Cortical inhibitory neurons and schizophrenia. *Nature Reviews Neuroscience, 6*(4), 312–324.

Luscher, B., Shen, Q., & Sahir, N. (2010). The GABAergic deficit hypothesis of major depressive disorder. *Molecular Psychiatry, 16*(4), 383–406.

Maddock, R. J., & Buonocore, M. H. (2012). MR spectroscopic studies of the brain in psychiatric disorders. *Current Topics in Behavioral Neuroscience* [Epub ahead of print].

Martin, D. L., & Barke, K. E. (1998). Are GAD65 and GAD67 associated with specific pools of GABA in brain? *Perspectives on Developmental Neurobiology, 5*(2–3), 119–129.

Martin, D. L., & Rimvall, K. (1993). Regulation of gamma-aminobutyric acid synthesis in the brain. *Journal of Neurochemistry, 60*(2), 395–407.

Mescher, M., Merkle, H., Kirsch, J., Garwood, M., & Gruetter, R. (1998). Simultaneous in vivo spectral editing and water suppression. *NMR in Biomedicine, 11*(6), 266–272.

Muthukumaraswamy, S. D., Edden, R. A., Jones, D. K., Swettenham, J. B., & Singh, K. D. (2009). Resting GABA concentration predicts peak gamma frequency and fMRI amplitude in response to visual stimulation in humans. *Proceedings of the National Academy of Sciences USA, 106*(20), 8356–8361.

Nitsche, M. A., & Paulus, W. (2000). Excitability changes induced in the human motor cortex by weak transcranial direct current stimulation. *Journal of Physiology, 527*(Pt 3), 633–639.

Northoff, G., Walter, M., Schulte, R. F., Beck, J., Dydak, U., Henning, A., et al. (2007). GABA concentrations in the human anterior cingulate cortex predict negative BOLD responses in fMRI. *Nature Neuroscience, 10*(12), 1515–1517.

Oberman, L., Ifert-Miller, F., Najib, U., Bashir, S., Woollacott, I., Gonzalez-Heydrich, J., et al. (2010). Transcranial magnetic stimulation provides means to assess cortical plasticity and excitability in humans with fragile x syndrome and autism spectrum disorder. *Front Synaptic Neurosci, 2*, 26.

Ongur, D., Prescot, A. P., Jensen, J. E., Cohen, B. M., & Renshaw, P. F. (2009). Creatine abnormalities in schizophrenia and bipolar disorder. *Psychiatry Research, 172*(1), 44–48.

Orth, M., & Rothwell, J. C. (2004). The cortical silent period: intrinsic variability and relation to the waveform of the transcranial magnetic stimulation pulse. *Clinical Neurophysiology, 115*(5), 1076–1082.

Petroff, O. A., & Rothman, D. L. (1998). Measuring human brain GABA in vivo: effects of GABA-transaminase inhibition with vigabatrin. *Molecular Neurobiology, 16*(1), 97–121.

Petroff, O. A. C. (2002). GABA and glutamate in the human brain. *The Neuroscientist, 8*(6), 562–573.

Petroff, O. A. C., Pan, J. W., & Rothman, D. L. (2002). Magnetic resonance spectroscopic studies of neurotransmitters and energy metabolism in epilepsy. *Epilepsia, 43*(Suppl. s1), 40–50.

Puts, N. A., & Edden, R. A. (2012). In vivo magnetic resonance spectroscopy of GABA: a methodological review. *Progress in Nuclear Magnetic Resonance Spectroscopy, 60*, 29–41.

Puts, N. A., Edden, R. A., Evans, C. J., McGlone, F., & McGonigle, D. J. (2011). Regionally specific human GABA concentration correlates with tactile discrimination thresholds. *Journal of Neuroscience, 31*(46), 16556–16560.

Reis, J., Swayne, O. B., Vandermeeren, Y., Camus, M., Dimyan, M. A., Harris-Love, M., et al. (2008). Contribution of transcranial magnetic stimulation to the understanding of cortical mechanisms involved in motor control. *Journal of Physiology, 586*(2), 325–351.

Rothman, D. L., Behar, K. L., Hetherington, H. P., & Shulman, R. G. (1984). Homonuclear 1H double-resonance difference spectroscopy of the rat brain in vivo. *Proceedings of the National Academy of Sciences USA, 81*(20), 6330–6334.

Rothman, D. L., Petroff, O. A., Behar, K. L., & Mattson, R. H. (1993). Localized 1H NMR measurements of gamma-aminobutyric acid in human brain in vivo. *Proceedings of the National Academy of Sciences USA, 90*(12), 5662–5666.

Sandrini, M., Umilta, C., & Rusconi, E. (2011). The use of transcranial magnetic stimulation in cognitive neuroscience: a new synthesis of methodological issues. *Neuroscience and Biobehavioral Reviews, 35*(3), 516–536.

Schousboe, A., Waagepetersen, H. S., Tepper, J. M., Abercrombie, E. D., & Bolam, J. P. (2007). *GABA: homeostatic and pharmacological aspects, Progress in Brain Research and the Basal Ganglia* (Vol. 160). Amsterdam: Elsevier.

Stagg, C. J., Bachtiar, V., & Johansen-Berg, H. (2011). The role of GABA in human motor learning. *Current Biology, 21*(6), 480–484.

Stagg, C. J., Bachtiar, V., & Johansen-Berg, H. (2011a). The role of GABA in human motor learning. *Current Biology, 21*(6), 480–484.

Stagg, C. J., Bachtiar, V., & Johansen-Berg, H. (2011b). What are we measuring with GABA magnetic resonance spectroscopy? *Communicative and Integrative Biology, 4*(5), 573–575.

Stagg, C. J., Bachtiar, V., O'Shea, J., Allman, C., Bosnell, R. A., Kischka, U., et al. (2011c). Cortical activation changes underlying stimulation-induced behavioural gains in chronic stroke. *Brain, 135*(Pt 1), 276–284.

Stagg, C. J., Best, J. G., Stephenson, M. C., O'Shea, J., Wylezinska, M., Kincses, Z. T., et al. (2009). Polarity-sensitive modulation of cortical neurotransmitters by transcranial stimulation. *Journal of Neuroscience, 29*(16), 5202–5206.

Stagg, C. J., Bestmann, S., Constantinescu, A. O., Moreno, L. M., Allman, C., Mekle, R., et al. (2011d). Relationship between physiological measures of excitability and levels of glutamate and GABA in the human motor cortex. *Journal of Physiology, 589*(Pt 23), 5845–5855.

Stinear, C. M., & Byblow, W. D. (2004). Impaired modulation of intracortical inhibition in focal hand dystonia. *Cereb Cortex, 14*, 555–561.

Streeter, C. C., Jensen, J. E., Perlmutter, R. M., Cabral, H. J., Tian, H., Terhune, D. B., et al. (2007). Yoga Asana sessions increase brain GABA levels: a pilot study. *Journal of Alternative and Complementary Medicine, 13*(4), 419–426.

Sumner, P., Edden, R. A., Bompas, A., Evans, C. J., & Singh, K. D. (2010). More GABA, less distraction: a neurochemical predictor of motor decision speed. *Nature Neuroscience, 13*(7), 825–827.

Tannan, V., Holden, J. K., Zhang, Z., Baranek, G. T., & Tommerdahl, M. A. (2008). Perceptual metrics of individuals with autism provide evidence for disinhibition. *Autism Research, 1*(4), 223–230.

Tkac, I., & Gruetter, R. (2005). Methodology of H NMR spectroscopy of the human brain at very high magnetic fields. *Applied Magnetic Resonance, 29*(1), 139–157.

Trepel, C., & Racine, R. J. (2000). GABAergic modulation of neocortical long-term potentiation in the freely moving rat. *Synapse, 35*(2), 120–128.

Valls-Sole, J., Pascual-Leone, A., Wassermann, E. M., & Hallett, M. (1992). Human motor evoked responses to paired transcranial magnetic stimuli. *Electroencephalography and Clinical Neurophysiology, 85*(6), 355–364.

Waddell, K. W., Avison, M. J., Joers, J. M., & Gore, J. C. (2007). A practical guide to robust detection of GABA in human brain by J-difference spectroscopy at 3 T using a standard volume coil. *Magnetic Resonance Imaging, 25*(7), 1032–1038.

Wassermann, E., Epstein, C., Ziemann, U., Walsh, V., Paus, T., & Lisanby, S. (2008). *Oxford handbook of Transcranial Stimulation*. Oxford, UK: Oxford University Press.

Ziemann, U., Muellbacher, W., Hallett, M., & Cohen, L. G. (2001). Modulation of practice-dependent plasticity in human motor cortex. *Brain, 124*(Pt 6), 1171–1181.

MRS in Development and Across the Life Span

Dallas Card[1], Margot J. Taylor[1,2,3,4] and John G. Sled[5,6]

[1]Department of Diagnostic Imaging and [2]Program of Neurosciences & Mental Health, Research Institute,
Hospital for Sick Children, Toronto, Ontario, Canada [3]Paediatrics and [4]Medical Imaging, University of Toronto,
Toronto, Ontario, Canada [5]Program of Physiology and Experimental Medicine, Research Institute, Hospital for Sick
Children, Toronto, Ontario, Canada [6]Department of Medical Biophysics, University of Toronto,
Toronto, Ontario, Canada

INTRODUCTION

It is estimated that the human brain contains from 2,000 to 20,000 unique metabolites (Schmidt, 2004). [1]H magnetic resonance spectroscopy (MRS) is able to provide a noninvasive metabolic snapshot of a handful of these metabolites. The information obtained from MRS is useful in clinical diagnosis, but is also of great interest for studying normal development, providing insight into infant brain development and the normal aging process, through both longitudinal and population studies.

The human brain goes through profound changes in the months leading up to birth and during the first few years of life. It is relatively stable in terms of anatomy, function, and metabolism from the third decade onward, although some changes are detected toward the end of life, in conjunction with decreased cognitive function. Not surprisingly, brain metabolism parallels this pattern of development and decline, with the most dramatic changes occurring in the months leading up to and following birth, and more subtle changes thereafter. As a result, the pattern of changes in infant brain metabolism is well established, while the available data on changes across the life span are more limited and in some cases inconsistent.

Part of the difficulty in interpreting the literature on MRS and aging is that, barring proper absolute quantification of metabolite concentrations, which is not generally feasible within reasonable time constraints, concentration estimates are subject to variation resulting from differences in protocols and analyses, as well as the influence of several characteristics of brain tissue, which also change throughout the life span.

This chapter reviews the literature related to MRS in aging, and brings together current understanding of changes in neural metabolite concentrations over the life span, focusing on the times of greatest age-related change, both in early brain development and toward the end of life. We also summarize parallel changes occurring in other parameters that factor into the quantification of MRS data. Finally, this chapter also contains a brief discussion of the repeatability of MRS, and the challenges of acquiring MRS data in infants.

OVERVIEW

Other chapters in this volume are dedicated to individual or groups of neural metabolites (see Chapters 2.1−2.5) so we focus here on those of primary interest in development. Although metabolites are often thought of as represented by individual spectral peaks, most metabolites actually give rise to multiple resonances, and these resonances tend to overlap. As a result, concentrations are typically reported for groups of metabolites. The most prominent and therefore most studied metabolic groups in the literature related to development and aging include: NAA (primarily N-acetylaspartate, a poorly understood but abundant amino acid in the central nervous system, but also N-acetylaspartylglutamate, both of which are found exclusively or primarily in neurons, immature oligodendrocytes, and their progenitors), CHO (a group of trimethylamine compounds involved in membrane synthesis and degradation, including glycophosphocholine, phosphocholine, and a small amount of free choline), CR (a combination of creatine and phosphocreatine, which are involved in the creatine kinase reaction, and are found in higher concentration in glial cells than in neurons), INS (*myo*-inositol, a pentose sugar involved in the inositol triphosphate intracellular second messenger system, which is also found in higher levels in glial cells than in neurons), lactate (a product of anaerobic glycolysis, which is not normally found in a healthy adult brain), and to a lesser extent GLX (overlapping resonances of glutamine and glutamate, the most abundant amino acid in the brain) (Pugash et al., 2009; Zhu & Barker, 2011; Gadin et al., 2012) (and references contained therein).

The details of acquiring and processing MRS data are covered elsewhere in this volume (see Chapters 1.1–1.5). In brief, however, in addition to the actual concentrations of metabolites, the MRS spectrum will be influenced by aspects of the imaging protocol, such as field strength, echo time, repetition time, acquisition type (single or multidimensional), localization scheme (PRESS/STEAM), and water-suppression technique, as well as the longitudinal (T_1) and transverse (T_2) relaxation times of the metabolites in the brain. With the exception of the relaxation times, these factors can be controlled, but differences need to be taken into account when comparing across sites and/or studies.

In addition, there are a wide variety of techniques available to estimate concentrations from an MRS spectrum, the choice of which will affect estimates, particularly for weak signals. Many of these sources of bias are avoided when reporting the ratios of two metabolite concentrations. While this approach has been widely applied in developmental studies, the absence of any suitable reference metabolites whose levels are stable across the life span complicates the interpretation of metabolite ratios. Compared to absolute quantitation approaches that typically make use of a reference water scan, corrections for the T_1 and T_2 relaxation times of water, water content of the brain, and the presence of cerebrospinal fluid (CSF) in the MRS voxel, reporting metabolite ratios greatly simplifies the analysis and facilitates large-scale studies.

As pointed out by Kreis et al. (2005), proper absolute quantification is virtually never carried out on a per subject basis, even in the research setting, as the time required to acquire sufficient information in each subject is prohibitive. While the needed model parameters can frequently be assumed to be stable across a study population, this is not necessarily a valid assumption in a long-term study. As will be discussed later, water content and relaxation times of water and individual metabolites change over the life span, and therefore have the potential to contribute to perceived differences in metabolite concentrations. Although the influence of some of these factors can be minimized through short echo time, long repetition time, and careful voxel selection, it is important to have an understanding of the issues involved to properly evaluate studies in the literature. For further information, see Chapter 1.5.

Measurement precision is an important consideration in life span studies, as the metabolite concentration changes that occur later in later life are small. There have been several studies using a variety of different approaches (Tedeschi et al., 1996; W. M. Brooks et al., 1999; Chard et al., 2002; Li et al., 2002; Geurts et al., 2004; Träber et al., 2006; Langer et al., 2007; Maudsley et al., 2010; Wijnen et al., 2010; Gasparovic et al., 2011; Kirov et al., 2012) that have examined reproducibility. In the best cases, groups have reported intrasubject coefficients of variation (CVs) on short timescales on the order of 5–10% for the major metabolites (W. M. Brooks et al., 1999; Geurts et al., 2004; Maudsley et al., 2010; Wijnen et al., 2010; Gasparovic et al., 2011; Kirov et al., 2012). A study employing a particularly rigorous methodology (Gasparovic et al., 2011) found CVs in the range of 5–7% for NAA, CR, and CHO, and 10–13% for INS and GLX, with interclass correlation coefficients in the range of 0.6–0.9 for all metabolites. In a 4 year longitudinal study of 10 healthy adults (Kirov et al., 2012), the authors similarly found CVs of ~7% for NAA, CR, CHO, and 10% for INS. By including both back-to-back and longitudinal sessions, the authors were able to analyze the source of variance, and determined that about half of the variance arose from "nonbiological" sources (i.e., were found in back-to-back scanning sessions).

In general, better reproducibility is to be expected from NAA, CR, and CHO than from INS, GLX, and lactate, the quantification of which is more subject to the influence of water suppression and baseline fitting. Based on the literature, in carefully controlled (experimental) settings, it is possible to get CVs on the order of 5–7% for the major metabolites at both 1.5 and 3 T. Although this is impressive, this still suggests that changes in metabolite concentrations on the order of 10% are necessary between two scanning sessions in one subject in order to be confidently detected. Additional sources of noise in the clinical setting (for example, patient motion) will result in ambiguity even at this level of difference.

In summary, reproducibility is influenced by a number of interacting factors, including field strength, field homogeneity, echo time, voxel size and location, signal-to-noise ratio (SNR), patient motion, and methods used in quantification. Of particular importance for longitudinal studies is the question of voxel placement, as metabolite concentrations have been shown to vary significantly across the brain in healthy adults (Gasparovic et al., 2011; Kirov et al., 2012). In addition, it is worth noting that all of these reproducibility studies were done in healthy adults, mostly aged 20–40, and the precise levels of variation cannot necessarily be assumed for different ages or pathologies.

Without full quantification, concentration estimates will be influenced by choices in MRS protocol and analysis, and cannot necessarily be directly compared across studies. As a result, relatively few numbers from the literature will be reported here. Rather the focus will be on how the values of interest change with age, and the extent of variation across the brain, between individuals, and across the life span. Readers are referred to the literature for additional details, as needed.

MRS IN EARLY BRAIN DEVELOPMENT

The human brain undergoes profound changes during intrauterine gestation. Differentiation of the neural tube occurs between 4 and 12 weeks. From 12 to 20 weeks, neurons proliferate and migrate to the cortex, climbing a scaffolding of glial cells. From 24 weeks gestation to 4 weeks after birth, a phase of extensive cell death takes place, with roughly half the neurons undergoing apoptosis (Lenroot & Giedd, 2006). Myelination begins in the brainstem at around 29 weeks gestation, and generally proceeds from the inferior to superior and posterior to anterior aspects. Sulcation and gyrification begin around 15 weeks gestation and are nearly complete by term (Lenroot & Giedd, 2006).

The third trimester of development can be visualized in detail with anatomical MRI scans, either *in utero*, or in infants born very preterm. Diffusion tensor imaging (DTI) and magnetization transfer ratio (MTR) sequences provide insight into the myelination process (Nossin-Manor et al., 2013). Quantitative T_1 and T_2 sequences reveal the changing relaxation times of water in the brain over this time frame and functional MRI is beginning to teach us about early brain activity.

MRS also has a role to play in understanding early human brain development. In brief, metabolite concentrations go through massive changes in the first year of life, especially around the time leading up to and following birth. As will be discussed in more detail later, there are high concentrations of INS and CHO in the fetal brain prior to birth, and these decrease with age. Conversely, there are initially very low concentrations of NAA and CR, and these increase with age. There are conflicting reports with respect to lactate as an injury marker, with some observations of lactate reported in the brains of otherwise healthy preterm infants. Furthermore, both water content in the brain and the T_1 and T_2 relaxation times of water decrease rapidly with age in newborns, along with small changes in the relaxation times of metabolites. Based on studies

of children, most metabolites observable with MRS reach stable concentrations in the brain between 1 and 4 years after birth.

A handful of studies have applied ^{1}H MRS *in utero* (Kok et al., 2002; Heerschap et al., 2003; Roelants-van Rijn et al., 2004; Girard et al., 2006; Charles-Edwards et al., 2010; Cetin et al., 2011). Fetal MRS presents unique difficulties, primarily due to the inability to prevent fetal motion. All of these studies relied on placing a single, large MRS voxel in the fetal brain. The earliest (Kok et al., 2002; Heerschap et al., 2003) included 36 healthy volunteers with healthy fetuses (as determined by ultrasound) in the range of 30–41 weeks gestational age. Using both long and short echo times, and two different analysis pipelines, the authors found NAA increased significantly with age with respect to CR and CHO, while the ratio of CHO/CR decreased significantly with age. There was also a trend toward a reduction of INS/CR with age.

A larger study (Girard et al., 2006), with data from 58 participants over a larger age range (22–40 weeks), also found that NAA increased significantly over this time frame. The authors reported that INS decreased with age (but with borderline significance), and CR increased (but only according to their short echo-time data), with no change in CHO or GLX, all referenced to internal water. However, there was no correction applied for relaxation times or CSF content, and although the trends are important, the absolute numbers cannot be taken as normative values.

Neither of the above studies observed lactate in the fetuses examined, but there have been a few isolated reports of lactate in fetal brains (Roelants-van Rijn et al., 2004; Charles-Edwards et al., 2010; Cetin et al., 2011). Two of these (Roelants-van Rijn et al., 2004; Cetin et al., 2011) based their findings on visual inspection of the spectra, and reported visible lactate in two of six fetuses with hydrocephalus, and in one of five intrauterine growth restricted fetuses, respectively. The third (Charles-Edwards et al., 2010) was more systematic, reporting values based on model fitting with the jMRUI software package, and found lactate in all three fetuses from which good quality spectra were obtained. This third paper also reported concentrations of NAA, CHO, and CR in these three infants. The authors applied a correction for CSF content, as well as for relaxation times and brain water content, using literature values. Limitations of this paper are that it only included these three infants, all of whom were growth restricted, and all the relevant literature values were taken from the postnatal literature. As such, there are no established normative values for metabolite concentrations in the fetal brain.

Further data on early brain development can be found from studies involving preterm infants. The earliest study of ^{1}H MRS in preterm infants (Hüppi et al., 1991) examined baseline *in vivo* metabolite concentrations in comparison to autopsy findings. Subsequent studies by other groups incorporated the additional parameters needed for absolute concentration estimates, including brain water content and relaxation times. An important paper by Kreis et al. (1993) examined 77 subjects ranging in age from 34.5 weeks gestation (born preterm) to 18 years. The authors reported T_1 and T_2 relaxation times, along with concentrations, for NAA, CR, CHO, and INS, as well as T_2 relaxation times for water and brain water content. The most important findings were that both brain water content and the T_2 of water decreased dramatically in the weeks leading up to and following term age. The authors estimated brain water content at 40 weeks gestation of 86 and 83% for parietal white matter and midline occipital, respectively. T_2 relaxation times at 40 weeks were estimated to be 177 ms for developing white matter and 158 ms for gray matter. Their data suggest that these continue to decrease gradually beyond the second year of life. Metabolite concentrations were found to change with age in ways that match with the fetal literature described above. NAA and CR increased rapidly in the first year of life, stabilizing around 4 years of age. CHO and INS both decreased rapidly. Metabolite T_2 relaxation times were found to trend toward longer values in newborns than in adults by $\sim$10–30%, but the differences were not significant. T_1 relaxation times were $\sim$10% longer in newborns than adults for CR and INS, with the opposite trend for NAA, and these differences were significant. However, these metabolite T_2 and T_1 relaxation times were measured in only six and seven infants, respectively. This paper has motivated a great deal of subsequent research.

A more recent paper (Williams et al., 2005) arrived at estimates of 94 and 90% water content in frontal white matter and frontal gray matter, respectively, in preterm infants, and 93 and 88% for the same tissue types in term infants. Several studies of preterm and/or term infants (Ferrie et al., 1999; Counsell et al., 2003; Ding, 2009; Leppert et al., 2009; and references therein) have confirmed at multiple field strengths that T_2 of water decreases dramatically in the first months of life, and more slowly beyond that. The largest of these included 114 healthy children aged 0–48 months (Leppert et al., 2009). The study reported mean T_2 values at birth of 404.4 ± 8.1 ms, 228.6 ± 3.6 ms, and 215.9 ± 3.2 ms in the white matter (major and minor forceps), corpus callosum, and deep gray matter (caudate nucleus and thalamus), respectively. In the older children, T_2 values in these locations were found to stabilize around 100–120 ms, 80–90 ms, and 90–100 ms, respectively, by $\sim$2 years, with only gradual decreases

beyond that. The decrease of T_2 with age is most likely a reflection of the reduction in free water in the brain, and may also be linked to myelination processes.

It has also been noted that quantitative T_1 and T_2 values in preterm infants are strongly correlated (Williams et al., 2005). T_1 relaxation times of water have been observed to vary significantly across the brain in preterm infants (Nossin-Manor et al., 2011), and to correlate in regionally varying ways with measurements from other modalities, such as MTR and DTI (Nossin-Manor et al., 2013), suggesting that no single modality provides a complete picture of how water content, myelination, and density vary across time and anatomical locations within the brain.

Three other papers (Toft et al., 1994; Cady et al., 1996; Kugel et al., 2003) have reported on metabolite relaxation times in infants at 1.5 and 2.4 T. The largest of these (Kugel et al., 2003) included 83 preterm infants scanned near term-equivalent age. The authors found relatively large intersubject variability, with standard deviations between 10 and 30% for the T_1 and T_2 relaxation times of NAA, CR, and CHO. T_1 values were within the range of previously published literature, as were the T_2 of NAA and CR, although the T_2 of CHO was lower than previous infant studies. Moreover, the authors of this paper were unable to confirm any previously reported age-dependent differences in metabolite relaxation times. By considering the effect that differing metabolite relaxation times would have on metabolite concentration estimates, the authors concluded that this particular source of uncertainty is less important than other factors. Interestingly, all three of these papers noted consistent observation of lactate in the preterm infants.

A follow-up paper to the Kreis et al. (1993) used LCModel (Provencher, 2001) to estimate concentrations of 22 metabolites in three locations in a cohort of 21 neonates, including both preterm and full-term infants (Kreis et al., 2002). Using parameters established from their earlier research, the authors demonstrated that no differences in metabolite concentrations could be found between intrauterine and extrauterine development, except for a possible difference in CR, which was slightly higher in those born preterm at term-equivalent age than in the full-term infants. Although there was a large amount of intersubject variability in the metabolite concentrations, the usual developmental patterns were found, with significant increases of NAA, GLX, and CR and significant decreases of INS and lactate with age; an exception was CHO, for which no difference was found between preterm and term scans of the preterm subjects. Also, the three regions studied showed significantly different metabolic profiles, with the thalamus having the highest concentrations of CR, NAA, CHO, and GLX, and INS much more concentrated in the occipital gray matter than the centrum semiovale. As expected, T_2 of water was highest in the preterm infants, and reduced at term-equivalent age.

Since then, no paper has demonstrated a convincing deviation from the findings of the previously mentioned publications, with the dramatic of increase of NAA/CHO in the first weeks of life as the most consistently replicated finding (Vigneron et al., 2001, 2006; Augustine et al., 2008; Limperopoulos et al., 2010; Xu & Vigneron, 2010; Xu et al., 2011). In a cohort of 99 infants born very preterm, (born at <32 weeks gestation), scanned within 2 weeks of birth and again at term-equivalent age, we have confirmed these trends in the basal ganglia, with both CR and NAA increasing rapidly relative to CHO, throughout the period from 28 to 46 weeks gestation. INS/CR showed the most dramatic rate of change, decreasing rapidly during the preterm period, and then more slowly around term-equivalent age. A small amount of lactate was present in most of this cohort, with large amounts of lactate in three infants, all of which had normal lactate levels at term-equivalent age (Card et al., 2013). Three of these metabolite ratios are shown in Fig. 3.9.1 from 20 preterm infants in this cohort that were scanned at three time points over the first 2 years of life.

Although the function of NAA is not well understood (Zhu & Barker, 2011), it does show decreases with neuron loss or dysfunction, and is often treated as a surrogate marker of neuronal activity and/or density. The reason for the decrease in CHO levels over time in infants is generally thought to be the result of it incorporated into cell membranes. Indeed, in preterm infants, the highest levels of NAA/CHO are seen in regions such as cortical spinal tracts, which mature the fastest (Xu et al., 2011). Lactate would not normally be detected in a healthy infant brain. It is seen most commonly in newborn full-term infants that have suffered a hypoxic-ischemic injury. Moreover, several studies have demonstrated that high levels of lactate and low levels of NAA indicate a poor prognosis in these infants. As described previously, several studies above have observed lactate in the brains of non-asphyxiated preterm infants. Although this is not always the case, the general consensus is that a small amount of lactate in the preterm brain is likely normal, and not indicative of pathology.

In a recent paper, Van Kooij et al. (2012) reported that cognitive scores at 2 years of age in a group of infants born preterm were significantly correlated with NAA/CHO in the cerebellum and cerebellar volume at term-equivalent age. Two other papers were unable to find any significant relationships between metabolite ratios and neurodevelopmental follow-up

at 6 months (Gadin et al., 2012) and 18–24 months (Augustine et al., 2008). In both cases, the infants were imaged near term-equivalent age. Although this avoids many of the difficulties of imaging preterm infants shortly after birth, our research discussed subsequently suggests that the most important predictors may only be visible in the first weeks after birth.

In agreement with Chau et al. (2009), the data from our cohort demonstrated that those preterm infants showing focal noncystic white matter abnormalities also had decreased NAA/CHO in the basal ganglia, suggesting that these white matter abnormalities are connected to diffuse change in metabolism, and possibly indicate neuronal loss. By term-equivalent age, however, the NAA/CHO ratios in these infants were not significantly different from the rest of the cohort. Similarly, preliminary results suggest that motor scores on the Bayley Scale of Infant Development at 2 years of age were significantly correlated with CHO/CR and INS/CR measured within 2 weeks of birth, but not from the same measures taken at term-equivalent age.

MR imaging (MRI) scanning of preterm infants within the first few days or weeks after birth requires significant additional preparations and precautions. Preterm infants are often highly unstable when born and require numerous interventions for a variety of conditions, including cardiopulmonary resuscitation, sepsis, patent ductus arteriosus, and necrotizing enterocolitis. Although they can in most cases be quickly brought to the point of stability, most still require monitoring and assistance with breathing and maintaining temperature. The only feasible solution is the use of an MRI-compatible incubator, which is similar in functionality to a conventional NICU incubator and is designed to be inserted directly into the bore of the magnet with the infant inside. Heart-rate and oxygen saturation can be continuously monitored and temperature and humidity controlled throughout the scanning session.

As with all participants, infants require hearing protection. Swaddling the infants reduces motion during the scan. In general, preterm infants are relatively immobile, limiting movement-related artifacts during the scan. Full-term infants, however, are prone to movement, and sedation can potentially assist in obtaining diagnostic-quality scans if clinically indicated.

With respect to MRS specifically, there are several challenges unique to imaging infants. The most obvious is the small size of the preterm brain. Given typical voxel volumes of $1-8 \text{ cm}^3$ needed to obtain sufficient SNR, it is not possible to place the voxel in a homogeneous tissue region. Multidimensional chemical shift imaging (CSI) provides a means to address this difficulty when combined with high-resolution anatomical scans to estimate the partial voxel contributions of

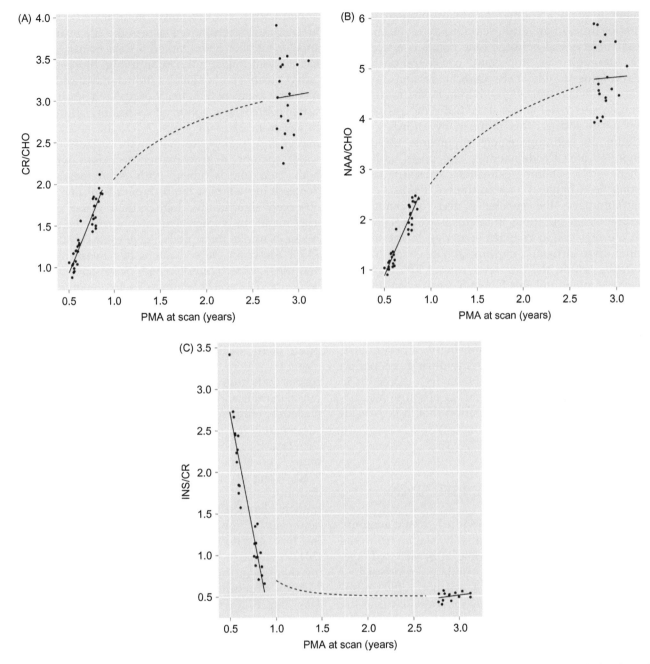

FIGURE 3.9.1 Developmental trends for CR/CHO (A), NAA/CHO (B), and INS/CR (C) with postmenstrual age (PMA) in the basal ganglia of 20 infants born very preterm and scanned at three time points: within 2 weeks of birth, at term-equivalent age, and at 2 years corrected age.

different tissue types to the CSI voxels. However, this approach requires accurate segmentation of the anatomical scans. Automated segmentation of the infant brain is an active area of research, as one needs to account for the reversal of gray/white matter contrast with respect to the adult brain as well as the conformation of the immature anatomy.

In addition to these issues, there is also the challenge of brain injury in preterm infants. Even in those infants that go on to have normal outcomes, brain injury is very common, with intraventricular hemorrhage (IVH) reported in ~20–25% of preterm infants and even higher rates of white matter abnormalities (Volpe, 2008, 2009). Injuries such as IVH, ventriculomegaly, and parenchymal infarctions may interfere with voxel selection in the desired location by distorting anatomy and by the abnormal presence of blood or CSF in various regions.

Finally, longitudinal studies involving infants present an additional challenge, primarily due to the change in brain anatomy that takes place over this period of time. In an adult, selecting an identical voxel across subjects and between time points is a relatively easy, although still important, consideration. When brain volume doubles between scan sessions, as may be the case when working with infants, the meaning of a homologous voxel is less clear. CSI protocols provide a means to address this problem by affording more flexibility in defining regions of interest (ROI). CSI is more technically demanding and poses additional challenges for obtaining estimates of absolute concentrations. See Chapter 1.3 for additional details.

In summary, the general pattern of changes in metabolite concentrations in infants is well established, with the most rapid changes occurring in the months leading up to birth, and most metabolite concentrations stabilizing within the first few years of life. However, as water content and the T_1 and T_2 relaxation times of water (and to a lesser extent, individual metabolites) are also changing with age during this time period, we must be cautious in interpreting absolute estimates of metabolite concentrations in newborns. Furthermore, due to the changing brain anatomy during this period and the high incidence of brain injury, especially in preterm infants, present estimates of absolute metabolite concentrations in this population should be considered preliminary.

MRS ACROSS THE LIFE SPAN

For the typical healthy individual, brain anatomy and composition remains relatively stable from the third decade onward. As people approach old age, however, the brain begins to undergo processes of decline, the reasons for which are not fully understood. The normal aging process manifests itself in the brain in several ways that are visible on MRI. The most consistent finding on MRI is a generalized atrophy of the brain, most pronounced in the frontal and temporal lobes (Minati et al., 2007; Dennis & Cabeza, 2008; Caserta et al., 2009). Postmortem findings confirm that white matter volume is decreased throughout the brain with aging, particularly in the frontal lobes, and DTI suggests a loss of white matter integrity in a number of areas, including frontal white matter tracts (Minati et al., 2007; Dennis & Cabeza, 2008; Caserta et al., 2009). One study found that 30% of adults over 60 show white matter hyperintensities on MRI, possibly related to local demyelination (Tumeh et al., 2007). Functional MRI is less specific, but the elderly tend to show smaller activations, with a reduction in the lateralization of function (Minati et al., 2007; Caserta et al., 2009).

Numerous studies have investigated changes in metabolite concentrations across the life span, while a smaller number have gathered data related to various factors that relate into quantifying those concentrations. Neeb et al. (2006) applied advanced imaging methods to study the effects of age and sex on cerebral water content in a cohort of 44 healthy adults ranging in age from 21 to 74 years. Averaging over total gray matter and total white matter, the authors found that water content in gray matter decreased with age in both men and women, with a sharper, nonlinear decrease in men past the fifth decade of life. They also observed significantly higher total water content in gray matter in women than men across the age range. As an example, their model gave estimates of 79.8 and 73.7% for brain water content in 60-year old women and men, respectively. No age- or sex-specific changes were noted in water content of white matter. A subsequent paper from the same group (Neeb et al., 2008) used a faster variant of the same imaging protocol and studied regional variation in water content in a group of 10 healthy volunteers aged 24—37 years. They observed water content in the range of 65—70% in the corpus callosum and frontal, occipital, and central white matter, and 80—85% in the head of the caudate nucleus, putamen, and prefrontal and visual cortex.

Several large studies have considered how T_1 and T_2 relaxation of water change with age in the human brain (Cho et al., 1997; Saito et al., 2009; Hasan et al., 2010; Wang et al., 2012). All have demonstrated that both transverse and longitudinal relaxation times continue to change throughout the life span, generally in a nonlinear fashion, although never so quickly as during the first months of life. Most recently, Wang et al. (2012) made use of nonparametric regression to examine changes in transverse relaxation rate ($R_2 = 1/T_2$) in 25 brain structures across the age range of 9—85 years. This paper revealed remarkable variation between structures in the pattern of change of R_2 with age. The gray matter structures all showed significant positive correlation with age over the range of 9—30 years of age. Past age 40, however, R_2 continued to increase in some structures and decreased in others. In contrast, R_2 in white matter tended to follow a more linear downward trend across the life span.

More extensive research has been done on metabolite relaxation times in adults than in infants (J. Brooks et al., 2001; Kreis et al., 2005; McIntyre et al., 2007; Zaaraoui et al., 2007; Kirov et al., 2008; and references contained therein). Relevant here is the way these relaxation times change as a function of age and location. Unfortunately, the published literature is somewhat inconsistent. The earliest study (J. Brooks et al., 2001) found no significant variation in the T_2 relaxation times of NAA, CR, or CHO across an age range of

20–70 years in a group of 50 males, in the cingulate gyrus and prefrontal cortex. A later study (Kreis et al., 2005) of a larger ROI in the centrum semiovale over a similar age range found that the T_1 of the methyl groups of NAA and CR decreased with age, while the T_2 of NAA increased. In contrast to these results, a third study (McIntyre et al., 2007) used 2D CSI in a somewhat older group (in the range of 50–90 years) and found that R_2 $(1/T_2)$ of NAA was positively correlated with age, with a similar trend for CR. Finally, a fourth study (Kirov et al., 2008) sought to resolve this uncertainty with even more comprehensive brain coverage, although the study only included 20 subjects in four age groups ranging from teenagers to elderly. In agreement with (McIntyre et al., 2007), this fourth paper found slight linear decreases in the transverse relaxation times of NAA, CR, and CHO in both white and gray matter. However, the authors noted that the changes over time were very small (equivalent to less than 1 ms/year). As such, the literature for adults suggests that the impact of age-related metabolite T_2 differences will be negligible compared to differences in metabolite concentrations between subjects and brain regions.

In summary, the relaxation times of metabolites do vary with age, but this variation can be safely neglected when estimating metabolite concentrations for healthy adults. In addition to the considerations described earlier, the effect of field strength on relaxation times (Ethofer et al., 2003; Oros-Peusquens et al., 2008) should be taken into account when using literature values for model parameters in MRS studies.

There have been a large number of studies examining aging by MRS; a tabulated summary can be found in Reyngoudt et al. (2012). Unfortunately, as the authors point out, there is little consistency in methodology, including field strength, age range of the participants, area of the brain studied, MRS sequence used, data processing, and rigor in quantification. Most of these papers examined multiple metabolites, sometimes in multiple brain regions, in some cases leading to dozens of comparisons, yet very few compensated for this potential source of type I error.

As mentioned previously, full absolute quantification is almost never performed. Of the studies tabulated in Reyngoudt et al. (2012) with more than 30 subjects, only one paper here measured metabolite relaxation times in their participants (J. Brooks et al., 2001), with a second using values from their previous research (Reyngoudt et al., 2012). In addition to these two studies, only one other measured the T_2 relaxation time of water in the participants (Chang et al., 2009). Some did not make a correction for CSF content when reporting absolute concentrations, and none measured the water content *in vivo*. As noted earlier, acquiring

this data in each subject, while theoretically possible, would be prohibitively time-consuming in practice. Moreover, in many cases, depending on the acquisition protocol used, correcting for these factors would likely only have a small impact. Nevertheless, the result is that making sense of this literature is a challenge.

The most consistent findings in the early studies was a reduction of NAA/CR with age in a variety of brain regions, including both gray and white matter (Fukuzako et al., 1997; Angelie et al., 2001; Grachev & Apkarian, 2001; Sijens et al., 2003), although this change was not always found in every region studied within each group. Other early studies that attempted absolute quantification were more likely to find trends toward CR increasing with age (Chang et al., 1996; Pfefferbaum et al., 1999; Leary et al., 2000; Harada et al., 2001), suggesting that the decrease in NAA/CR is at least partially attributable to an increase in CR. However, two of these did not make any corrections for CSF or relaxation times, and the trends in the ones that did correct for CSF content (Chang et al., 1996; Harada et al., 2001) would likely not be significant if corrected for multiple comparisons. Moreover, there were exceptions to this pattern. Saunders et al. (1999) found no change with age for any NAA, CR, CHO, or INS. Kadota et al. (2001) only reported NAA/CHO, and found that this decreased significantly with age. Finally, by far the most methodologically rigorous of the early studies (J. Brooks et al., 2001) found a significant decrease in NAA with age, quantified with respect to an external phantom, with no change in CR or CHO.

These discrepancies have continued in the more recent literature. Three recent studies (Charlton et al., 2007; McIntyre et al., 2007; Sailasuta et al., 2008; Chang et al., 2009; Raininko & Mattsson, 2010) have used LCModel for quantification, which has the advantage of being more easily comparable across studies. Two papers based on one of these studies (Charlton et al., 2007; McIntyre et al., 2007), which did correct for CSF content, reported a significant increase in CR with age, with no change in NAA. One which did not correct for CSF (Raininko & Mattsson, 2010) found a significant decrease in NAA with age, but no change in CR. The fourth was published and then revised (Sailasuta et al., 2008; Chang et al., 2009), and studied four brain regions. The only age-effect found among CR, CHO, and NAA, was a significant decrease in CR in the basal ganglia, even without correcting for multiple comparisons.

The pattern of change of CHO is usually reported, but has been found to be not significant, or only borderline significant, either up or down, in most cases. INS has been much less studied, but was found to increase significantly with age in three fairly rigorous studies (Chang et al., 1996; Raininko & Mattsson, 2010; Reyngoudt et al., 2012). Three papers examined glutamate/glutamine (Grachev & Apkarian, 2001; Chang et al., 2009; Raininko & Mattsson, 2010), with one finding a nonlinear pattern of change with age (Raininko & Mattsson, 2010). However, without additional evidence, drawing any conclusions about changes in glutamate and glutamine with age would be premature.

In general, the most noticeable feature in looking at these papers is the large intersubject variability. Based on the research, there does seem to be a trend toward increasing CR with age, and possibly decreasing NAA and increasing INS, but the effect sizes are small compared to the variability that will be found within the population at any given time point. This variability is most notable in the largest of these studies (Sijens et al., 2003), which is also the only longitudinal study referenced here, including 271 adults at two time points. Comparing these time points, both CHO and NAA were found to decrease with respect to CR, again suggesting an increase in CR over time. Unfortunately, this paper does not comment on precautions that were taken to ensure identical voxel placement at the follow-up scan.

Because NAA is found primarily in neurons, a decrease with age is often interpreted as either a loss of neurons or neuronal dysfunction. Although aging is associated with volume loss in the brain, this does not necessarily involve loss of neurons, and the dysfunction hypothesis should not be discounted. In contrast, increases in CR and INS could be related to reactive gliosis, the proliferation of astrocytes in the brain, as both of these metabolites are found in higher concentrations in glial cells than in neurons (Minati et al., 2007). Further support for altered mitochondrial metabolism with aging can be found in studies that have combined ^{13}C and ^{1}H MRS, such as Boumezbeur et al. (2010), which reported highly significant correlations between the neuronal tricarboxylic acid cycle rate and both NAA and glutamate concentrations in healthy elderly subjects. The similarity of these correlations may also help to explain some of the intersubject variability described earlier.

Alzheimer's disease (AD) is the leading cause of dementia in older adults. Although it is distinct from the normal aging, it does in some ways accentuate the aging process, and is interesting to consider from the perspective of MRS. Most studies of MRS in AD report concordant findings of decreased NAA and increased INS. Moreover, the progression of this pattern seems to parallel the progression of the disease in terms of the regions of the brain that are affected. These findings are well supported by research involving cognitive measures and support hypotheses related to AD, particularly the loss of neurons, and the process of gliosis. Moreover, many studies report findings that suggest that mild cognitive impairment is midway between AD and healthy elderly individuals, metabolically speaking (Kantarci, 2007; Griffith et al., 2009).

The metabolic changes associated with aging are far from definitive, but it seems that there is a possible concordance of decreasing NAA and increasing INS, although the trend is more pronounced and apparent in AD. Although most studies of normal aging were careful to only include healthy adults, the AD literature suggests that the metabolic changes observable with MRS precede the development of AD, thus it is possible that in some cases this pattern of change, when found in normal aging, is perhaps related to a process of cognitive decline in a subset of the study population. Conversely, it is possible that it is a part of a process of normal aging, which is exaggerated in degenerative disorders. Either way, it will be important for further research into AD, particularly longitudinal studies, to consider the trend toward increasing CR with age in healthy individuals, as well as the various factors involved in quantification of MRS data.

THE WAY FORWARD

MRS has added considerably to our understanding the early maturation and aging processes, and is a valuable source of information for certain disease conditions. Going forward, however, additional technical developments are needed. More basic research is required to establish normative parameters such as T_1 and T_2 relaxation parameters in developing populations such as preterm infants. In addition, MRS is one area where making raw data publicly available has enormous potential for furthering the understanding of aging, AD, and other diseases. Although there will always be limitations to combining data from different acquisition protocols, variation in analyses are a huge barrier to comparing results from various studies. It is only by sharing data and subjecting them to identical analysis pipelines that age-related differences will be understood. Standardized analysis packages such as LCModel are a step in the right direction, but any such analysis package still obscures details of the original data, which are potentially necessary in understanding the results. Only by making data public and encouraging large-scale analyses will this hurdle be overcome.

References

Angelie, E., Bonmartin, A., Boudraa, A., Gonnaud, P. M., Mallet, J. J., & Sappey-Marinier, D. (2001). Regional differences and metabolic changes in normal aging of the human brain: proton MR spectroscopic imaging study. *American Journal of Neuroradiology*, 22(1), 119–127.

Augustine, E. M., Spielman, D. M., Barnes, P. D., Sutcliffe, T. L., Dermon, J. D., Mirmiran, M., et al. (2008). Can magnetic resonance spectroscopy predict neurodevelopmental outcome in very low birth weight preterm infants? *Journal of Perinatology*, 28(9), 611–618.

Boumezbeur., F., Mason, G. F., de Graaf, R. A., Behar, K. L., Cline, G. W., Shulman, G. I., et al. (2010). Altered brain mitochondrial metabolism in healthy aging as assessed by *in vivo* magnetic resonance spectroscopy. *Journal of Cerebral Blood Flow and Metabolism*, 30(1), 211–221.

Brooks, J., Roberts, N., Kemp, G., Gosney, M. A., Lye, M., & Whitehorse, G. H. (2001). A proton magnetic resonance spectroscopy study of age-related changes in frontal lobe metabolite concentrations. *Cerebral Cortex*, 11(7), 598–605.

Brooks, W. M., Friedman, S. D., & Stidley, C. A. (1999). Reproducibility of ^{1}H-MRS *in vivo*. *Magnetic Resonance in Medicine*, 41(1) 193–197.

Cady, E. B., Penrice, J., Amess, P. N., Lorek, A., Wylezinska, M., Aldridge, R. F., et al. (1996). Lactate, N-acetylaspartate, choline and creatine concentrations, and spin-spin relaxation in thalamic and occipito-parietal regions of developing human brain. *Magnetic Resonance in Medicine*, 36(6), 878–886.

Card, D., Nossin-Manor, R., Moore, A. M., Raybaud, C., Sled, J. G., & Taylor, M. J. (2013). Brain metabolite concentrations associated with illness severity scores and white matter abnormalities in very preterm infants. *Pediatric Research*, 74, 75–81.

Caserta, M. T., Bannon, Y., Fernandez, F., Giunta, B., Schoenberg, M. R., & Tan, J. (2009). *Normal brain aging clinical, immunological, neuropsychological, and neuroimaging features*, (1st ed.). *International Review of Neurobiology*, (Vol. 84). Amsterdam: Elsevier.

Cetin, I., Barberis, B., Brusati, V., Brighina, E., Mandia, L., Arighi, A., et al. (2011). Lactate detection in the brain of growth-restricted fetuses with magnetic resonance spectroscopy. American Journal of Obstetrics and Gynecology, 205, 4(350), e1–e7.

Chang, L., Ernst, T., Poland, R. E., & Jenden, D. J. (1996). *In vivo* proton magnetic resonance spectroscopy of the normal aging human brain. *Life Sciences*, 58(22), 2049–2056.

Chang, L., Jiang, C. S., & Ernst, T. (2009). Effects of age and sex on brain glutamate and other metabolites. *Magnetic Resonance Imaging*, 27(1), 142–145.

Chard, D. T., McLean, M. A., Parker, G. J. M., MacManus, D. G., & Miller, D. H. (2002). Reproducibility of *in vivo* metabolite quantification with proton magnetic resonance spectroscopic imaging. *Journal of Magnetic Resonance Imaging*, 15(2), 219–225.

Charles-Edwards, G. D., Jan, W., To, M., Maxwell, D., Keevil, S. F., & Robinson, R. (2010). Non-invasive detection and quantification of human foetal brain lactate in utero by magnetic resonance spectroscopy. *Prenatal Diagnosis*, 30(3), 260–266.

Charlton, R., McIntyre, D., Howe, F., Morris, R., & Markus, H. (2007). The relationship between white matter brain metabolites and cognition in normal aging: the GENIE study. *Brain Research*, 1164, 108–116.

Chau, V., Poskitt, K. J., McFadden, D. E., Bowen-Roberts, T., Synnes, A., Brant, R., et al. (2009). Effect of chorioamnionitis on brain development and injury in premature newborns. *Annals of Neurology*, 66(2), 155–164.

Cho, S., Jones, D., Reddick, W. E., Ogg, R. J., & Steen, R. G. (1997). Establishing norms for age-related changes in proton T1 of human brain tissue *in vivo*. *Magnetic Resonance Imaging*, 15(10), 1133–1143.

Counsell, S. J., Kennea, N. L., Herlihy, A. H., Allsop, J. M., Harrison, M. C., Cowan, F. M., et al. (2003). T2 relaxation values in the developing preterm brain. *American Journal of Neuroradiology*, 24(8), 1654–1660.

Dennis, N. A., & Cabeza, R. (2008). Neuroimaging of healthy cognitive aging. In F. Craik, & T. Salthouse (Eds.), *Handbook of Aging and Cognition* (3rd ed., pp. 1–54). Mahwah, NJ: Lawrence Erlbaum.

Ding, X. -Q. (2009). T2 relaxometry of maturing brains. *Journal of Magnetic Resonance Imaging*, 30(4), 911 author reply 912

Ethofer, T., Mader, I., Seeger, U., Helms, G., Erb, M., Grodd, W., et al. (2003). Comparison of longitudinal metabolite relaxation times in different regions of the human brain at 1.5 and 3 Tesla. *Magnetic Resonance Medicine*, 50(6), 1296–1301.

Ferrie, J., Barantin, L., Saliba, E., Akoka, S., Tranquart, F., Sirinelli, D., et al. (1999). MR assessment of the brain maturation during the perinatal period: quantitative T 2 MR study in premature newborns. *Magnetic Resonance Imaging*, 17(9), 1275–1288.

Fukuzako, H., Hashiguchi, T., Sakamoto, Y., Okamura, H., Doi, W., Takenouchi, K., et al. (1997). Metabolite changes with age measured by proton magnetic resonance spectroscopy in normal subjects. *Psychiatry and Clinical Neurosciences*, 51(4), 261–263.

Gadin, E., Lobo, M., Paul, D. A., Sem, K., Steiner, K. V., Mackley, A., et al. (2012). Volumetric MRI and MRS and early motor development of infants born preterm. *Pediatric Physical Therapy*, 24(1), 38–44.

Gasparovic, C., Bedrick, E. J., Mayer, A. R., Yeo, R. A., Chen, H., Damaraju, E., et al. (2011). Test-retest reliability and reproducibility of short-echo-time spectroscopic imaging of human brain at 3 T. *Magnetic Resonance in Medicine*, 66(2), 324–332.

Geurts, J. J. G., Barkhof, F., Castelijns, J. A., Uitdehaag, B. M. J., Polman, C. H., & Pouwels, P. J. W. (2004). Quantitative ^{1}H-MRS of healthy human cortex, hippocampus, and thalamus: metabolite concentrations, quantification precision, and reproducibility. *Journal of Magnetic Resonance Imaging*, 20(3), 366–371.

Girard, N., Gouny, S. C., Viola, A., Le Fur, Y., Viout, P., Chaumoitre, K., et al. (2006). Assessment of normal fetal brain maturation in utero by proton magnetic resonance spectroscopy. *Magnetic Resonance in Medicine*, 56(4), 768–775.

Grachev, I. D., & Apkarian, A. V. (2001). Aging alters regional multichemical profile of the human brain: an *in vivo* ^{1}H-MRS study of young versus middle-aged subjects. *Journal of Neurochemistry*, 76(2), 582–593.

Griffith, H. R., Stewart, C. C., & den Hollander, J. A. (2009). Proton magnetic resonance spectroscopy in dementias and mild cognitive impairment, (1st ed.). *International Review of Neurobiology*, (Vol. 84). Amsterdam: Elsevier.

Harada, M., Miyoshi, H., Otsuka, H., Nishitani, H., & Uno, M. (2001). Multivariate analysis of regional metabolic differences in normal ageing on localised quantitative proton MR spectroscopy. *Neuroradiology*, 43(6), 448–452.

Hasan, K. M., Walimuni, I. S., Kramer, L. A., & Frye, R. E. (2010). Human brain atlas-based volumetry and relaxometry: application to healthy development and natural aging. *Magnetic Resonance in Medicine*, 64(5), 1382–1389.

Heerschap, A., Kok, R. D., & van den Berg, P. P. (2003). Antenatal proton MR spectroscopy of the human brain *in vivo*. *Child's Nervous System*, 19(7–8), 418–421.

Hüppi, P. S., Posse, S., Lazeyras, F., Burri, R., Bossi, E., & Herschkowitz, N. (1991). Magnetic resonance in preterm and term newborns: [1]H-spectroscopy in developing human brain. *Pediatric Research*, 30(6), 574–578.

Kadota, T., Horinouchi, T., & Kuroda, C. (2001). Development and aging of the cerebrum: assessment with proton MR spectroscopy. *American Journal of Neuroradiology*, 22(1), 128–135.

Kantarci, K. (2007). [1]H magnetic resonance spectroscopy in dementia. *British Journal of Radiology*, 80(Spec No 2), S146–S152.

Kirov, I. I., Fleysher, L., Fleysher, R., Patil, V., Liu, S., & Gonen, O. (2008). Age dependence of regional proton metabolites T2 relaxation times in the human brain at 3 T. *Magnetic Resonance in Medicine, 60*(4), 790–795.

Kirov, I. I., George, I. C., Jayawickrama, N., Babb, J. S., Perry, N. N., & Gonen, O. (2012). Longitudinal inter- and intra-individual human brain metabolic quantification over 3 years with proton MR spectroscopy at 3 T. *Magnetic Resonance in Medicine, 67*(1), 27–33.

Kok, R. D., van den Berg, P. P., van den Bergh, A. J., Nijland, R., & Heerschap, A. (2002). Maturation of the human fetal brain as observed by ^{1}H MR spectroscopy. *Magnetic Resonance in Medicine, 48*(4), 611–616.

Kreis, R., Ernst, T., & Ross, B. D. (1993). Development of the human brain: *in vivo* quantification of metabolite and water content with proton magnetic resonance spectroscopy. *Magnetic Resonance in Medicine, 30*(4), 424–437.

Kreis, R., Hofmann, L., Kuhlmann, B., Boesch, C., Bossi, E., & Hüppi, P. S. (2002). Brain metabolite composition during early human brain development as measured by quantitative *in vivo* [1]H magnetic resonance spectroscopy. *Magnetic Resonance Medicine, 48*(6), 949–958.

Kreis, R., Slotboom, J., Hofmann, L., & Boesch, C. (2005). Integrated data acquisition and processing to determine metabolite contents, relaxation times, and macromolecule baseline in single examinations of individual subjects. *Magnetic Resonance in Medicine, 54*, 761–768.

Kugel, H., Roth, B., Pillekamp, F., Kru, K., Schulte, O., Gontard, A. V., et al. (2003). Proton spectroscopic metabolite signal relaxation times in preterm infants: a prerequisite for quantitative spectroscopy in infant brain. *Journal of Magnetic Resonance Imaging, 17*, 634–640.

Langer, D. L., Rakaric, P., Kirilova, A., Jaffray, D. A., & Damyanovich, A. Z. (2007). Assessment of metabolite quantitation reproducibility in serial 3D-(1)H-MR spectroscopic imaging of human brain using stereotactic repositioning. *Magnetic Resonance in Medicine, 58*(4), 666–673.

Leary, S. M., Brex, P. A., MacManus, D. G., Parker, G. J., Barker, G. J., Miller, D. H., et al. (2000). A (1)H magnetic resonance spectroscopy study of aging in parietal white matter: implications for trials in multiple sclerosis. *Magnetic Resonance Imaging, 18*(4), 455–459.

Lenroot, R. K., & Giedd, J. N. (2006). Brain development in children and adolescents: insights from anatomical magnetic resonance imaging. *Neuroscience and Biobehavioral Reviews, 30*(6), 718–729.

Leppert, I. R., Almli, C. R., McKinstry, R. C., Mulkern, R. V., Pierpaoli, C., Rivkin, M. J., et al. (2009). T(2) relaxometry of normal pediatric brain development. *Journal of Magnetic Resonance Imaging, 29*(2), 258–267.

Li, B. S. Y., Babb, J. S., Soher, B. J., Maudsley, A. A., & Gonen, O. (2002). Reproducibility of 3D proton spectroscopy in the human brain. *Magnetic Resonance in Medicine, 47*(3), 439–446.

Limperopoulos, C., Tworetzky, W., McElhinney, D. B., Newburger, J. W., Brown, D. W., Robertson, R. L., et al. (2010). Brain volume and metabolism in fetuses with congenital heart disease: evaluation with quantitative magnetic resonance imaging and spectroscopy. *Circulation, 121*(1), 26–33.

Maudsley, A. A., Domenig, C., & Sheriff, S. (2010). Reproducibility of serial whole-brain MR spectroscopic imaging. *NMR in Biomedicine, 23*(3), 251–256.

McIntyre, D. J. O., Charlton, R. A., Markus, H. S., & Howe, F. A. (2007). Long and short echo time proton magnetic resonance spectroscopic imaging of the healthy aging brain. *Journal of Magnetic Resonance Imaging, 26*(6), 1596–1606.

Minati, L., Grisoli, M., & Bruzzone, M. G. (2007). MR spectroscopy, functional MRI, and diffusion-tensor imaging in the aging brain: a conceptual review. *Journal of Geriatric Psychiatry and Neurology, 20*(1), 3–21.

Neeb, H., Ermer, V., Stocker, T., & Shah, N. J. (2008). Fast quantitative mapping of absolute water content with full brain coverage. *NeuroImage, 42*(3), 1094–1109.

Neeb, H., Zilles, K., & Shah, N. J. (2006). Fully-automated detection of cerebral water content changes: study of age- and gender-related H2O patterns with quantitative MRI. *NeuroImage, 29*(3), 910–922.

Nossin-Manor, R., Card, D., Morris, D., Noormohamed, S., Shroff, M. M., Whyte, H. E., et al. (2013). Quantitative MRI in the very preterm brain: assessing tissue organization and myelination using magnetization transfer, diffusion tensor and T(1) imaging. *NeuroImage, 64*, 505–516.

Nossin-Manor, R., Chung, A. D., Morris, D., Soares-Fernandes, J. P., Thomas, B., Cheng, H.-L. M., et al. (2011). Optimized T_1- and T_2-weighted volumetric brain imaging as a diagnostic tool in very preterm neonates. *Pediatric Radiology, 41*(6), 702–710.

Oros-Peusquens, A. M., Laurila, M., & Shah, N. J. (2008). Magnetic field dependence of the distribution of NMR relaxation times in the living human brain. *MAGMA, 21*(1–2), 131–147.

Pfefferbaum, A., Adalsteinsson, E., Spielman, D., Sullivan, E. V., & Lim, K. O. (1999). *In vivo* spectroscopic quantification of the N-acetyl moiety, creatine, and choline from large volumes of brain gray and white matter: effects of normal aging. *Magnetic Resonance in Medicine, 41*(2), 276–284.

Provencher, S. W. (2001). Automatic quantitation of localized *in vivo* [1]H spectra with LCModel. *NMR in Biomedicine, 14*(4), 260–264.

Pugash, D., Krssak, M., Kulemann, V., & Prayer, D. (2009). Magnetic resonance spectroscopy of the fetal brain. *Prenatal Diagnosis, 29*(4), 434–441.

Raininko, R., & Mattsson, P. (2010). Metabolite concentrations in supraventricular white matter from teenage to early old age: A short echo time ^{1}H magnetic resonance spectroscopy (MRS) study. *Acta Radiologica, 51*(3), 309–315.

Reyngoudt, H., Claeys, T., Vlerick, L., Verleden, S., Acou, M., Deblaere, K., et al. (2012). Age-related differences in metabolites in the posterior cingulate cortex and hippocampus of normal ageing brain: a ^{1}H-MRS study. *European Journal of Radiology, 81*(3), e223–e231.

Roelants-van Rijn, A. M., Groenendaal, F., Stoutenbeek, P., & van der Grond, J. (2004). Lactate in the foetal brain: detection and implications. *Acta Paediatrica, 93*(7), 937–940.

Sailasuta, N., Ernst, T., & Chang, L. (2008). Regional variations and the effects of age and gender on glutamate concentrations in the human brain. *Magnetic Resonance Imaging, 26*(5), 667–675.

Saito, N., Sakai, O., Ozonoff, A., & Jara, H. (2009). Relaxo-volumetric multispectral quantitative magnetic resonance imaging of the brain over the human lifespan: global and regional aging patterns. *Magnetic Resonance Imaging, 27*(7), 895–906.

Saunders, D. E., Howe, F. A., van den Boogaart, A., Griffiths, J. R., & Brown, M. M. (1999). Aging of the adult human brain: *in vivo* quantitation of metabolite content with proton magnetic resonance spectroscopy. *Journal of Magnetic Resonance Imaging, 9*(5), 711–716.

Schmidt, C. W. (2004). Metabolomics: what's happening downstream of DNA. *Environmental Health Perspectives, 112*(7), A410–A415.

Sijens, P. E., den Heijer, T., Origgi, D., Vermeer, S. E., Breteler, M. M. B., Hofman, A., et al. (2003). Brain changes with aging: MR spectroscopy at supraventricular plane shows differences between women and men. *Radiology, 226*(3), 889–896.

Tedeschi, G., Bertolino, A., Campbell, G., Barnett, A. S., Duyn, J. H., Jacob, P. K., et al. (1996). Reproducibility of proton MR spectroscopic imaging findings. *American Journal of Neuroradiology, 17*(10), 1871–1879.

Toft, P. B., Leth, H., Lou, H. C., Pryds, O., & Henriksen, O. (1994). Metabolite concentrations in the developing brain estimated with proton MR spectroscopy. *Journal of Magnetic Resonance Imaging*, 4(5), 674–680.

Träber, F., Block, W., Freymann, N., Gür, O., Kucinski, T., Hammen, T., et al. (2006). A multicenter reproducibility study of single-voxel ¹H-MRS of the medial temporal lobe. *European Radiology*, 16(5), 1096–1103.

Tumeh, P. C., Alavi, A., Houseni, M., Greenfield, A., Chryssikos, T., Newberg, A., et al. (2007). Structural and functional imaging correlates for age-related changes in the brain. *Seminars in Nuclear Medicine*, 37(2), 69–87.

Van Kooij, B. J. M., Benders, M. J. N. L., Anbeek, P., Van Haastert, I. C., De Vries, L. S., & Groenendaal, F. (2012). Cerebellar volume and proton magnetic resonance spectroscopy at term, and neurodevelopment at 2 years of age in preterm infants. *Developmental Medicine and Child Neurology*, 54(3), 260–266.

Vigneron, D. B. (2006). Magnetic resonance spectroscopic imaging of human brain development. *Neuroimaging Clinics of North America*, 16(1), 75–85.

Vigneron, D. B., Barkovich, A. J., Noworolski, S. M., von dem Bussche, M., Henry, R. G., Lu, Y., et al. (2001). Three-dimensional proton MR spectroscopic imaging of premature and term neonates. *American Journal of Neuroradiology*, 22(7), 1424–1433.

Volpe, J. J. (2008). *Neurology of the Newborn* (5th ed.). Philadelphia, PA: WB Saunders.

Volpe, J. J. (2009). Brain injury in premature infants: a complex amalgam of destructive and developmental disturbances. *Lancet Neurology*, 8(1), 110–124.

Wang, J., Shaffer, M. L., Eslinger, P. J., Sun, X., Weitekamp, C. W., Patel, M. M., et al. (2012). Maturational and aging effects on human brain apparent transverse relaxation. *PloS One*, 7(2), e31907.

Wijnen, J. P., van Asten, J. J. A., Klomp, D. W. J., Sjobakk, T. E., Gribbestad, I. S., Scheenen, T. W. J., et al. (2010). Short echo time ¹H MRSI of the human brain at 3 T with adiabatic slice-selective refocusing pulses; reproducibility and variance in a dual center setting. *Journal of Magnetic Resonance Imaging*, 31(1), 61–70.

Williams, L., Gelman, N., Picot, P. A., Lee, D. S., Ewing, J. R., Han, V. K., et al. (2005). Neonatal brain: regional variability of *in vivo* MR imaging relaxation rates at 3.0 T–initial experience. *Radiology*, 235(2), 595–603.

Xu, D., Bonifacio, S. L., Charlton, N. N., Vaughan, P. C., Lu, Y., Ferriero, D. M., et al. (2011). MR spectroscopy of normative premature newborns. *Journal of Magnetic Resonance*, 33(2), 306–311.

Xu, D., & Vigneron, D. (2010). Magnetic resonance spectroscopy imaging of the newborn brain–a technical review. *Seminars in Perinatology*, 34(1), 20–27.

Zaaraoui, W., Fleysher, L., Fleysher, R., Liu, S., Soher, B. J., & Gonen, O. (2007). Human brain-structure resolved T(2) relaxation times of proton metabolites at 3 Tesla. *Magnetic Resonance in Medicine*, 57(6), 983–989.

Zhu, H., & Barker, P. B. (2011). MR Spectroscopy and Spectroscopic Imaging of the Brain. In M. Modo, & J. W. M. Bulte (Eds.), *Magnetic Resonance Neuroimaging* (Vol. 711, pp. 203–226). Totowa, NJ: Humana Press.

Hormonal Influences on Magnetic Resonance Spectroscopy Measures

Jennifer Brawn[1] *and Katy Vincent*[1,2]

[1]Functional Magnetic Resonance Imaging of the Brain Centre, University of Oxford, UK

[2]Nuffield Department of Obstetrics and Gynaecology, University of Oxford, UK

INTRODUCTION

Hormones have long been known to have important physiological influences on the body. However, an increasing body of literature now also documents their effects on the brain (McEwen et al., 2012). Moreover, it is not just the hormones themselves that influence neurobiology; both their precursors and derivatives also play an important role. These compounds have been observed to alter brain function through a variety of mechanisms including regional volumetric changes (Woolley & McEwen, 1993) and altering neurotransmitter binding affinity (Majewska et al., 1986). Unfortunately, the extent to which they alter neurochemistry is still not fully understood. Clearly hormonal factors are of particular interest to researchers considering sex differences and menstrual cycle influences on brain function; however, this chapter highlights the possible confounds that may be introduced if they are not considered in all experimental designs. We will begin by giving a brief overview of the synthesis and functions of the hormones of interest and will then review the research to date demonstrating an influence on magnetic resonance spectroscopy (MRS) measures.

OVERVIEW OF HORMONE BIOLOGY

A detailed review of the endocrinology of the hormones relevant to this topic is beyond the scope of this chapter; however, a brief overview is given here to put the following discussion in context. For a more detailed review see *Johnson & Everitt's Essential Reproduction* (Johnson & Everitt, 2007).

Synthesis and Regulation

Several steroid hormones have been the subject of interest in MRS research, including cortisol, estradiol, and progesterone (see Tables 3.10.1 and 3.10.2). Cortisol, a glucocorticoid, is central to the stress response. It is synthesized in the adrenal cortex and is regulated through the hypothalamic–pituitary–adrenal (HPA) axis. Production of cortisol is modulated through negative feedback, inhibiting further production. Cortisol levels experience diurnal fluctuation (for review, see Greenstein & Wood, 2006). However, rates of cortisol synthesis are not consistent across the population. One study found that despite similar mean cortisol levels, production was greater in males than in females (Vierhapper et al., 1998). Additionally, differences in the timing of cortisol release have been reported between females with premenstrual dysphoric disorder (PMDD) and healthy individuals (Parry et al., 2000). Furthermore, both basal levels of cortisol and the amount released in response to a stressor are altered in a number of conditions, including major depression, post-traumatic stress disorder (PTSD), and a variety of chronic pain states (Holsboer, 2001; Strohle et al., 2008; Galli et al., 2009).

Estradiol and progesterone are important female reproductive hormones that fluctuate over the menstrual cycle (see Fig. 3.10.1). They are primarily synthesized in the ovaries and are regulated by the hypothalamus and anterior pituitary (for review, see Greenstein & Wood, 2006). Estradiol can be produced through two different chemical pathways: aromatizing testosterone or reducing estrone. Pregnenolone is the precursor to progesterone, and allopregnanolone is derived from progesterone (for review, see Stoffel-Wagner, 2003). During the menstrual cycle, increases in estradiol trigger

TABLE 3.10.1   Influence of Cortisol on Neurochemicals

Authors	Subject type	Region of interest	Neurochemicals measured	Results
Neylan et al. (2003)	PTSD Healthy	Hippocampus	NAA	PTSD and Healthy: positive relationship between NAA and cortisol
Colla et al. (2009)	Bipolar Healthy	Hippocampus	NAA Glutamate	Bipolar and Healthy: negative relationship between neurochemicals (NAA and glutamate) and cortisol
Wang et al. (2012)	MDD Healthy	Hippocampus	NAA Choline Creatine	MDD: no relationship between neurochemicals (NAA/creatine and choline/creatine) and cortisol

TABLE 3.10.2   Influence of Estradiol and Progesterone on Neurochemicals

Authors	Subject type	Region(s) of interest	Neurochemicals measured	Results
Rasgon et al. (2001)	PMDD Healthy	Parietal WM Frontal GM	Choline NAA Myo-inositol Creatine	PMDD and Healthy: WM choline/creatine ↑ across the menstrual cycle; GM NAA/creatine ↓ across the menstrual cycle
Epperson et al. (2002)	PMDD Healthy	Occipital cortex	GABA	PMDD: GABA ↑ across menstrual cycle[a] Healthy: GABA ↓ across menstrual cycle[b]
Epperson et al. (2005)	Smokers Healthy	Occipital cortex	GABA	Healthy: GABA ↓ across menstrual cycle
Epperson et al. (2006)	PPD Healthy Postpartum Healthy	Occipital cortex	GABA	GABA was higher in healthy females compared to postpartum females[c]
Batra et al. (2008)	PMDD Healthy	Medial prefrontal cortex	Glutamate	PMDD and Healthy: glutamate/creatine ↓ across menstrual cycle
Harada et al. (2011)	Healthy	LN FL AC	GABA	Healthy: GABA ↓ across menstrual cycle (in LN and FL, not AC)
McEwen et al. (2012)	PPD Healthy	Medial prefrontal cortex	Glutamate NAA Choline Creatine	Glutamate was lower in healthy females than those with PPD

[a]Positive correlation between GABA and estradiol and progesterone values.
[b]Negative correlation between GABA and estradiol and progesterone and allopregnanolone values.
[c]No correlation between GABA and estradiol, progesterone, allopregnanolone, and pregnenolone values.
WM, white matter; GM, gray matter; LN, Lentiform nucleus; FL, frontal lobe; AC, anterior cingulate.

secretion of luteinizing hormone (LH) via positive feedback to the hypothalamus and anterior pituitary. This peak in LH promotes ovulation, increasing progesterone production. Both estradiol and progesterone levels remain high until just before menses (for review, see Greenstein & Wood, 2006). There is, however, notable variation in estradiol and progesterone within and between individuals. In one study, researchers observed that in healthy, fertile women their profiles of one or more of estradiol, progesterone, and LH deviated from established normal means in over 70% of the cycles (Alliende, 2002). Estradiol and progesterone are also present in males, with the testes and adrenal cortex responsible for their synthesis (for review, see Greenstein & Wood, 2006).

Testosterone is the major sex steroid hormone in men, with LH promoting its synthesis in the testes. Increasing testosterone concentrations feed back negatively to the hypothalamus and anterior pituitary. Testosterone is also present in females with synthesis taking place in the ovaries and adrenal cortex (for review, see Greenstein & Wood, 2006). Testosterone

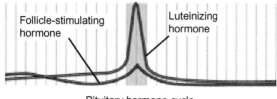

Pituitary hormone cycle

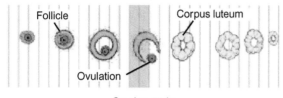

Ovarian cycle

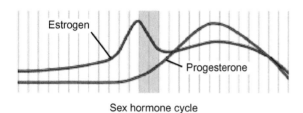

Sex hormone cycle

Endometrial cycle

FIGURE 3.10.1 Physiological changes over the human menstrual cycle. This figure is reproduced in color in the color plate section. *(From Porter, R. (2013). The Merck Manual Home Health Handbook, edited by Robert Porter. Copyright (2013) by Merck Sharp & Dohme Corp., a subsidiary of Merck & Co., Inc., Whitehouse Station, NJ. Available at: http://www.merckmanuals.com/home/index.html.)*

Quantifying Hormone Levels

There are several methods available for direct hormonal measurement, including salivary and blood assays. Salivary measurements have a significant advantage in that they reflect only biologically active hormones; however, these measurements are less sensitive to biological changes (for review, see Hofman, 2001). In addition, it has been reported that there is notable variation between individuals with regard to free estradiol in serum and salivary measures, highlighting a possible limitation (Gann et al., 2001). Blood sampling is the most effective method of capturing real-time hormonal changes (for review, see Riley et al., 1999). Unfortunately, measurement of serum levels reflects both protein-bound and free hormones (Slaunwhite & Sandberg, 1959). Only unbound hormones are of interest since they have the potential to be biologically active (for review, see Greenstein & Wood, 2006). There are methods available for estimating the ratio of free to bound hormones, but they are complicated and obviously lack the specificity that an actual measurement provides (Södergård et al., 1982). To further complicate the situation, hormones themselves can alter the concentration of binding proteins and thereby the level of free hormone (for review, see Anderson, 1974).

While it is assumed that serum levels of hormones reflect those in brain tissue, transport of hormones across the blood–brain barrier depends on a number of factors (Pardridge, 1981). However, ethical issues prevent a direct measurement of brain hormone concentration in human studies. This may be a particular confound when subjects using exogenous hormones are included (e.g., in the combined oral contraceptive pill), as these compounds can dramatically alter rates of synthesis of binding proteins. Furthermore, neurosteroids including estradiol, testosterone, and allopregnanolone can also be synthesized *de novo* in the central nervous system (for review, see Stoffel-Wagner, 2003). In rodents, researchers found that allopregnanolone levels in the blood were not necessarily reflective of those in the brain (Barbaccia et al., 1997), and it is conceivable that concentrations may also vary between specific brain regions.

NEUROCHEMICALS: MALES VERSUS FEMALES

Sex-specific differences in neurochemistry have been a topic of interest in MRS studies. In healthy males and females, some studies report differing neurochemical concentrations (Wilkinson et al., 1997) while others observe no differences at all (Safriel et al.,

levels are important to account for in both males and females since they vary between people within each gender (Meikle et al., 1986; Dabbs & de La Rue, 1991) and fluctuate seasonally (Stanton et al., 2011) and throughout the day (Dabbs, 1990). Additionally, testosterone fluctuates over the course of the menstrual cycle (Dabbs, 1990). To date, however, there have not been any MRS studies directly evaluating the role of testosterone on brain chemistry.

2005). Gender differences have also been reported in psychiatric conditions such as schizophrenia (Tayoshi et al., 2009) and depression (Sanacora et al., 1999). While this does not offer information on the influence of individual hormones, it indicates that sex-specific biology may play a role in neurochemical regulation.

Influence of Glucocorticoids on Neurochemicals

In healthy individuals, increasing cortisol concentrations have been associated with both increasing (Neylan et al., 2003) and decreasing N-acetylaspartic acid (NAA; Colla et al., 2009). Additionally, a negative relationship between glutamate and cortisol has been described (Colla et al., 2009).

Abnormal HPA axis regulation has been a subject of interest in mood disorder research (Kudielka & Kirschbaum, 2005). Individuals with depression exhibit abnormal cortisol levels, which have been attributed to malfunctioning feedback loops within the axis (for review, see Pariante & Lightman, 2008). Some MRS studies of these patients have reported decreased glutamate/glutamine and GABA levels in various brain regions, although these studies were not specifically interested in the impact of glucocorticoids on neurochemicals (for review, see Hasler 2010). One MRS study evaluating major depressive disorder (MDD) directly addressed the possibility that cortisol might play a role in neurochemical regulation. However, no correlation was observed between cortisol and hippocampal ratios of NAA/creatine and choline/creatine (Wang et al., 2012).

The relationship between cortisol and neurochemicals has also been explored in other psychiatric disorders. In bipolar patients, researchers have observed that both hippocampal NAA and glutamate were negatively correlated with cortisol (Colla et al., 2009). In patients with post-traumatic stress disorder (PTSD), the opposite relationship between NAA and cortisol was observed: NAA in the left hippocampus was positively correlated with cortisol (Neylan et al., 2003). These results suggest that cortisol may play an important role in regulating NAA, which is used as a measure of neuronal integrity (Gazdzinski et al., 2010). However, there are few studies and the results are contradictory, thus limiting the extent to which conclusions can be drawn on the nature of this relationship (see Table 20.1).

Female Sex Steroidal Hormones and Neurochemical Changes

Female biology offers an excellent opportunity to study the impact of sex steroidal hormones, progesterone and estradiol, on neurochemical regulation. Estradiol and progesterone have been implicated in increasing and decreasing dendritic spine density, respectively (Woolley & McEwen, 1993). As described earlier, the most common and predictable fluctuation in these hormones occurs during the menstrual cycle, where estradiol and progesterone levels fluctuate over approximately 28 days (for review, see Greenstein & Wood, 2006). The bulk of research evaluating sex steroidal hormones and neurochemistry takes advantage of the menstrual cycle (Rasgon et al., 2001; Epperson et al., 2002, 2005; Batra et al., 2008; Harada et al., 2011). Pregnancy is another important biological event, with large increases and postpartum decreases in progesterone and estradiol. Two studies have used pregnancy as a marker for hormonal changes and collected neurochemical data (Epperson et al., 2006; McEwen et al., 2012).

Much of the research in this field is centered on understanding the impact of hormones on changes in psychological health, such as PMDD and postpartum depression (PPD; Rasgon et al., 2001; Epperson et al., 2002, 2006; Batra et al., 2008; McEwen et al., 2012). This is a logical approach since there is a substantial body of research supporting differences in neurochemicals between healthy individuals and those with psychological ailments (Auer et al., 2000; Bhagwagar et al., 2008).

Influence of Estradiol and Progesterone on Neurochemicals

In the domain of MRS and hormones, estradiol and progesterone, are the most heavily studied. Researchers have examined various neurochemicals including myo-inositol, choline, NAA, γ-aminobutyric acid (GABA) and glutamate/glutamine (see Table 20.2).

NAA, Choline, and Myo-inositol

In healthy females, Rasgon and colleagues (2001) observed an increase in parietal white matter choline/creatine ratios from the follicular to luteal phase. In frontal gray matter, the NAA/creatine ratio decreased from the follicular to luteal phase. Myo-inositol levels were not observed to change. The same trends seen in healthy females were also reported in those with PMDD. Although there were no statistically significant differences between subject groups, in the parietal white matter PMDD females demonstrated slightly higher luteal phase myo-inositol/creatine ratios than healthy controls (Rasgon et al., 2001). This was the first reported observation of neurochemicals changing over the menstrual cycle.

GABA

The GABA system is well known for being influenced by ovarian hormones. Progesterone has been shown to increase sensitivity of the GABA system through its derivative, allopregnanolone, which increases the binding affinity of GABA to the GABA$_A$ receptor (Majewska et al., 1986). Conversely, estradiol decreases binding affinity to the GABA$_A$ receptor (Smith et al., 2002). There is substantial evidence supporting hormonally induced GABAergic changes and several studies suggesting these changes include neurotransmitter regulation (Epperson et al., 2002, 2005).

CHANGES IN GABA OVER THE MENSTRUAL CYCLE

GABA is the most heavily studied of all the neurochemicals over the menstrual cycle (see Table 20.2). In healthy females, GABA levels in the occipital cortex decreased across the menstrual cycle (Epperson et al., 2002, 2005). In a different study examining the lentiform nucleus and frontal lobe, GABA levels decreased from the follicular phase to the luteal phase. The anterior cingulate also experienced changes in GABA concentrations; however, the results were not significant (Harada et al., 2011). In females with PMDD, changes in GABA were opposite to that of healthy females with increasing concentrations from the follicular to luteal phase (Epperson et al., 2002).

These results suggest that in healthy females GABA concentrations decrease as estradiol, progesterone, and their metabolites increase during the luteal phase (Epperson et al., 2002, 2005; Harada et al., 2011). However, only Epperson and colleagues (2002) compared GABA to hormonal measures—observing that estradiol, progesterone, and allopregnanolone were negatively correlated with cortical GABA in healthy females. In females with PMDD, conversely, estradiol and progesterone were positively correlated with cortical GABA, and allopregnanolone was nonsignificant (Epperson et al., 2002).

CHANGES IN GABA POSTPARTUM

GABA levels have also been examined after pregnancy. In comparing two groups of 6 month postpartum females, Epperson and colleagues (2006) found that those with PPD had significantly higher estradiol levels than the healthy postpartum females (no differences in progesterone, allopregnanolone, and pregnenolone). Healthy women who had not recently been pregnant were also included in the study. As would be expected, these women had significantly higher estradiol levels during their follicular phase than the healthy postpartum females. Allopregnanolone was also significantly higher in the healthy females when compared to the postpartum groups. Cortical GABA was significantly higher in the healthy follicular phase women compared to both healthy and depressed postpartum groups. The females with PPD had higher GABA levels in the occipital cortex than the healthy postpartum females; however, this difference was not statistically significant (Epperson et al., 2006). This study is more difficult to interpret in terms of hormonal impact on neurochemicals since groups varied by psychiatric condition, pregnancy history, and presence of active menstrual cycle.

GABA appears to be regulated by hormones and their derivatives, but the exact nature of the relationship is still unclear. Epperson and colleagues (2002) hypothesized that hormones, such as estradiol and progesterone, might play a role in GABA regulation. In healthy individuals, it has been suggested that in the presence of GABA$_A$ binding agonists, like allopregnanolone, GABA synthesis might decrease in response (Epperson et al., 2002, 2005). Pathologies like PMDD might potentially reverse this relationship (Epperson et al., 2002). These observations highlight the complexity of neurotransmitter regulation. This is further emphasized by the fact that estradiol and progesterone appeared to regulate GABA in a similar manner, despite their opposing influences on the system as a whole, which raises more questions about this complex process (Epperson et al., 2002). The challenge in future research is to untangle the individual impacts of estradiol, progesterone, and their metabolites on GABA. Despite the confusion, the literature on GABA offers the most complete picture of hormonal regulation of neurotransmitters. MRS research on glutamate, GABA's opposing force, highlights the complex relationship between these systems (Batra et al., 2008).

Glutamine and Glutamate

Estradiol and progesterone have also been observed to influence the glutamatergic system. In rodents, estradiol increases glutamate's binding affinity to receptors (Woolley et al., 1997), while progesterone reduces activity in the glutamatergic system (Smith et al., 1987). To date, only one study has measured glutamate over the menstrual cycle.

GLUTAMATE OVER THE MENSTRUAL CYCLE

Batra and colleagues (2008) observed that in healthy females the glutamate/creatine ratio decreased from the follicular to luteal phase. The same trend was observed in females with PMDD. While the PMDD results were as predicted, the researchers had not anticipated that glutamate concentrations in the healthy females would follow the same trend (Batra et al., 2008).

CHANGES IN GLUTAMATE POSTPARTUM

Changes in glutamate have also been observed postpartum. McEwen and colleagues (2012) examined the medial prefrontal cortex, observing that glutamate levels were higher in females with PPD than in healthy postpartum females, possibly linking glutamate to PPD. Changes in other neurochemicals were not significant (McEwen et al., 2012). While there is only a small body of literature dedicated to hormonal influences on glutamate, there does appear to be a regulatory relationship (see Table 20.2).

SUMMARY OF ESTRADIOL AND PROGESTERONE

Considering the research on GABA, hormonal data was collected in all the studies to verify cycle phase or potential differences in subject groups (Epperson et al., 2002, 2005). However, only two studies have compared GABA to hormonal values independent of menstrual phase, with one finding a negative correlation in healthy females and a positive correlation in females with PMDD (Epperson et al., 2002) and the other observing no correlation between GABA and the hormones (Epperson et al., 2006). The latter study examined postpartum females and healthy females in the follicular phase only once, rather than multiple times over menstrual cycle, so study design could potentially account for this difference. Nonetheless, these results highlight that hormonal measures alone may not be sufficient and, as suggested by several studies (Epperson et al., 2002, 2005; Batra et al., 2008), a more sophisticated relationship between hormones and neurochemicals potentially exists.

As previously mentioned, in healthy females glutamate demonstrates similar trends to GABA, with decreasing concentrations in the luteal phase compared with the follicular phase of the menstrual cycle (Batra et al., 2008). The researchers hypothesized that this might reflect a regulatory relationship between glutamate and GABA. In females with PMDD, however, glutamate demonstrated the opposite trend found in GABA, with decreasing concentrations across the menstrual cycle. It was postulated that these results reflect possible pathological changes in neurochemical regulation in females with PMDD. The researchers did highlight that these relationships may not hold when both GABA and glutamate are measured in the same location (Batra et al., 2008). As observed in depression research, the relationship between GABA, glutamate, and glutamine varies with brain region (Bhagwagar et al., 2008). Researchers should also explore how the relationship between GABA and glutamate is mediated

with fluctuating estradiol and progesterone. Before this relationship can be understood under the umbrella of hormones, their relationship to glutamate alone needs to be researched further.

MALE SEX STEROIDAL HORMONES AND NEUROCHEMICAL CHANGES

MRS research has not specifically considered the role of hormones on neurochemical regulation in males. This could be attributed to the lack of hormonal fluctuation, a characteristic inherent to female biology. Nonetheless, literature in this domain suggests that MRS might be a useful tool in evaluating the impact of testosterone and its derivatives on neurochemistry. As previously discussed, estradiol can be derived from testosterone and estradiol has already been shown to have an impact on neurochemistry. Additionally, testosterone can be reduced to form dihydrotestosterone, which is a precursor to 3β-androstanediol—a chemical observed to influence the GABA system (Reddy, 2004).

In a surgical, non-MRS study using castrated rats, researchers observed that GABA levels decreased in the septal area and amygdala after castration. However, in the midbrain GABA levels increased. Researchers attributed these changes to decreased testosterone levels. When the rodents were treated with estradiol, GABA concentrations were found to increase in all three regions (Earley & Leonard, 1978). These types of studies are useful but, for obvious reasons, cannot be replicated in humans. However, they do suggest that it may be wise to consider testosterone levels in future human MRS studies.

CONCLUSIONS

While many excellent studies exist examining the role of hormones on brain neurochemistry, they do not provide enough information to paint the full biological picture. The current body of research varies in region of interest, neurochemicals studied, and hormones measured. It is clear that more studies are needed to corroborate previous findings as well as clarify current contradictions. Moving forward, researchers should try to better define how hormones differentially affect brain regions since fluctuations in neurotransmitters, such as GABA, have been found to vary (Harada et al., 2011).

Nonetheless, even for researchers not specifically interested in hormones, it can be seen that they are an important variable to consider. As highlighted in a review by Sherman & LeResche (2006), for studies enrolling females, menstrual cycle phase should be verified and consistent for all subjects, which is not common practice, and ideally serum hormone concentrations obtained. Furthermore, it is important to determine whether subjects have been or are using hormonal medications. Oral contraceptives, for example, are popular among females of reproductive age, not only for birth control but also as treatment for a variety of conditions (including dysmenorrhea, endometriosis, and acne; Guillebaud, 2008). Identifying these medications will help ensure the acquisition of quality data. This is especially crucial in the field of neuroimaging where sample sizes remain relatively small. While not all neurochemical levels experience drastic changes, small shifts could compromise study results if not taken into account.

References

Alliende, M. E. (2002). Mena versus individual hormonal profiles in the menstrual cycle. *Fertility and Sterility, 78*(1), 90–95.

Anderson, D. C. (1974). Sex-hormone-binding globulin. *Clinical Endocrinology, 3*(1), 69–96.

Auer, D. P., Putz, B., et al. (2000). Reduced glutamate in the anterior cingulate cortex in depression: an in vivo proton magnetic resonance spectroscopy study. *Biological Psychiatry, 47*(4), 305–313.

Barbaccia, M. L., Roscetti, G., Trabucchi, M., Purdy, R. H., Mostallino, M. C., Concas, A., et al. (1997). The effects of inhibitors of GABAergic transmission and stress on brain and plasma allopregnanolone concentrations. *British Journal of Pharmacology, 120*(8), 1582–1588.

Batra, N. A., Seres-Mailo, J., et al. (2008). Proton magnetic resonance spectroscopy measurement of brain glutamate levels in premenstrual dysphoric disorder. *Biological Psychiatry, 63*(12), 1178–1184.

Bhagwagar, Z., Wylezinska, M., et al. (2008). Low GABA concentrations in occipital cortex and anterior cingulate cortex in medication-free, recovered depressed patients. *International Journal of Neuropsychopharmacology, 11*(2), 255–260.

Colla, M., Schubert, F., et al. (2009). Glutamate as a spectroscopic marker of hippocampal structural plasticity is elevated in long-term euthymic bipolar patients on chronic lithium therapy and correlates inversely with diurnal cortisol. *Molecular Psychiatry, 14*(7), 696–704 647

Dabbs, J. M., Jr. (1990). Salivary testosterone measurements: reliability across hours, days, and weeks. *Physiology and Behavior, 48*(1), 83–86.

Dabbs, J. M., & de La Rue, D. (1991). Salivary testosterone measurements among women: relative magnitude of circadian and menstrual cycles. *Hormone Research, 35*(5), 182–184.

Earley, C. J., & Leonard, B. E. (1978). GABA and gonadal hormones. *Brain Research, 155*(1), 27–34.

Epperson, C. N., Haga, K., et al. (2002). Cortical gamma-aminobutyric acid levels across the menstrual cycle in healthy women and those with premenstrual dysphoric disorder: a proton magnetic resonance spectroscopy study. *Archivevs of General Psychiatry, 59*(9), 851–858.

Epperson, C. N., Gueorguieva, R., et al. (2006). Preliminary evidence of reduced occipital GABA concentrations in puerperal women: a 1H-MRS study. *Psychopharmacology (Berl), 186*(3), 425–433.

Epperson, C. N., O'Malley, S., et al. (2005). Sex, GABA, and nicotine: the impact of smoking on cortical GABA levels across the menstrual cycle as measured with proton magnetic resonance spectroscopy. *Biological Psychiatry, 57*(1), 44–48.

Galli, U., Gaab, J., et al. (2009). Enhanced negative feedback sensitivity of the hypothalamus-pituitary-adrenal axis in chronic myogenous facial pain. *European Journal of Pain, 13*(6), 600–605.

Gann, P. H., Giovanazzi, S., Van Horn, L., Branning, A., & Chatterton, R. T., Jr. (2001). Saliva as a medium for investigating intra- and interindividual differences in sex hormone levels in premenopausal women. *Cancer Epidemiology, Biomarkers & Prevention: A Publication of the American Association for Cancer Research, Cosponsored by the American Society of Preventive Oncology, 10*(1), 59–64.

Gazdzinski, S., Millin, R., et al. (2010). BMI and neuronal integrity in healthy, cognitively normal elderly: a proton magnetic resonance spectroscopy study. *Obesity (Silver Spring), 18*(4), 743–748.

Greenstein, B., & Wood, D. F. (2006). *The Endocrine System at a Glance*. Malden, MA: Blackwell Publishers.

Guillebaud, J. (2008). *Contraception: Your Questions Answered*. New York: Churchill Livingstone.

Harada, M., Kubo, H., et al. (2011). Measurement of variation in the human cerebral GABA level by in vivo MEGA-editing proton MR spectroscopy using a clinical 3 T instrument and its dependence on brain region and the female menstrual cycle. *Hum Brain Mapp, 32*(5), 828–833.

Hasler, G. (2010). Pathophysiology of depression: do we have any solid evidence of interest to clinicians? *World Psychiatry, 9*(3), 155–161.

Hofman, L. F. (2001). Human saliva as a diagnostic specimen. *Journal of Nutrition, 131*(5), 1621S–1625S.

Holsboer, F. (2001). Stress, hypercortisolism and corticosteroid receptors in depression: implications for therapy. *Journal of Affective Disorders, 62*(1-2), 77–91.

Johnson, M. H., & Everitt, B. J. (2007). *Johnson & Everitt's Essential Reproduction*. Oxford, UK: Blackwell Publishers.

Kudielka, B. M., & Kirschbaum, C. (2005). Sex differences in HPA axis responses to stress: a review. *Biological Psychology, 69*(1), 113–132.

Majewska, M. D., Harrison, N. L., et al. (1986). Steroid hormone metabolites are barbiturate-like modulators of the GABA receptor. *Science, 232*(4753), 1004–1007.

McEwen, A. M., Burgess, D. T., et al. (2012). Increased glutamate levels in the medial prefrontal cortex in patients with postpartum depression. *Neuropsychopharmacology, 37*(11), 2428–2435.

Meikle, A. W., Bishop, D. T., Stringham, J. D., & West, D. W. (1986). Quantitating genetic and nongenetic factors that determine plasma sex steroid variation in normal male twins. *Metabolism: Clinical and Experimental, 35*(12), 1090–1095.

Neylan, T. C., Schuff, N., et al. (2003). Cortisol levels are positively correlated with hippocampal N-acetylaspartate. *Biological Psychiatry, 54*(10), 1118–1121.

Pardridge, W. M. (1981). Transport of protein-bound hormones into tissues in vivo. *Endocrinological Review, 2*(1), 103–123.

Pariante, C. M., & Lightman, S. L. (2008). The HPA axis in major depression: classical theories and new developments. *Trends in Neuroscience, 31*(9), 464–468.

Parry, B. L., Javeed, S., et al. (2000). Cortisol circadian rhythms during the menstrual cycle and with sleep deprivation in premenstrual dysphoric disorder and normal control subjects. *Biological Psychiatry, 48*(9), 920–931.

Porter, R. (Ed.), (2013). *The Merck Manual Home Health Handbook* Whitehouse Station, NJ: Merck Sharp & Dohme. Available at <http://www.merckmanuals.com/home/index.html>. March 7, 2013.

Rasgon, N. L., Thomas, M. A., et al. (2001). Menstrual cycle-related brain metabolite changes using 1H magnetic resonance spectroscopy in premenopausal women: a pilot study. *Psychiatry Research*, 106(1), 47–57.

Reddy, D. S. (2004). Anticonvulsant activity of the testosterone-derived neurosteroid 3alpha-androstanediol. *Neuroreport*, 15(3), 515–518.

Riley, J. L., III, Robinson, M. E., Wise, E. A., & Price, D. D. (1999). A meta-analytic review of pain perception across the menstrual cycle. *Pain*, 81(3), 225–235.

Safriel, Y., Pol-Rodriguez, M., et al. (2005). Reference values for long echo time MR spectroscopy in healthy adults. *American Journal of Neuroradiology*, 26(6), 1439–1445.

Sanacora, G., Mason, G. F., Rothman, D. L., Behar, K. L., Hyder, F., Petroff, O. A., et al. (1999). Reduced cortical gamma-aminobutyric acid levels in depressed patients determined by proton magnetic resonance spectroscopy. *Archives of General Psychiatry*, 56(11), 1043–1047.

Sherman, J. J., & LeResche, L. (2006). Does experimental pain response vary across the menstrual cycle? A methodological review. *American Journal of Physiology, Regulatory, Integrative and Comparative Physiology*, 291(2), R245–R256.

Slaunwhite, W. R., Jr, & Sandberg, A. A. (1959). Transcortin: a corticosteroid-binding protein of plasma. *Journal of Clinical Investigation*, 38(2), 384–391.

Smith, S. S., Waterhouse, B. D., Chapin, J. K., & Woodward, D. J. (1987). Progesterone alters GABA and glutamate responsiveness: a possible mechanism for its anxiolytic action. *Brain Research, 400*: 353–359.

Smith, M. J., Adams, L. F., et al. (2002). Effects of ovarian hormones on human cortical excitability. *Annals of Neurology*, 51(5), 599–603.

Södergård, R., Bäckström, T., Shanbhag, V., & Carstensen, H. (1982). Calculation of free and bound fractions of testosterone and estradiol-17 beta to human plasma proteins at body temperature. *Journal of Steroid Biochemistry*, 16(6), 801–810.

Stanton, S. J., Mullette-Gillman, O. A., & Huettel, S. A. (2011). Seasonal variation of salivary testosterone in men, normally cycling women, and women using hormonal contraceptives. *Physiology and Behavior*, 104(5), 804–808.

Stoffel-Wagner, B. (2003). Neurosteroid biosynthesis in the human brain and its clinical implications. *Annals of the New York Academy of Sciences*, 1007, 64–78.

Strohle, A., Scheel, M., et al. (2008). Blunted ACTH response to dexamethasone suppression-CRH stimulation in posttraumatic stress disorder. *Journal of Psychiatric Research*, 42(14), 1185–1188.

Tayoshi, S., Sumitani, S., Taniguchi, K., Shibuya-Tayoshi, S., Numata, S., Iga, J., et al. (2009). Metabolite changes and gender differences in schizophrenia using 3-Tesla proton magnetic resonance spectroscopy (1H-MRS). *Schizophrenia Research*, 108(1–3), 69–77.

Vierhapper, H., Nowotny, P., & Waldhäusl, W. (1998). Sex-specific differences in cortisol production rates in humans. *Metabolism: Clinical and Experimental*, 47(8), 974–976.

Wang, Y., Jia, Y., Chen, X., et al. (2012). Hippocampal N-acetylaspartate and morning cortisol levels in drug-naive, first-episode patients with major depressive disorder: effects of treatment. *Journal of Psychopharmacology*, 26(11), 1463–1470.

Wilkinson, I. D., Paley, M. N., et al. (1997). Cerebral volumes and spectroscopic proton metabolites on MR: is sex important? *Magnetic Resonance Imaging*, 15(2), 243–248.

Woolley, C. S., & McEwen, B. S. (1993). Roles of estradiol and progesterone in regulation of hippocampal dendritic spine density during the estrous cycle in the rat. *Journal of Comparative Neurology*, 336(2), 293–306.

Woolley, C. S., Weiland, N. G., et al. (1997). Estradiol increases the sensitivity of hippocampal CA1 pyramidal cells to NMDA receptor-mediated synaptic input: correlation with dendritic spine density. *Journal of Neuroscience*, 17(5), 1848–1859.

Magnetic Resonance Spectroscopy in Neuroenergetics and Neurotransmission

Nicola R. Sibson[1] and Kevin L. Behar[2]

[1]CR-UK/MRC Gray Institute for Radiation Oncology and Biology, Department of Oncology, University of Oxford, Oxford, UK [2]Department of Psychiatry and Yale Magnetic Resonance Research Center, Yale University School of Medicine, New Haven, CT, USA

A key advantage of magnetic resonance spectroscopy (MRS) is that reaction kinetics, and hence metabolic rates, can be measured noninvasively *in vivo*. Through the use of isotopically labeled precursors, such as glucose, it is possible to measure the movement of the isotopic label from the precursor into a variety of metabolite pools, thus enabling quantitative measurement of the associated metabolic fluxes. This ability of MRS lends it to biochemical studies of the brain, which are largely inaccessible *in vivo* by other methodologies. ^{13}C MRS, in particular, has been used extensively to measure the rate of cerebral glucose oxidation in the tricarboxylic acid (TCA) cycle, as well as the rates of the neuron-glia neurotransmitter cycles subserving the glutamatergic and GABAergic systems. The term "neuronal activity" encompasses a spectrum of energy-requiring processes, including action potential propagation; restoration and maintenance of membrane potentials; and neurotransmitter release, uptake, and recycling. Consequently, it is not surprising that neuronal activity and energy metabolism are tightly coupled in the brain, a concept first proposed over a century ago (Roy & Sherrington, 1890). It is only with the recent development of methods enabling *in vivo* metabolic measurements that the energetic cost of neuronal activity has become accessible. This relationship between neuronal activity and energy metabolism is of considerable importance for the interpretation of data from functional neuroimaging studies, in which surrogate markers, such as glucose consumption, oxygen consumption, or blood flow are used to infer changes in neuronal activity. In this chapter, we discuss the ways through which *in vivo* ^{13}C MRS in combination with ^{13}C isotopically labeled substrates can be used to explore major pathways of brain energy metabolism and function, while probing the elusive nature of metabolic compartmentation and neuron-astrocyte interactions. *In vivo* ^{13}C MRS studies of the brain now date back about 20 years. During this time substantial advances have been made in measurement technology, data quality, and the sophistication and understanding of interpretative metabolic models, providing the framework for a quantitative understanding of the neuroenergetics of neurotransmission. Moreover, with the recent introduction of hyperpolarized ^{13}C MRS methods (Marjanska et al., 2010), new vistas in metabolic mapping are becoming possible. We will discuss both the early animal work in which the use of ^{13}C MRS approaches for measuring neuroenergetics and neurotransmission was validated, and the more recent translation to human studies.

^{13}C MRS MEASUREMENTS OF CEREBRAL ENERGY METABOLISM

Glucose is the primary fuel for energy metabolism in the brain (Siesjo, 1978). Each glucose molecule is metabolized through the glycolytic pathway to two molecules of pyruvate, which are subsequently oxidized to CO_2 via the TCA cycle. The oxidative steps of glucose metabolism (from pyruvate to CO_2) are generally considered to contribute 32 to 36 high-energy ATP molecules generated during metabolism of a single glucose molecule, while just two ATP molecules are contributed by the glycolytic (nonoxidative) pathway. In an alternative to glycolysis, a small amount of glucose ($\sim$3–5%) is metabolized through the pentose

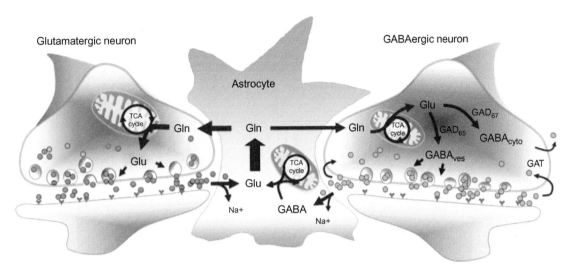

FIGURE 3.11.1 Idealized depiction of glutamate/GABA—glutamine (Gln) cycling between glutamatergic neurons, GABAergic neurons, and astrocytes. Glutamate (Glu) and GABA released from neurons during neural activity are cleared by astrocytes via glutamate and GABA membrane transporters. Some of the GABA may return directly to GABAergic terminals via reuptake. In astrocytes glutamate is converted to glutamine and released for reuptake into neurons for resynthesis of glutamate by glutaminase, followed by packaging into synaptic vesicles in preparation for release. GABA metabolism in astrocytes is indirect, involving the TCA cycle and conversion to succinate following a two-step reaction with initial transamination by α-ketoglutarate, producing glutamate, which can then proceed to glutamine. Following uptake of glutamine by GABAergic neurons and its conversion to glutamate by glutaminase, GABA is synthesized by glutamate decarboxylase (GAD) and loaded into synaptic vesicles in preparation for release.

phosphate pathway (hexose monophosphate shunt). Approximately 5—10% of glucose that undergoes glycolysis is converted to lactate and does not enter the TCA cycle, although this may be balanced under certain conditions by a corresponding uptake and oxidative metabolism of ketone bodies.

A number of techniques by which the rate of cerebral glucose metabolism can be measured have been available for some time, from snapshot *ex vivo* techniques like autoradiography to *in vivo* techniques such as arteriovenous difference measurements and positron emission tomography (PET). However, these approaches cannot differentiate metabolic fluxes associated with specific pathways (e.g., glycolysis vs. TCA cycle) or between specific cell populations in the brain, and it is at this level that *in vivo* ^{13}C MRS excels. Two main factors contribute to this. First, the chemical shift of each ^{13}C peak identifies a specific carbon position within a particular molecule, allowing the specific pathways of metabolism to be distinguished. Second, the restricted localization of certain synthetic enzymes and membrane transporters in specific neural cell populations leads to high concentrations of certain amino acids with major roles in neurotransmission and energy metabolism, which can be measured by MRS.

Glutamate is the major excitatory neurotransmitter in the mammalian brain, while γ-aminobutyric acid (GABA) is the primary inhibitory neurotransmitter. In contrast, glutamine is synaptically inert, yet plays a key role in the metabolism of both neurotransmitters.

The major brain amino acid pools of glutamate, GABA, and glutamine are highly concentrated within glutamatergic neurons, GABAergic neurons, and astrocytes, respectively, reflecting both the localization of their synthetic enzymes, as well as other aspects of cellular and functional specialization. The amino acid pools are not static, but undergo dynamic turnover following neuronal release and resynthesis. Astrocytes have a major role in the clearing of released glutamate and GABA from the synapse, and in the synthesis of precursors, mainly glutamine, required for their replenishment. Together, the pathways of release and replenishment of neurotransmitters is referred to collectively as the glutamate/GABA—glutamine cycle (Fig. 3.11.1). ^{13}C MRS can be used to measure the neuroenergetics requirements of these cell populations, and their coupled neurotransmitter cycles, as discussed in the following sections.

Neuronal Energy Metabolism

The approach adopted to measure metabolic rates by ^{13}C MRS involves intravenous infusion of a ^{13}C-labeled substrate (e.g., glucose, acetate, etc.) that will readily cross the blood—brain barrier and be metabolized within the brain. Subsequently, a number of metabolite pools within the brain become enriched with ^{13}C, and these can be detected using ^{13}C MRS or, alternatively, the ^{13}C nucleus can be detected indirectly

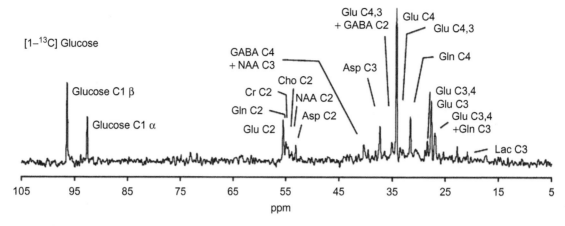

FIGURE 3.11.2 ^{13}C MRS spectrum of the human brain acquired from a healthy subject during an intravenous infusion of [1-^{13}C]glucose. The spectrum was acquired over a 60 min period using ^{1}H-decoupled, NOE-enhanced ^{13}C MRS. The numerous peaks correspond to the ^{13}C-labeled carbon atoms of different brain amino acids and metabolite products of glucose metabolism. *(Modified from Mason et al. 2007.)*

using ^{1}H-[^{13}C] MRS (de Graaf et al., 2011). This ^{1}H-[^{13}C] MRS method takes advantage of the higher sensitivity of ^{1}H MRS to detect ^{13}C nuclei via the protons (^{1}H nuclei) that are directly bonded to them. Thus, it is possible to detect the same ^{13}C-labeled metabolites as using direct ^{13}C detection, but with enhanced sensitivity. In a typical ^{1}H-[^{13}C] MRS experiment, ^{1}H MRS spectra are acquired alternately in the absence and presence of a ^{13}C radiofrequency (RF) pulse that inverts the phase of ^{1}H resonances coupled to ^{13}C nuclei. When the two spectra are subtracted, the ^{1}H resonances coupled to ^{13}C are retained; whereas protons bonded to unlabeled (^{12}C atoms) are removed. To reduce spectral complexity arising from the ^{13}C-^{1}H couplings (multiplets), both spectra are acquired with ^{13}C RF decoupling, collapsing the multiplets while increasing the signal-to-noise ratio. An additional advantage of this approach over direct ^{13}C MRS is that both total concentration (sum of the ^{13}C-labeled and unlabeled carbons bound to ^{1}H) and the ^{13}C-labeled quantity of a particular metabolite is measured together in the same experiment, permitting fractional enrichment to be determined. A caveat to this approach is the lower spectral resolution of ^{1}H MRS, which leads to the overlap of certain resonances of interest, for example, glutamate and glutamine C4 resonances in the "^{13}C-edited" ^{1}H NMR spectrum. At low magnetic field strengths (<3 T) glutamate (Glu) and glutamine (Gln) are poorly resolved so that the combined signal, Glx, is often reported. Interestingly, the earliest MRS studies of brain metabolism employing ^{13}C labeling *in vivo* were conducted with the ^{1}H-[^{13}C] MRS technique at the relatively high magnetic field strength of 8.4 T (Rothman et al., 1985). Since that time many advances in magnetic field homogenization (shimming), water suppression, pulse sequence, and

hardware developments have demonstrated the utility of ^{1}H-[^{13}C] MRS, particularly at higher magnetic field strengths where spectral separations are enhanced (Xin et al., 2010; de Graaf et al., 2011). With the development of multicompartment metabolic models it has become possible to determine absolute metabolic rates from the time courses of isotopic labeling in the brain obtained using either direct ^{13}C or ^{1}H-[^{13}C] MRS.

The most commonly used isotopic precursor for both ^{13}C and ^{1}H-[^{13}C] MRS studies is [1-^{13}C]glucose, although a number of ^{13}C-labeled substrates (e.g., lactate, acetate, β-hydroxybutyrate, octanoate) have been employed. The number of isotopically labeled metabolites that can be detected depends on several factors, including the dimensions of the volume of interest, field strength, coil dimensions and performance, and temporal resolution. A typical spectrum from human brain obtained at the end of a 2 h infusion of [1-^{13}C] glucose is shown in Fig. 3.11.2, in which ^{13}C labeling in five different amino acids can be observed. The study by Fitzpatrick et al. (1990), in which MRS measurements of metabolic fluxes in the brain *in vivo* were reported for the first time, focused on the TCA cycle and glucose oxidation. In this work ^{1}H-[^{13}C] MRS was used to follow the flux of ^{13}C isotope from [1-^{13}C]glucose primarily into glutamate. The metabolic pathways involved are depicted in Fig. 3.11.3. The [1-^{13}C]glucose is initially metabolized to pyruvate via the glycolytic pathway, which results in labeling of pyruvate at C3. The label is then transferred to the TCA cycle by the sequential actions of pyruvate dehydrogenase (PDH) and citrate synthase. When the label reaches α-ketoglutarate C4 it undergoes rapid exchange with glutamate C4, because of the high activity of the amino acid transaminases and mitochondrial/cytosolic transporters. Further metabolism of α-ketoglutarate C4 through

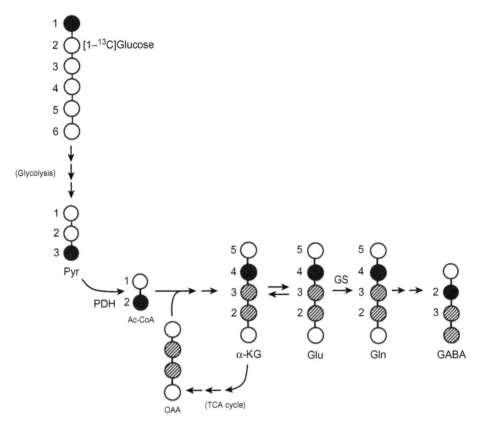

FIGURE 3.11.3 Major pathways of [1-^{13}C]glucose metabolism and ^{13}C labeling in brain amino acids. Following uptake of [1-^{13}C]glucose into the brain from the blood, the glucose is converted by glycolysis to pyruvate (Pyr) labeled at C3, which enters the mitochondria, labeling acetyl-coenzyme A (CoA) at C2 catalyzed by pyruvate dehydrogenase (PDH). Ac-CoA condenses with oxaloacetate (OAA) to form citrate C4, and eventually α-ketoglutarate (α-KG) labeled at C4. α-KG undergoes rapid exchange with glutamate (Glu) via aminotransferases and mitochondrial transporters, labeling glutamate at C4. Glutamate serves as precursor for glutamine (Gln) and GABA, catalyzed by glutamine synthetase (GS) and glutamate decarboxylase, respectively. Subsequent turns of the TCA cycle result in the labeling of additional carbon atom positions (shown as hatched circles), with eventual loss as CO_2.

the TCA cycle leads to the labeling of glutamate C3, C2, and C1. In practice, measurements of both glutamate C4 and C3 permit accurate assessments of TCA cycle flux. Thus, the flux of ^{13}C isotope from [1-^{13}C] glucose into glutamate enables quantitative determination of the TCA cycle rate (Mason et al., 1992, 1995, 1999; Gruetter et al., 1994, 2001; Rothman et al., 1999; Shen et al., 1999). Since the TCA cycle is intrinsically linked to mitochondrial oxidative phosphorylation and the synthesis of adenosine triphosphate (ATP), and glucose is the primary fuel of oxidative metabolism in the brain, the measurements of the TCA cycle may be converted to measurements of glucose oxidation using known stoichiometries (Mason et al., 1992, 1995).

The measurements described previously reflect a mixture of the metabolic rates in the different cell populations of the brain, all of which contain the necessary enzymes in the pathways of glycolysis, the TCA cycle, and oxidative phosphorylation. Consequently, one might assume that the rate of oxidative glucose metabolism obtained by this measurement is an average of the metabolic rates of all cell types. However, since the measurement is made by following the flux of the ^{13}C label into glutamate, it will in fact be weighted to different cell populations by virtue of their relative glutamate pool sizes. The existence of more than one glutamate pool in the brain was determined several decades ago in ^{14}C tracer studies (van den Berg & Garfinkel, 1971), and initially two primary glutamate pools were identified: "large-pool" and "small-pool" glutamate having slower and faster turnover rates, respectively. Based on kinetic and immunohistochemical staining studies, large-pool glutamate is believed to correspond to the glutamate pools in glutamatergic (and GABAergic) neurons (Ottersen et al., 1992; Conti & Minelli, 1994; Mason et al., 1995), while small-pool glutamate is associated mainly with glial specific enzymes and pathways. These glutamate pools differ in size by an order of magnitude and, consequently, the glutamate pool observed by ^{13}C MRS from a [1-^{13}C] glucose precursor is generally attributed to large-pool glutamate within glutamatergic neurons (although large-pool glutamate includes GABAergic neurons, their glutamate concentration is believed to be relatively low at <1 mM). Therefore, the ^{13}C measurement of the TCA cycle rate (and, hence, oxidative glucose consumption) using ^{13}C MRS with [1-^{13}C]glucose as the isotopic precursor, is strongly weighted toward the glutamatergic neuronal compartment. In contrast, the choice of a precursor that is selectively oxidized in astroglia, such as ^{13}C-labeled acetate, allows selective measurement of the astrocytic TCA cycle rate.

Since the initial study in 1990, the rate of glucose oxidation in glutamatergic neurons has been determined in numerous animal studies using both ^{13}C and ^{1}H-[^{13}C] MRS (Fitzpatrick et al., 1990; Mason et al., 1992; van Zijl et al., 1993, 1997; Hyder et al., 1996, 1997, 1999; Sibson et al., 1997, 1998b, 2001; de Graaf et al., 2004; Patel et al., 2004, 2005; Chowdhury et al., 2007; van Eijsden et al., 2010). Similarly, analogous studies in humans have demonstrated the potential for translation not only to normal human brain (Mason et al., 1992, 1995, 1999, 2007; Gruetter et al., 1994, 1998, 2001; Shen et al., 1999; Pan et al., 2000; Chen et al., 2001; Chhina et al., 2001; Boumezbeur et al., 2010; Henry et al., 2010; for review, see Rothman et al., 2011 and Chapter 1.1) but also to human studies of neurological disease (Rothman et al., 1991; Bluml et al., 2001; Petroff et al., 2002; Lin et al., 2003; Wijnen et al., 2010). Although the majority of animal studies have been conducted under anesthesia, broad agreement between the values of oxidative metabolism in animals and humans is evident, with rates for neuronal glucose oxidation ranging from 0.25 to 0.50 μmol/min/g. Moreover, these ^{13}C MRS measurements of neuronal glucose metabolism are consistent with results published previously using conventional arteriovenous difference, ^{14}C-2-deoxyglucose autoradiography, and PET measurements of total glucose metabolism (Rothman et al., 2003; Boumezbeur et al., 2005). Together, these data indicate that the major fraction (60–90%) of total glucose oxidation is associated with glutamatergic neurons in both the rat and human cerebral cortex.

Contribution of Astrocytes to Cerebral Energy Metabolism

However, as mentioned earlier, glutamate is present in all brain cells including astrocytes and GABAergic neurons. Although the concentration of glutamate in these other cell types is considerably lower than in glutamatergic neurons, all brain cells will contribute to some degree to cerebral glucose metabolism. Considerable controversy has surrounded measurements of glucose oxidation in astrocytes for several decades. Early estimates ranged from 10% to >50% of

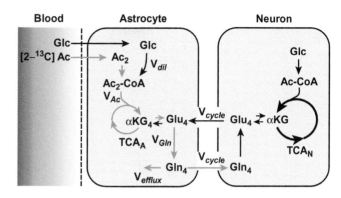

FIGURE 3.11.4   [2-^{13}C]acetate is metabolized mainly by astroglia resulting in preferential labeling of glutamine. Glutamate–glutamine cycling moves glutamine ^{13}C label from astrocytes to neurons resulting in labeling of glutamate C4 and GABA-C2 (not shown). Continuous metabolism of other unlabeled substrates, mainly by glucose, results in dilution of the acetyl-CoA pool, reducing the apparent enrichment of amino acids labeled from [2-^{13}C]acetate. Dilution fluxes must be incorporated into the metabolic model used for the calculation of absolute fluxes. *(From Patel et al., 2010)*.

total glucose oxidation (Siesjo, 1978). Calculations of astrocytic glucose oxidation from early *in vivo* [1-^{13}C] glucose MRS experiments in human cortex yielded a tighter range of values (5–15% of total glucose oxidation), but with some uncertainties because of the complex metabolic modeling (Shen et al., 1999; Gruetter et al., 2001). However, owing to the specific localization of the enzyme glutamine synthetase to astrocytes (Martinez-Hernandez et al., 1977), and the introduction of alternatively labeled glial-specific isotopic precursors, it has become possible to measure astrocytic glucose oxidation *in vivo* by ^{13}C MRS.

The use of alternative precursors to [1-^{13}C]glucose, in combination with either ^{13}C or ^{1}H-[^{13}C] MRS, has been common practice since the 1990s in studies performed *in vitro* or *ex vivo* (Bachelard et al., 1998; Cruz & Cerdan, 1999). One isotopic precursor that has been used extensively to study astrocyte metabolism is [2-^{13}C]acetate, because of the substantially greater transport of acetate into astrocytes than neurons (Waniewski & Martin, 1998). From [2-^{13}C]acetate, the ^{13}C label enters the astrocytic TCA cycle via acetyl-CoA, passes into the astrocytic glutamate pool, and, subsequently, into glutamine (Fig. 3.11.4). Comparison of labeling patterns following infusion of [1-^{13}C]glucose and [2-^{13}C]acetate has provided valuable information about cellular compartmentation and neuronal-glial interactions (Cerdan et al., 1990; Badar-Goffer et al., 1992; Sonnewald et al., 1993; Bachelard et al., 1995; Hassel & Sonnewald, 1995; Hassel et al., 1995; Brand et al., 1997; Haberg et al., 1998). Although few of these studies have yielded absolute metabolic rates, the contribution of astrocytic glucose oxidation to total glucose oxidation

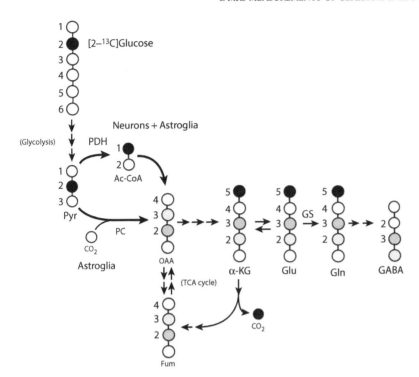

FIGURE 3.11.5 Major pathways of [2-^{13}C]glucose metabolism and ^{13}C labeling in brain amino acids. [2-^{13}C]pyruvate generated from [2-^{13}C]glucose by glycolysis enters the TCA cycles of neurons and astrocytes through pyruvate dehydrogenase (PDH), labeling α-ketoglutarate (α-KG), glutamate (Glu), and glutamine (Gln) at C5, which is lost as CO_2. Alternatively, [2-^{13}C]pyruvate can be metabolized through the anaplerotic pathway in astrocytes (pyruvate carboxylase, PC), labeling the methylene carbon of oxaloacetate (OAA) at C3 (and C2 and C1 by fumarase exchange and further TCA cycle turns), and subsequently, α-KG at C3 (and C2). Further metabolism leads to Glu (and Gln) labeled at C3 (and C2), and GABA at C3 and C1.

was estimated in one review to be 20–30% (Cruz & Cerdan, 1999). This estimate is in agreement with the *in vivo* studies described previously, with ~70–80% of total glucose oxidation attributed to the neuronal compartment.

Despite the long-standing use of alternative isotopic precursors *in vitro*, it was only relatively recent that the use of [2-^{13}C]acetate was translated to the *in vivo* setting. A number of studies have been conducted in rats using [2-^{13}C]acetate as the infused substrate (Chowdhury et al., 2007; Hassel et al., 1997; Patel et al., 2005, 2010; Serres et al., 2008), and where metabolic rates have been calculated glucose oxidation in astrocytes was found to account for approximately 20% of total glucose oxidation (Patel et al., 2010). These findings are in accord not only with the previous *in vitro* findings, but also with [2-^{13}C]acetate studies in human cerebral cortex, in which astrocytic glucose oxidation has been found to be equal to 15–20% of total glucose oxidation (Lebon et al., 2002; Boumezbeur et al., 2010), with similar rates estimated from ^{13}C-labeled bicarbonate production using [1-^{13}C]acetate (Bluml et al., 2002; Sailasuta et al., 2010).

It is also possible to use [2-^{13}C]glucose as the isotopic precursor to measure oxidative metabolism in astrocytes (Kanamatsu & Tsukada, 1999; Sibson et al., 2001). Although [2-^{13}C]glucose will be metabolized by both astrocytes and neurons, this precursor acts as an astrocyte-specific precursor owing to the anaplerotic pyruvate carboxylase pathway, which is localized exclusively to astrocytes in the adult brain (Yu et al.,

1983; Shank, et al., 1985; Brand et al., 1993). Via this pathway, label from [2-^{13}C]glucose is transferred to the C3 and C2 positions of the small astrocytic glutamate pool (Brand et al., 1993; Taylor et al., 1996; Kanamatsu & Tsukada, 1999; Sibson et al., 2001), while label flux through either the neuronal or astrocytic PDH pathway does not contribute to labeling in these positions (see Fig. 3.11.5). In practice, the ^{13}C label is first observed in glutamine (C3 and C2) because of the small glutamate pool in astrocytes and high glutamine synthetase activity and, therefore, the flux of label from [2-^{13}C]glucose to glutamine can be used to obtain measurements of astrocytic metabolism.

In humans, studies employing [2-^{13}C]glucose infusions have reported on the contribution of anaplerosis to glutamine synthesis in healthy subjects (Mason et al., 2007), as well as findings of reduced glutamine synthesis and glutamate/glutamine cycling measured *ex vivo* in brain tissue removed during neurosurgery to control intractable seizures in individuals with temporal lobe epilepsy (Petroff et al., 2002). Human studies have been limited thus far to measurements of steady-state ^{13}C enrichment, due to the relatively low amount of label incorporation into glutamate and glutamine methylene carbons (compared to carbonyl carbons), and thus the rate of anaplerosis. This can be readily appreciated by comparing human brain ^{13}C MR spectra measured at isotopic steady state following infusion of [2-^{13}C]glucose or [1-^{13}C]glucose (Fig. 3.11.6).

In rodents, [2-^{13}C]glucose has been used in studies of brain tissue extracts *ex vivo* to probe both the role of

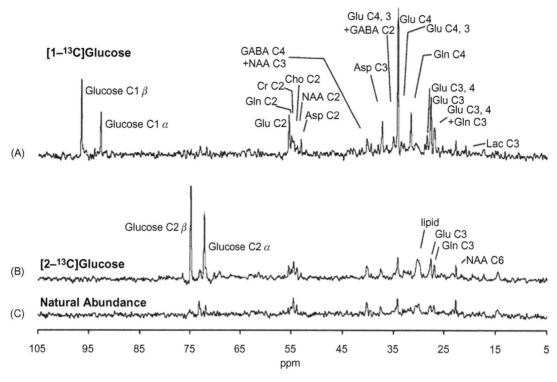

FIGURE 3.11.6 ^{13}C MRS spectra depicting metabolism of [2-^{13}C]glucose compared with [1-^{13}C]glucose in the human brain. (A) Spectrum acquired over 60 min during intravenous infusion of [2-^{13}C]glucose. (B) Spectrum acquired over 60 min during intravenous infusion of [2-^{13}C] glucose. (C) Background natural abundance (1.1%) ^{13}C spectrum acquired over the same time interval. The differences in ^{13}C-labeling patterns of glutamate and glutamine reflect effects of compartmentation of metabolism in neurons and astrocytes as discussed in the text. *(Modified from Mason et al., 2006.)*

glutamine as a precursor of GABA (Patel et al., 2001) and the role of anaplerosis in activity-dependent glutamate/glutamine cycling (Patel et al., 2005). The low level of isotopic labeling in brain glutamine from [2-^{13}C]glucose seen under normal conditions (Sibson et al., 2001), is increased substantially by raising blood ammonia levels. Hyperammonemia increases the astrocytic glutamine pool approximately threefold, and, consequently, the amount of label incorporated into brain metabolites is proportionately higher. Under normal levels of blood ammonia anaplerosis comprised about one-quarter of glutamine synthesis, but during hyperammonemia this contribution was increased by 23−68%.

MRS MEASUREMENTS OF NEUROTRANSMITTER FLUXES

The metabolism of glutamatergic neurons, GABAergic neurons, and astrocytes is coupled by neurotransmitter cycles. The concept of such a cycle between glutamatergic neurons and astrocytes was first postulated in the early 1970s by van den Berg and colleagues (van den Berg & Garfinkel, 1971), based on

data from ^{14}C-labeling studies (Lajtha et al., 1959; Berl et al., 1961). This cycle enables rapid removal of neurotransmitter glutamate from the synaptic cleft by astrocytes, while preventing depletion of the nerve terminal glutamate pool by recycling via glutamine. Although glutamate transporters have been found on both presynaptic and postsynaptic nerve terminals (Bergles et al., 1999), it is now generally accepted that the majority of glutamate released from nerve terminals is taken up by surrounding astrocytes (Rothstein et al., 1996; Bergles & Jahr, 1998; Bergles et al., 1999). As mentioned earlier, glutamate is converted to glutamine, by glutamine synthetase, exclusively within astrocytes. Subsequently, the synaptically inert glutamine is transported into the extracellular space, taken up by neurons and converted back to glutamate by phosphate-activated glutaminase (Kvamme et al., 1985). Thus, a "glutamate−glutamine cycle" between neurons and astrocytes is formed (Fig. 3.11.1). Similarly, GABA released into the synaptic cleft also participates in a neuronal-astrocytic cycle, although the metabolism of GABA after its uptake into astrocytes differs from glutamate. Whereas glutamate can be directly converted to glutamine after uptake in astrocytes, GABA is first processed in the mitochondria in a transamination reaction with α-ketoglutarate producing succinic semialdehyde and glutamate. The glutamate formed contains the nitrogen from GABA but not its carbon skeleton; thus the ^{13}C enrichment of glutamine carbons arising indirectly through GABA catabolism will reflect the ^{13}C enrichment of acetyl-CoA entering the astrocytic TCA cycle. When glucose labeled at [1-^{13}C] or [1,6-^{13}C] is the substrate, glutamine C4 labeling will reflect the rate of GABA catabolism in the astrocytic mitochondria. Although the synthesis of GABA from glutamine was the earliest neurotransmitter cycle proposed (glutamate's role as an excitatory neurotransmitter was proven only in the 1970s, and long after the recognition of GABA's role in inhibition), GABA is also removed by reuptake into GABAergic terminals. MRS studies conducted by our group using [2-^{13}C]glucose or [2-^{13}C]acetate with high-resolution analysis of brain tissue extracts have shown relatively high rates of GABA synthesis from astrocytic glutamine (Patel et al., 2005, 2010), approaching 20% of the total glutamate and GABA cycling between neurons and astrocytes, and much higher than previously believed.

Since the initial proposal of a glutamate–glutamine cycle between neurons and astrocytes, this concept has gained much support from a variety of *in vitro* studies, including enzyme localization studies, isotope labeling studies in cells and brain slices, and immunohistochemical studies of the cellular distribution of glutamate and glutamine (for review, see Erecinska & Silver, 1990). However, ^{13}C MRS is currently the only methodology by which this cycle can be measured noninvasively *in vivo*. In the following section the neurochemical and conceptual basis of the MRS measurement of glutamate–glutamine cycling is discussed.

Measuring the Glutamate–Glutamine Cycle with [1-^{13}C]glucose

As discussed previously, ^{13}C label from [1-^{13}C]glucose rapidly labels the large neuronal pool of glutamate. Subsequently, according to the glutamate–glutamine cycle described earlier, synaptic release of glutamate followed by uptake and conversion to glutamine in astrocytes will transfer label into astrocytic glutamine. In line with this concept, rapid labeling of glutamine from [1-^{13}C]glucose was clearly demonstrated in the earliest ^{13}C MRS studies of human occipital/parietal cortex (Gruetter et al., 1994; Mason et al., 1995). On this basis, it was hypothesized that the rate of glutamine synthesis and, consequently, the rate of the glutamate–glutamine cycle could be determined using ^{13}C MRS *in vivo*. The first measurement of glutamine synthesis in human brain (Mason et al., 1995) was based on ^{13}C MRS data acquired previously (Gruetter et al.,

1994). A relatively simple metabolic model was used in that work, and it was concluded that the measurement contained a high degree of uncertainty. Subsequently, considerable refinement of the metabolic model has markedly increased the confidence of the measurement and has validated the use of glutamine synthesis as a measure of glutamate–glutamine cycling.

One potential confound to this approach is the contribution of any other significant fluxes through the glutamine synthetase pathway, which would contribute to labeling of the glutamine pool. Glutamine synthesis is also known to act as an important detoxification pathway for blood-borne ammonia entering the brain (Cooper & Plum, 1987; Fig. 3.11.7); thus, under conditions of increased blood ammonia, an additional contribution to glutamine synthesis occurs. Indeed, it was originally thought that ammonia detoxification was the primary role of glutamine synthesis in the brain. However, the degree to which ammonia detoxification contributes to total glutamine synthesis is, in fact, dependent on the rate of net ammonia transport into the brain (Cooper & Plum, 1987; Shen et al., 1998; Sibson et al., 1998b), as well as potential endogenous production through the purine nucleotide cycle (Cooper, 2012).

Because of the mass balance constraints, nitrogen influx to the brain in the form of ammonia must be balanced by nitrogen efflux in glutamine (Cooper & Plum, 1987; Fig. 3.11.7). At the same time, loss of

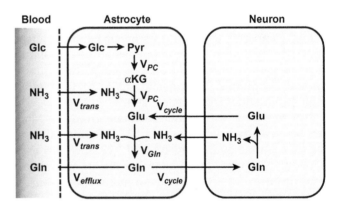

FIGURE 3.11.7 Glutamine synthesis in astrocytes plays important roles in ammonia detoxification and glutamate–glutamine cycling. Ammonia transported into the brain from blood is incorporated mainly as glutamine amide nitrogen (N5) through glutamine synthetase. Under conditions of more profound ammonia elevation, reductive amination of α-KG by glutamate dehydrogenase can occur, resulting in labeling of glutamine amine nitrogen (N2). In astrocytes, branched-chain amino acids such as leucine may contribute significantly to net glutamate formation from α-ketoglutarate (α-KG) during anaplerosis, altering the apparent labeling rate of glutamine amino relative to amide nitrogen. The glutamine synthesis flux represents the sum of the rates of glutamate–glutamine cycling (V_{cycle}) and the removal of blood-borne ammonia, resulting in net glutamine efflux from the brain. Glutamine efflux is balanced by anaplerosis involving flux through pyruvate carboxylase (V_{PC}).

carbon skeletons from the brain in glutamine must be matched by net synthesis (anaplerosis) of carbon skeletons in astrocytes (Sibson et al., 1998b, 2001). Thus, the total rate of glutamine synthesis will be equal to the sum of glutamate and GABA neurotransmitter cycling and anaplerotic glutamine synthesis. To differentiate the relative contributions of ammonia detoxification and glutamate—glutamine cycling several strategies can be used. In the first case, glutamine synthesis can be determined by ^{13}C MRS using [1-^{13}C]glucose as the substrate in rats for different levels of plasma ammonia. In one such study, increased glutamine synthesis was found on comparing hyperammonemic (0.4—0.5 mM plasma NH$_4$) with normoammonemic ($\sim$0.05 mM plasma NH$_4$) conditions (Sibson et al., 1997). This study demonstrated a relationship between glutamine synthesis and plasma ammonia levels, it also revealed a significant flux through the glutamine synthetase pathway even under conditions of minimal plasma ammonia. These findings indicate that under normal conditions glutamate—glutamine cycling is the predominant role of glutamine synthesis.

A second approach to differentiating between ammonia detoxification and glutamate—glutamine cycling is to measure the anaplerotic flux through the astroglial enzyme, pyruvate carboxylase, in relation to increased levels of blood ammonia. Using [2-^{13}C]glucose, it is possible to directly observe increased anaplerosis by the appearance of ^{13}C labeling in glutamate and glutamine C2 and C3, as shown in Fig. 3.11.5, which was substantially increased during hyperammonemia compared to normoammonemia (Sibson et al., 2001). Compared to hyperammonemia, there is significantly less flux through the anaplerotic pathway under normal conditions, comprising $\sim$20% of total glutamine production (Sibson et al., 2001).

Net ammonia influx into the brain from the blood can be measured directly using ^{15}N MRS by following the time course of accumulation of ^{15}N label into brain pools of glutamate and glutamine during an intravenous infusion of ^{15}N-labeled ammonia (Kanamori & Ross, 1993; Kanamori, et al., 1993; Shen et al., 1998; Cudalbu et al., 2012). Under hyperammonemic conditions, such measures of ammonia fixation have been found to correlate closely with the increases in glutamine synthesis and anaplerosis measured between normoammonemic and hyperammonemic conditions (Shen et al., 1998). The good agreement between all of these findings supports the concept that ammonia detoxification by glutamine synthesis is determined, in large part, by the rate of net ammonia transport into the brain. Collectively these experiments demonstrated that under normal conditions glutamate—glutamine cycling dominates ($\sim$80%) glutamine synthesis in the anesthetized rat cerebral cortex. Similar findings were

reported for awake rats infused with [1-^{13}C]glucose and H^{14}CO$_3$ and measured *ex vivo* (71—80%; Oz et al., 2004). Strong support for this conclusion also comes from extracellular measurements of ^{13}C and ^{15}N-labeled glutamine and glutamate by microdialysis and mass spectrometry following [2,5-^{13}C$_2$]glucose and ^{15}N-ammonium acetate infusion (Kanamori et al., 2002), finding that glial uptake of extracellular glutamate released through neurotransmission accounted for 80—90% of glutamine synthesis. Studies of the human cerebral cortex using ^{13}C MRS also support this concept, indicating that 70—90% of glutamine synthesis subserves glutamate—glutamine cycling (Gruetter et al., 2001; Mason et al., 2007). On this basis it is now generally agreed that the measurement of glutamine synthesis by ^{13}C MRS largely reflects glutamate neurotransmitter trafficking.

The previous findings have led to the proposal that the rate of glutamate—glutamine cycling can be used as a measure of glutamatergic neuronal activity. To validate this proposal, the cycling rate was measured under different conditions of neuronal activity, with the hypothesis that as neuronal activity increased so should the cycling rate. Thus, ^{13}C MRS was used to measure the rate of glutamine synthesis in the rat cerebral cortex at three levels of electrocortical activity; isoelectric electroencephalogram induced by high-dose pentobarbital anesthesia, and two milder levels of anesthesia (Sibson et al., 1998b). Under isoelectric conditions, at which minimal glutamate release takes place, almost no glutamine synthesis was measured (0.04 μmol/min/g). Above isoelectricity, the rate of glutamine synthesis increased with increasing electrical activity, indicating a close relationship between glutamate—glutamine cycling and glutamatergic neuronal activity. These findings also supported the hypothesis that the ^{13}C MRS measurement of glutamine synthesis primarily reflects glutamate—glutamine cycling rather than internal exchange of ^{13}C label within astrocytes, which would not be expected to change with the level of neuronal activity. As discussed in Chapter 4.3, since the initial study by Sibson et al., (1998a) the rates of the glutamate—glutamine cycle and the neuronal TCA cycle have been measured at different levels of brain activity using ^{13}C MRS by several groups, and the measurements have shown excellent agreement with the original findings (Fig. 3.11.8).

Measuring the Glutamate—Glutamine Cycle with Alternative ^{13}C-Labeled Precursors

A further approach to validating the ^{13}C MRS measurement of glutamate—glutamine cycling is to use alternative isotopically labeled precursors that enter

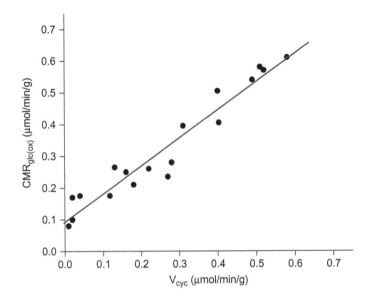

FIGURE 3.11.8 The relationship between the rates of neuronal glucose oxidation and glutamate–glutamine cycling with increasing activity in rat brain. Above isoelectricity, where the rate of glutamate–glutamine cycling (V_{cyc}) equals zero, V_{cyc} and neuronal glucose oxidation ($CMR_{glc(ox)}$) follow a 1:1 relationship. These data represent values from eleven published studies ranging from isoelectricity to awake conditions as described in Rothman et al. (2011).

the metabolic pathways of the brain via astrocytes. If label is introduced specifically into astrocytic metabolite pools, then subsequent appearance of label in neuronal metabolites provides direct evidence of substrate trafficking between these cells. As discussed in previously sections, both [2-^{13}C]acetate and [2-^{13}C]glucose can be utilized as an astrocyte-specific precursor, from which the isotopic label is first observed in glutamine. If there was significant cycling of labeled glutamine from the astrocyte to the neuron (as predicted by the glutamate–glutamine cycle), label would subsequently appear in neuronal glutamate at the rate of the cycle. In accord with this hypothesis, labeling of neuronal glutamate has been demonstrated using either [2-^{13}C] acetate or [2-^{13}C]glucose in both rat and human brain (Hassel et al., 1997; Sibson et al., 2001; Lebon et al., 2002; Patel et al., 2005, 2010; Chowdhury et al., 2007; Mason et al., 2007; Serres et al., 2008; Boumezbeur et al., 2010). A number of other pathways of neurotransmitter replenishment in astrocytes use TCA cycle intermediates to return carbon to neurons. Since the [2-^{13}C]glucose/acetate experiment does not differentiate between label transferred in either glutamine or any other TCA cycle intermediate (e.g., α-ketoglutarate), the flux of label into glutamate reflects the sum of *all* substrate trafficking pathways from astrocytes to neurons. In contrast, in the [1-^{13}C]glucose experiment flux of label from neuronal glutamate to astrocytic glutamine reflects glutamate–glutamine cycling alone. Nevertheless, close agreement has been found between the rates determined using [1-^{13}C]glucose to measure glutamate–glutamine cycling, and those measured using glial-specific substrates, which take into account all cycling pathways. These findings indicate that the glutamate–glutamine cycle is the primary pathway of

neurotransmitter glutamate recycling *in vivo* under normal conditions in both rodent and man.

Measuring the Glutamate–Glutamine Cycle with ^{15}N MRS

A third approach to validating the measurement of glutamate–glutamine cycling is to use ^{15}N MRS to measure glutamine synthesis through label incorporation from ^{15}N-labeled ammonia into the amide position of cerebral glutamine (Kanamori & Ross, 1993; Kanamori et al., 1993, 1996; Shen et al., 1998). The rates of glutamine synthesis as reported in these studies differ, likely due to differences in the metabolic models and assumed parameters used to fit the data, as well as differences in blood ammonia concentration. It has been shown that using the same metabolic model to fit both the ^{13}C and ^{15}N MRS data obtained under similar experimental conditions yields similar values of the rate of glutamate–glutamine cycling (Shen et al., 1998).

The ^{15}N MRS measurements have played an important role in the validation of the interpretative brain metabolic models used in the determination of absolute metabolic rates from the ^{13}C enrichment time courses. However, ^{15}N has significant limitations as an isotopic tracer compared to ^{13}C in the quantitative assessment of absolute metabolic rates *in vivo*. Ammonia is a toxic end product of metabolism, and when infused at supranormal levels, significantly alters the metabolic fluxes involved in ammonia fixation and detoxification, namely glutamine synthesis and anaplerosis, thus limiting the technique to hyperammonemic conditions. Furthermore, the extensive degree of α-nitrogen exchange (side reactions) catalyzed by amino acid transaminases, principally involving the branched-chain amino acids, such as leucine, can significantly confound a straightforward rate interpretation of ^{15}N labeling. In addition the ^{15}N enrichment of ammonia at the intracellular sites of glutamine (γ-amide nitrogen) or glutamate (α-amino nitrogen) synthesis is not known, adding uncertainty to the derived metabolic rates. Because of these limitations, along with the lower inherent sensitivity of ^{15}N MRS compared to ^{13}C MRS, absolute metabolic rate assessments in brain *in vivo* have employed mostly ^{13}C-labeled substrates with either direct or indirect ^{13}C detection.

Together, the ^{13}C and ^{15}N MRS studies strongly support the existence of a glutamate–glutamine cycle between neurons and astrocytes *in vivo*, and indicate that ^{13}C MRS may be used *in vivo* to measure the rate of glutamatergic neuronal activity, in the form of glutamate–glutamine cycling. Similar rates of glutamate–glutamine cycling have been measured in rodent (0.2–0.6 µmol/min/g) (Sibson et al., 1997, 1998a, 2001; de Graaf et al., 2004; Patel et al., 2004, 2005; Chowdhury et al., 2007; van Eijsden et al., 2010) and human (0.2–0.3 µmol/min/g) cortex (Gruetter et al., 1998; Shen et al., 1999; Gruetter et al., 2001; Lebon et al., 2002; Boumezbeur et al., 2010), and in both cases this cycle provides the major contribution ($\sim$80%) to total glutamine synthesis. These findings indicate that the glutamate–glutamine cycle is a major metabolic pathway in the mammalian cortex, and the predominant route by which neuronal glutamate pools are replenished. Moreover, these studies highlight the importance of astrocytes in maintaining synaptic glutamate homeostasis, which has long been a source of controversy. The significance of astrocytic glutamate uptake can be readily appreciated by considering the high rate of glutamate–glutamine cycling, which in the awake rat cortex transports over 0.5 µmol/g of glutamate per minute (Wang et al., 2010) from neurons to astrocytes through the synaptic extracellular space. Complete interruption of astrocytic glutamate uptake would lead to a rapid increase in extracellular glutamate, from a normally low level of ≤ 1 µM to excitotoxic levels of >10 µM in a fraction of 1 s (assuming that extracellular space occupies 20% of brain volume). Because the actual synaptic volume is highly localized, and much less than the total extracellular volume, the magnitude and speed of the glutamate rise in this smaller space would be many times greater.

Energetic Requirements of Neurotransmission

Neuronal activity requires energy, which is provided almost exclusively by oxidation of glucose supplied continuously via the circulation (Siesjo, 1978).

This vascular supply is regulated locally and dynamically to meet the increased energetic demand of functional activation. Functional imaging utilizes the coupling between increased neuronal activity and energetic demand, by measuring changes in either blood flow, glucose utilization, or oxygen metabolism and delivery as a surrogate marker of neuronal activity (Raichle, 1998). Despite the rapidly expanding use of these imaging tools in both basic and clinical applications, the neurobiological processes responsible for these surrogate imaging signals remain to be fully elucidated. It is now broadly agreed that glutamate release may trigger both vascular and metabolic responses via different signaling processes, at least in some brain regions (for review, see Bonvento et al., 2002). Thus, glutamate may be a key co-coordinator of the physiological responses underlying the signal changes observed in brain imaging.

^{13}C MRS has provided a means by which the relationship between glutamatergic neurotransmission and energy metabolism can be tested *in vivo*. In some of the earliest ^{13}C MRS studies in rat brain the rates of glutamate–glutamine cycling and neuronal glucose oxidation in the cerebral cortex were measured simultaneously across a range of neuronal activity (Sibson et al., 1998a). As described earlier, electrocortical activity was varied using differing levels of anesthesia, and when neuronal glucose oxidation was plotted against the rate of glutamate–glutamine cycling a linear relationship was obtained. Since those early studies, numerous measurements have been made of these two metabolic rates using ^{13}C MRS. A recent review of the published literature (Rothman et al., 2011) indicates that there is good agreement regarding the 1:1 incremental flux relationship originally reported (Fig. 3.11.8). This graph, which plots the rate of glucose oxidation against the rate of glutamate–glutamine cycling, shows that the relationship is linear and above isoelectricity and the relationship between the two rates is $\sim$1:1, that is, for every molecule of glucose oxidized by neurons, one molecule of neuronally released glutamate is cycled to glutamine. At isoelectricity, the rate of glutamate–glutamine cycling falls to zero (y-intercept on the graph), revealing a basal level of glucose oxidation not related to synaptic activity. This so-called "housekeeping" activity reflects $\sim$15% of the awake resting rate of neuronal glucose oxidation, and is likely to be related to basic cellular processes not invoked during acute activity, such as protein, lipid, and nucleotide synthesis. Based on *in vitro* studies and energy budget modeling the majority of the energy demands in neurons relates to the activity of the sodium/potassium ATPase and the restoration of ionic balance across presynaptic and postsynaptic membranes (Attwell & Laughlin, 2001).

Although there is good agreement between the various studies of rodents regarding the relationship between glucose oxidation and glutamate–glutamine cycling (Hertz, 2011; Rothman et al., 2011), controversy exists over the actual mechanism underlying the relationship between these fluxes. A discussion of the issues surrounding potential mechanisms can be found in Rothman et al. (2011).

APPLICATION OF ^{13}C MRS IN HUMAN DISEASE

The importance of both neurotransmitter metabolism and neuroenergetics in neurological disease is becoming increasingly clear. Changes in neurotransmitter concentration measured by ^{1}H MRS have been reported in a variety of neurological diseases over many years. However, such steady-state concentration measurements, although useful, do not provide information on changes in flux through specific metabolic pathways. ^{13}C MRS has the potential to address this issue, but historically its application has been limited for a number of reasons, including technical and experimental complexity, low sensitivity, high substrate costs, and the need for complex mathematical modeling (for review, see Ross et al., 2003). Nevertheless, initial studies have proven to be of considerable value in understanding the neuroenergetics and neurotransmitter abnormalities associated with various neuropathologies, including stroke, brain cancer, hepatic encephalopathy, Alzheimer's disease, and epilepsy. In stroke, for example, enhanced accumulation of ^{13}C label from [1-^{13}C]glucose into lactate, detected using ^{1}H-[^{13}C] MRS, has been observed both acutely and chronically. However, in the two cases the underlying cause was found to be different—enhanced glycolytic metabolism acutely (Rothman et al., 1991) and high metabolism in infiltrating macrophages chronically (Petroff et al., 1992). Elevated lactate production has also been measured in primary brain tumors, compared to normal brain, together with reduced TCA cycle flux using direct ^{13}C MRS both in animals (Terpstra et al., 1998) and, very recently, in man (Wijnen et al., 2010). Similar direct ^{13}C MRS studies in patients with either hepatic encephalopathy (Bluml et al., 2001) or Alzheimer's disease (Lin et al., 2003) have reported reduced glucose oxidation and impairment of glutamate–glutamine cycling.

Where neurosurgical specimens are likely to be available, ex vivo ^{13}C MRS studies can also be considered. For example, neurosurgical samples obtained from epilepsy patients after intravenous infusion of [2-^{13}C]glucose have been analyzed ex vivo by high-resolution ^{13}C MRS (Petroff et al., 2002). In this study marked impairment of glutamate–glutamine cycling was evident in epileptogenic tissue with sclerosis and glial proliferation compared with more histologically normal tissue. A second study found that this decrease in cycling might be a secondary result of reduced glutamine synthetase activity, suggesting this as a potential therapeutic target in epilepsy (Eid et al., 2004, 2012). It seems likely that with continued improvements in both hardware and sequence design, together with higher field human MR imaging scanners and new developments such as hyperpolarized ^{13}C (Bhattacharya et al., 2007; Marjanska et al., 2010; Park et al., 2010; Day et al., 2011), the application of ^{13}C MRS in neurological patients will become a more practical possibility in time.

SUMMARY

The application of MRS to the study of neurotransmitter and energy metabolism in the brain has provided several new insights into the relationship between brain metabolism and function. Glutamate release and recycling has been shown to be a major metabolic pathway in the cerebral cortex. Consequently, steady-state measurements of neurotransmitter levels may reflect alterations in regional brain activity through feedback between neurotransmitter release and resynthesis. The glutamate–glutamine cycle appears to be the predominant route by which the neurotransmitter glutamate pool in neurons is replenished, and demonstrates the importance of astrocytes in maintaining synaptic glutamate homeostasis. Interestingly, the glutamate–glutamine cycle constitutes a significant metabolic flux in the brains of both awake humans and anesthetized rats, indicating that there is considerable neuronal activity even under "nonstimulated" conditions. Moreover, the 1:1 coupling between neurotransmission and neuroenergetics (above isoelectricity) provides a link between functional imaging and specific neuronal processes.

References

Attwell, D., & Laughlin, S. B. (2001). An energy budget for signaling in the grey matter of the brain. *Journal of Cerebral Blood Flow and Metabolism, 21*(10), 1133–1145.

Bachelard, H. (1998). Landmarks in the application of ^{13}C-magnetic resonance spectroscopy to studies of neuronal/glial relationships. *Developmental Neuroscience, 20*(4-5), 277–288.

Bachelard, H., Morris, P., Taylor, A., & Thatcher, N. (1995). High-field MRS studies in brain slices. *Magnetic Resonance Imaging, 13*(8), 1223–1226.

Badar-Goffer, R. S., Ben-Yoseph, O., Bachelard, H. S., & Morris, P. G. (1992). Neuronal-glial metabolism under depolarizing conditions. A ^{13}C-n.m.r. study. *Biochemical Journal, 282*(Pt 1), 225–230.

Bergles, D. E., Diamond, J. S., & Jahr, C. E. (1999). Clearance of glutamate inside the synapse and beyond. *Current Opinion in Neurobiology*, 9(3), 293–298.

Bergles, D. E., & Jahr, C. E. (1998). Glial contribution to glutamate uptake at Schaffer collateral- commissural synapses in the hippocampus. *Journal of Neuroscience*, 18(19), 7709–7716.

Berl, S., Lajhta, A., & Waelch, H. (1961). Amino acid and protein metabolism VI. Cerebral compartments of glutamic acid metabolism. *Journal of Neurochemistry*, 7, 186–192.

Bhattacharya, P., Chekmenev, E. Y., Perman, W. H., Harris, K. C., Lin, A. P., Norton, V. A., et al. (2007). Towards hyperpolarized ^{13}C-succinate imaging of brain cancer. *Journal of Magnetic Resonance*, 186(1), 150–155.

Bluml, S., Moreno-Torres, A., & Ross, B. D. (2001). [1-^{13}C]glucose MRS in chronic hepatic encephalopathy in man. *Magnetic Resonance in Medicine*, 45(6), 981–993.

Bluml, S., Moreno-Torres, A., Shic, F., Nguy, C. H., & Ross, B. D. (2002). Tricarboxylic acid cycle of glia in the in vivo human brain. *NMR in Biomedicine*, 15(1), 1–5.

Bonvento, G., Sibson, N., & Pellerin, L. (2002). Does glutamate image your thoughts? *Trends in Neuroscience*, 25(7), 359–364.

Boumezbeur, F., Besret, L., Valette, J., Gregoire, M. C., Delzescaux, T., Maroy, R., et al. (2005). Glycolysis versus TCA cycle in the primate brain as measured by combining ^{18}F-FDG PET and ^{13}C-NMR. *Journal of Cerebral Blood Flow and Metabolism*, 25(11), 1418–1423.

Boumezbeur, F., Mason, G. F., de Graaf, R. A., Behar, K. L., Cline, G. W., Shulman, G. I., et al. (2010). Altered brain mitochondrial metabolism in healthy aging as assessed by in vivo magnetic resonance spectroscopy. *Journal of Cerebral Blood Flow and Metabolism*, 30(1), 211–221.

Brand, A., Richter-Landsberg, C., & Leibfritz, D. (1993). Multinuclear NMR studies on the energy metabolism of glial and neruonal cells. *Developmental Neurology*, 15, 289–298.

Brand, A., Richter-Landsberg, C., & Leibfritz, D. (1997). Metabolism of acetate in rat brain neurons, astrocytes and cocultures: metabolic interactions between neurons and glia cells, monitored by NMR spectroscopy. *Cellular and Molecular Biology (Noisy-le-grand)*, 43(5), 645–657.

Cerdan, S., Kunnecke, B., & Seelig, J. (1990). Cerebral metabolism of [1,2-^{13}C$_2$]acetate as detected by in vivo and in vitro ^{13}C NMR. *Journal of Biological Chemistry*, 265(22), 12916–12926.

Chen, W., Zhu, X. H., Gruetter, R., Seaquist, E. R., Adriany, G., & Ugurbil, K. (2001). Study of tricarboxylic acid cycle flux changes in human visual cortex during hemifield visual stimulation using ^{1}H-[^{13}C] MRS and fMRI. *Magnetic Resonance Medicine*, 45(3), 349–355.

Chhina, N., Kuestermann, E., Halliday, J., Simpson, L. J., Macdonald, I. A., Bachelard, H. S., et al. (2001). Measurement of human tricarboxylic acid cycle rates during visual activation by ^{13}C magnetic resonance spectroscopy. *Journal of Neuroscience Research*, 66(5), 737–746.

Chowdhury, G. M., Patel, A. B., Mason, G. F., Rothman, D. L., & Behar, K. L. (2007). Glutamatergic and GABAergic neurotransmitter cycling and energy metabolism in rat cerebral cortex during postnatal development. *Journal of Cerebral Blood Flow and Metabolism*, 27(12), 1895–1907.

Conti, F., & Minelli, A. (1994). Glutamate immunoreactivity in rat cerebral cortex is reversibly abolished by 6-diazo-5-oxo-L-norleucine (DON), an inhibitor of phosphate-activated glutaminase. *Journal of Histochemistry and Cytochemistry*, 42(6), 717–726.

Cooper, A. J. (2012). The role of glutamine synthetase and glutamate dehydrogenase in cerebral ammonia homeostasis. *Neurochemical Research*, 37(11), 2439–2455.

Cooper, A. J., & Plum, F. (1987). Biochemistry and physiology of brain ammonia. *Physiology Review*, 67(2), 440–519.

Cruz, F., & Cerdan, S. (1999). Quantitative ^{13}C NMR studies of metabolic compartmentation in the adult mammalian brain. *NMR in Biomedicine*, 12(7), 451–462.

Cudalbu, C., Lanz, B., Duarte, J. M., Morgenthaler, F. D., Pilloud, Y., Mlynarik, V., et al. (2012). Cerebral glutamine metabolism under hyperammonemia determined in vivo by localized ^{1}H and ^{15}N NMR spectroscopy. *Journal of Cerebral Blood Flow and Metabolism*, 32(4), 696–708.

Day, S. E., Kettunen, M. I., Cherukuri, M. K., Mitchell, J. B., Lizak, M. J., Morris, H. D., et al. (2011). Detecting response of rat C6 glioma tumors to radiotherapy using hyperpolarized [1-^{13}C]pyruvate and ^{13}C magnetic resonance spectroscopic imaging. *Magnetic Resonance in Medicine*, 65(2), 557–563.

de Graaf, R. A., Mason, G. F., Patel, A. B., Rothman, D. L., & Behar, K. L. (2004). Regional glucose metabolism and glutamatergic neurotransmission in rat brain in vivo. *Proceedings of the National Academy of Sciences USA*, 101(34), 12700–12705.

de Graaf, R. A., Rothman, D. L., & Behar, K. L. (2011). State of the art direct ^{13}C and indirect ^{1}H-[^{13}C] NMR spectroscopy in vivo. A practical guide. *NMR in Biomedicine*, 24(8), 958–972.

Eid, T., Behar, K., Dhaher, R., Bumanglag, A. V., & Lee, T. S. (2012). Roles of glutamine synthetase inhibition in epilepsy. *Neurochemical Research*, 37(11), 2339–2350.

Eid, T., Thomas, M. J., Spencer, D. D., Runden-Pran, E., Lai, J. C., Malthankar, G. V., et al. (2004). Loss of glutamine synthetase in the human epileptogenic hippocampus: possible mechanism for raised extracellular glutamate in mesial temporal lobe epilepsy. *Lancet*, 363(9402), 28–37.

Erecinska, M., & Silver, I. A. (1990). Metabolism and role of glutamate in mammalian brain. *Progress in Neurobiology*, 35, 245–296.

Fitzpatrick, S. M., Hetherington, H. P., Behar, K. L., & Shulman, R. G. (1990). The flux from glucose to glutamate in the rat brain in vivo as determined by ^{1}H-observed, ^{13}C-edited NMR spectroscopy. *Journal of Cerebral Blood Flow and Metabolism*, 10(2), 170–179.

Gruetter, R., Novotny, E. J., Boulware, S. D., Mason, G. F., Rothman, D. L., Shulman, G. I., et al. (1994). Localized ^{13}C NMR spectroscopy in the human brain of amino acid labeling from D-[1-^{13}C] glucose. *Journal of Neurochemistry*, 63(4), 1377–1385.

Gruetter, R., Seaquist, E. R., Kim, S., & Ugurbil, K. (1998). Localized in vivo ^{13}C-NMR of glutamate metabolism in the human brain: initial results at 4 tesla. *Developmental Neuroscience*, 20(4-5), 380–388.

Gruetter, R., Seaquist, E. R., & Ugurbil, K. (2001). A mathematical model of compartmentalized neurotransmitter metabolism in the human brain. *American Journal of Physiology. Endocrinology and Metabolism*, 281(1), E100–112.

Haberg, A., Qu, H., Haraldseth, O., Unsgard, G., & Sonnewald, U. (1998). In vivo injection of [1-^{13}C]glucose and [1,2-^{13}C]acetate combined with ex vivo ^{13}C nuclear magnetic resonance spectroscopy: a novel approach to the study of middle cerebral artery occlusion in the rat. *Journal of Cerebral Blood Flow and Metabolism*, 18, 1223–1232.

Hassel, B., Bachelard, H., Jones, P., Fonnum, F., & Sonnewald, U. (1997). Trafficking of amino acids between neurons and glia in vivo. Effects of inhibition of glial metabolism by fluoroacetate. *Journal of Cerebral Blood Flow and Metabolism*, 17(11), 1230–1238.

Hassel, B., & Sonnewald, U. (1995). Glial formation of pyruvate and lactate from TCA cycle intermediates: implications for the inactivation of transmitter amino acids? *Journal of Neurochemistry*, 65(5), 2227–2234.

Hassel, B., Sonnewald, U., & Fonnum, F. (1995). Glial-neuronal interactions as studied by cerebral metabolism of [2-^{13}C]acetate and [1-^{13}C]glucose: an *ex vivo* ^{13}C NMR spectroscopic study. *Journal of Neurochemistry*, 64(6), 2773–2782.

Henry, P. G., Criego, A. B., Kumar, A., & Seaquist, E. R. (2010). Measurement of cerebral oxidative glucose consumption in patients with type 1 diabetes mellitus and hypoglycemia unawareness using ^{13}C nuclear magnetic resonance spectroscopy. *Metabolism, 59*(1), 100−106.

Hertz, L. (2011). Astrocytic energy metabolism and glutamate formation--relevance for ^{13}C-NMR spectroscopy and importance of cytosolic/mitochondrial trafficking. *Magnetic Resonance Imaging, 29*(10), 1319−1329.

Hyder, F., Chase, J. R., Behar, K. L., Mason, G. F., Siddeek, M., Rothman, D. L., et al. (1996). Increased tricarboxylic acid cycle flux in rat brain during forepaw stimulation detected with ^{1}H [^{13}C]NMR. *Proceedings of the National Academy of Sciences USA, 93* (15), 7612−7617.

Hyder, F., Renken, R., & Rothman, D. L. (1999). In vivo carbonedited detection with proton echo-planar spectroscopic imaging (ICED PEPSI): [3,4-[13]CH₂]glutamate/glutamine tomography in rat brain. *Magnetic Resonance in Medicine, 42*(6), 997−1003.

Hyder, F., Rothman, D. L., Mason, G. F., Rangarajan, A., Behar, K. L., & Shulman, R. G. (1997). Oxidative glucose metabolism in rat brain during single forepaw stimulation: a spatially localized [1]H [^{13}C] nuclear magnetic resonance study. *Journal of Cerebral Blood Flow and Metabolism, 17*(10), 1040−1047.

Kanamatsu, T., & Tsukada, Y. (1999). Effects of ammonemia on the anaplerotic pathway and amino acid metabolism in the brain an *ex vivo* ^{13}C NMR spectroscopic study of rats after administering [2-^{13}C]glucose with of without ammonium acetate. *Brain Research, 841*, 11−19.

Kanamori, K., Parivar, F., & Ross, B. D. (1993). A ^{15}N NMR study of *in vivo* cerebral glutamine synthesis in hyperammonemic rats. *NMR in Biomedicine, 6*(1), 21−26.

Kanamori, K., & Ross, B. D. (1993). [15]N n.m.r. measurement of the in vivo rate of glutamine synthesis and utilization at steady state in the brain of the hyperammonaemic rat. *Biochem J, 293*(Pt 2), 461−468.

Kanamori, K., Ross, B. D., Chung, J. C., & Kuo, E. L. (1996). Severity of hyperammonemic encephalopathy correlates with brain ammonia level and saturation of glutamine synthetase in vivo. *Journal of Neurochemistry, 67*(4), 1584−1594.

Kanamori, K., Ross, B. D., & Kondrat, R. W. (2002). Glial uptake of neurotransmitter glutamate from the extracellular fluid studied in vivo by microdialysis and ^{13}C NMR. *Journal of Neurochemistry, 83*(3), 682−695.

Kvamme, E., Torgner, I. A., & Svenneby, G. (1985). Glutaminase from mammalian tissues. *Methods in Enzymology, 113*, 241−256.

Lajtha, A., Berl, S., & Waelch, H. (1959). Amino acid and protein metabolism of the brain IV. The metabolism of glutamic acid. *Journal of Neurochemistry, 3*, 322−332.

Lebon, V., Petersen, K. F., Cline, G. W., Shen, J., Mason, G. F., Dufour, S., et al. (2002). Astroglial contribution to brain energy metabolism in humans revealed by ^{13}C nuclear magnetic resonance spectroscopy: elucidation of the dominant pathway for neurotransmitter glutamate repletion and measurement of astrocytic oxidative metabolism. *Journal of Neuroscience, 22*(5), 1523−1531.

Lin, A. P., Shic, F., Enriquez, C., & Ross, B. D. (2003). Reduced glutamate neurotransmission in patients with Alzheimer's disease-an in vivo ^{13}C magnetic resonance spectroscopy study. *MAGMA, 16* (1), 29−42.

Marjanska, M., Iltis, I., Shestov, A. A., Deelchand, D. K., Nelson, C., Ugurbil, K., et al. (2010). In vivo ^{13}C spectroscopy in the rat brain using hyperpolarized [1-^{13}C]pyruvate and [2-^{13}C]pyruvate. *Journal of Magnetic Resonance, 206*(2), 210−218.

Martinez-Hernandez, A., Bell, K. P., & Norenberg, M. D. (1977). Glutamine synthetase: glial localization in brain. *Science, 195* (4284), 1356−1358.

Mason, G. F., Gruetter, R., Rothman, D. L., Behar, K. L., Shulman, R. G., & Novotny, E. J. (1995). Simultaneous determination of the rates of the TCA cycle, glucose utilization, α-ketoglutarate/glutamate exchange, and glutamine synthesis in human brain by NMR. *Journal of Cerebral Blood Flow and Metabolism, 15*(1), 12−25.

Mason, G. F., Pan, J. W., Chu, W. J., Newcomer, B. R., Zhang, Y., Orr, R., et al. (1999). Measurement of the tricarboxylic acid cycle rate in human grey and white matter in vivo by [1]H-[^{13}C] magnetic resonance spectroscopy at 4.1T. *Journal of Cerebral Blood Flow and Metabolism, 19*(11), 1179−1188.

Mason, G. F., Petersen, K. F., de Graaf, R. A., Shulman, G. I., & Rothman, D. L. (2007). Measurements of the anaplerotic rate in the human cerebral cortex using ^{13}C magnetic resonance spectroscopy and [1-^{13}C] and [2-^{13}C] glucose. *Journal of Neurochemistry, 100*(1), 73−86.

Mason, G. F., Rothman, D. L., Behar, K. L., & Shulman, R. G. (1992). NMR determination of the TCA cycle rate and α-ketoglutarate/glutamate exchange rate in rat brain. *Journal of Cerebral Blood Flow and Metabolism, 12*(3), 434−447.

Ottersen, O. P., Zhang, N., & Walberg, F. (1992). Metabolic compartmentation of glutamate and glutamine: morphological evidence obtained by quantitative immunocytochemistry in rat cerebellum. *Neuroscience, 46*(3), 519−534.

Oz, G., Berkich, D. A., Henry, P. G., Xu, Y., LaNoue, K., Hutson, S. M., et al. (2004). Neuroglial metabolism in the awake rat brain: CO_2 fixation increases with brain activity. *Journal of Neuroscience, 24*(50), 11273−11279.

Pan, J. W., Stein, D. T., Telang, F., Lee, J. H., Shen, J., Brown, P., et al. (2000). Spectroscopic imaging of glutamate C4 turnover in human brain. *Magnetic Resonance in Medicine, 44*(5), 673−679.

Park, I., Larson, P. E., Zierhut, M. L., Hu, S., Bok, R., Ozawa, T., et al. (2010). Hyperpolarized ^{13}C magnetic resonance metabolic imaging: application to brain tumors. *Neuro-Oncology, 12*(2), 133−144.

Patel, A. B., de Graaf, R. A., Mason, G. F., Kanamatsu, T., Rothman, D. L., Shulman, R. G., et al. (2004). Glutamatergic neurotransmission and neuronal glucose oxidation are coupled during intense neuronal activation. *Journal of Cerebral Blood Flow and Metabolism, 24*(9), 972−985.

Patel, A. B., de Graaf, R. A., Mason, G. F., Rothman, D. L., Shulman, R. G., & Behar, K. L. (2005). The contribution of GABA to glutamate/glutamine cycling and energy metabolism in the rat cortex in vivo. *Proceedings of the National Academy of Sciences USA, 102* (15), 5588−5593.

Patel, A. B., de Graaf, R. A., Rothman, D. L., Behar, K. L., & Mason, G. F. (2010). Evaluation of cerebral acetate transport and metabolic rates in the rat brain in vivo using ^{1}H-[^{13}C]-NMR. *Journal of Cerebral Blood Flow and Metabolism, 30*(6), 1200−1213.

Patel, A. B., Rothman, D. L., Cline, G. W., & Behar, K. L. (2001). Glutamine is the major precursor for GABA synthesis in rat neocortex in vivo following acute GABA-transaminase inhibition. *Brain Research, 919*(2), 207−220.

Petroff, O. A., Errante, L. D., Rothman, D. L., Kim, J. H., & Spencer, D. D. (2002). Glutamate-glutamine cycling in the epileptic human hippocampus. *Epilepsia, 43*(7), 703−710.

Petroff, O. A., Graham, G. D., Blamire, A. M., al-Rayess, M., Rothman, D. L., Fayad, P. B., et al. (1992). Spectroscopic imaging of stroke in humans: histopathology correlates of spectral changes. *Neurology, 42*(7), 1349−1354.

Raichle, M. E. (1998). Behind the scenes of functional brain imaging: a historical and physiological perspective. *Proceedings of the National Academy of Sciences USA, 95*(3), 765−772.

Ross, B., Lin, A., Harris, K., Bhattacharya, P., & Schweinsburg, B. (2003). Clinical experience with ^{13}C MRS in vivo. *NMR in Biomedicine, 16*(6-7), 358−369.

Rothman, D. L., Behar, K. L., Hetherington, H. P., den Hollander, J. A., Bendall, M. R., Petroff, O. A., et al. (1985). [1]H-Observe/^{13}C-decouple spectroscopic measurements of lactate and glutamate in the rat brain *in vivo. Proceedings of the National Academy of Sciences USA, 82*(6), 1633–1637.

Rothman, D. L., Behar, K. L., Hyder, F., & Shulman, R. G. (2003). In vivo NMR studies of the glutamate neurotransmitter flux and neuroenergetics: implications for brain function. *Annual Review of Physiology, 65*, 401–427.

Rothman, D. L., De Feyter, H. M., de Graaf, R. A., Mason, G. F., & Behar, K. L. (2011). ^{13}C MRS studies of neuroenergetics and neurotransmitter cycling in humans. *NMR in Biomedicine, 24*(8), 943–957.

Rothman, D. L., Howseman, A. M., Graham, G. D., Petroff, O. A., Lantos, G., Fayad, P. B., et al. (1991). Localized proton NMR observation of [3-^{13}C]lactate in stroke after [1-^{13}C]glucose infusion. *Magnetic Resonance in Medicine, 21*(2), 302–307.

Rothman, D. L., Sibson, N. R., Hyder, F., Shen, J., Behar, K. L., & Shulman, R. G. (1999). In vivo nuclear magnetic resonance spectroscopy studies of the relationship between the glutamate-glutamine neurotransmitter cycle and functional neuroenergetics. *Philosophical Transactions of the Royal Society B: Biological Sciences, 354*(1387), 1165–1177.

Rothstein, J. D., Dykes-hoberg, M., Pardo, C. A., Bristol, L. A., Jin, L., Kuncl, R. W., et al. (1996). Knockout of glutamate transporters reveals a major role for astroglial transport in excit otoxicity and clearance of glutamate. *Neuron, 16*, 675–686.

Roy, C. S., & Sherrington, C. S. (1890). On the regulation of the blood-supply of the brain. *Journal of Physiology, 11*(1-2), 85–158 117.

Sailasuta, N., Tran, T. T., Harris, K. C., & Ross, B. D. (2010). Swift Acetate Glial Assay (SAGA): an accelerated human ^{13}C MRS brain exam for clinical diagnostic use. *Journal of Magnetic Resonance, 207*(2), 352–355.

Serres, S., Raffard, G., Franconi, J. M., & Merle, M. (2008). Close coupling between astrocytic and neuronal metabolisms to fulfill anaplerotic and energy needs in the rat brain. *Journal of Cerebral Blood Flow and Metabolism, 28*(4), 712–724.

Shank, R. P., Bennett, G. S., Freytag, S. O., & Campbell, G. L. (1985). Pyruvate carboxylase: an astrocyte-specific enzyme implicated in the replenishment of amino acid neurotransmitter pools. *Brain Research, 329*, 364–367.

Shen, J., Petersen, K. F., Behar, K. L., Brown, P., Nixon, T. W., Mason, G. F., et al. (1999). Determination of the rate of the glutamate/glutamine cycle in the human brain by *in vivo* ^{13}C NMR. *Proceedings of the National Academy of Sciences USA, 96*(14), 8235–8240.

Shen, J., Sibson, N. R., Cline, G., Behar, K. L., Rothman, D. L., & Shulman, R. G. (1998). 15N-NMR spectroscopy studies of ammonia transport and glutamine synthesis in the hyperammonemic rat brain. *Developmental Neuroscience, 20*(4-5), 434–443.

Sibson, N. R., Dhankhar, A., Mason, G. F., Behar, K. L., Rothman, D. L., & Shulman, R. G. (1997). *In vivo* ^{13}C NMR measurements of cerebral glutamine synthesis as evidence for glutamate-glutamine cycling. *Proceedings of the National Academy of Sciences USA, 94*(6), 2699–2704.

Sibson, N. R., Dhankhar, A., Mason, G. F., Rothman, D. L., Behar, K. L., & Shulman, R. G. (1998a). Stoichiometric coupling of brain glucose metabolism and glutamatergic neuronal activity. *Proceedings of the National Academy of Sciences USA, 95*(1), 316–321.

Sibson, N. R., Mason, G. F., Shen, J., Cline, G. W., Herskovits, A. Z., Wall, J. E., et al. (2001). *In vivo* ^{13}C NMR measurement of neurotransmitter glutamate cycling, anaplerosis and TCA cycle flux in rat brain during [2-^{13}C]glucose infusion. *Journal of Neurochemistry, 76*(4), 975–989.

Sibson, N. R., Shen, J., Mason, G. F., Rothman, D. L., Behar, K. L., & Shulman, R. G. (1998b). Functional energy metabolism: in vivo ^{13}C-NMR spectroscopy evidence for coupling of cerebral glucose consumption and glutamatergic neuronal activity. *Developmental Neuroscience, 20*(4-5), 321–330.

Siesjo, B. (1978). *Brain energy metabolism.* New York: John Wiley and Sons.

Sonnewald, U., Westergaard, B., Hassel, B., Miller, T. B., Unsgard, G., Fonnum, F., et al. (1993). NMR spectroscopic studies of ^{13}C acetate and ^{13}C glucose metabolism in neocortical astrocytes: evidence for mitochondrial heterogeneity. *Developmental Neuroscience, 15*, 351–358.

Taylor, A., Mclean, M., Morris, P., & Bachelard, H. (1996). Approaches to studies on neruonal/glial relationships by ^{13}C-MRS analysis. *Developmental Neuroscience, 18*, 434–442.

Terpstra, M., Gruetter, R., High, W. B., Mescher, M., DelaBarre, L., Merkle, H., et al. (1998). Lactate turnover in rat glioma measured by in vivo nuclear magnetic resonance spectroscopy. *Cancer Research, 58*(22), 5083–5088.

van den Berg, C. J., & Garfinkel, D. (1971). A stimulation study of brain compartments. Metabolism of glutamate and related substances in mouse brain. *Biochemistry Journal, 123*(2), 211–218.

van Eijsden, P., Behar, K. L., Mason, G. F., Braun, K. P., & de Graaf, R. A. (2010). *In vivo* neurochemical profiling of rat brain by 1H-[13C] NMR spectroscopy: cerebral energetics and glutamatergic/GABAergic neurotransmission. *Journal of Neurochemistry, 112*(1), 24–33.

van Zijl, P. C., Chesnick, A. S., DesPres, D., Moonen, C. T., Ruiz-Cabello, J., & van Gelderen, P. (1993). In vivo proton spectroscopy and spectroscopic imaging of [1-13C]- glucose and its metabolic products. *Magnetic Resonance in Medicine, 30*(5), 544–551.

van Zijl, P. C., Davis, D., Eleff, S. M., Moonen, C. T., Parker, R. J., & Strong, J. M. (1997). Determination of cerebral glucose transport and metabolic kinetics by dynamic MR spectroscopy. *American Journal of Physiology, 273*(6 Pt 1), E1216–1227.

Wang, J., Jiang, L., Jiang, Y., Ma, X., Chowdhury, G. M., & Mason, G. F. (2010). Regional metabolite levels and turnover in the awake rat brain under the influence of nicotine. *Journal of Neurochemistry, 113*(6), 1447–1458.

Waniewski, R. A., & Martin, D. L. (1998). Preferential utilization of acetate by astrocytes is attributable to transport. *Journal of Neuroscience, 18*(14), 5225–5233.

Wijnen, J. P., Van der Graaf, M., Scheenen, T. W., Klomp, D. W., de Galan, B. E., Idema, A. J., et al. (2010). *In vivo* ^{13}C magnetic resonance spectroscopy of a human brain tumor after application of ^{13}C-1-enriched glucose. *Magnetic Resonance Imaging, 28*(5), 690–697.

Xin, L., Mlynarik, V., Lanz, B., Frenkel, H., & Gruetter, R. (2010). ^{1}H-[^{13}C] NMR spectroscopy of the rat brain during infusion of [2-^{13}C] acetate at 14.1 T. *Magnetic Resonance in Medicine, 64*(2), 334–340.

Yu, A. C. H., Drejer, J., Hertz, L., & Schousboe, A. (1983). Pyruvate carboxylase activity in primary cultures of astrocytes and neurons. *Journal of Neurochemistry, 41*, 1484–1487.

APPLICATIONS OF NON-PROTON MRS

Quantitative Metabolic Magnetic Resonance Imaging of Sodium, Oxygen, Phosphorus and Potassium in the Human Brain: A Rationale for Bioscales in Clinical Applications

Keith R. Thulborn and Ian C. Atkinson

Center for Magnetic Resonance Research, University of Illinois at Chicago, USA

INTRODUCTION

The high cost of magnetic resonance (MR) imaging in a cost-conscious medical climate demands that it supply high quality, clinically relevant information that impacts on patient care to improve outcome. The goal of cost containment is even more daunting if the quality of medical care is not to be compromised. The need to do more for less without loss of quality suggests that medical care needs to refocus on disease prevention, early diagnosis, and prompt treatment of diseases earlier in their progression. Treatments of catastrophic diseases in late stages are expensive and the outcome is often unsatisfactory. The goal of earlier treatment implies the need for methods for earlier diagnosis and to measure disease progression and response to treatment. If we can measure disease progression, then we have a means to evaluate interventions appropriate for these earlier stages. Even if such interventions do not currently exist, a tool that is sensitive to early disease is essential for the development of such therapies. Although genomics has promised improved insight into disease, it is now appreciated that, despite having decoded the complete human genome for more than a decade, the genome is not the whole story. Its expression by translation into proteins is just as important and as complicated. The functional output of these proteins is the basis of metabolomics, the many small molecules expressed in the bodily fluids. Although changes in concentration of these molecules have been advocated as biomarkers of disease, care must be taken to establish the validity of this linkage (Ioannidis & Panagiotou, 2011). A point to be made is that assessment of such molecules is usually remote from the site of the disease with these markers appearing in blood, urine, and cerebrospinal fluid (CSF) only after local disease has progressed sufficiently to release measurable amounts systemically.

The desire to detect earlier disease in regions of the body that are not readily accessible suggests a role for imaging. The use of MR imaging to fill this role can be rationalized if this noninvasive methodology can be used not only to monitor the disease site anatomically but also to provide objective pertinent information on disease progression and therapeutic response. Conventional clinical MR imaging is unlikely to fulfill these requirements. Clinical MR imaging of the human brain, as it is performed today, is based on the proton signal from hydrogen in water. It is the modality of choice for neuroimaging because of the exquisite high-resolution anatomy that can be obtained in a short time. However, this is possible only because the high concentration ($\sim 80\,M$) of water protons in brain tissue. The signal contrast is a reflection of dipole–dipole interactions that determine the longitudinal (T_1) and transverse (T_2) relaxation times as well as the acquisition parameters and the scanner performance rather than fundamental biological properties. Water reflects the tissue milieu, but not the many intricately coupled metabolic reactions that make up the complex biology of the human brain. It is the non-proton elements of sodium, potassium, phosphorus, carbon, oxygen, and nitrogen that make up metabolism. Although these elements have MR signals, the concentrations and MR sensitivity are all significantly reduced compared to hydrogen. The simple solution is to increase sensitivity by increasing the magnetic field strength. Human imaging has now been routinely performed at 3 T for more than two decades, at 7.0 T for over one decade, and at 9.4 T for almost one decade. Moving to these high (3 T) and ultrahigh (>3 T) static magnetic fields does not completely meet all of the challenges of imaging non-proton signals. Non-proton signals have lower concentrations and may have much shorter relaxation times than water proton signals, making efficient data acquisition at a sufficient signal-to-noise ratio (SNR) still a challenge. The method of acquisition including pulse sequence design, image quantification, and display must all be tailored to the nuclear properties of the nucleus of interest.

In this chapter, sodium, oxygen, potassium, and phosphorus will be discussed. Sodium (^{23}Na), oxygen (^{17}O), and potassium (^{39}K) are quadrupolar nuclei (^{23}Na, ^{39}K, I $= 3/2$; ^{17}O, I $= 5/2$) with very short longitudinal and transverse relaxation characteristics; thus they require very different imaging parameters compared to protons (I $= 1/2$). In contrast, phosphorus is spin $1/2$ like protons with relatively long relaxation parameters but with a multiple resonance spectrum in which all of the resonances are of similar intensity. Because of the very low concentrations of the small mobile phosphorus metabolites in brain (<5 mM), special strategies are required to improve acquisition efficiency of the phosphorus resonances of clinical interest.

JUSTIFICATION FOR QUANTIFICATION OF MR SIGNALS

Quantification of an MR image is challenging and conventionally not performed for a number of reasons. The spatially encoded MR signal is usually displayed as a relative gray scale image. The intensity reflects not just the tissue properties of spin density but also the nuclear relaxation rates (as measured by the relaxation times T_1 and T_2) and the acquisition parameters that balance these rates to generate image contrast. The inhomogeneity of the main magnetic field, B_0, caused by insertion of the patient causes localized spatial encoding errors unless corrected. The radiofrequency (RF) field, B_1, generated by the RF coil is non-uniform for both the excitation (B_1^+) and reception (B_1^-) fields over the field of view (FOV) producing variations in signal intensity. The imperfections in performance of the imaging encoding gradients and power supplies can cause image distortions

and spatially varying voxel dimensions. The scanner electronics and the environment, including the quality of Faraday cage of the room in which the magnet must reside, all contribute to the SNR performance, which determines the relative magnitude and variance of the signal to be quantified. Given the multitude of these challenges, the incentive for image quantification must be justified.

To meet the demands of the managed healthcare initiative to contain costs without compromise of quality, diseases must be treated earlier with less expensive solutions, hopefully leading to better outcomes. An example is useful to illustrate this point. The long-term sequel of chronic hypertension is congestive heart failure. Control of hypertension early in its development, detected by measuring blood pressure in units of millimeters of mercury (mmHg) by a simple blood pressure cuff and stethoscope, can reduce the ultimate morbidity and mortality of cardiovascular disease (CVD; Levy et al., 1996). CVD including stroke is a $298 billion a year disease in the United States alone (Writing Group, 2012).

An example of a target disease for quantitative MR imaging is Alzheimer's disease (AD). This disease has an estimated annual cost in 2012 of $200 billion in the United States (Alzheimer's Association, 2012) and the increasing aging population will continue to amplify this cost. Although the cause of AD remains unknown, pathology has established that β-amyloid deposition in the interstitial space and tau (τ)-protein accumulation in neurons occur initially in the entorhinal cortex and hippocampus and later become more widespread throughout the cortex of the brain. The neuronal cell death from these brain regions results in tissue loss (Murray, 2012). Current pharmacological treatments are targeted at slowing progression of the clinical manifestations of the disease, yet the pathology starts decades before symptoms are apparent. Although genomics continues to provide biomarkers (e.g., APO-E alleles) for increased risk of the disease, the development of new interventions for use prior to symptoms will require a means for measuring pathological progression *in vivo* in humans prior to clinically apparent disease. The current use of the biomarkers of β-amyloid and τ-protein measured remotely in blood and CSF are unlikely to be sufficiently early indicators and may be insensitive to disease progression. The imaging of morphological changes in the hippocampus (Schuff et al., 2009) is also a late sign, more apparent after the disease has significantly progressed and possibly not useful for clinical trials of interventions targeted at preclinical disease. An MR imaging measurement of cell density may be postulated as a potential parameter of use in this application and the details will be discussed later (see the section, Clinical applications of

TABLE 4.1.1 Properties of a Bioscale for Quantitative Metabolic Imaging in Humans

#	Bioscale property	Implication
1	Spatially resolved	Imaging based parameter
2	Precisely and accurately measured parameter	Quantification
3	Small biological variance	Highly conserved in normal
4	Mechanistically related to specific metabolic pathway	High sensitivity to disturbance
5	Disease is linked to disruption of that specific metabolic pathway	Valid surrogate for disease

quantitative sodium imaging). This chapter emphasizes such biologically based MR imaging measurements beyond anatomy and image contrast and the methodologies are presented with this goal in mind.

The properties of an imaging parameter that would allow direct access to the site of the disease and be useful for assessment of an early stage of pathology are tabulated in Table 4.1.1. These properties extend well beyond the National Institutes of Health definition of the term *biomarker*—"a characteristic that is *objectively measured* and evaluated as an *indicator* of normal biologic processes, pathogenic processes, or pharmacologic responses to a therapeutic intervention"—to require a new term, *bioscale*, which refers to spatially resolved biochemistry captured by quantitative metabolic imaging. Bioscales, by definition, are quantitative imaging parameters of highly conserved metabolic processes that are therefore sensitive to the earliest stages of human disease. The challenge of developing a useful bioscale is to meet the goal of having an early sensitive means of monitoring disease progression in humans. Such a bioscale would enable clinical trials of early interventions to be undertaken on short timescales and powered with small numbers of subjects. The Prentice criterion for surrogate markers of clinical outcome must be met by such parameters (Prentice, 1989; Berger, 2004). This statement requires that the parameter must be sensitive to the pathological process and not just a correlated change so that it is valid to conclude that lack of progression of the bioscale implies interruption of the disease process (Thulborn et al., 2011a; Atkinson et al., 2012; Thulborn & Atkinson, 2012).

The remainder of this chapter will focus on illustrating the bioscales for sodium, oxygen, and phosphorus MR imaging and only briefly discuss the existing challenges that remain for human potassium MR imaging.

QUANTIFICATION OF MR SIGNALS

23-Sodium (and Potentially 39-Potassium) MR Imaging

The MR signal arising from the mobile sodium ions in human brain tissue is a single resonance made up of the signal coming from the intracellular, interstitial, and CSF compartments. Sodium ions (Na^{23}) and potassium ions (K^{39}) have natural abundances of 100 and 93%, respectively, removing the possibility of any further enrichment strategies. The concentrations of sodium ions in these significant compartments in normal tissue are about 12, 145, and 150 mM, respectively. The corresponding tissue potassium concentrations are 145, 4, and 3 mM, respectively. The vascular compartment is only a few percent of the total brain volume and, for simplicity, can be considered to be a part of the interstitial compartment. Because of the similarities of sodium and potassium MR properties, sodium will be used as the prototype for detailed discussion. The much lower intrinsic MR sensitivity of potassium and the fact that human brain potassium imaging has not yet been achieved makes it less significant in the context of this chapter focused on bioscales in human brain. The low sensitivity of potassium implies that the achievable spatial resolution is likely to be poor in acceptable imaging times, resulting in large partial volume effects that will negate any sensitivity for regional effects. Thus, current MR technology is unlikely to provide a useful ^{39}K-based bioscale in the near future.

As a quadrupolar nucleus, the tissue sodium T_2 value is biexponential with very fast relaxation rates that compromise conventional Cartesian Fourier MR imaging if quantification is required. Although T_2 signal loss can be compensated if the T_2 is known, the loss of SNR further compromises accuracy. The measurement of T_2 is also time-consuming. The preferred approach is to use projection encoding under conditions of full T_1 relaxation and minimal T_2 relaxation. A number of sequences that meet these conditions are available (Boada et al., 1997; Gurney et al., 2006; Nagel et al., 2009; Lu et al., 2010; Thulborn et al., 2011a; Atkinson et al., 2012). Conventional projection imaging uses radial projections from the center of k-space so that encoding starts immediately after the generation of the transverse magnetization by the RF pulse. This minimizes T_2 loss but still allows T_2 blurring, i.e., increased point spread function (PSF), from the nonzero readout time of the k-space trajectory during which the signal decays. The spherical k-space coverage also increases the PSF relative to comparable cubic k-space coverage of Cartesian k-space trajectories. Thus, the actual spatial resolution is not given by the nominal voxel dimension, but should be specified by the PSF when partial volume effects are to be

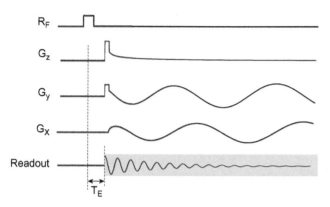

FIGURE 4.1.1   3D flexTPI pulse sequence showing the hard RF pulse; spatial encoding gradients G_x, G_y, and G_z; and the readout of the detected signal. The gradients are switched without violating the constraints of the maximum gradient slew rates. The time, T_E, from the center of the hard RF pulse of duration 0.5 ms to the start of the readout is minimized to about 0.26 ms to avoid signal loss for nuclei with short T2 relaxation times.

corrected during quantification The T_1 value of sodium is short and allows rapid repetition of projections while still maintaining full longitudinal relaxation to simplify quantification. However, since conventional projection imaging with radial trajectories requires a large number of projections to critically sample k-space, the total acquisition time can be unacceptably long. The proposed techniques reduce the total acquisition time by using projections that twist in three dimensions. The pulse sequence, flexible twisted projection imaging (flexTPI), used in this chapter is shown schematically in Fig. 4.1.1. The efficiency of projection spatial encoding is enhanced using flexTPI as the radial projections from the over-sampled center of k-space transition into a twisted trajectory to effectively encode multiple radial projections in a single trajectory (Boada et al., 1997; Gurney et al., 2006; Lu et al., 2010). Obviously this extends the duration of the readout with additional T_2 blurring with resultant loss of resolution. However, the total acquisition time can be reduced significantly and the flexTPI acquisition parameters can be optimized to maximize resolution subject to a total acquisition time (Atkinson et al., 2011).

Projection encoding without echoes is sensitive to eddy currents and gradient performance and care must be taken to determine the actual encoding gradients to ensure that high-fidelity images are obtained with accurate quantification (Lu et al., 2011). As a requested gradient is not the same as that realized in practice due to eddy currents and system delays, determining and correcting the eddy current characteristics and system timing is required and straightforward (Atkinson et al., 2009).

To minimize T_2 relaxation during excitation, the shortest RF pulse is desired for imaging. This implies a nonselective (e.g., "hard") RF pulse. However, for the short repetition times used for quadrupolar nuclei, the specific absorption rate (SAR) limit set by the Food and Drug Administration (FDA) guidelines is quickly approached when using very short RF pulses. Longer RF pulses of the same shape are required to stay within the SAR guideline. However, longer RF pulses allow more T_2 decay during the pulse before spatial encoding with signal acquisition can begin. Correction for T_2 signal losses should be measured from the center of the RF pulse. In practice, however, quantitative imaging with a repetition time of at least four times the T_1 value to avoid T_1 saturation effects allows for reasonably short RF pulses while remaining well within the SAR guidelines (Atkinson et al., 2007).

The static magnetic field (B_0) can be made very homogeneous with a spherical water phantom, but the insertion of the human head into the field greatly distorts the effective B_0 field. Room temperature shims can be used to apply first-order and higher order shim gradients to improve the uniformity. This is important, but becomes increasingly difficult at higher magnetic fields as the B_1 excitation field becomes more distorted when the RF wavelength approaches the FOV. This is one of the challenges of ultrahigh field for proton imaging in that as the sensitivity increases, the B_1 uniformity becomes more compromised making quantification more challenging. Fortunately, the metabolic signals of sodium and other non-proton nuclei are at much lower frequencies than protons and so are more easily quantified even at ultrahigh field. The increased sensitivity at ultrahigh field allows for the shimming to be done on the sodium signal, where the B_1 field is more homogeneous compared to that of protons.

The transmission and reception fields of an RF coil, normally termed B_1^+ and B_1^-, respectively, become unequal at higher frequencies. Although the transmission field can be mapped, methods for mapping the reception field are not yet available without assumptions that cannot be readily tested _in vivo_. This issue is less contentious for quantification of non-proton signals where the frequencies are much lower than for protons.

Calibration of the MR signal as a concentration requires an external calibration phantom of known concentrations that can be imaged under the same conditions as a human head or an internal structure of known concentration (e.g., CSF). The use of phantoms within the same FOV as the human head has proven to be unsatisfactory as the usual cylindrical shape of the phantom produces susceptibility artifacts that compromise signal intensity. The close proximity of the human head also produces magnetic susceptibility artifacts over the phantoms. Additionally, because the phantoms are placed around the head, they are close to the RF coil where B_1 non-uniformity is greatest.

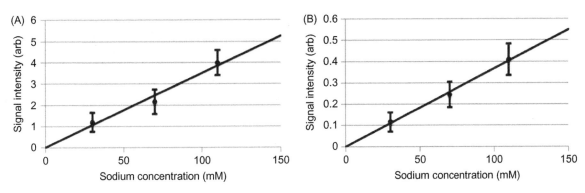

FIGURE 4.1.2 Linearity of the arbitrary sodium MR signal intensity as a function of concentration is obtained at the SNR attained at (A) 9.4 T for voxel dimensions of $3.5 \times 3.5 \times 3.5 mm^3$ and (B) 3 T for voxel dimensions of $5 \times 5 \times 5 mm^3$ as used for human brain MR imaging. The phantom with concentrations of 30, 70, and 110 mM has the same electrical loading of the RF coil as a human head.

We have found that a spherical phantom with the same electrical loading as a human head and placed in the identical position as the head provides the most accurate means of calibration. This phantom can also be used for normalization of the B_1 field. This ratio method is similar to that first proposed almost three decades ago using the proton signal as the reference (Thulborn & Ackerman, 1983). The calibration phantom must also have B_0 optimization and have adequate SNR for accurate quantification. The MR signal intensity is linearly related to sodium concentration over the biological concentration range for the SNR levels attained by quantitative sodium MR imaging. Linear calibration curves are produced at 3.0 and 9.4 T as shown in Fig. 4.1.2 when all of these quantification steps are used. The resulting quantified maps of tissue sodium concentration (TSC) are shown in Fig. 4.1.3. The quantification algorithm for 9.4 T is shown in Table 4.1.2 along with the acquisition times for each step. The total acquisition time for the patient is about 30 min. (for application for this 30 min procedure, see the section, Clinical applications of quantitative sodium imaging). The quantification described previously is for the signal coming from the single quantum transitions of the sodium nuclei. Although higher order transitions can be observed using multiple quantum filtered acquisitions (Hancu et al., 1999; Fiege et al., 2012), these are weaker and require much longer acquisition times to obtain an SNR level appropriate for quantification. Additional information is available from these more complex experiments using, for example, triple quantum filter acquisitions. Some have discussed relationships to intracellular and extracellular compartments, although the interpretations remain limited (Hancu et al., 1999; Fiege et al., 2012). Because the relationship between these nuclear transitions and biological processes remains obscure and the still clinically unacceptable acquisition times, they will not be discussed further. Similarly, the use of sodium MR imaging for non-quantitative anatomical contrast also will not be discussed (Nagel et al., 2011).

17-Oxygen MR Imaging

Oxygen has three stable isotopes of which only 17-oxygen (^{17}O) has an MR signal. Although ^{17}O has a low natural abundance of 0.038%, the high water content of the human brain makes the effective ^{17}O concentration approximately 16 mM in brain tissue. This is about half the concentration of sodium ions, although the low gyromagnetic ratio reduces the intrinsic sensitivity of ^{17}O by another factor of two compared to that of sodium. However, as ^{17}O has a higher spin quantum number ($I = 5/2$), the short T_1 relaxation times ($\sim 0.02s$) allow for efficient signal averaging without compromise of quantification under full T_1 relaxation. The T_2 relaxation times are also slightly shorter so that quantification under conditions of maximum magnetization demands the use of similar projection imaging techniques as for sodium. The low natural abundance allows use of an enrichment strategy for improving SNR for imaging while also obtaining biologically relevant information.

An important property of the human brain is its obligatory use of aerobic respiration as an efficient supply of metabolic energy in the form of adenosine triphosphate (ATP) for the multitude of cellular processes. Over 60% of the energy is used to maintain the ionic gradients across the semipermeable cell membrane that then become the potential energy that is coupled to many other cellular transport processes including action potentials and neurotransmitter activity (Attwell & Laughlin, 2001; Fahmeed Hyder et al., 2013). Thus, the cerebral metabolic rate of oxygen consumption ($CMRO_2$) becomes a fundamental parameter of the health and workload of the brain. $CMRO_2$ can be estimated using positron emission tomography

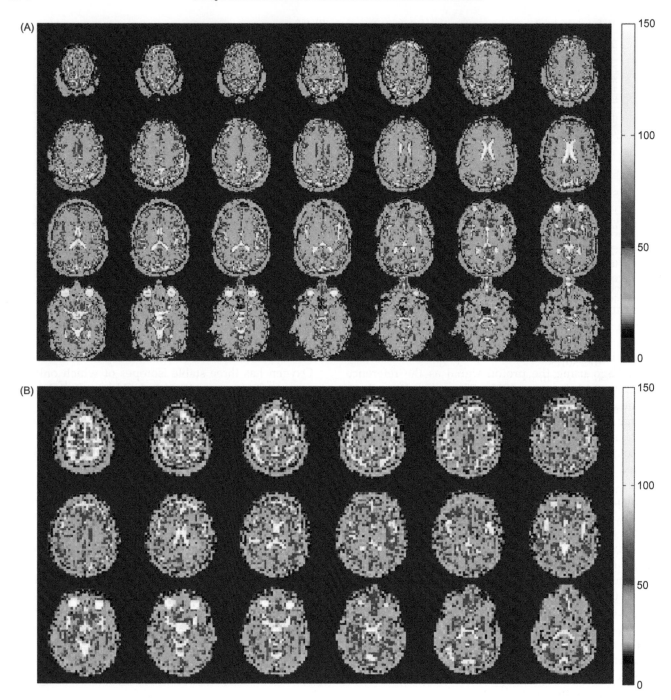

FIGURE 4.1.3   Representative TSC maps from quantitative sodium MR imaging of a normal human head at **(A)** 9.4 T at a voxel dimension of $3.5 \times 3.5 \times 3.5mm^3$ in 10 min and **(B)** 3.0 T at a voxel size of $5 \times 5 \times 5mm^3$ in 10 min. The color scale is in units of mM.

(PET) from a series of separate measurements (oxygen extraction, blood flow, and blood volume), using ^{15}O radioisotopic tracers in the form of oxygen gas, water, and carbon monoxide. As ^{15}O is a short-lived radioisotope (~ 2 min half-life), it must be made on site using a cyclotron. There are few sites in the world capable of this type of PET measurement.

Despite the challenge of SNR, ^{17}O MR imaging offers a viable alternative methodology that simplifies the measurement and uses a stable isotope. The PET

TABLE 4.1.2 Algorithm for Quantification of Tissue Sodium Concentration in the Human Head

Steps	^{23}Na MRI steps for phantom	Acquisition parameters	Acquisition time/processing
1	Shimming on ^{23}Na free induction decay	TR/TE = 500/0.26 ms, flip angle <90°	3 min, no processing
2	^{23}Na B_0 map (flexTPI)	TR/TE = 160/1.26 ms, flip angle = 90°	10 min, steps 2 and 3 give B_0 map
3	Quantitative ^{23}Na acquisition (flexTPI)	TR/TE = 160/0.26 ms, flip angle = 90°	10 min, B_0, and step 3 give calibration
	Steps for human brain		
4	Shimming on ^{23}Na free induction decay	TR/TE = 500/0.26 ms, flip angle <90°	3 min, no processing
5	^{23}Na B_0 map (flexTPI)	TR/TE = 160/1.26 ms, flip angle = 90°	10 min, steps 5 and 6 give B_0 map
6	Quantitative ^{23}Na acquisition (flexTPI)	TR/TE = 160/0.26 ms, flip angle = 90°	10 min, step 6, B_0, and calibration give TSC

This was done using a phantom and head in separate acquisitions with B_0 and B_1 corrections using full longitudinal relaxation and minimizing transverse relaxation using the flexTPI pulse sequence.

technology measures ^{15}O in all of its chemical forms as the detection is of gamma rays emitted from the decay of positrons. Each chemical form must be accounted for and so must be measured separately, hence the multiple measurements with different ^{15}O tracers. In contrast, ^{17}O gas is not visible to MR imaging and so only its conversion to ^{17}O-enriched water as the final step in oxidative phosphorylation produces a measurable MR signal. Introducing ^{17}O-enriched oxygen gas modulates the production of MR-visible $H_2{}^{17}O$, which leads to a corresponding change in signal intensity (McLaughlin et al., 1992). As ^{17}O behaves chemically like ^{16}O, enrichment does not disturb the metabolism and acts like a tracer, albeit at higher concentrations. Rather than use the PET modeling for MR imaging data (Zhu & Chen, 2011), a simpler model of conservation of mass balance between ^{17}O-labeled water entering from arterial blood, the conversion of ^{17}O enriched oxygen gas to ^{17}O-enriched water in the tissue, and any washout of ^{17}O-enriched water from the tissue into the venous blood or chemical conversion can be used to determine CMRO2 (Atkinson & Thulborn, 2010). This model is summarized schematically in Fig. 4.1.4 and is described mathematically in the following equation:

$$\frac{dM_V^{H_2{}^{17}O}(t)}{dt} = 2 \cdot CMRO_2 \cdot A^{17}O(t) - K_L \cdot M_V^{H_2{}^{17}O}(t) + K_G \cdot B^{H_2{}^{17}O}(t)$$

(22.1)

The possible formation of other products from the enriched water does not complicate the single resonance of ^{17}O-enriched water as the very large chemical shift range ensures that there is no contamination of the ^{17}O water resonance used for the image.

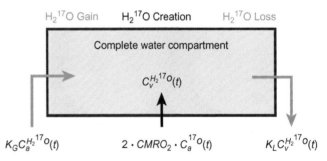

FIGURE 4.1.4 Model for generation of ^{17}O-labeled water from inhaled ^{17}O-enriched oxygen gas in a single imaging voxel (solid black line). $M_V^{H_2{}^{17}O}(t)$, $A^{17}O(t)$, and $B^{H_2{}^{17}O}(t)$ are the moles of ^{17}O-labeled water, the fraction of ^{17}O-labeled arterial oxygen gas, and the relative amount of ^{17}O-labeled water in the blood, respectively, each in excess of natural abundance. The rate constants K_L and K_G are the loss and gain of ^{17}O-labeled water within the voxel, respectively. CMRO$_2$ is the cerebral metabolic rate of oxygen consumption that is to be determined. The total amount of ^{17}O-labeled water in the voxel depends on metabolically generated water (blue), ^{17}O-labeled water gained by inward diffusion from the blood (green), and ^{17}O-labeled water lost due to outward diffusion or chemical conversion to other intermediates (brown). The color scale is in units of mM.

Imaging is performed as a dynamic process in which the subject is imaged continuously through a period of breathing room air as a baseline, inhaling ^{17}O-enriched oxygen gas for a fixed period, and finally, rebreathing room air again during a washout period (Atkinson & Thulborn, 2010; Hoffmann et al., 2011). When the imaging is performed at full T_1 relaxation (as required to limit SAR) and minimal T_2 relaxation by using projection-based imaging, the change in signal intensity can be quantified as a direct measure of

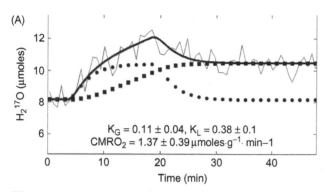

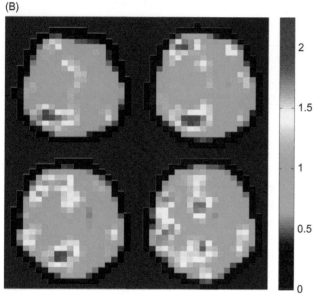

FIGURE 4.1.5 (A) Representative ^{17}O time course for a single gray matter voxel. The three-phase metabolic model of water production (thick solid line) accurately describes the experimental ^{17}O MR data (thin gray line) to yield $CMRO_2$ values with K_G and K_L constants shown. The signal contribution (black squares) from $H_2{}^{17}O$ generated throughout the body, transported by the blood, and diffusing into the tissue reaches a plateau when the $H_2{}^{17}O$ gain from wash-in and $H_2{}^{17}O$ loss from washout and chemical conversion are balanced. The signal contribution (black circles) from local oxygen metabolism reaches a maximum during inhalation and returns to baseline as $H_2{}^{17}O$ loss due to washout and chemical conversion occurs. $CMRO_2 = 1.37 \pm 0.39 \mu mol\ g^{-1}\ min^{-1}$ in agreement for age-matched ^{15}O PET measurements for gray matter (Siciliano et al., 1995). (B) Four axial partitions from a full 3D dataset of the $CMRO_2$ bioscale through a human head. The color scale at right is in units of $\mu mol\ g^{-1}\ min^{-1}$. Total acquisition time is 48 min.

the $CMRO_2$ at rest. An example of results in a normal human brain is shown in Fig. 4.1.5. As ^{17}O is a natural isotope, the FDA has no concerns with the use of ^{17}O-enriched gas for human applications. ^{17}O-enriched gas is expensive today but only because of its low demand. Manufacturing processes are already in place as ^{17}O-enriched water is obtained as a byproduct from the manufacturing process of ^{18}O water, which is used

as the substrate in cyclotrons for the formation of ^{18}F for PET agents. Increased demand from potential clinical applications, as will be discussed later, would be expected to greatly reduce this cost.

31-Phosphorus MR Imaging

Unlike the single MR resonances of sodium, potassium, and oxygen in biological tissues, the phosphorus spectrum has multiple resonances from several mobile low molecular weight molecules containing phosphate (Qiao et al., 2006). The most intense resonances are from the three high-energy phosphates of ATP and the high-energy phosphate of phosphocreatine (PCr) and then lower intensity resonances from sugar phosphates, lipid phosphates, and inorganic phosphate. The concentrations of these metabolites in human muscle (PCr 25 mM; ATP, 5 mM) are higher than in brain (PCr, ATP ~3 mM) and with very different proportions. This reflects the different metabolic strategies of brain (obligatorily aerobic with the substrate of glucose) and muscle (predominately anaerobic with non-glucose substrates). The high concentrations in muscle surrounding the calvarium require that imaging be performed at a spatial resolution that can separate brain from muscle. Albeit at much lower concentrations, the nuclear properties of phosphorus (spin $= 1/2$) are similar to hydrogen with long transverse and longitudinal relaxation times. The T_1 of PCr is as long as 3s and that of ATP is about 1s. These long T_1 values are an enormous obstacle, restricting the data-acquisition efficiency for quantification if full longitudinal magnetization is demanded as used for the sodium MR bioscales. The long T_2 means more time for spatial encoding, but the low concentrations already restrict the achievable resolution in a reasonable time acceptable for human imaging.

The conventional approach is to use chemical shift imaging (CSI; Brown et al., 1982; Pykett & Rosen, 1983) in which the entire chemical shift range is acquired in each voxel in a qualitative manner in which SNR is optimized in preference to quantification. The T_1 saturation and T_2 loss effects can, in principle, be corrected if measured, but this is rarely done in the setting of disease. The spectra become fingerprints of normal and disease, but this methodology has not reached clinical practice despite having been available for decades. The lack of specificity and sensitivity for biological assessments are handicaps that do not as yet warrant the challenge of its complexity on a clinical service.

Although such CSI acquisitions are more efficient by SNR criteria, the short TE of the flexTPI sequence

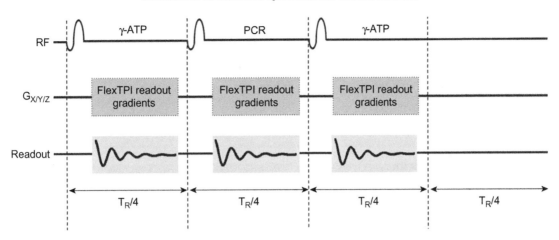

FIGURE 4.1.6 SIMPLE flexTPI pulse sequence for interleaved imaging of ATP and PCr. The flexTPI readout gradients, $G_{x/y/z}$, are shown in Fig. 4.1.1, which are repeated three times in each TR to separately and identically encode the PCr and ATP resonances. The selective RF pulses are also identical in shape and magnitude but shifted to match the appropriate resonance frequency of each metabolite. The detected signal of each resonance is shown for the readout.

has the advantage of minimizing T_2 losses as well as the effects of B_0 inhomogeneity. The important clinical question of the energy status of the tissue does not require the full spectral information. As such, the relevant information is given by the concentrations of ATP and PCr and, in fact, by the ratio of these two metabolic concentrations. The flexTPI pulse sequence (Fig. 4.1.1) has been modified so that the phosphorus resonance of each metabolite can be acquired separately but within a single acquisition using a migrating selective excitation RF pulse (Fig. 4.1.6). The long T_1 of PCr allows two acquisitions of the gamma resonance of ATP to improve the acquisition efficiency for its lower concentration. The simultaneous acquisition of both PCr and ATP signals ensures near perfect coregistration. Longer acquisitions (33 min) than for sodium MR imaging are required to reach a nominal resolution of 15 mm in the human brain at 9.4 T (Lu et al., 2013). This long acquisition and low spatial resolution limits potential clinical applications. The increasing concern about B_1 inhomogeneities at the higher phosphorus frequency is counteracted by the use of the PCr/ATP ratio as the bioscale. By using the ratio of the two signals acquired with almost full T_1 and minimal T_2 relaxation allows this ratio to be independent of B_1 effects once a reasonable SNR is reached. The SNR necessary will depend on how the final bioscale is to be analyzed, but a minimum ratio of ~20:1 is needed to have a 95% probability of the measured bioscale being within ±10% of the true value (Atkinson et al., 2011). These SNR requirements for quantification are more severe for a ratio of two measurements. The longer acquisitions will be compromised by almost inevitable head motion. However, the lower resolution tolerates some motion as does the projection-based acquisition technique. Representative

^{1}H MR images at 3 T and the PCr/ATP bioscale from 9.4 T from an adult patient with a rare manifestation of systemic lupus erythematosus (SLE), which results in diffusion brain inflammation with edema, are shown in Fig. 4.1.7 (A. Lu, personal communication). The rationale for this PCr/ATP bioscale is as a measure of ATP metabolic demand. The cytosolic PCr acts as a local source of high-energy phosphate to convert the adenosine diphosphate (ADP) from ATP catabolism back to ATP. This reaction is catalyzed by phosphocreatine kinase. This local cytoplasmic response to resupply ATP is faster than oxidative phosphorylation in the mitochondria. Thus, the ratio of PCr to ATP concentrations may be expected to be a more sensitive reflection of the rate of ATP utilization than a direct measurement of the ATP concentration. Although not shown by this cognitively normal patient, diseases compromising energy metabolism could, in principle, be monitored with this bioscale. The algorithm for measuring the PCr/ATP bioscale is provided in Table 4.1.3. No phantom calibration image is needed for the PCr/ATP ratio. Prior shimming can be performed with sodium MR imaging without moving the subject.

CLINICAL APPLICATIONS OF QUANTITATIVE SODIUM IMAGING

Aging and Neurodegenerative Disease in Humans

Now that the sodium bioscale methodology in humans has been introduced, initial clinical applications will be discussed in association with the model used for interpretation.

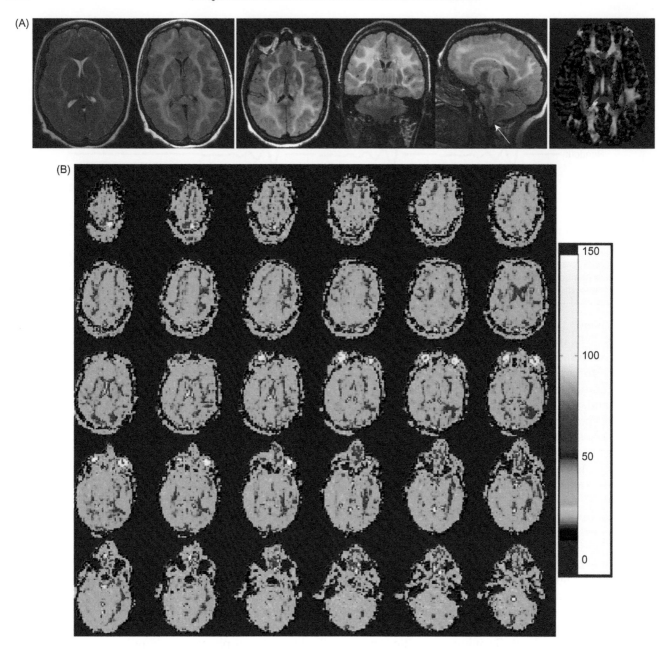

FIGURE 4.1.7   A patient with a rare manifestation of SLE with diffusion brain edema with mass effect and brain herniation through the foramen magnum. **(A)** ^{1}H imaging at 3 T showing marked T_2 hyperintense signal throughout the white matter of T_2-weighted fast spin-echo, T_2-weighted FLAIR (left partition), in three planes of T_2-weighted FLAIR CUBE images showing herniation (white arrow) of the foramen magnum (center partition), and orientation map from diffusion tensor imaging showing intact white matter tracts. **(B)** ^{23}Na image of an abnormal human brain with diffuse cerebral edema at 9.4 T. **(C)** PCr ^{31}P image at a nominal isotropic spatial resolution of 15 mm, **(D)** similar ATP ^{31}P image acquired simultaneously with the PCr image, and **(E)** PCr/ATP bioscale at 9.4 T. Patient shows PCr/ATP = 1.5, not significantly different from normal of 1.4. This figure is reproduced in color in the color plates section. *(Images provided courtesy of Dr. Aiming Lu, personal communication.)*

Normal brain tissue has a high cell density (~80%) with a small interstitial space (~20% of tissue volume), which has a tightly controlled ionic environment of low potassium and high sodium concentrations (~4 and ~145 mM, respectively) (Syková & Nicholson, 2008). Sodium ion homeostasis requires large numbers of ATP-consuming sodium/potassium ion pumps (Na$^+$/ K$^+$ ATPases) at the endothelial, neuronal, and glial cell membranes to maintain the ionic concentration gradients across these semipermeable cell membranes. At cell death, the intracellular volume at low intracellular sodium concentration converts to extracellular space at

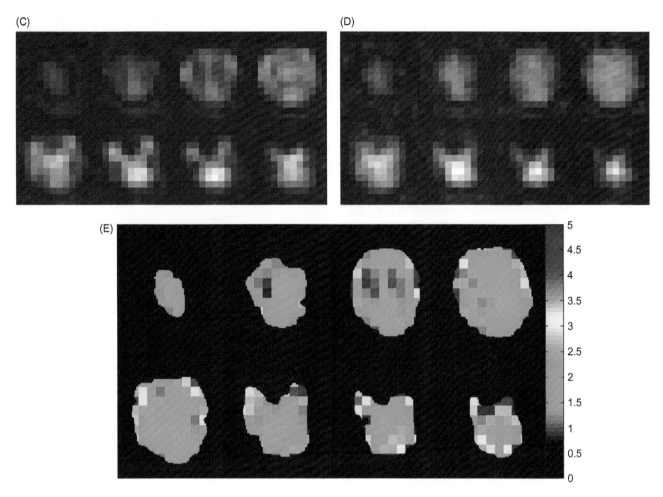

FIGURE 4.1.7 (*Continued*)

TABLE 4.1.3 Algorithm for Measurement of the PCr/ATP Bioscale in the Human Brain

Steps	PCr/ATP in humans ^{23}Na/^{31}P MR imaging	Acquisition parameters	Acquisition time
1	^{23}Na B_0 shimming Free induction decay	TR/TE = 500/ 0.2 ms, flip angle <90°	5 min
2	^{31}P SIMPLE TPI acquisition Selective RF pulses for PCr and γ-ATP 2γ-ATP RF pulses per PCr RF pulse for each TR	TR/TE = 8000/ 0.26 ms, flip angle = 90°	~16 min/ repeated twice for a total of 33 min

This was done using the Simultaneous Imaging of Multiple spectral Peaks with interLeaved Excitations and Flexible Twisted Projection Imaging Readout Trajectories (SIMPLE TPI) pulse sequence. The ^{23}Na MR imaging from Table 4.1.2 is usually done for each patient having ^{31}P MR imaging.

high sodium ion concentration. Although the initial redistribution of ions would not change the local TSC, ionic concentrations of the interstitial space are highly controlled and so the expanded space rapidly leads to increased TSC. Unless the tissue contracts to maintain cell density, the interstitial space expands and TSC increases.

A biological model for TSC has been proposed that involves two compartments: extracellular (C_e) and intracellular (C_i). The sodium concentration in each compartment in normal tissue is $C_e \sim 145$ mM and $C_i \sim 12$ mM, respectively (Lu et al., 2010; Thulborn et al., 2011a; Atkinson et al., 2012). As the vascular compartment is small ($\sim 2\%$ of brain volume) and has a similar sodium concentration to the interstitial compartment, it is considered to be part of the extracellular compartment. TSC measured by quantitative sodium MR imaging reflects the volume fraction weighted sum of the intracellular and extracellular sodium concentrations, respectively. Each imaging voxel within brain tissue encloses intracellular and extracellular spaces with relative volumes that depend on the tissue cell fraction (TCF), which is defined as the fraction of the intracellular volume in the total voxel volume. As shown in Fig. 4.1.8, TSC can be expressed mathematically as follows:

$$TSC = TCF * C_i + (1 - TCF) * C_e \qquad (22.2)$$

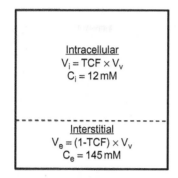

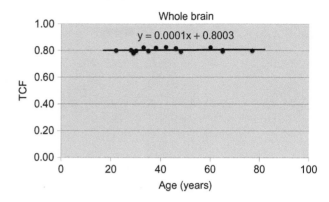

FIGURE 4.1.8 Two-compartment model of a single voxel (solid black line) showing that the tissue sodium concentration (TSC) measured within voxel volume V_V is divided between the intracellular volume V_i and interstitial volume V_e based on the TCF. TSC is the volume fraction weighted sum of the products of the compartment volume and its sodium concentration where C_i and C_e are the intracellular (~ 12 mM) and extracellular (~ 145 mM) sodium concentrations, respectively, as given in Equation 22.2. TCF is derived from TSC using Equation 22.3.

FIGURE 4.1.9   Hippocampal TCF measured at 9.4 T as a function of age (years) in the cognitively normal subjects ($N = 16$). The fitted line has near-zero linear trend, indicating that there is no age dependence for TCF in the hippocampus of cognitively normal individuals. This trend is also true for other regions of the brain.

that can be rearranged to give TCF as follows:

$$TCF = (TSC - C_e)/(C_i - C_e) \qquad (22.3)$$

For normal brain, TSC is measured at 9.4 T (and 3 T) as 37.1 $\pm$ 0.9 mM to give a TCF of 0.81 $\pm$ 0.01, in agreement with the recent literature (Syková & Nicholson, 2008). The large difference between intracellular and extracellular sodium concentrations means that small differences in cell density produce large increases in TSC. Thus, TSC is sensitive to small changes in cell density with positive contrast in the setting of disease or treatments that kill cells. TSC can be measured with a realistic accuracy of $\sim 5\%$, suggesting that a change in TCF of 2% can be readily detected, assuming known CSF and intracellular sodium concentrations. The calculation is relatively insensitive to the intracellular sodium concentration as it is so much smaller than the interstitial sodium concentration.

Fig. 4.1.9 uses the model from Fig. 4.1.8 to demonstrate that TCF in cognitively normal adults across a wide age range (20–77 years) have a narrow distribution, i.e., a small range in cell density. This result also shows that there is only a small variation in cell density across the brain and across the population, and it is slightly lower in gray matter than white matter. The highly conserved feature of cell density for normal cognitive function across normal aging, emphasized by the narrow distribution of TCF for normal subjects (Fig. 4.1.9), suggests that the reason for brain shrinkage with age is to maintain cell density as cells are lost with increasing age. Hence, the loss of brain volume with age should be considered an expected physiological process that compensates for cell loss to maintain cell density and normal function rather than a pathological process. If the normal contraction process is

disrupted, possibly by deposition of extracellular debris such as β-amyloid protein, the expanded interstitial space may also compromise function. It remains to be established if TCF can detect such changes reliably in subjects with AD pathology (Thulborn et al., 2011b).

The importance of this sodium bioscale can be rationalized from another perspective based on the resting membrane potential V_m of neuronal cell membranes. This potential is determined by the ion gradients across the semipermeable cell membrane, as given by the Goldman–Hodgkin–Katz equation as follows:

$$V_m = (RT/F) \ln(\Sigma P_c[C^-]_e + \Sigma P_A[A^+]_i)/(\Sigma P_c[C^-]_i + \Sigma P_A[A^+]_e)$$
$$(22.4)$$

where each of the terms are P permeability for cations C and anions A in the intracellular (i) and extracellular (e) compartments, respectively, and R, T, and F are the gas constant, absolute temperature, and Faraday constant, respectively. As potassium is the most permeable ion, it is the permeability and intracellular and extracellular concentrations of the potassium ion that largely determine the resting V_m. However as potassium and sodium ion concentrations are tightly linked by the Na$^+$/K$^+$ ATPase, the sodium measurements of TSC and TCF reflect the equivalent potassium measurements. Once a cell membrane has been perturbed from its rest state, such as after an action potential with systematic temporally ordered changes in selective ion permeabilities, the membrane potential must return to the resting V_m. This requires that the ion permeability and ion concentrations return to normal to close the voltage-sensitive ion channels. Expansion of the extracellular volume demands that more ions be pumped to produce the same concentration gradient to return to the normal V_m. This increased interstitial space requires more energy to be expended to achieve that same concentration gradient and resting V_m. In the absence of sufficient energy, this recovery process takes longer and function must decline as action potentials fail to initiate in a timely fashion. Although this hypothesis remains to be tested *in vivo*, this argument rationalizes why cell density measured as TCF is an important structural design parameter for the brain that remains constant with normal aging.

It remains to be tested if the AD pathology can be detected with TCF. The long latency of AD offers the opportunity for early intervention to prevent progression to extensive brain damage. The location and small size of the hippocampus demand an imaging approach with suitable spatial resolution at acquisition times acceptable for human imaging. The bioscale of TCF would appear to be suitable for detecting this pathology and quantifying its progression, but its sensitivity for early preclinical detection remains to be tested. The criticism that there are no early interventions begs the question as early interventions cannot be developed or evaluated without such a tool.

Real-Time Treatment Responsiveness of Human Brain Tumors

Although high-grade brain tumors are not a significant financial burden on the healthcare system compared to neurodegenerative disease, they do represent a disease in which modern medical care has failed abysmally. Older individuals with high-grade brain tumors have very short disease progression-free intervals and a grim prognosis that is only slightly better in younger patients. The multimodality treatment involves surgical resection and fractionated radiation with simultaneous low-dose chemotherapy followed by multiple cycles of high-dose chemotherapy. This standard of care has been established by multicenter trials over many years across thousands of patients using survival as the clinical outcome measure. Standard clinical assessment and routine MR imaging are insensitive measures of disease progression. Using survival as an outcome measure provides no opportunity to tailor treatment to the responsiveness of each tumor. Standard protocols are based on population statistics, far removed from personalized healthcare. An early indicator of treatment response would be of significant use in triaging patients to new treatments when a tumor is rapidly found to be unresponsive to the initial treatment.

As treatment response is really a question of changes in cell density, we have used the sodium bioscale to measure treatment response in terms of changes in TCF on a weekly basis across the 6 weeks of fractionated radiation treatment (60 Gy) in high-grade brain tumors. The responses for two representative cases are shown in Figs. 4.1.10 and 4.1.11. Case 1 of a very vascular grade III oligodendroglioma in a young man shows a good response to radiation treatment in that ultimately 60% of the voxels in the tumor showed significant changes, yet the magnitude of the cell kill was small. The tumor cell density changed from 0.55 to 0.45 and the tumor blood volume from dynamic susceptibility contrast MR perfusion imaging remained elevated until completion of 12 cycles of standard chemotherapy with Temodar. This suggests that radiation is not as successful as might be hoped and as generally believed in high-grade brain tumors. This lack of responsiveness is clearly emphasized in case 2 for a grade IV glioneuroma in which no response was elicited by the radiation treatment. Again, there was a response to chemotherapy with anatomical changes but the tumor blood volume remains elevated consistent with a yet incomplete result. Even the tumors that show a response do not show a spatially uniform response; instead they appear to show marked regional variations in response (Fig. 4.1.12). Such information could be used to adapt the treatment plan to produce a better response or to triage patients with radiation-unresponsive tumors to more appropriate treatment with chemotherapy rather than wasting valuable resources and the time and effort of patients with an ineffective and costly treatment. The sodium MR imaging-based TCF bioscale also becomes an efficient way to evaluate therapies as they become available. The question of prediction of outcome is meaningless in the setting of high-grade brain tumors, given the grim prognosis today. A better goal is to measure the magnitude of the early success (or not) of a therapy. A high cell kill (large decrease in TCF within the tumor) reflects a good therapeutic response that is presumed to help the patient whereas no cell kill (no change in TCF) reflects wasted resources without benefit to the patient. Whether a good response is predictive of prolonged disease-free survival is still to be proven.

Real-Time Viability Detection in Acute Stroke

The question of whether or not to treat acute stroke is currently based on the time from onset of symptoms and the absence of hemorrhage. The intervention of choice if symptom onset is within 4.5 h is intravenous thrombolysis of the clot. If time is beyond the time window, the onset is unknown, or there are contraindications to the use of thrombolysis, then endovascular

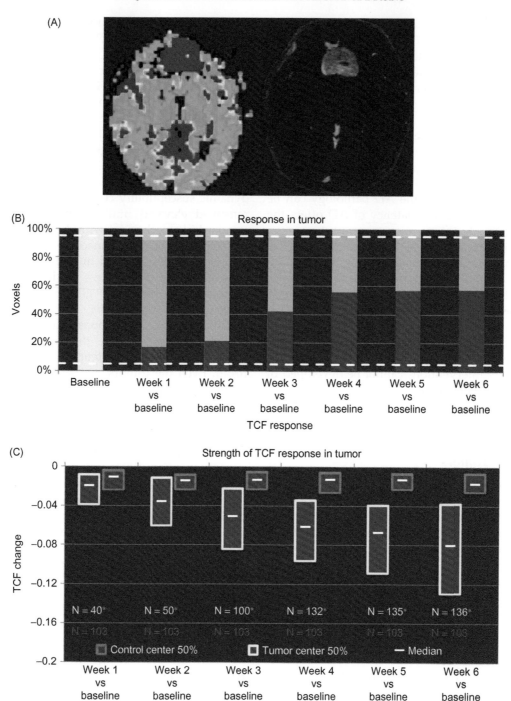

FIGURE 4.1.10   **(A)** Blood volume map and contrast enhanced T_1-weighted image through a grade III oligodendroglioma. **(B)** Percentage of voxels with significant changes in tumor accumulated weekly during radiation treatment. Cell density changes are colorized as decreased (magenta, increasing cell kill), increased (blue, decreasing edema), or unchanged (green, unresponsive). **(C)** Accumulated weekly median change (white line) in TCF within the tumor (yellow box) compared to control region (brown box).

clot retrieval has been shown to be effective (Bosel et al., 2012; Wood, 2012).

The concern is that reperfusion can result in reperfusion transformation to a hemorrhagic stroke, which happens in about 10% of patients with resultant worsening prognosis. The question that is left unanswered is whether the tissue within the affected region of brain distal to the clot is viable. The concept of penumbra and its conversion into a clinically useful and measurable parameter of the perfusion–diffusion

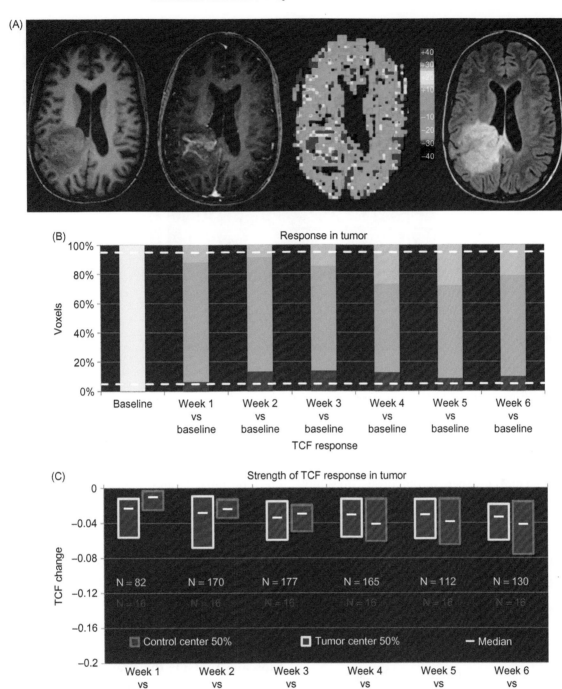

FIGURE 4.1.11 (A) Blood volume and contrast enhanced T_1-weighted images of grade IV glioneuroma in right parietal lobe prior to radiation. (B) Percentage of voxels in tumor accumulated weekly during radiation treatment in which cell density decreases (magenta, increasing cell kill), increases (blue, decreasing edema), or remains unchanged (green, unresponsive). (C) Accumulated weekly change in TCF within the tumor. No change in TCF in any voxels is observed in this tumor.

mismatch has dominated stroke thinking for many years now (Warach, 2003; Chen & Ni, 2012). If TSC-reflecting ion homeostasis is used as the operational definition of viability, then increasing TSC is the metabolic clock that provides the pertinent clinical answer. As shown in Fig. 4.1.13 for a non-human primate model of embolic stroke, TSC shows a relatively linear increase with time. Modifying the water correction for TSC values from literature values (Thulborn et al., 1999), TSC values of 36 mM are normal but TSC over 54 mM is indicative of completed infarction while some data suggest that values below 44 mM may be

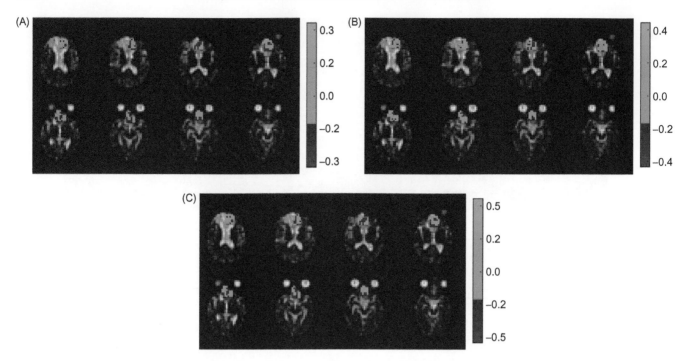

FIGURE 4.1.12　Cumulative spatial variation in TCF response for the case in Fig. 4.1.11 across the course of fractionated radiation treatment at week 1 **(A)**, week 3 **(B)**, and week 6 **(C)**. Some regions are responsive (magenta) while other regions are nonresponsive (green). Areas of resolving edema (blue) are minimal for this case. Note that the color scale expands across weeks consistent with increasing cell kill in some regions while some regions show no change. This suggests that radiation response is not random or uniform even in uniformly vascular tumors.

reversible. The rates of change of TSC in this animal model are 3–5 mM/h when thrombolysis does not occur. As the expansion of the interstitial compartment comes about from loss of cellular integrity, the sodium ions not only redistribute within the infarcted tissue but are supplemented by sodium ions from the rest of the body. The local TSC increases because systemic ion homeostasis maintains the extracellular sodium concentration everywhere at ~145 mM. Even when tissue perfusion drops to very low levels in a stroke-like setting, there is still sufficient perfusion to allow ion exchange and certainly diffusion from adjacent tissue along the initial concentration gradients that maintain the uniform sodium concentration of this space. The rate of change of TSC locally may well reflect these ion distribution processes as well as loss of cell ion homeostasis. When recanalization is achieved before all of the tissue is infarcted, TSC does not continue to increase and infarction does not progress. Although it is not ethical to delay patient care to make the full quantitative TSC measurement, it is feasible to use a TSC index as a ratio of the signal intensities from equivalent regions of the affected and unaffected cerebral hemispheres within 10 min. The patient can be started on intravenous thrombolysis as soon as the diagnosis of non-hemorrhagic stroke is confirmed with diffusion-weighted and T_2*weighted gradient-echo ^1H MR

imaging. The additional time in the scanner does not preclude rapid treatment by a dedicated stroke management team. This new information that may indicate viable tissue is present may also be useful in making the decision of whether to proceed with mechanical removal of the clot for patients at longer than the 4.5 h time window. If the tissue is already infarcted based on a TSC index ratio of 50%, reperfusing dead tissue may be counterproductive.

Other Potential Applications of Sodium Bioscales Outside the Brain

Although this chapter has focused on quantitative metabolic MR imaging and its bioscales in the human brain, such MR methodologies must be extended to other body applications for a viable business plan of a clinical service. Such applications are already developing, although quantification has not yet been rigorously applied.

Probably the best example of a musculoskeletal application is the use of sodium MR imaging to define the surface charge density of cartilage as an early marker of degenerative joint disease. Sodium is the counter ion for the negatively charged sulfate groups and carboxy residues on the glycosaminoglycan side

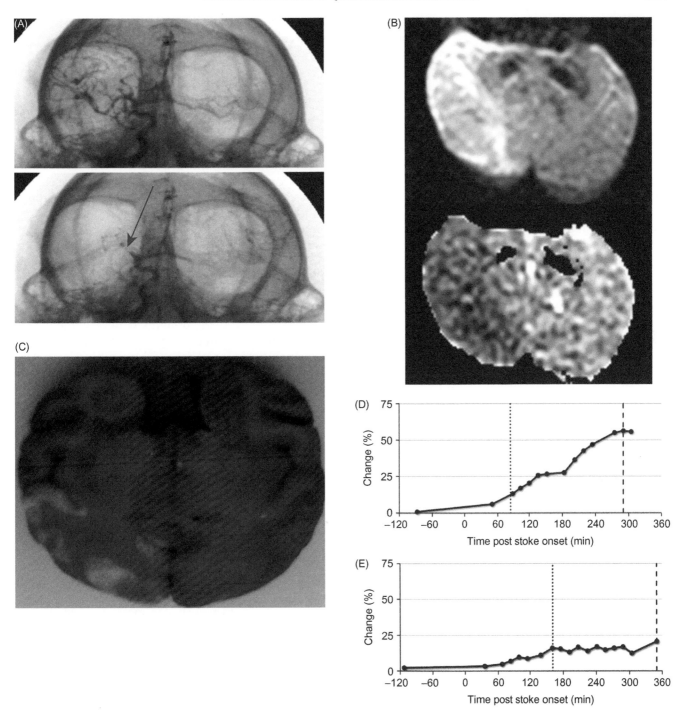

FIGURE 4.1.13 Non-human primate model of embolic ischemic stroke. (A) Catheter angiogram before (top) and after (bottom) emboliza-tion of autologous clot into the right internal carotid artery showing loss of the right middle cerebral artery branches (red arrow). (B) Diffusion-weighted ^{1}H image (upper) and apparent diffusion coefficient map (lower) of the monkey brain after stroke induction showing right hemispheric stroke with increased signal intensity with depressed apparent diffusion coefficient, corresponding to (C) pathological tissue slice stained with vital stain showing the stroke as the nonstaining white regions in the right cerebral hemisphere (shown in the same orientation as the MR images). (D, E) Time courses for two different animals of percentage change in the ratio of the difference in signal intensities in the stroke region and contralateral hemisphere to that signal intensity in the contralateral normal hemisphere are shown for (D) an animal that did not respond to a single thrombolysis treatment (vertical dotted line) and (E) an animal that did respond to two treatments of thrombolysis (vertical dotted line) with recanalization demonstrated by magnetic resonance angiography. Dashed vertical line indicates the time of animal death. The methodology is given by Warach (2003). Although the TSC was quantified in this animal model, full quantification is too time-consuming for application in the urgent acute human stroke and so a ratio comparison to the contralateral normal brain provides an internal parameter that is quickly measured. This index would be applicable to following human stroke in the early acute and subacute stages to deter-mine whether viable but threatened tissue is salvageable.

4. APPLICATIONS OF NON-PROTON MRS

groups of the proteoglycans that provide the high hydration level of cartilage. These charged groups provide the fixed charge density that results in electrostatic repulsion that causes cartilage to swell. This is opposed by collagen fibers that provide tensile strength (Borthakur et al., 2006; Staroswiecki et al., 2010). Thus, as the sodium concentration plays a central role in cartilage integrity and function, the TSC bioscale may have a role as an early surrogate for cartilage degeneration. As the cost of osteoarthritis in the United States is estimated to be $185.5 billion, this disease is also an excellent target for evaluating drug interventions using this methodology (Kotlarz et al., 2009).

Other clinical applications in the body include evaluation of renal function where sodium concentration gradients through the medulla of the kidney determine its concentrating function (Haneder et al., 2011). Such broader applications will need to be proven of clinical value if sodium MR imaging and its metabolic parameters are to become accepted into the medical management of patients.

POTENTIAL APPLICATIONS OF QUANTITATIVE 17-OXYGEN MR IMAGING

The measurement of $CMRO_2$ in humans using the inhalation of ^{17}O-enriched oxygen gas that is now possible on 7 and 9.4 T ultrahigh field scanners opens the possibility of providing this bioscale to the clinical service for application in cerebrovascular disease. $CMRO_2$ has been promised as a clinical parameter by ^{15}O PET for more than three decades (Frackowiak et al., 1980; Herscovitch et al., 1983; Mintun et al., 1984), but has failed to enter clinical practice due to its need for an onsite cyclotron for ^{15}O production and the time-consuming complexity of the multiple measurements required by this methodology. Despite simplifications to avoid arterial sampling and the use of relative rather than absolute values (Ibaraki et al., 2004), the ^{15}O PET method remains a research tool in only a few PET centers with cyclotrons (Bremmer et al., 2011).

The dynamic ^{17}O MR method requires no arterial sampling and is straightforward to apply in cooperative subjects. The study requires about 45 min for the dynamic scan, a baseline of 5 min of breathing room air, up to 10 min of inhalation of ^{17}O-enriched gas, and 30 min of washout again breathing room air. Stationary head position must be maintained during this long dynamic scan. A head fixation frame could be used to help the subject with this requirement, as is used for PET. The cost of ^{17}O-enriched oxygen gas is comparable to PET costs and remains a hurdle to clinical implementation until the usefulness of the results in clinical

management is established. Such studies are in progress in centers with ultrahigh field MR scanners.

POTENTIAL APPLICATIONS OF QUANTITATIVE 31-PHOSPHORUS MR IMAGING

As high-energy phosphate metabolites involve the central bioenergetic pathways of the cell, *in vivo* ^{31}P MR spectroscopy (MRS) has been suggested to have clinical applications in observing alterations of the proportions of these compounds in disease states. This was first demonstrated in the clinical setting of McArdle's syndrome decades ago (Ross et al., 1981; Siciliano et al., 1995). However, despite considerable research effort, ^{31}P MRS has had no significant clinical impact. Even ^{1}H MRS is no longer reimbursed and rarely found to contribute to clinical management. The low sensitivity at current clinical field strengths requires large voxels to be used to achieve adequate SNR in acceptable acquisition times for patients. The resulting large partial volume effects dilute regional spectral changes producing large biological variances that limit the sensitivity and specificity for distinguishing different pathologies.

These limitations can be at least partially overcome by using ultrahigh magnetic field scanners designed for humans (Thulborn, 2006). ^{31}P MR signals can be interrogated selectively using the imaging approach described earlier in which only the metabolic signals of interest are imaged. Quantification requires a reasonable SNR value (>10). The type of pathology determines the required spatial resolution and determines the total acquisition time. Whether the resultant parametric map, e.g., PCr/ATP, may reflect underlying pathology to become useful clinically remains to be established.

Although the PCr/ATP parameter is evaluated in the setting of chronic cerebrovascular disease where aerobic energy metabolism may be compromised, as of this time there are currently no practical clinical applications of quantitative ^{31}P MR imaging in the human brain. Even at 9.4 T, the spatial resolution is limited to a nominal 15 mm isotropic voxel size (i.e., $15 \times 15 \times 15 mm^3$) in a 33 min acquisition. Such numbers suggest limited clinical potential unless further sensitivity improvements can be found.

APPLICATIONS OF QUANTITATIVE POTASSIUM MR IMAGING

Quantum potassium MR imaging has never been performed in the human brain because of the low sensitivity and extraordinary long acquisition times that

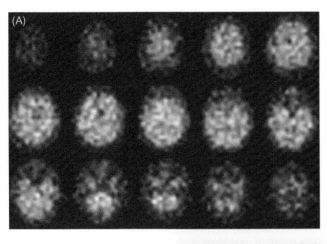

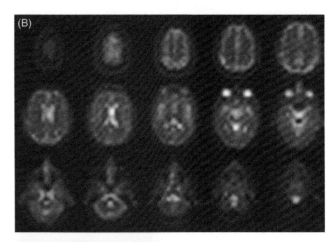

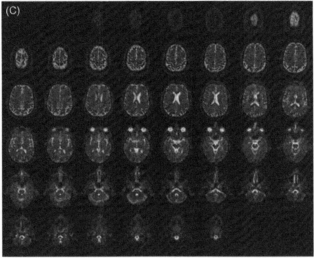

FIGURE 4.1.14 (A) ^{39}K image at a nominal spatial resolution of $10 \times 10 \times 10$ mm^3 of the normal human brain acquired in 40 min at 9.4 T using TPI. (B) Co-registered ^{23}Na images reconstructed at the same resolution as the ^{39}K images in (A) from the high-resolution images in (C). (C) Co-registered ^{23}Na image at a nominal spatial resolution of $3.23 \times 3.25 \times 3.25$ mm^3 acquired in 10 min.

would be expected to achieve useful anatomic resolution. As an effort to make this chapter as comprehensive as possible, a first attempt has been made at ^{39}K MR imaging of the human brain at 9.4 T. The same strategies that were developed for sodium imaging have been used. A volume quadrature RF coil and the flexTPI pulse sequence produced the images shown in Fig. 4.1.14, which reflect a nominal isotropic spatial resolution of 10 mm in 40 min with an SNR of 5.2. This is not an optimized acquisition method as yet, but the image provides feasibility to strive for quantifiable ^{39}K images in human brains. Quantification with acceptable accuracy will require an SNR of >10.

CONCLUSIONS

Quantitative metabolic MR imaging of sodium and oxygen bioscales, especially at ultrahigh field, offers new

assessment parameters that go beyond anatomical changes and interrogate metabolic aspects of the human brain function and dysfunction. The fundamental nature of these processes, as suggested by the small biological variance, increases the sensitivity of these bioscales for detection of perturbations caused by disease. At ultrahigh fields, these nuclei achieve an imaging resolution that can be used to correct for the partial volume averaging that dilutes such sensitivity. These properties suggest that bioscales may contribute toward the development and evaluation of new therapies for earlier stages of important neurodegenerative diseases such as dementia and CVD that have very long latencies and other chronic degenerative diseases such as osteoarthritis outside the brain.

Although phosphorus MR imaging can be performed, its low sensitivity gives a pessimistic view for its future clinical applications. The quantification of potassium MR imaging remains a dream for future strategies of sensitivity enhancement.

Acknowledgments

The authors acknowledge financial support from National Institutes of Health Grant RO1 CA129553

References

Alzheimer's Association. (2012). Alzheimer's disease facts and figures report. Amsterdam: Elsevier.

Atkinson, I. C., & Thulborn, R. (2010). Feasibility of mapping the tissue mass corrected bioscale of cerebral metabolic rate of oxygen consumption using 17-oxygen and 23-sodium MR imaging in a human brain at 9.4 T. *Neuroimage, 51*, 723–733.

Atkinson, I. C., Lu, A., & Thulborn, K. R. (2012). Quantitative metabolic MR imaging of human brain using 17O and 23Na. In R. K. Harris, & R. E. Wasylishen (Eds.), *Encyclopedia of magnetic resonance*. Chichester, UK: John Wiley.

Atkinson, I. C., Lu, A., & Thulborn, K. R. (2009). Characterization and correction of system delays and eddy currents for MR imaging with ultrashort echo-time and time-varying gradients. *Magnetic Resonance in Medicine, 62*(2), 532–537.

Atkinson, I. C., Lu, A., & Thulborn, K. R. (2011). Clinically constrained optimization of flexTPI acquisition parameters for the tissue sodium concentration bioscale. *Magnetic Resonance in Medicine, 66*(4), 1089–1099.

Atkinson, I. C., Renteria, L., Burd, H., Pliskin, N. H., & Thulborn, K. R. (2007). Safety of human MRI at static fields above the FDA 8T guideline: sodium imaging at 9.4T does not affect vital signs or cognitive ability. *Journal of Magnetic Resonance Imaging, 26*, 1222–1227.

Attwell, D., & Laughlin, S. B. (2001). An energy budget for signaling in the grey matter of the brain. *Journal of Cerebral Blood Flow and Metabolism, 21*, 1133–1145.

Berger, V. W. (2004). Does the Prentice criterion validate surrogate endpoints? *Statistics in Medicine, 23*, 1571–1578.

Boada, F. E., Gillen, J. S., Shen, G. X., Chang, S. Y., & Thulborn, K. R. (1997). Fast three dimensional sodium imaging. *Magnetic Resonance in Medicine, 37*, 706–715.

Borthakur, A., Mellon, E., Niyogi, S., Witschey, W., Kneeland, J. B., & Reddy, R. (2006). Sodium and T1rho MRI for molecular and diagnostic imaging of articular cartilage. *NMR in Biomedicine, 19*(7), 781–821.

Bosel, J., Hacke, W., Bendszus, M., & Rohde, S. (2012). Treatment of acute ischemic stroke with clot retrieval devices. *Current Treatment Options in Cardiovascular Medicine, 14*, 260–272.

Bremmer, J. P., van Berckel, B. N., Persoon, S., Kappelle, L. J., Lammertsma, A. A., Kloet, R., et al. (2011). Day-to-day test-retest variability of CBF, CMRO2, and OEF measurements using dynamic 15O PET studies. *Molecular Imaging in Biology, 13*(4), 759–768.

Brown, T., Kincaid, B., & Ugurbil, K. (1982). NMR chemical shift imaging in three dimensions. *Proceedings of the National Academy of Sciences USA, 79*, 3523–3526.

Chen, F., & Ni, Y. -C. (2012). Magnetic resonance diffusion-perfusion mismatch in acute ischemic stroke: an update. *World Journal of Radiology, 4*(3), 63–74.

Fahmeed Hyder, F., Rothman, D. L., Maxwell, R., & Bennett, M. R. (2013). Cortical energy demands of signaling and nonsignaling components in brain are conserved across mammalian species and activity levels. *Proceedings of the National Academy of Sciences USA, 110*, 3549–3554.

Fiege, D. P., Romanzetti, S., Mirkes, C. C., Brenner, D., & Shah, N. J. (2012). Simultaneous single-quantum and triple-quantum-filtered MRI of 23Na (SISTINA). *Magnetic Resonance in Medicine, 69*(6), 1691–1696.

Frackowiak, R. S., Lenzi, G. L., Jones, T., & Heather, J. D. (1980). Quantitative measurement of regional cerebral blood flow and oxygen metabolism in man using 15O and positron emission tomography: theory, procedure, and normal values. *Journal of Computer Assisted Tomography, 4*, 727–736.

Gurney, P. T., Hargreaves, B. A., & Nishimura, D. G. (2006). Design and analysis of a practical 3D cones trajectory. *Magnetic Resonance in Medicine, 55*, 575–582.

Hancu, I., Boada, F. E., & Shen, G. X. (1999). Three-dimensional triple-quantum-filtered (23)Na imaging of in vivo human brain. *Magnetic Resonance in Medicine, 42*(6), 1146–1154.

Haneder, S., Konstandin, S., Morelli, J. N., Nagel, A. M., Zoellner, F. G., Schad, L. R., et al. (2011). Quantitative and qualitative (23)Na MR imaging of the human kidneys at 3 T: before and after a water load. *Radiology, 260*(3), 857–865.

Herscovitch, P., Markham, J., & Raichle, M. E. (1983). Brai006E blood flow measured with intravenous H215O: I. theory and error analysis. *Journal of Nuclear Medicine, 24*, 782–789.

Hoffmann, S. H., Begovatz, P., Nagel, A. M., Umathum, R., Schommer, K., Bachert, P., et al. (2011). A measurement setup for direct 17O MRI at 7T. *Magnetic Resonance in Medicine, 66*, 1109–1115.

Ibaraki, M., Eku Shimosegawa, E., Miura, S., Kazuhiro Takahashi, K., Ito, H., Kanno, I., et al. (2004). PET measurements of CBF, OEF, and CMRO2 without arterial sampling in hyperacute ischemic stroke: method and error analysis. *Annals of Nuclear Medicine, 18*(1), 35–44.

Ioannidis, J. P. A., & Panagiotou, O. A. (2011). Comparison of effect sizes associated with biomarkers reported in highly cited individual articles and in subsequent meta-analyses. *JAMA, 305*(21), 2200–2210.

Kotlarz, H., Gunnarsson, C. L., Fang, H., & Rizzo, J. A. (2009). Insurer and out-of-pocket costs of osteoarthritis in the US: evidence from national survey data. *Arthritis and Rheumatism, 60*(12), 3546–3553.

Levy, D., Larson, M. G., Vasan, R. S., Kannel, W. B., & Ho, K. K. (1996). The progression from hypertension to congestive heart failure. *JAMA, 275*(20), 1557–1562.

Lu, A., Atkinson, I. C., & Thulborn, K. R. (2011). Factors Influencing the accuracy of sodium concentration quantification from sodium flexible twisted projection MR imaging. *Magnetic Resonance in Medicine, 213*(1), 176–181.

Lu, A., Atkinson, I. C., Claiborne, T., Damen, F., & Thulborn, K. R. (2010). Quantitative sodium imaging with a flexible twisted projection pulse sequence. *Magnetic Resonance in Medicine, 63*, 1583–1593.

Lu, A., Atkinson, I. C., Zhou, X. J., & Thulborn, K. R. (2013). PCr/ATP ratio mapping of the human head by simultaneously imaging of multiple spectral peaks with interleaved excitations and flexible twisted projection imaging readout trajectories at 9.4 T. *Magnetic Resonance in Medicine, 69*(2), 538–544.

McLaughlin, A. C., Pekar, J., Ligeti, L., Zoltan, R., Lyon, R., Sinnwell, T., et al. (1992). In vivo measurement of cerebral blood flow and oxygen consumption using 17O magnetic resonance imaging. In S. Zackery (Ed.), *Imaging in Alcohol Research* (pp. 273–286). Washington DC: U.S. Government Press.

Mintun, M. A., Raichle, M. E., Martin, W. R. W., & Heroscovitch, P. (1984). Brain oxygen utilization measured with O-15 radiotracers and positron emission tomography. *Journal of Nuclear Medicine, 25*, 177–187.

Murray, A. D. (2012). Imaging approaches for dementia. *American Journal of Neuroradiology, 33*, 1836–1844.

Nagel, A. M., Bock, M., Hartmann, C., Gerigk, L., Neumann, J. O., Weber, M. A., et al. (2011). The potential of relaxation-weighted sodium magnetic resonance imaging as demonstrated on brain tumors. *Investigative Radiology, 46*(9), 539−547.

Nagel, A. M., Laun, F. B., Weber, M. A., Matthies, C., Semmler, W., & Schad, L. R. (2009). Sodium-MRI using a density-adapted 3D radial acquisition technique. *Magnetic Resonance in Medicine, 62*(6), 1565−1573.

Prentice, R. I. (1989). Surrogate endpoints in clinical trials: definition and operational criteria. *Statistics in Medicine, 8*, 431−440.

Pykett, I., & Rosen, B. (1983). Nuclear magnetic resonance: in-vivo proton chemical shift imaging. *Radiology, 149*, 197−201.

Qiao, H., Zhang, X., Zhu, X. -H., Du, F., & Chen, W. (2006). In vivo ^{31}P MRS of human brain at high/ultrahigh fields: a quantitative comparison of NMR detection sensitivity and spectral resolution between 4 T and 7 T. *Magnetic Resonance Imaging, 24*(10), 1281−1286.

Ross, B. D., Radda, G. K., Gadian, D. G., Rocker, G., Esiri, M., & Falconer-Smith, J. C. (1981). Examination of a case of suspected McArdle's syndrome by 31P nuclear magnetic resonance. *New England Journal of Medicine, 304*(22), 1338−1342.

Schuff, N, Woerner, N, Boreta, L, Kornfield, T, Shaw, LM, & Trojanowski, JQ (2009). MRI of hippocampal volume loss in early Alzheimer's disease in relation to ApoE genotype and biomarkers. *Brain, 132*(4), 1067−1077.

Siciliano, G., Rossi, B., Martini, A., Angelini, C., Martinuzzi, A., Lodi, R., et al. (1995). Myophosphorylase deficiency affects muscle mitochondrial respiration as shown by 31P-MR spectroscopy in a case with associated multifocal encephalopathy. *Journal of Neurological Sciences, 128*(1), 84−91.

Staroswiecki, E., Bangerter, N. K., Gurney, P. T., Grafendorfer, T., Gold, G. E., & Hargreaves, B. A. (2010). In vivo sodium imaging of human patellar cartilage with a 3D cones sequence at 3 T and 7 T. *Journal of Magnetic Resonance Imaging, 32*(2), 446−451.

Syková, E., & Nicholson, C. (2008). Diffusion in brain extracellular space. *Physiology Review, 88*, 1277−1340.

Thulborn K. R. & Atkinson I. C. (2013). From standardization to quantification: beyond biomarkers towards bioscales as neuro MR imaging surrogates of clinical endpoints. *Neurographics*, in press.

Thulborn, K. R. (2006). The challenges of integrating a 9.4T MR scanner for human brain imaging. In P. -M. Robitaille, & L. J. Berliner (Eds.), *Ultra High Field Magnetic Resonance Imaging* (pp. 105−126). New York: Springer Science and Business Media.

Thulborn, K. R., & Ackerman, J. H. H. (1983). Absolute molar concentrations by NMR in inhomogeneous B1: a scheme for analysis of *in vivo* metabolites. *Journal of Magnetic Resonance, 55*, 357−371.

Thulborn, K. R., Atkinson, I. C., & Lu, A. (2011a). Metabolic magnetic resonance imaging: a case for bioscales in medicine. In S. H. Faro, & F. B. Mohamed (Eds.), *Functional Neuroradiology: Principles And Clinical Applications* (pp. 911−928). New York: Springer.

Thulborn K.R., Atkinson I.C., Lu A., Ganin H., Shah R., Bennett D. A., et al. (2011b). Tissue sodium concentration biosca les from sodium MR imaging: application to aging and Alzheimer's disease. In: *Proceedings of 49th Annual Meeting, American Society of Neuroradiology, 2011, Paper 106.*

Thulborn, K. R., Gindin, T. S., Davis, D., & Erb, P. (1999). Comprehensive MRI protocol for stroke management: tissue sodium concentration as a measure of tissue viability in a non-human primate model and clinical studies. *Radiology, 139*, 26−34.

Warach, S. (2003). Measurement of the ischemic penumbra with MRI: it's about time. *Stroke, 34*, 2533−2534.

Wood, H. (2012). New mechanical clot retrieval devices show superiority in patients with acute ischaemic stroke. *Nature Reviews Neurology, 8*, 531 Published online September 18, 2012.

Writing Group. Heart disease and stroke statistics-2012 update: a report from the American Heart Association. *Circulation*, 2012; 125:e2-e220.

Zhu, X. -H., & Chen, W. (2011). *In vivo* oxygen-17 NMR for imaging brain oxygen metabolism at high field. *Progress in Nuclear Magnetic Resonance Spectroscopy, 59*(4), 319−335.

Carbon (^{13}C) MRS

Douglas L. Rothman and Henk M. De Feyter

Departments of Diagnostic Radiology, Magnetic Resonance Research Center, Yale University School of Medicine, New Haven, CT, USA

INTRODUCTION

In this chapter we review the current state of ^{13}C magnetic resonance spectroscopy (MRS) as it is used to study neuroenergetics and neurotransmitter cycling in humans. We focus primarily on the present status of the measurement (pathways and spatial resolution) and recent findings, leaving descriptions of the experimental methodology to earlier chapters. We finish by reviewing the results of initial applications of ^{13}C MRS and ^1H-$[^{13}C]$ MRS to study human disease and potential improvements in sensitivity, cost, and ease of performing studies.

^{13}C MRS is presently the only method that provides noninvasive measurements of neuroenergetics and neurotransmitter cycling in human brain. The ability to use ^{13}C MRS to study cell-specific neuroenergetics and neurotransmitter cycling is due to the localization of key enzymes and metabolite pools in neurons and glia and the specificity of ^{13}C-labeled precursors to specific cell types. Fig. 4.2.1 shows a diagram of neuronal and astrocyte (a form of glial cell) cell metabolism and the interplay of neuronal and astrocyte metabolism via the glutamate/glutamine cycle. Both neurons and astrocytes can take up glucose and oxidize it in their mitochondria via the tricarboxylic acid (TCA) cycle. As will be discussed later, neurons and astrocytes in addition to glucose can oxidize lactate and β-hydroxybutyrate (BHB) while astrocytes can also oxidize acetate and fatty acids. Excitatory glutamatergic neurons, which account for over 80% of the neurons and synapses in the cerebral cortex (Shephard, 1994), release glutamate as a neurotransmitter, most of which is taken up by the astrocytes (Rothstein et al., 1996; Bergles et al., 1999) and converted to glutamine or oxidized (Sibson et al., 2001; Hertz et al., 2007). Neurons lack the enzymes required for *de novo* synthesis of glutamate, and therefore depend on the astrocytes to provide substrates for the synthesis of glutamate lost during neurotransmission (Yu et al., 1983). The neuron then converts glutamine to glutamate via phosphate-activated glutaminase. The complete series of steps from neuronal glutamate release to resynthesis of glutamate from glutamine is called the glutamate/glutamine cycle.

Fig. 4.2.2 shows spectra obtained at 4 T from human brain localized to the midline occipital parietal lobe during infusions of three different isotopic-labeled substrates—99% enriched [1-^{13}C]glucose, [3-^{13}C]lactate, and [2-^{13}C]acetate—and shows labeling in the brain pools of aspartate, GABA, glutamine, and glutamate. The brain pools of glutamate, GABA, and glutamine have been shown to be localized within glutamatergic neurons, GABAergic neurons, and glia, respectively (under nonpathological conditions). By following the flow of ^{13}C label from glucose, acetate, and other precursors into these metabolites, MRS, in combination with metabolic modeling, allows the measurement of the TCA cycle rate in glutamatergic neurons, GABAergic neurons, and glia, as well as glutamate and GABA neurotransmitter cycles between neurons and astrocytes (Mason & Rothman, 2002; Rothman et al., 2003). When expressed as total substrate oxidation, the rates determined by MRS are found to be in excellent agreement with earlier methods, including positron emission tomography (PET; Rothman et al., 2003; Boumezbeur et al., 2005; Hyder et al., 2006; Chaumeil et al., 2009). However, *in vivo* MRS is unique among other techniques in its measurement of cell type-specific energetics and neuronal/glial neurotransmitter cycles.

STUDIES IN ANIMAL AND CELL MODELS OF THE GLUTAMATE/GLUTAMINE CYCLE AND NEURONAL AND GLIAL ENERGETICS

Although this chapter will primarily focus on human studies, we briefly review here some relevant

312

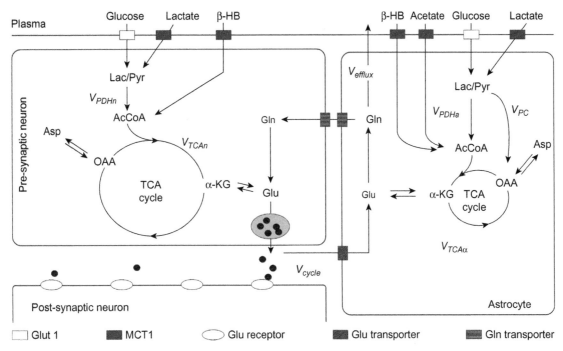

FIGURE 4.2.1   Diagram of the glutamate/glutamine cycle. The top shows a schematic of metabolic pathways within glutamatergic neurons and surrounding astroglial cells. Glucose and lactate will enter both the glial (V_{TCAa}) and neuronal TCA cycles (V_{TCAn}) via pyruvate dehydrogenase (V_{pdh}), BHB is directly incorporated into the neuronal and astroglial TCA cycles while acetate is near exclusively incorporated into the glial TCA cycle. Neuronal glutamate (Glu) that is released via neurotransmission will be taken up by astroglial cells and converted by glutamine synthetase to glutamine at a rate proportional to the glutamate/glutamine cycle. The synthesis of glutamine is believed to be exclusively within astroglia and other glial cells. In addition to neurotransmitter cycling glutamine may be synthesized *de novo* starting with the PC reaction (V_{PC}). Glutamine synthesized via PC can replace neurotransmitter glutamate oxidized in the astrocyte or elsewhere (and be recycled back to the neuron) or leave the brain (V_{efflux}) to remove ammonia and maintain nitrogen balance (Cooper & Plum, 1987; Sibson et al., 2001; Mason et al., 2007). To measure the rates of these pathways ^{13}C-labeled substrates are used and the flow of ^{13}C isotope into glutamate and glutamine measured using ^{13}C MRS. (For detailed descriptions of how these pathways are tracked using ^{13}C MRS and isotopically labeled substrates and rates then calculated by metabolic modeling, see Mason et al., 1995, 2007; Gruetter et al., 2001; Lebon et al., 2002; Mason & Rothman, 2004; Shestov et al., 2007; Shen et al., 2008.)

studies in animal and cell models that have helped validate ^{13}C MRS measurements of neuroenergetics and neurotransmitter cycling as well as identify key questions to address in human research.

Glutamate Neurotransmitter Cycling is the Main Pathway of Cerebral Cortex Glutamine Synthesis

Although the metabolic pathways of glial glutamate uptake and the glutamate/glutamine cycle were well established from ^{14}C radiotracer and cellular studies, they were not considered relevant to whole-brain neuroenergetics prior to *in vivo* studies using MRS (Van den Berg et al., 1969; Hertz, 1979, 2007). Because the neurotransmitter glutamate was shown to be packaged in small vesicles, the predominant concept arose of a small, non-metabolic "transmitter" pool that did not interact with the large "metabolic" glutamate pool (Maycox et al., 1990; Nicholls & Attwell, 1990).

This concept was brought into question by one of the first ^{13}C MRS studies of human brain, which found a high rate of glutamine labeling from [1-^{13}C]glucose in the human occipital parietal lobe (Gruetter et al., 1994). At the time of the study it was unclear whether this high labeling was due to the glutamate/glutamine cycle or due to glutamine synthesis to remove ammonia from the brain, with the latter then believed to be its major role (Cooper & Plum, 1987). As pointed out by Sibson and coworkers in 1997, these pathways could be distinguished because glutamine that leaves the brain must be replaced by anaplerosis, which occurs in glial cells (Sibson et al., 1997). Furthermore, due to mass balance constraints the glutamine synthesized for this purpose must match the efflux of glutamine and uptake of ammonia and CO_2 by the brain as measured by arteriovenous (AV) difference (Sibson et al., 1997, 2001). To distinguish these possibilities glutamine synthesis was measured in rat cortex during hyperammonemia. When blood ammonia levels were extrapolated to a physiologically normal and low level, anaplerosis was

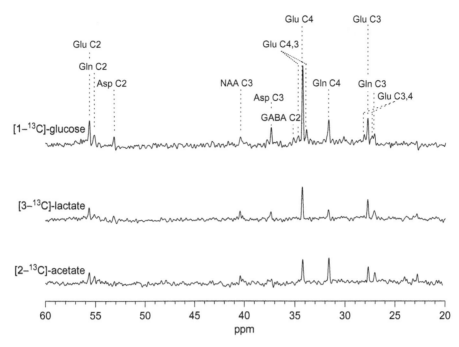

FIGURE 4.2.2　Localized ^{13}C MR spectra acquired at 4 T from the midline occipitoparietal lobe of a volunteer infused with ^{13}C-labeled glucose, lactate, or acetate. Upper spectrum: acquired during the last 18 min of a 2 h [1-^{13}C]glucose infusion. Middle spectrum: acquired during the last 18 min of a 2 h [3-^{13}C]lactate infusion ([Lac]$_{Plasma}$ ~1.5 mmol/L and ^{13}C-fractional enrichment, ~30%). Lower spectrum: acquired during the last 18 min of a 2 h [2-^{13}C]acetate infusion. Spectra are scaled to NAA C3 to exhibit the differences in ^{13}C-fractional enrichment reached for glutamate (Glu) and glutamine (Gln) and aspartate. The highest fractional enrichment is attained with glucose as label precursor. For glucose or lactate as precursor the majority of labeling appears in glutamate C4, consistent with the majority of brain metabolism of these substrates occurring in the neurons, which contain the majority of glutamate under normal conditions (Lebon et al., 2002). In contrast label from [2-^{13}C]acetate is highly enriched in glutamine C4, consistent with the localization of acetate metabolism in the astrocyte TCA cycle as shown in Fig. 4.2.1, resulting in preferential labeling of glutamine C4. Glu, glutamate; Gln, glutamine; Asp, aspartate; NAA, *N*-acetylaspartate; GABA, γ-aminobutyric acid.

found to account for approximately 20% of glutamine synthesis (Sibson et al., 1997). Measurements of anaplerotic glutamine synthesis using precursors that label this pathway directly, [2-^{13}C]glucose, ^{15}N ammonia, and ^{14}CO$_2$, have found that ~80% of glutamine synthesis is devoted to neurotransmitter cycling (Sibson et al., 1997; Shen et al., 1998; Lieth et al., 2001; Oz et al., 2004; Patel et al., 2005b). Analysis of ^{13}C-labeled extracellular glutamate measured by microdialysis and mass spectrometry has led to a similar conclusion that neurotransmitter cycling is the major source of glutamine (Kanamori et al., 2003). Similar conclusions have been obtained from studies performed in human brain using [1-^{13}C]glucose, [2-^{13}C]acetate, and [2-^{13}C]glucose as labeled substrates (Shen et al., 1999; Gruetter et al., 2001; Lebon et al., 2002; Mason et al., 2007).

The Glutamate/Glutamine Cycle is a Major Metabolic Pathway and is Directly Coupled to Neuroenergetics

To determine the relationship between the glutamate/glutamine cycle and cerebral cortex neuroenergetics,

^{13}C MRS was used to measure the relationship of neuronal glucose oxidation and the glutamate/glutamine cycle (V_{cyc}) in rat cerebral cortex (Siesjö, 1978). Cortical activity was modulated through anesthesia ranging from an isoelectric electroencephalogram (EEG) to higher EEG activity at two lower doses of anesthesia. With increasing electrical activity the rates of the glutamate/glutamine cycle and neuronal glucose oxidation via the TCA cycle (expressed as CMR$_{glc(ox)}$ in Sibson et al., 1998) increased linearly with a slope of 1.0 ± 0.1. Subsequent studies have confirmed this relationship (for review, see Hyder et al., 2006). Fig. 4.2.3 shows a plot of measurements in the rat cerebral cortex of the rate of the neuronal TCA cycle (V_{TCAn}) plotted versus the rate of the glutamate/glutamine cycle (V_{cyc}) taken from 11 published research articles at different levels of brain electrical activity ranging from isoelectricity to awake. As reported originally by Sibson and coworkers (1998) the relationship between V_{cyc} and $0.5*V_{TCAn}$ is linear with a slope 0.89. (We note that in Sibson et al. (1998) $0.5*V_{TCAn}$ was taken as equivalent to neuronal glucose oxidation, which will be the case under the hyperglycemic conditions of the study under which glucose is the only net fuel for neuronal oxidation (Siesjö, 1978)). Furthermore comparison of the

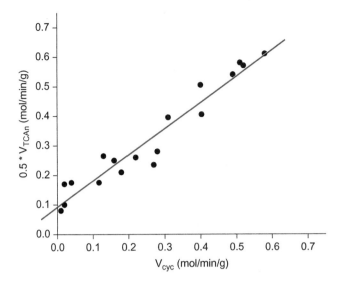

FIGURE 4.2.3 Approximately 1:1 relationship between the neuronal TCA cycle ($0.5*V_{TCAn}$) and the glutamate/glutamine cycle (V_{cyc}) with increasing electrical activity in the rat cerebral cortex. The plot shows the mean values of $0.5*V_{TCAn}$ (equivalent to $CMR_{glc(ox)N}$ in Sibson et al., 1998) plotted versus V_{cyc} reported from 11 published studies at activity levels ranging from awake to isoelectricity (Sibson et al., 1998; Choi et al., 2002; de Graaf et al., 2004; Oz et al., 2004; Patel et al., 2004, 2005b; Yang & Shen, 2005; Chowdhury et al., 2007; Serres et al., 2008; van Eijsden et al., 2010; Wang et al., 2010). Regression analysis yields a slope of 0.89 ($R^2 = 0.92$) and an intercept of $0.5*V_{TCAn}$ of 0.09 at isoelectricity ($V_{cyc} \sim 0$), values similar to those found in the original 1998 study by Sibson et al. (1998). In the case of reference (Serres et al., 2008) for both anesthetized and awake state, values of V_{TCAn} were calculated from the time constants reported for glutamate turnover during a glucose infusion. The ratio of glutamate to glutamine steady-state fractional enrichment during [2-^{13}C]acetate infusion was used to calculate V_{cyc} using the equation described in Lebon et al. (2002).

intercept at isoelectricity versus the values of V_{TCAn} and V_{cyc} in the awake state supports that over 80% of neuronal oxidative ATP production is coupled to neuronal signaling (as measured by V_{cyc}) even in the absence of stimulation. Thus the rate of V_{cyc} in the awake state is close to the rate of neuronal glucose oxidation and constitutes a major metabolic flux. As described later, recent ^{13}C MRS results from human cerebral cortex are consistent with this finding.

There are several molecular models that have been proposed to explain the near stoichiometric relation between changes in the flux of neuronal glucose oxidation and the glutamate/glutamine cycle. The relationship has been shown to be consistent with a model in which the energy for taking neurotransmitter glutamate up into the astrocyte is provided using glycolytic ATP production from glucose or glycogen (Magistretti et al., 1999; Shulman et al., 2001). Alternatively, it has been shown that the observed slope can be explained

based upon redox shuttling requirements between the neuronal cytosol and mitochondria in order to oxidize glutamine taken back up from the glial cells (Hertz et al., 2007). Determination of the actual molecular mechanism may have important implications for understanding brain disease since any dysfunction in this mechanism would severely impact the ability to sustain glutamate neurotransmission. In addition the measured coupling between neurotransmission and neuroenergetics has provided key data for detailed models of the energy budget of the brain for supporting signaling and information transfer (Attwell & Laughlin, 2001; Jolivet et al., 2009; Occhipinti et al., 2009; Strelnikov, 2010).

Validation of Measurements of Neurotransmitter Cycling and Anaplerosis Using Alternate Substrates and Labeling Strategies

The ability to measure bulk glutamate neurotransmission (via the glutmate/glutamine cycle) is unique to MRS. Because there is no gold standard to compare with, validation strategies have focused on the consistency of results using alternate labels and observation of the impact on pharmacological and physiological interventions that have been shown on an individual neuron level to increase or decrease neuronal glutamate release and electrical activity. A labeling strategy that has been used to validate the glutamate/glutamine cycle measurement is to use alternate ^{13}C- and ^{15}N-labeled substrates that are incorporated specifically in astrocytes. The subsequent flow of label from astrocyte glutamine (or other potential trafficking substrates) into neuronal glutamate then provides an independent measure of the rate of the glutamate/glutamine cycle from studies using [1-^{13}C]glucose, which labels the neuronal glutamate pool to a greater degree than the glial pool. Animal studies employing this strategy have used as label sources ^{15}N ammonia (Shen et al., 1999), [2-^{13}C]glucose (Sibson et al., 2001), ^{14}CO$_2$ (Lieth et al., 2001; Oz et al., 2004), and [2-^{13}C] acetate (Hassel et al., 1997; Patel et al., 2005a; Chowdhury et al., 2007; Serres et al., 2008; Patel et al., 2010) and found results consistent with a high rate of glutamate neurotransmitter trafficking. Similar results have been reported in studies of human subjects using [2-^{13}C]acetate (Lebon et al., 2002; Boumezbeur et al., 2010a) and [2-^{13}C]glucose as tracers (Mason et al., 2007). In addition analysis of ^{15}N labeling of glutamine obtained from extracellular fluid also supported the majority of glutamine derived from glutamate neurotransmitter cycling (Kanamori et al., 2003). The extracellular fluid measurement in principle is a more direct assessment of the pools relevant to neurotransmission than the whole-tissue MRS measurement.

In addition to the glutamate/glutamine cycle there are several other potential pathways of neurotransmitter repletion by the astrocytes including the glutamate/glutamine cycle and other cycles that use TCA cycle intermediates to return carbon to the neurons (Lebon et al., 2002; Maciejewski & Rothman, 2008). However, the agreement found between the rates determined for the glutamate/glutamine cycle measured by [1-^{13}C]glucose and the rates measured using glial-specific substrates (which take into account all cycling pathways) suggests that the glutamate/glutamine cycle is the major pathway under normal conditions in rodents and humans *in vivo* (Shen et al., 1998; Sibson et al., 2001; Lebon et al., 2002; Oz et al., 2004; Boumezbeur et al., 2010a).

Controversies Regarding the Relationship between Neuronal Energetics and the Glutamate/Glutamine Cycle

Despite the good agreement between findings by different investigators (see Fig. 4.2.3 and Table 4.2.1),

there has been considerable controversy regarding the relationship between the neuronal TCA cycle and the glutamate/glutamine cycle rate. The two major areas of debate have been the proposed molecular mechanism, and the slope of the relationship due to questions regarding the accuracy of measuring V_{TCAn} and V_{cyc} (Magistretti et al., 1999; Hertz et al., 2007; Jolivet et al., 2009; DiNuzzo et al., 2010). In the following sections the controversies over the accuracy of determining V_{TCAn} and V_{cyc} are discussed.

The Fraction of Glutamine Synthesis due to Anaplerosis via Pyruvate Carboxylase as Opposed to Neurotransmitter Cycling

As shown in Fig. 4.2.1, in addition to neurotransmitter cycling glutamine synthesis is used to replace glutamine that leaves the brain for ammonia detoxification and maintenance of nitrogen balance across the blood–brain barrier (Cooper & Plum, 1987; Sibson et al., 2001). Glutamine synthesis used to maintain nitrogen balance derives from anaplerosis via pyruvate carboxylase (PC), which under normal conditions appears to exclusively take place in astrocytes (and glial cells in general). The controversy regarding anaplerosis has largely been settled due to

TABLE 4.2.1   Experimental Mean and SD of V_{cyc}, V_{TCAn}, V_{TCAa}, V_{PC}, V_{cyc}/V_{gln}, and $V_{cyc}/0.5*V_{TCAn}$ in the Resting Awake Human Midline Occipital/Parietal Lobe from ^{13}C and ^{1}H-[^{13}C] MRS Studies

Reference	$V_{TCAtotal}$	V_{TCAn}	V_{TCAa}	V_{cyc}	V_{PC}	$V_{cyc}/0.5*V_{TCAn}$	V_{cyc}/V_{gln}
Mason et al., 1995[a]		0.73					
Gruetter et al., 1998a		0.74		0.32	0.08	0.86	0.80
Shen et al., 1999	0.77	0.71	0.06	0.32	0.04	0.90	0.95
Pan et al., 2000[b]		0.66					
Chen et al., 2001[a]		0.83					
Blüml et al., 2002	0.70		0.13				
Lebon et al., 2002			0.12*	0.28*		0.78	
Chhina et al., 2001		0.75		0.29			
Gruetter et al., 2001	0.63	0.57	0.06	0.17	0.09	0.60	0.65
Mason et al., 2007		0.72			0.02	0.73	0.93
Boumezbeur et al., 2010a	0.65	0.53	0.13	0.16		0.64	
Sailasuta et al., 2010a			0.09				
Henry et al., 2010[b]		0.79					
Mean ± SD	0.69 ± 0.06	0.70 ± 0.09	0.09 ± 0.04	0.26 ± 0.08	0.06 ± 0.03	0.75 ± 0.12	0.83 ± 0.14

Measured steady-state ratios converted to rates using the value of V_{TCAn} from Shen et al., 1999.
[a]*One-compartment model for the neuron used. We assume the derived TCA rate most closely reflects V_{TCAn}.*
[b]*Average of white and gray matter rates which were measured separately.*

As in the rat brain, the majority of human cortical glutamine synthesis is due to the glutamate/glutamine cycle as shown by the average value of V_{cyc}/V_{gln} of 0.83. Similarly the ratio of $V_{cyc}/0.5*V_{TCAn}$ of 0.75 is consistent with the coupling between V_{cyc} and V_{TCAn} measured in the rat cerebral cortex and indicates that the majority of neuronal energy production in the resting awake human brain is likely to be devoted to supporting neuronal activity. Based on the relative values of V_{TCAa} and V_{TCAn} and V_{PC}, ~20% of brain ATP production occurs in astrocytes.

a convergence of results in animal models (Lieth et al., 2001; Sibson et al., 2001; Kanamori et al., 2003; Oz et al., 2004; Hyder et al., 2006) and similar findings in human brain (Gruetter et al., 2001; Mason et al., 2007; see the section, *In vivo* ^{13}C MRS studies of human brain). There is now general consensus that in rat cerebral cortex a minimum of 80% of glutamine synthesis supports neurotransmitter cycling under normal conditions and between 70 and 90% in humans. Of the remaining 20% of glutamine synthesized by anaplerosis the majority is likely also used to replete neurotransmitter glutamate that is oxidized in the glial cells (see later) as opposed to ammonia detoxification although this still remains to be definitely established (Sibson et al., 2001; Mason et al., 2007).

The Effect of a Slow Rate of the Mitochondrial Glutamate Exchange, V_x, on Calculating Neuronal TCA Cycle Rate, V_{TCAn}

Another factor that may influence the measured relationship is the rate of exchange of label from mitochondrial α-ketoglutarate to cytosolic glutamate, often termed V_x in the literature. If this exchange is not much faster than the TCA cycle rate it may cause an underestimate of V_{TCAn} unless it is incorporated in the metabolic modeling through measurement of the C2 and/or C3 positions of glutamate (Gruetter et al., 2001; Shestov et al., 2007). Interestingly, it has been noted that independent of whether multiple glutamate positions were measured, very little difference has been found in the calculated rate of V_{TCAn} or V_{cyc} in studies of human brain (see Hyder et al., 2006). Based on numerical simulations it has been shown that the accuracy of measuring V_x in the brain using ^{13}C MRS is highly dependent on signal to noise and any internal label dilutions (Mason et al., 1995; Shestov et al., 2007), which most likely explains the extended controversy on this issue. Recently, Yang et al. (2009), using an elegant saturation transfer method, showed that V_x is at minimum several times greater than V_{TCAn} in the brain, explaining why it has not impacted measurements of rates of the neuronal TCA cycle. Despite the controversy it can be shown that if the C4 and C2/C3 positions of glutamate are measured, as is presently standard in the field, the values of V_{TCAn} and V_{cyc} calculated are relatively insensitive to the range of reported V_x values.

In addition to the consistency of results between different studies and labs the rates of V_{TCAn} measured in rat and human cerebral cortex are consistent with results previously published using ^{14}C-2-deoxyglucose autoradiography, AV difference, and PET (Hyder et al., 2006; Rothman et al., 2003). Recently two studies have directly compared PET measurements in non-human primates with ^{13}C MRS and found excellent

agreement between the total rate of glucose metabolism measured (Boumezbeur et al., 2005; Chaumeil et al., 2009).

Effects of Isotopic Dilution of Glutamine on the Calculated Rate of Neurotransmitter Cycling, V_{cyc}

Shestov and coworkers (2007) published the results of simulation studies in which they reported much poorer precision measuring the rate of the glutamate/glutamine cycle using a [1-^{13}C]glucose precursor than reported in experimental papers. Shen and coworkers (2008) were able to explain this discrepancy by showing that when isotopic dilution of glutamine was taken into account, as had been done in most previous experimental studies but not in the simulations by Shestov et al. (2007), the theoretical precision for the V_{cyc} measurement was similar to that reported experimentally. A similar conclusion regarding the importance of including the glutamine dilution in metabolic modeling was arrived at by Oz and coworkers (2004) when comparing rates calculated using [1-^{13}C]glucose and ^{14}C CO_2 as precursors. We note that when astrocyte specific labels such as [2-^{13}C]acetate are used to determine V_{cyc}, alone or in combination with [1-^{13}C]glucose, considerably higher precision for measuring V_{cyc} is obtained (Patel et al., 2005a; Boumezbeur et al., 2010a).

Oxidation of Neurotransmitter Glutamate

Glutamate released by neurons and taken up into astroglia can undergo oxidation as well as being converted to glutamine. The oxidized glutamate is then replaced by anaplerosis and cycled back to the neuron as glutamine (Hertz et al., 2007). This scenario of oxidation and replacement by anaplerosis must occur in order to maintain constant levels of TCA cycle intermediates and glutamate-derived neurotransmitters, since transport of necessary five-carbon precursors from the blood are comparatively minimal. The presence of glutamate oxidation has been argued as being in contradiction to the measured relationship between cycling and energetics (McKenna, 2007). However, contrary to these criticisms, it has been shown that presence of glutamate oxidation has no impact on the MRS measurement of the glutamate/glutamine cycle using a glial-specific labeled precursor such as [2-^{13}C]acetate because the oxidized glutamate is replaced by *de novo* glutamine synthesis, which is cycled back to the neuron (Sibson et al., 2001; Lebon et al., 2002; Mason et al., 2007). When [1-^{13}C]glucose is used as the precursor, replacement of oxidized glutamate will be included in the anaplerotic contribution to glutamine synthesis, unless it is distinguished from glutamine synthesis related to ammonia removal (detoxification) based on other measurements, and therefore will not impact the measurement of Vcyc.

IN VIVO ^{13}C MRS STUDIES OF HUMAN BRAIN

In the following sections we review results from ^{13}C and ^{1}H-[^{13}C] MRS studies of human brain, focusing primarily on studies that report metabolic rates or labeling. Following initial studies of the animal brain in the 1980s (Rothman et al., 1985; Behar et al., 1986; Fitzpatrick et al., 1990) the availability of high-field human MR systems and improvements in B$_0$ shimming (Gruetter, 1993) led to the first ^{13}C and ^{1}H-[^{13}C] MRS studies of humans (Beckmann et al., 1991; Gruetter et al., 1992, 1994; Rothman et al., 1992). While the use of ^{13}C MRS in humans has been relatively limited (see the section, Future prospects for ^{13}C MRS studies in humans), ^{13}C MRS has already made important contributions to understanding human brain energetics and neurotransmitter cycling and how alterations in these pathways may contribute to a range of human diseases.

^{13}C MRS Measurements of the Rate of the Neuronal and Astrocyte TCA Cycle and V$_{cyc}$ in Human Brain

Table 4.2.1 shows a compilation of studies from different groups measuring the rates of V$_{TCAn}$, V$_{TCAa}$, V$_{PC}$, and V$_{cyc}$ in the human midline occipital lobe. As illustrated there is very good agreement in the rates derived by different studies, with most of the difference explainable by different volume fractions of white matter (which has an approximately 3–4 times lower rate of V$_{TCAn}$ than gray matter; Mason et al., 1999; Pan et al., 2000). As discussed earlier the rates of V$_{TCAn}$ are similar whether the modeling used the C4, C3, and C2 positions of glutamate and glutamine or just the C4 positions. For the measurement of V$_{TCAa}$ there is good agreement between three independent label strategies using [1-^{13}C]glucose, [2-^{13}C]acetate, and ^{13}C bicarbonate as precursors. In the human studies the rate of the neuronal TCA cycle largely reflects glutamatergic neurons since it is derived from fitting the isotopic turnover of the large glutamate pool. Although the rate of the GABAergic neuron TCA cycle has not yet been determined, labeling of GABA during infusion of [1-^{13}C]glucose has been reported at 4 T (Gruetter et al., 1998a, 2001). Results in animal models suggest that on the order of 10% of cerebral cortex energy consumption may be due to GABAergic neurons (Patel et al., 2005b; van Eijsden et al., 2010).

The Relationship between Neuronal Energetics and the Glutamate/Glutamine Cycle in Human Brain and Implications for Resting Brain Functional Activity

^{13}C MRS studies by several groups have found a ratio of V$_{TCAn}$ to V$_{cyc}$ that is highly consistent with the relationship found in studies of rats. Table 4.2.1 shows the ratio of V$_{cyc}$/0.5*V$_{TCAn}$ derived in human studies (half the value of V$_{TCAn}$ is used to convert the units into the rate of glucose oxidation in the TCA cycle). The values range from 0.6 to 0.9 with an average of 0.75 ± 0.12. This average is similar to the value of V$_{cyc}$/0.5*V$_{TCAn}$ predicted from animal studies using the best fit of the relationship between V$_{cyc}$ and V$_{TCAn}$ in Fig. 4.2.2. The variation in the ratio measured in humans is largely due to variation in the measurement of V$_{PC}$. However, based upon AV measurements in humans the majority of V$_{PC}$ is for replacement of oxidized glutamate and therefore reflects glutamine synthesis that is cycled back to the neuron (Mason et al., 2007). Overall these studies show that functional neuronal activity is extremely high in the awake resting human brain and accounts for the majority of neuronal glucose consumption. Furthermore, the energy devoted to neuronal activity in the resting state is much higher than the changes in activity that occur during standard activation paradigms such as cognitive challenges and visual stimulation (Shulman & Rothman, 1998). These findings have contributed to the recent surge in interest in studying resting brain activity by functional MRI (fMRI) and other methods and form part of the basis of several theories of resting brain function (Shulman & Rothman, 1998; Raichle, 2009).

Measurements of the Rate of Glutamine Synthesis via PC in Human Cerebral Cortex

Due to the astrocyte localization of PC, anaplerosis occurs only in the glia and is used both to synthesize glutamine that leaves the brain to maintain nitrogen balance and to replace released neurotransmitter glutamate oxidized in the astrocytes. In order to address the question of what fraction of glutamine synthesis is due to the glutamate/glutamine cycle versus anaplerosis via PC, several studies in human brain have measured this rate. As shown in Table 4.2.1, based on these measurements the fraction of glutamine synthesis due to the glutamate/glutamine cycle (V$_{cyc}$/V$_{gln}$) has been reported to range between 0.65 and 0.93 in human cerebral cortex with a mean value of rate of 0.83 ± 0.14 (Shen et al., 1999; Gruetter et al., 2001; Mason et al., 2007). A complication in using [1-^{13}C] glucose precursor to measure this ratio is that the label enters the inner positions of glutamate both via pyruvate dehydrogenase and PC. To eliminate the complications arising from [1-¹³C]glucose as precursor, Mason and coworkers (2007) measured ¹³C incorporation into glutamate and glutamine in the midline occipital/parietal lobe of human volunteers from infused [2-¹³C]glucose, which labels the C2 and C3 positions of glutamine and glutamate primarily via PC. Labeling in glutamate C4 was used to assess the rate of pyruvate recycling coupled to glutamate oxidation. Metabolic modeling of the labeling data indicated that PC flux (V_{PC}) ranges from 6 to 10% of the rate of glutamine synthesis (0.02–0.03 μmol/g/min). Comparison of the measurements of V_{PC} in humans to date with AV difference measurements of human brain glutamine efflux suggests that the majority of the PC flux is used for replacing glutamate lost by oxidation in glia and possibly elsewhere, and therefore can be considered to support neurotransmitter cycling (Mason et al., 2007). However, the direct demonstration of glutamate oxidation in the human brain remains to be performed.

Studies of Substrate Oxidation and Transport

Because of its ability to distinguish a substrate from its metabolic products ¹³C MRS can be used to independently assess the rate of transport of a substrate and the rate of its metabolism. Furthermore, it can be uniquely used to determine cell type-specific metabolism. Glucose has long been known to be the primary fuel for brain metabolism (Siesjö, 1978). However, the brain can also consume alternate substrates including acetate, BHB, lactate, and fatty acids. BHB is a particularly important substrate during development and under conditions of fasting where AV difference methods have revealed its capacity to supply 40–60% of the fuel oxidized by the brain (Owen et al., 1967). Similar high rates of utilization of lactate has been reported under conditions of elevated plasma lactate, such as during exercise (Smith et al., 2003; van Hall et al., 2009). Although total usage and oxidation of these substrates have been determined for humans by AV difference methods, and to some extent by PET, the ¹³C MRS studies reviewed next have provided the first information on the cell-type specificity of substrate usage, as well as revealing new insights into blood-to-brain transport of these substrates.

Glucose

Due to the commercial availability of [1-¹³C]glucose, and the high rate of brain glucose metabolism, the majority of metabolic ¹³C MRS studies have been focused on the measurement of neuronal and glial glucose metabolism (see the section, ¹³C MRS measurements of the rate of the neuronal and astrocyte TCA cycle and V_{cyc} in human brain). ¹³C MRS has been used to measure glucose transport parameters (K_T and T_{max}) in the human midline occipital/parietal lobe (Gruetter et al., 1992). Subsequent studies of brain glucose transport in humans have used ¹H MRS for higher sensitivity. These studies have provided support for the blood–brain barrier to be the rate-limiting step for human brain glucose transport (Gruetter et al., 1996), which is best described by a reversible, Michaelis–Menten transport model (as opposed to the nonreversible model used previously to interpret most PET glucose studies; Heiss et al., 1984; Blomqvist et al., 1991; Gruetter et al., 1998b; de Graaf et al., 2001). In this model glucose transport is described by transporters with reversible Michaelis–Menten kinetics across the membranes of the capillary endothelial cells that make up the blood–brain barrier (Gruetter, et al. 1998b; de Graaf et al., 2001). Based on *in vivo* kinetic and isolated transporter studies the glial and neuronal glucose transporters have a relatively much higher activity and can to a first order be neglected in the kinetic modeling. These results have been used to develop and test kinetic models of glucose transport and metabolism (Simpson et al., 2007), and may have potential value for assessing whether impaired substrate delivery may impact brain function in disease (Simpson et al., 2007).

Acetate

Studies in animal models and neural cell culture have found that acetate is almost exclusively transported into and metabolized by the astroglia (Künnecke & Cerdan, 1989; Badar-Goffer et al., 1990; Cerdán et al., 1990; Hassel et al., 1997; Waniewski & Martin, 1998). Lebon and coworkers (2002) studied healthy human subjects infused intravenously with [2-¹³C]acetate while monitoring ¹³C labeling in the midline occipital/parietal lobe with ¹³C MRS. The concentration of brain acetate was ~10-fold lower than the plasma concentration indicating that acetate transport was primarily unidirectional. Analysis of the steady-state ¹³C-labeling pattern of glutamine and glutamate, as shown in Fig. 4.2.2, as well as the kinetics of glutamate and glutamine labeling, were consistent with acetate metabolism localized to glial cells (Lebon et al., 2002). Furthermore the steady-state labeling patterns were in agreement with findings from [1-¹³C]glucose of a high rate of glutamate/glutamine cycling (Lebon et al., 2002; Boumezbeur et al., 2010a). Similar conclusions were obtained by Blüml et al. (2002) using [1-¹³C]acetate as a precursor. Although normal plasma levels of acetate in humans are relatively low, the levels can be elevated to ~1 mM or more by alcohol consumption, becoming a major source of oxidative energy for the astrocyte (Blüml et al., 2002; Lebon et al., 2002; Mason et al., 2006; Boumezbeur et al., 2010a). Acetate may be considered to be the shortest chain fatty acid and the ability of the astrocytes to oxidize acetate may reflect a high capacity for fatty acid oxidation in general. Evidence for this possibility is the substantial dilution of glutamine labeling relative to glutamate labeling when a labeled glucose precursor is used in animal models and humans (Shen et al., 2008).

BHB

BHB is a substrate critical for brain function during fasting. BHB enters the brain via facilitated diffusion using a monocarboxylate carrier at the blood–brain barrier (Simpson et al., 2007). Although brain BHB consumption had been studied extensively using AV difference methods, it was not known whether BHB was preferentially consumed in neurons or astrocytes, or whether the blood–brain barrier was limiting for its metabolism (Siesjö, 1978). To answer these questions localized ^{13}C MRS measurements were performed during an infusion of [2,4-^{13}C]BHB in healthy subjects and the entry and metabolism of BHB was measured in the medial occipital/parietal cortex (Pan et al., 2002). During the 2 h infusion study, ^{13}C label was detected in the BHB resonance positions at a time resolution of 5 min and in the amino acid pools of glutamate, glutamine, and aspartate. The pattern of the ^{13}C labeling at the steady-state period (0–120 min) was very different from that resulting from infusions of ^{13}C acetate, but was broadly similar to that of [1-^{13}C]glucose, indicating a predominant neuronal consumption of this substrate. The cortical BHB concentration (0.18 mM) was much lower than in plasma (2 mM), indicating that transport across the blood–brain barrier limits brain BHB metabolism. Consumption of BHB accounted for ~6 % of total brain oxidative metabolism in nonfasted volunteers, consistent with earlier reports using AV difference methods (Siesjö, 1978). The study demonstrated that ^{13}C MRS has the potential to study BHB usage under clinical conditions (for example, the ketogenic diet used in childhood epilepsy) and to answer basic questions regarding its importance in brain development and fasting.

Lactate

Studies over the last decade have provided evidence that lactate may be an important metabolic fuel for the brain, including proposals that an astrocyte-to-neuron lactate shuttle may exist in order to provide neurons with fuel during periods of enhanced activity (Magistretti et al., 1999; Jolivet et al., 2009). In addition AV difference and PET studies of humans after blood

lactate elevation by exercise have reported that when elevated lactate can provide a significant fraction of oxidative fuel to the brain (Smith et al., 2003; van Hall et al., 2009). To determine the conditions under which plasma lactate might contribute as a significant fuel for human brain energy metabolism, Boumezbeur and coworkers (2010b) infused [3-^{13}C]lactate and measured by ^{13}C MRS the entry and utilization of lactate in the midline occipital/parietal cortex of healthy human volunteers. During the 2 h infusion study, ^{13}C incorporation in the amino acid pools of glutamate and glutamine were measured every 5 min. With a plasma concentration of lactate ([Lac]$_P$) in the 0.8–2.8 mmolL^{-1} range, the brain tissue lactate concentration ([Lac]$_B$) was assessed as well as the fractional contribution of lactate to brain energy metabolism (CMR$_{lac}$). By fitting the measured relationship between unidirectional lactate influx (V$_{in}$) and plasma and brain lactate concentrations, the lactate transport constants were calculated using a model in which the rate-limiting step was assumed to be based on previous work lactate transport at the blood–brain barrier. The transporters at the blood–brain barrier were modeled as reversible Michaelis–Menten transporters similar to what has been done with glucose transport. The results showed that in the physiological range of plasma lactate concentration, the unidirectional rate of transport and concentration of brain lactate rose linearly with plasma concentration. The maximum potential contribution of plasma lactate to brain metabolism was 10% for basal plasma lactate concentration of ~1.0 mM, and possibly as much as 60% at supraphysiological plasma lactate concentrations when the transporters are saturated (assuming lactate oxidation is limited only by transport). Based on the similarity of the steady-state pattern of ^{13}C labeling, as shown in Fig. 4.2.2, it was concluded that the relative consumption of plasma lactate between neurons and astrocytes is similar to that of glucose (Boumezbeur et al., 2010b). The calculation of the lactate metabolic capacity is in good agreement with recent AV difference studies using isotopically labeled lactate as a tracer, further confirming the potential importance of plasma lactate as a substrate for brain metabolism (van Hall et al., 2009).

Use of ^{1}H-[^{13}C] MRS to Study the Energetics of Brain Tissue Types (White/Gray Matter) and Sensory Stimulation

As described in the section, Future prospects for ^{13}C MRS studies in humans, the sensitivity and spatial resolution limitations of ^{13}C MRS can be partially overcome by using the more sensitive ^{1}H nucleus to measure the ^{13}C enrichment of bound carbon atoms.

These inverse MRS methods take advantage of the J-coupling between ^{1}H and ^{13}C nuclei (Rothman et al., 1985; de Graaf et al., 2011). By combining ^{1}H-[^{13}]C MRS with spectroscopic imaging and gray/white matter segmentation Pan and coworkers (2000) reported the rates of V_{TCAn} in gray and white matter finding a $\sim$4 times higher rate of metabolism in gray matter. The higher resolution of ^{1}H-[^{13}]C MRS has been used to address the question of whether glycolytic or oxidative ATP production provides most of the incremental energy for brain function during activation (Fox et al., 1988; Prichard et al., 1991; Dienel & Hertz, 2001; Hyder et al., 2006; Mangia et al., 2007). Using this technique Chen and coworkers (2001) reported a 25% increase in V_{TCAn} during visual stimulation. This finding is consistent with recent calibrated fMRI measurements of $CMRO_2$ (Marrett & Gjedde, 1997; Hoge et al., 1999; Kim et al., 1999), and indicates that ATP produced oxidatively is the major source of energy for the incremental neuronal activity during sensory stimulation.

Application of ^{13}C MRS to Study Neuroenergetics and Neurotransmission in Human Brain Disease

The important role of neuroenergetics, and the glutamate/GABA neurotransmitter cycles, in the pathogenesis of brain disease is being increasingly recognized. Changes in the concentrations of GABA, glutamate, and glutamine have been measured by ^{1}H MRS in a wide range of neurological and psychiatric diseases including aging (Haga et al., 2009), depression and related disorders (Goddard et al., 2001; Epperson et al., 2002; Gruber et al., 2003; Dager et al., 2004; Sanacora et al., 2004; Hasler et al., 2007), epilepsy (Novotny et al., 1999; Petroff et al., 2000; Kuzniecky et al., 2002), genetic disorders of metabolism (Novotny et al., 2003), hepatic encephalopathy (Ross et al., 1994), and neurodegenerative disorders (Martin, 2007). However, concentration measurements while informative are not specific for the alterations in metabolic fluxes or cellular neurochemical distributions responsible for the change. The measurement of metabolic rates in human by ^{13}C MRS may potentially be of great value in studying the pathogenesis and treatment of brain disease. However, its application to disease has been limited by several factors, including the technical complexity of conducting ^{13}C MRS experiments, which is exacerbated by the lack of such study support with most clinical scanners. Furthermore there is the need for a support team to perform the infusion and analysis of substrates labeled with ^{13}C isotope, the relatively low sensitivity and volume resolution of ^{13}C MRS compared with ^{1}H MRS (and especially MRI),

availability and cost of ^{13}C-labeled substrates, radiofrequency (RF) heating concerns due to the need to decouple the J-interaction of ^{13}C resonances with bound protons, and the need to perform sophisticated kinetic analysis to extract metabolic rate information from the MRS data (see Ross et al., 2003 for an informative review on clinical ^{13}C MRS studies in humans and the obstacles in performing them). In the section, Future prospects for ^{13}C MRS studies in humans, we speculate on how some of these barriers may be lowered through a range of developments, including hyperpolarized ^{13}C. Despite these challenges the initial applications of ^{13}C MRS in studies of human brain disease and dysfunction have been highly informative, which are briefly reviewed in the following sections.

Application of ^{13}C MRS to Study Stroke and Tumors

The initial application of ^{13}C MRS to clinical brain disease was to assess the source of chronic lactate elevation in stroke. In this study ^{1}H MRS was used to measure lactate ^{13}C fractional enrichment in an infarct during infusion of [1-^{13}C]glucose. ^{1}H MRS was used due to its severalfold higher sensitivity for measuring ^{13}C enrichment than direct ^{13}C MRS (Novotny et al., 1990). The lactate was found to rapidly incorporate label from glucose indicating active metabolic production even long after the initial infarct event (Rothman et al., 1991). Subsequent ^{1}H MRS and histological assessment indicated that most of the lactate elevation in chronic stroke was likely to be due to macrophage metabolic activity and infiltration (Petroff et al., 1992). A similar strategy was used in animal models of brain cancer by Terpstra and coworkers (1998) to assess the metabolic source of lactate in tumors. Recently ^{13}C MRS was used to measure lactate turnover in a human brain tumor (Wijnen et al., 2010).

Application of ^{13}C MRS to Study Hepatic Encephalopathy and Genetic Diseases of Ammonia Metabolism

Studies by Ross and coworkers (Butterworth, 1993; Behar et al., 1999; Kanamori et al., 2003; Ross et al., 2003) have established ^{1}H MRS measurements of glutamine and glutamate as one of the best ways to assess the severity of hepatic encephalopathy, a disease of the brain that is caused by chronic exposure to elevated ammonia in the blood due to liver failure. Animal studies using conventional methods, as well as ^{13}C and ^{15}N MRS, showed that ammonia led to increased anaplerosis and glutamine synthesis in astrocytes, as well as disruption of the glutamate/glutamine cycle (Cooper & Plum, 1987; Behar & Fitzpatrick, 1989; Fitzpatrick et al., 1989a,b; Kanamori & Ross, 1997; Shen et al., 1999; Sibson et al., 2001). To test whether similar metabolic alterations were present in humans Blüml and cowor-kers (2001b) studied patients with diagnosed hepatic encephalopathy during infusion of [1-^{13}C] glucose at 1.5 T. The studies found disrupted neuroenergetics with increasing disease severity, including evidence for impairment in the glutamate/glutamine cycle. More recently Gropman and coworkers (2009) have used ^{13}C MRS to demonstrate abnormalities in glutamate metab-olism in patients with ornithine transcarbamylase deficiency.

Application of ^{13}C MRS to Study Alzheimer's Disease and Healthy Aging

Mitochondrial dysfunction has been implicated in the loss of brain function in neurodegenerative disease and normal aging (Lin & Beal, 2006). Studies using PET have found decreased rates of brain oxygen con-sumption and glucose consumption in Alzheimer's disease and in healthy aging (Rapoport, 1999; Kalpouzos et al., 2009). In a pioneering study on Alzheimer's disease, Ross and coworkers infused two patients with [1-^{13}C]glucose and found a reduction in ^{13}C labeling of C4 glutamate, consistent with an impairment in the TCA cycle (Lin et al., 2003). Recently, Boumezbeur and coworkers (2010a), using combined infusions of [1-^{13}C]glucose and [2-^{13}C]ace-tate with ^{13}C MRS, compared occipital lobe metabolic rates in a healthy group of elderly subjects with young adult controls. The elderly subjects showed decreased rates of the neuronal TCA cycle (V$_{TCAn}$) and gluta-mate/glutamine cycle along with an increased rate of the astroglial TCA cycle, changes that were indepen-dent of the relatively small age-dependent loss of brain tissue volume in the occipital lobe. The decrease in the neuronal TCA cycle rate correlated highly with decreases in N-acetylaspartate (NAA) and glutamate concentrations (Fig. 4.2.4) indicating that the reduced metabolic rates were associated with cellular level changes as opposed to differences in sensory input or subject wakefulness during the study. These findings are consistent with the theory that mitochondria lose oxidative capacity with advancing age leading to loss of brain function. Overall, the ability to study aging and associated dementias with ^{13}C MRS provides a unique opportunity to study the role of mitochondria in the pathogenesis process and how this process can be slowed or ceased through treatment.

Application of ^{13}C MRS to Study Hypoglycemic Unawareness in Type 1 Diabetes

A major complication in insulin therapy for type 1 dia-betes is hypoglycemia, the frequency of which is wors-ened due to the phenomenon of hypoglycemic unawareness (Cryer, 1994, 2004). Among the theories to explain this phenomenon is that repeated hypoglycemic

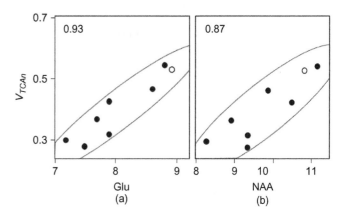

FIGURE 4.2.4 Comparison of V$_{TCAn}$ versus glutamate and NAA concentrations in the midline occipitoparietal lobe of healthy elderly subjects. The results show a strong correlation between the rate of the neuronal TCA cycle and the concentrations of glutamate (Glu) and NAA, both of which have been associated with cellular dysfunc-tion and chronically reduced mitochondrial activity in other studies. Pearson correlation coefficients appear in upper left corners (a, 0.93 and b, 0.87). Closed circles, values measured for the individual elderly subjects (n = 7); open circles, average values for the respective metabolite concentrations from a young cohort (n = 7). Fluxes and metabolite concentrations are expressed as μmol.g^{-1}min^{-1} and μmolg^{-1}, respectively.

episodes in type 1 diabetics may lead to metabolic adap-tations that allow improved function during periods of mild hypoglycemia. Using [2-^{13}C]acetate as a tracer, Mason and coworkers (2006) tested the hypothesis that patients with type 1 diabetes have upregulated blood-to-brain transport and metabolism of monocarboxylic acids (e.g., acetate, BHB, and lactate), supporting heightened brain function during hypoglycemia. In their study of the medial occipital/parietal cortex, type 1 diabetics showed increased metabolism of acetate, which was secondary to increased acetate transport. An example of the higher ^{13}C labeling attained in the patients with type 1 diabetes is shown in Fig. 4.2.5. At a blood concentration of 1 mM acetate was found to provide on average ~20% of astro-cyte oxidative needs in control subjects and ~35% in patients with type 1 diabetes, which would theoretically be sufficient to compensate for the decrease in glucose transport anticipated under moderate hypoglycemia.

In addition to studying alternate substrate use ^{13}C MRS has been used to study metabolism of glucose and glycogen in type 1 diabetes under normal and hypoglycemic conditions. Oz and coworkers (2004) used ^{13}C MRS to show that brain glycogen may be a significant fuel source during hypoglycemia and that hypoglycemia led to elevated glycogen synthesis upon restoration of normal glucose levels (119). Very recently Van de Ven and coworkers (2013) directly looked at glucose metabolism in patients with type 1 diabetes under hypoglycemic conditions using ^{13}C MRS.

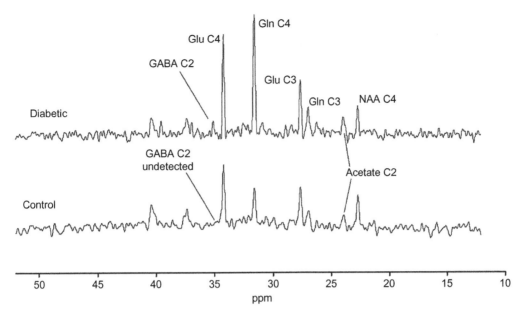

FIGURE 4.2.5 Comparison of steady-state ^{13}C MRS spectra during [2-^{13}C]acetate infusion from a type 1 diabetic with a healthy control subject. Brain ^{13}C MRS spectra were averaged over the final 45 min of a hypoglycemic period during infusion of [2-^{13}C]acetate. The diabetic subject (top spectrum) had significantly greater labeling in glutamate (Glu) and glutamine (Gln) C4 than the control (bottom spectrum). The acetate C2 signal was also greater in the diabetic subject. Other resonances labeled in the figure include NAA C4, GABA C2, and Glu C3.

They found that glucose metabolism in patients with type 1 diabetes was minimally impacted by hypoglycemia while subjects without diabetes showed a significant decrease in glucose metabolism. The combination of increased alternate fuel consumption capacity and resistance of glucose metabolism to downregulation may explain why patients with type 1 diabetes and frequent hypoglycemia are often unaware of being mild to moderately hypoglycemic.

Application of ^{13}C MRS to Study Epilepsy

Epilepsy has been studied extensively by ^{1}H MRS and there is considerable evidence from PET, ^{1}H MRS, and ^{31}P MRS of hypometabolism in brain regions affected by epilepsy that may be secondary to a failure in neuroenergetics (Pan et al., 2008). Furthermore, in medial temporal lobe epilepsy chronically elevated extracellular glutamate has been found by microdialysis in epileptogenic sclerotic tissue, possibly contributing to the hyperexcited state of the tissue (Cavus et al., 2005). In order to test whether the chronically elevated extracellular glutamate was due to an impairment in glial glutamate uptake and cycling, Petroff and coworkers (2002) obtained neurosurgical specimens from patients intravenously infused with [2-^{13}C]glucose and analyzed the labeling *ex vivo* using high-resolution ^{13}C MRS. In the epileptogenic tissue from the hippocampus with sclerosis and glial proliferation there was marked impairment in glutamate/glutamine cycling compared with more histologically normal tissue (Petroff et al., 2002). A subsequent study showed that this impairment in glutamate/glutamine cycling may be secondary to reduced activity in glutamine synthetase establishing this step in the pathophysiology as a potential therapeutic target (Eid et al., 2004).

Application of ^{13}C MRS to Study Pediatric Disease

The increasing concerns over radiation dosage in PET scans of pediatric patients have provided additional motivation for noninvasive application of ^{13}C MRS with this vulnerable group. Studies of infants and young children with ^{13}C MRS, however, are complicated by the need for extended infusion times increasing the time spent in the magnet. To assess the feasibility of pediatric studies Blüml and colleagues (2001a) performed ^{13}C MRS on 17 children and pediatric patients receiving [1-^{13}C]glucose either orally or intravenously. They observed marked differences in ^{13}C-labeling patterns in premature brain and pediatric patients with leukodystrophies and mitochondrial disorders. This study demonstrated the significant potential of ^{13}C MRS applications to pediatric disease, particularly with the improvements in sensitivity discussed in the following section.

FUTURE PROSPECTS FOR ^{13}C MRS STUDIES IN HUMANS

As discussed in the previous section, there are several major challenges that must be met for ^{13}C MRS to become a routine tool in the study of human brain disease and treatment. Next, we briefly discuss these limitations and how they may be overcome through future technological developments.

Improvements in the Sensitivity and Spatial Resolution of the ^{13}C MRS Measurement

The primary limitation for the study of human brain disease by ^{13}C MRS is its low sensitivity, with typical volume resolution on the order of 25–100 cm^3. Substantial improvements have been achieved by detecting ^{13}C labeling indirectly via the J-scalar coupling to bound protons (Rothman et al., 1991, 1992), enhancing spatial resolution to several cm^3 obtained at 4 T (Pan et al., 2000; Chen et al., 2001). However, due to the limited spectral resolution of ^{1}H MRS only labeling of glutamate C4, the combined resonances of glutamate and glutamine C3 and lactate C3 have been reported, limiting the rates that can be measured to the neuronal TCA cycle, or in cases of elevated lactate to glycolysis. With the advent of ultrahigh field human MRS systems (7 T and above), in principle it should be possible to measure resonances of glutamine and GABA, as has been demonstrated in animal studies (Pfeuffer et al., 1999; de Graaf et al., 2004; van Eijsden et al., 2010), although increased heating associated with decoupling at higher fields may limit this application.

An alternate possibility, which would retain the high spectral resolution and information of direct ^{13}C MRS and provide much higher spatial resolution, is the use of hyperpolarized ^{13}C MRS, which is covered in detail in Chapter 4.3. There are also several promising initial reports in animal models (Bhattacharya et al., 2007; Cudalbu et al., 2010; Marjańska et al., 2010). Hyperpolarized ^{13}C MRS obtains fractions of spin polarization on the order of 10,000 or more times greater than equilibrium values by prepolarizing a ^{13}C-containing compound at very low temperature. When the compound is removed and dissolved in the aqueous vehicle to be injected it rapidly loses its excess polarization with a characteristic time constant of T_1. The two major limitations for using hyperpolarized ^{13}C MRS for studying brain metabolism are the slow rate of substrate transport into the brain, which limits the rate of label entry, and several enzymatic steps between the substrates that can be labeled (e.g., acetate, lactate, glucose) and the compounds of interest such as glutamate, glutamine, and GABA. For example, to measure the rate of the glutamate/glutamine cycle from hyperpolarized ^{13}C acetate the acetate must first be transported into the glial cells, then converted successively to acetyl-CoA, citrate, isocitrate,

α-ketoglutarate, and glutamate before being converted by glutamine synthetase into glutamine. Based on the concentration of the precursor pools and metabolic rate of acetate metabolism, it would take on the order of 1–2 min for the immediate precursor glial glutamate to be labeled sufficiently to measure the glutamine synthesis rate, during which time there will be significant loss of hyperpolarized magnetization due to T_1 relaxation. These issues and possible solutions are discussed in more detail in Chapter 4.3. Measurement of the glial and neuronal TCA cycle and anaplerosis may be feasible by directly looking at TCA cycle intermediates (e.g., citrate) from precursors such as [2-^{13}C] acetate and [2-^{13}C]lactate, which label TCA cycle intermediates in one or two enzymatic steps. An alternate approach is to directly hyperpolarize TCA cycle intermediates themselves, the feasibility of which has been demonstrated in extracts (Bhattacharya et al., 2007).

Improvements in Shimming and Reduction of RF Heating to Allow Multivolume ^{13}C MRS

To date the majority of human brain ^{13}C MRS studies have been performed in the midline occipital or occipital/parietal lobe, due largely to the relative ease of shimming to improve B_0 homogeneity in this region and the distance from the eyes, which are believed to be more sensitive than the brain to heating from the decoupling B_1 field. Over the last decade limitations due to shimming have been greatly reduced based on improvements in shim coil strengths and advanced field mapping and shim calculation and updating methods, allowing well-shimmed spectra to be obtained from multiple volumes within the human brain even at ultrahigh fields (Gruetter, 1993; Hetherington et al., 2006; Koch et al., 2007; Juchem et al., 2010).

A continuing limitation is heating that results from the applied RF energy to the protons bound to ^{13}C needed to decouple the J-interaction. It has been shown that there are theoretical limits on the minimum decoupling power (de Graaf, 2005), which even at 4 T are close to the allowable power deposition limits mandated by the United States Food and Drug Administration (FDA; Collins et al., 2004). Although advances in RF coil design allow human brain ^{13}C studies to be performed safely even up to 4 T (Adriany & Gruetter, 1997; Klomp et al., 2006), concerns remain about RF heating of the eyes, which may be more vulnerable than the brain due to areas of restricted circulation. A recently developed alternate approach to circumvent the RF heating is to observe ^{13}C labeling of the carboxyl groups of glutamate and glutamine that require no (or low-power) decoupling (Li et al., 2007; Sailasuta et al., 2010a). This approach takes advantage of the turnover kinetics of glutamate (Glu) C5 from exogenous [2-^{13}C]glucose, which is identical to the turnover of Glu C4 from exogenous [1-^{13}C]glucose (Li et al., 2009). The carboxylic carbons are only coupled to protons via very weak long-range ^{1}H-[^{13}C] scalar couplings so that they can be effectively decoupled at low RF power. An additional advantage of this strategy is the lack of contamination from subcutaneous lipids because there are no overlapping fat signals in the vicinity of the glutamate C5 and glutamine C5 peaks. An example showing the feasibility of this strategy at 3 T is the work of (Li et al. 2009; Fig. 4.2.6). High-quality spectra can be obtained with a maximum regional power deposition in the brain below 2 W/kg, several times below the FDA limit, even using a ^{1}H resonator to deliver the RF decoupling field (Li et al., 2010). The ability to deliver RF decoupling from a volume coil further opens up the possibility of multivolume whole brain ^{13}C MRS.

An alternate approach to reduce RF heating would be to use hyperpolarized ^{13}C MRS without decoupling. The higher sensitivity of hyperpolarized ^{13}C would, in principle, make decoupling unnecessary. However, due to the blood−brain barrier restricting the ability to isotopically label brain metabolites from plasma, ^{13}C-labeled substrates decoupling may be necessary even for hyperpolarized ^{13}C MRS applications.

Improvements in ^{13}C Infusion Protocols

A third major limitation in ^{13}C MRS studies is the requirement for a continuous infusion of the isotopically labeled substrate with venous sampling for fractional enrichment determination. This infusion must occur over a time period (typically 2 h) to capture sufficient kinetic information from spectral time courses for absolute rate estimation using metabolic modeling (Mason et al., 1995; Gruetter et al., 2001; Mason & Rothman, 2004). However several studies have shown it is possible to obtain considerable information on metabolism using simplified infusion schemes or oral ingestion (Moreno et al., 2001; Mason et al., 2003; van de Ven et al., 2010; Sailasuta et al., 2010b). Given that the majority of information on absolute and relative rates is derived from the early and steady-state portions of the time course, a significant reduction in the time required for a subject to be in the scanner may be possible (Mason & Rothman, 2004).

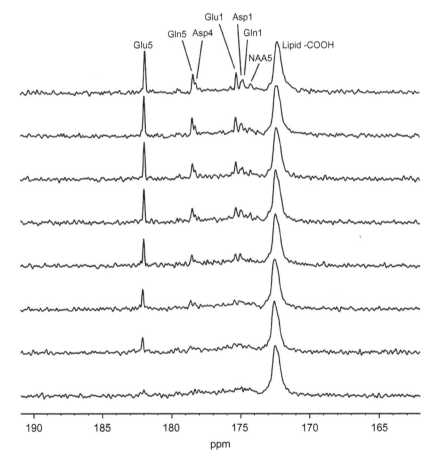

FIGURE 4.2.6 ^{13}C MRS time course spectra of glutamate, glutamine, and aspartate turnover detected in the occipital lobe during intravenous infusion of [2-^{13}C]glucose. Lorentz−Gauss transformation (LB = 3 Hz, GB = −0.3) was applied. The time-averaged decoupling power was 1.46 W. Each spectrum corresponds to 8.5 min of signal averaging (128 scans). Glu C5 (182.0 ppm) and C1 (175.4 ppm), Gln C5 (178.5 ppm) and C1 (174.9 ppm), Asp C4 (178.3 ppm) and C1 (175.0 ppm), as well as NAA C5 (174.3 ppm) were detected. No baseline corrections were made. Glu, glutamate; Gln, glutamine; Asp, aspartate; NAA, N-acetylaspartate.

SUMMARY AND CONCLUSIONS

Work over the past two decades has established ^{13}C MRS studies of the brain in animal models and humans as the only noninvasive method for measuring neuronal and glial energy metabolism and glutamate and GABA neurotransmitter cycling. Although some debates regarding metabolic modeling remain, much of our present knowledge of the brain energy budget (glutamatergic neurons, GABAergic neurons, astrocytes) and the relationship between neuroenergetics and neurotransmission has been obtained from *in vivo* ^{13}C MRS studies. ^{13}C MRS studies have also played an important role in delineating how alternate substrates such as acetate, ketone bodies, and lactate support neuronal and astrocyte energetics. The application of ^{13}C MRS to study human disease faces considerable obstacles, particularly cost, the need for ^{13}C substrate infusions and monitoring, decoupling heating, and the low sensitivity of ^{13}C MRS and lack of technical capability of most MR systems. Despite these difficulties, ^{13}C MRS has been successfully applied to study a variety of neurological and psychiatric diseases as well as diabetes and healthy aging. The increasing availability of high-field MR magnets, which allow higher sensitivity indirect detection methods, and the development of hyperpolarized ^{13}C have the potential of greatly increasing the sensitivity of the method leading to the possibility of using ^{13}C MRS for metabolic imaging of the human brain. These technological developments, along with further improvements in ^{13}C infusion protocols to minimize patient time in the magnet, have the potential of greatly expediting clinical and research studies.

References

Adriany, G., & Gruetter, R. (1997). A half-volume coil for efficient proton decoupling in humans at 4 tesla. *Journal of Magnetic Resonance, 125*(1), 178–184.

Attwell, D., & Laughlin, S. B. (2001). An energy budget for signaling in the grey matter of the brain. *Journal of Cerebral Blood Flow and Metabolism, 21*(10), 1133–1145.

Badar-Goffer, R. S., Bachelard, H. S., & Morris, P. G. (1990). Cerebral metabolism of acetate and glucose studied by 13C-n.m.r. spectroscopy. A technique for investigating metabolic compartmentation in the brain. *Biochemical Journal, 266*(1), 133–139.

Beckmann, N., Turkalj, I., Seelig, J., & Keller, U. (1991). 13C NMR for the assessment of human brain glucose metabolism in vivo. *Biochemistry, 30*(26), 6362–6366.

Behar, K. L., & Fitzpatrick, S. M. (1989). Effects of hypercarbia and porta-caval shunting on amino acids and high energy phosphates of the rat brain: a 1H and 31P NMR study. In R. F. Butterworth, & G. P. Layrargues (Eds.), *Hepatic Encephalopathy* (Vol. 22, pp. 189–200). New York: Humana Press.

Behar, K. L., Petroff, O. A., Prichard, J. W., Alger, J. R., & Shulman, R. G. (1986). Detection of metabolites in rabbit brain by 13C NMR spectroscopy following administration of [1-13C]glucose. *Magnetic Resonance In Medicine, 3*(6), 911–920.

Behar, K. L., Rothman, D. L., Petersen, K. F., Hooten, M., Delaney, R., Petroff, O. A., et al. (1999). Preliminary evidence of low cortical GABA levels in localized ^{1}H-MR spectra of alcohol-dependent and hepatic encephalopathy patients. *American Journal of Psychiatry, 156*(6), 952–954.

Bergles, D. E., Diamond, J. S., & Jahr, C. E. (1999). Clearance of glutamate inside the synapse and beyond. *Current Opinion in Neurobiology, 9*(3), 293–298.

Bhattacharya, P., Chekmenev, E. Y., Perman, W. H., Harris, K. C., Lin, A. P., Norton, V. A., et al. (2007). Towards hyperpolarized ^{13}C-succinate imaging of brain cancer. *Journal of Magnetic Resonance, 186*(1), 150–155.

Blomqvist, G., Gjedde, A., Gutniak, M., Grill, V., Widén, L., Stone-Elander, S., et al. (1991). Facilitated transport of glucose from blood to brain in man and the effect of moderate hypoglycaemia on cerebral glucose utilization. *European Journal of Nuclear Medicine, 18*(10), 834–837.

Blüml, S., Moreno, A., Hwang, J. H., & Ross, B. D. (2001a). 1-^{13}C glucose magnetic resonance spectroscopy of pediatric and adult brain disorders. *NMR in Biomedicine, 14*(1), 19–32.

Blüml, S., Moreno-Torres, A., & Ross, B. D. (2001b). [1-^{13}C]glucose MRS in chronic hepatic encephalopathy in man. *Magnetic Resonance in Medicine, 45*(6), 981–993.

Blüml, S., Moreno-Torres, A., Shic, F., Nguy, C. -H., & Ross, B. D. (2002). Tricarboxylic acid cycle of glia in the in vivo human brain. *NMR in Biomedicine, 15*(1), 1–5.

Boumezbeur, F., Besret, L., Valette, J., Gregoire, M. -C., Delzescaux, T., Maroy, R., et al. (2005). Glycolysis versus TCA cycle in the primate brain as measured by combining ^{18}F-FDG PET and ^{13}C-NMR. *Journal of Cerebral Blood Flow and Metabolism, 25*(11), 1418–1423.

Boumezbeur, F., Mason, G. F., de Graaf, R. A., Behar, K. L., Cline, G. W., Shulman, G. I., et al. (2010a). Altered brain mitochondrial metabolism in healthy aging as assessed by in vivo magnetic resonance spectroscopy. *Journal of Cerebral Blood Flow and Metabolism, 30*(1), 211–221.

Boumezbeur, F., Petersen, K. F., Cline, G. W., Mason, G. F., Behar, K. L., Shulman, G. I., et al. (2010b). The contribution of blood lactate to brain energy metabolism in humans measured by dynamic 13C nuclear magnetic resonance spectroscopy. *Journal of Neuroscience, 30*(42), 13983–13991.

Butterworth, R. F. (1993). Portal-systemic encephalopathy: a disorder of neuron-astrocytic metabolic trafficking. *Developmental Neuroscience, 15*(3-5), 313–319.

Cavus, I., Kasoff, W. S., Cassaday, M. P., Jacob, R., Gueorguieva, R., Sherwin, R. S., et al. (2005). Extracellular metabolites in the cortex and hippocampus of epileptic patients. *Annals of Neurology, 57*(2), 226–235.

Cerdán, S., Künnecke, B., & Seelig, J. (1990). Cerebral metabolism of [1,2-13C2]acetate as detected by in vivo and in vitro 13C NMR. *Journal of Biological Chemistry, 265*(22), 12916–12926.

Chaumeil, M. M., Valette, J., Guillermier, M., Brouillet, E., Boumezbeur, F., Herard, A. -S., et al. (2009). Multimodal neuroimaging provides a highly consistent picture of energy metabolism, validating ^{31}P MRS for measuring brain ATP synthesis. *Proceedings of the National Academy of Sciences USA, 106*(10), 3988–3993.

Chen, W., Zhu, X. H., Gruetter, R., Seaquist, E. R., Adriany, G., & Ugurbil, K. (2001). Study of tricarboxylic acid cycle flux changes in human visual cortex during hemifield visual stimulation using ^{1}H-[^{13}C] MRS and fMRI. *Magnetic Resonance in Medicine, 45*(3), 349–355.

Chhina, N., Kuestermann, E., Halliday, J., Simpson, L. J., Macdonald, I. A., Bachelard, H. S., et al. (2001). Measurement of human tricarboxylic acid cycle rates during visual activation by (13)C magnetic resonance spectroscopy. *Journal of Neuroscience Research*, 66(5), 737–746.

Choi, I. -Y., Lei, H., & Gruetter, R. (2002). Effect of deep pentobarbital anesthesia on neurotransmitter metabolism in vivo: on the correlation of total glucose consumption with glutamatergic action. *Journal of Cerebral Blood Flow and Metabolism*, 22(11), 1343–1351.

Chowdhury, G. M. I., Patel, A. B., Mason, G. F., Rothman, D. L., & Behar, K. L. (2007). Glutamatergic and GABAergic neurotransmitter cycling and energy metabolism in rat cerebral cortex during postnatal development. *Journal of Cerebral Blood Flow and Metabolism*, 27(12), 1895–1907.

Collins, C. M., Liu, W., Wang, J., Gruetter, R., Vaughan, J. T., Ugurbil, K., et al. (2004). Temperature and SAR calculations for a human head within volume and surface coils at 64 and 300 MHz. *Journal of Magnetic Resonance Imaging*, 19(5), 650–656.

Cooper, A. J., & Plum, F. (1987). Biochemistry and physiology of brain ammonia. *Physiological Reviews*, 67(2), 440–519.

Cryer, P. E. (1994). Banting Lecture. Hypoglycemia: the limiting factor in the management of IDDM. *Diabetes*, 43(11), 1378–1389.

Cryer, P. E. (2004). Diverse causes of hypoglycemia-associated autonomic failure in diabetes. *New England Journal of Medicine*, 350 (22), 2272–2279.

Cudalbu, C., Comment, A., Kurdzesau, F., van Heeswijk, R. B., Uffmann, K., Jannin, S., et al. (2010). Feasibility of in vivo ^{15}N MRS detection of hyperpolarized 15N labeled choline in rats. *Physical Chemistry Chemical Physics*, 12(22), 5818–5823.

Dager, S. R., Friedman, S. D., Parow, A., Demopulos, C., Stoll, A. L., Lyoo, I. K., et al. (2004). Brain metabolic alterations in medication-free patients with bipolar disorder. *Archives of General Psychiatry*, 61(5), 450–458.

de Graaf, R. A. (2005). Theoretical and experimental evaluation of broadband decoupling techniques for in vivo nuclear magnetic resonance spectroscopy. *Magnetic Resonance in Medicine*, 53(6), 1297–1306.

de Graaf, R. A., Mason, G. F., Patel, A. B., Rothman, D. L., & Behar, K. L. (2004). Regional glucose metabolism and glutamatergic neurotransmission in rat brain in vivo. *Proceedings of the National Academy of Sciences of the USA*, 101(34), 12700–12705.

de Graaf, R. A., Pan, J. W., Telang, F., Lee, J. H., Brown, P., Novotny, E. J., et al. (2001). Differentiation of glucose transport in human brain gray and white matter. *Journal of Cerebral Blood Flow and Metabolism*, 21(5), 483–492.

de Graaf, R. A., Rothman, D. L., & Behar, K. L. (2011). State of the art direct ^{13}C and indirect 1H-[13C] NMR spectroscopy in vivo. A practical guide. *NMR in Biomedicine*, 24(8), 958–972.

Dienel, G. A., & Hertz, L. (2001). Glucose and lactate metabolism during brain activation. *Journal of Neuroscience Research*, 66(5), 824–838.

DiNuzzo, M., Mangia, S., Maraviglia, B., & Giove, F. (2010). Changes in glucose uptake rather than lactate shuttle take center stage in subserving neuroenergetics: evidence from mathematical modeling. *Journal of Cerebral Blood Flow and Metabolism*, 30(3), 586–602.

Eid, T., Thomas, M. J., Spencer, D. D., Rundén-Pran, E., Lai, J. C. K., Malthankar, G. V., et al. (2004). Loss of glutamine synthetase in the human epileptogenic hippocampus: possible mechanism for raised extracellular glutamate in mesial temporal lobe epilepsy. *Lancet*, 363(9402), 28–37.

Epperson, C. N., Haga, K., Mason, G. F., Sellers, E., Gueorguieva, R., Zhang, W., et al. (2002). Cortical gamma-aminobutyric acid levels across the menstrual cycle in healthy women and those with premenstrual dysphoric disorder: a proton magnetic resonance spectroscopy study. *Archives of General Psychiatry*, 59(9), 851–858.

Fitzpatrick, S. M., Behar, K. L., & Shulman, R. G. (1989a). In vivo NMR spectroscopy studies of cerebral metabolism in rats after

portal–caval shunting. In R. F. Butterworth, & G. P. Layrargues (Eds.), *Hepatic Encephalopathy* (Vol. 22, pp. 177–187). New York: Humana Press.

Fitzpatrick, S. M., Hetherington, H. P., Behar, K. L., & Shulman, R. G. (1989b). Effects of acute hyperammonemia on cerebral amino acid metabolism and pHi in vivo, measured by ^{1}H and ^{31}P nuclear magnetic resonance. *Journal of Neurochemistry*, 52(3), 741–749.

Fitzpatrick, S. M., Hetherington, H. P., Behar, K. L., & Shulman, R. G. (1990). The flux from glucose to glutamate in the rat brain in vivo as determined by ^{1}H-observed, ^{13}C-edited NMR spectroscopy. *Journal of Cerebral Blood Flow and Metabolism*, 10(2), 170–179.

Fox, P. T., Raichle, M. E., Mintun, M. A., & Dence, C. (1988). Nonoxidative glucose consumption during focal physiologic neural activity. *Science*, 241(4864), 462–464.

Goddard, A. W., Mason, G. F., Almai, A., Rothman, D. L., Behar, K. L., Petroff, O. A., et al. (2001). Reductions in occipital cortex GABA levels in panic disorder detected with [1]H-magnetic resonance spectroscopy. *Archives of General Psychiatry*, 58(6), 556–561.

Gropman, A. L., Sailasuta, N., Harris, K. C., Abulseoud, O., & Ross, B. D. (2009). Ornithine transcarbamylase deficiency with persistent abnormality in cerebral glutamate metabolism in adults. *Radiology*, 252(3), 833–841.

Gruber, S., Frey, R., Mlynárik, V., Stadlbauer, A., Heiden, A., Kasper, S., et al. (2003). Quantification of metabolic differences in the frontal brain of depressive patients and controls obtained by ^{1}H-MRS at 3 Tesla. *Investigative Radiology*, 38(7), 403–408.

Gruetter, R. (1993). Automatic, localized in vivo adjustment of all first- and second-order shim coils. *Magnetic Resonance in Medicine*, 29(6), 804–811.

Gruetter, R., Novotny, E. J., Boulware, S. D., Mason, G. F., Rothman, D. L., Shulman, G. I., et al. (1994). Localized ^{13}C NMR spectroscopy in the human brain of amino acid labeling from D-[1-13C] glucose. *Journal of Neurochemistry*, 63(4), 1377–1385.

Gruetter, R., Novotny, E. J., Boulware, S. D., Rothman, D. L., Mason, G. F., Shulman, G. I., et al. (1992). Direct measurement of brain glucose concentrations in humans by ^{13}C NMR spectroscopy. *Proceedings of the National Academy of Sciences of the USA*, 89(3), 1109–1112.

Gruetter, R., Novotny, E. J., Boulware, S. D., Rothman, D. L., & Shulman, R. G. (1996). ^{1}H NMR studies of glucose transport in the human brain. *Journal of Cerebral Blood Flow and Metabolism*, 16 (3), 427–438.

Gruetter, R., Seaquist, E. R., Kim, S., & Ugurbil, K. (1998a). Localized in vivo ^{13}C-NMR of glutamate metabolism in the human brain: initial results at 4 tesla. *Developmental Neuroscience*, 20(4-5), 380–388.

Gruetter, R., Seaquist, E. R., & Ugurbil, K. (2001). A mathematical model of compartmentalized neurotransmitter metabolism in the human brain. *American Journal of Physiology Endocrinology and Metabolism*, 281(1), E100–E112.

Gruetter, R., Ugurbil, K., & Seaquist, E. R. (1998b). Steady-state cerebral glucose concentrations and transport in the human brain. *Journal of Neurochemistry*, 70(1), 397–408.

Haga, K. K., Khor, Y. P., Farrall, A., & Wardlaw, J. M. (2009). A systematic review of brain metabolite changes, measured with ^{1}H magnetic resonance spectroscopy, in healthy aging. *Neurobiology of Aging*, 30(3), 353–363.

Hasler, G., van der Veen, J. W., Tumonis, T., Meyers, N., Shen, J., & Drevets, W. C. (2007). Reduced prefrontal glutamate/glutamine and gamma-aminobutyric acid levels in major depression determined using proton magnetic resonance spectroscopy. *Archives of General Psychiatry*, 64(2), 193–200.

Hassel, B., Bachelard, H., Jones, P., Fonnum, F., & Sonnewald, U. (1997). Trafficking of amino acids between neurons and glia in vivo. Effects of inhibition of glial metabolism by fluoroacetate. *Journal of Cerebral Blood Flow and Metabolism, 17*(11), 1230–1238.

Heiss, W. D., Pawlik, G., Herholz, K., Wagner, R., Göldner, H., & Wienhard, K. (1984). Regional kinetic constants and cerebral metabolic rate for glucose in normal human volunteers determined by dynamic positron emission tomography of [18F]-2-fluoro-2-deoxy-D-glucose. *Journal of Blood Flow and Metabolism, 4*(2), 212–223.

Henry, P. -G., Criego, A. B., Kumar, A., & Seaquist, E. R. (2010). Measurement of cerebral oxidative glucose consumption in patients with type 1 diabetes mellitus and hypoglycemia unawareness using ^{13}C nuclear magnetic resonance spectroscopy. *Metabolism: Clinical and Experimental, 59*(1), 100–106.

Hertz, L. (1979). Functional interactions between neurons and astrocytes I. Turnover and metabolism of putative amino acid transmitters. *Progress in Neurobiology, 13*(3), 277–323.

Hertz, L., Peng, L., & Dienel, G. A. (2007). Energy metabolism in astrocytes: high rate of oxidative metabolism and spatiotemporal dependence on glycolysis/glycogenolysis. *Journal of Cerebral Blood Flow and Metabolism, 27*(2), 219–249.

Hetherington, H. P., Chu, W. -J., Gonen, O., & Pan, J. W. (2006). Robust fully automated shimming of the human brain for high-field ^{1}H spectroscopic imaging. *Magnetic Resonance in Medicine, 56*(1), 26–33.

Hoge, R. D., Atkinson, J., Gill, B., Crelier, G. R., Marrett, S., & Pike, G. B. (1999). Linear coupling between cerebral blood flow and oxygen consumption in activated human cortex. *Proceedings of the National Academy of Sciences of the USA, 96*(16), 9403–9408.

Hyder, F., Patel, A. B., Gjedde, A., Rothman, D. L., Behar, K. L., & Shulman, R. G. (2006). Neuronal-glial glucose oxidation and glutamatergic-GABAergic function. *Journal of Cerebral Blood Flow and Metabolism, 26*(7), 865–877.

Jolivet, R., Magistretti, P. J., & Weber, B. (2009). Deciphering neuron-glia compartmentalization in cortical energy metabolism. *Frontiers in Neuroenergetics, 1*, 4.

Juchem, C., Nixon, T. W., McIntyre, S., Rothman, D. L., & de Graaf, R. A. (2010). Magnetic field homogenization of the human prefrontal cortex with a set of localized electrical coils. *Magnetic Resonance in Medicine, 63*(1), 171–180.

Kalpouzos, G., Chételat, G., Baron, J. -C., Landeau, B., Mevel, K., Godeau, C., et al. (2009). Voxel-based mapping of brain gray matter volume and glucose metabolism profiles in normal aging. *Neurobiology of Aging, 30*(1), 112–124.

Kanamori, K., Kondrat, R. W., & Ross, B. D. (2003). 13C enrichment of extracellular neurotransmitter glutamate in rat brain--combined mass spectrometry and NMR studies of neurotransmitter turnover and uptake into glia in vivo. *Cellular and Molecular Biology, 49*(5), 819–836.

Kanamori, K., & Ross, B. D. (1997). Glial alkalinization detected in vivo by 1H-15N heteronuclear multiple-quantum coherence-transfer NMR in severely hyperammonemic rat. *Journal of Neurochemistry, 68*(3), 1209–1220.

Kim, S. G., Rostrup, E., Larsson, H. B., Ogawa, S., & Paulson, O. B. (1999). Determination of relative CMRO2 from CBF and BOLD changes: significant increase of oxygen consumption rate during visual stimulation. *Magnetic Resonance in Medicine, 41*(6), 1152–1161.

Klomp, D. W. J., Renema, W. K. J., van der Graaf, M., de Galan, B. E., Kentgens, A. P. M., & Heerschap, A. (2006). Sensitivity-enhanced 13C MR spectroscopy of the human brain at 3 Tesla. *Magnetic Resonance in Medicine, 55*(2), 271–278.

Koch, K. M., Sacolick, L. I., Nixon, T. W., McIntyre, S., Rothman, D. L., & de Graaf, R. A. (2007). Dynamically shimmed multivoxel 1H magnetic resonance spectroscopy and multislice magnetic resonance spectroscopic imaging of the human brain. *Magnetic Resonance in Medicine, 57*(3), 587–591.

Kuzniecky, R., Ho, S., Pan, J., Martin, R., Gilliam, F., Faught, E., et al. (2002). Modulation of cerebral GABA by topiramate, lamotrigine, and gabapentin in healthy adults. *Neurology, 58*(3), 368–372.

Künnecke, B., & Cerdan, S. (1989). Multilabeled 13C substrates as probes in in vivo ^{13}C and ^{1}H NMR spectroscopy. *NMR in Biomedicine, 2*(5-6), 274–277.

Lebon, V., Petersen, K. F., Cline, G. W., Shen, J., Mason, G. F., Dufour, S., et al. (2002). Astroglial contribution to brain energy metabolism in humans revealed by ^{13}C nuclear magnetic resonance spectroscopy: elucidation of the dominant pathway for neurotransmitter glutamate repletion and measurement of astrocytic oxidative metabolism. *Journal of Neuroscience, 22*(5), 1523–1531.

Li, S., Yang, J., & Shen, J. (2007). Novel strategy for cerebral ^{13}C MRS using very low RF power for proton decoupling. *Magnetic Resonance in Medicine, 57*(2), 265–271.

Li, S., Zhang, Y., Wang, S., Araneta, M. F., Johnson, C. S., Xiang, Y., et al. (2010). ^{13}C MRS of occipital and frontal lobes at 3 T using a volume coil for stochastic proton decoupling. *NMR in Biomedicine, 23*(8), 977–985.

Li, S., Zhang, Y., Wang, S., Yang, J., Araneta, M. F., Farris, A., et al. (2009). In vivo ^{13}C magnetic resonance spectroscopy of human brain on a clinical 3 T scanner using [2-^{13}C] glucose infusion and low-power stochastic decoupling. *Magnetic Resonance in Medicine, 62*(3), 565–573.

Lieth, E., LaNoue, K. F., Berkich, D. A., Xu, B., Ratz, M., Taylor, C., et al. (2001). Nitrogen shuttling between neurons and glial cells during glutamate synthesis. *Journal of Neurochemistry, 76*(6), 1712–1723.

Lin, A. P., Shic, F., Enriquez, C., & Ross, B. D. (2003). Reduced glutamate neurotransmission in patients with Alzheimer's disease -- an in vivo (13)C magnetic resonance spectroscopy study. *MAGMA, 16*(1), 29–42.

Lin, M. T., & Beal, M. F. (2006). Mitochondrial dysfunction and oxidative stress in neurodegenerative diseases. *Nature, 443*(7113), 787–795.

Maciejewski, P. K., & Rothman, D. L. (2008). Proposed cycles for functional glutamate trafficking in synaptic neurotransmission. *Neurochemistry international, 52*(4-5), 809–825.

Magistretti, P. J., Pellerin, L., Rothman, D. L., & Shulman, R. G. (1999). Energy on demand. *Science, 283*(5401), 496–497.

Mangia, S., Tkác, I., Gruetter, R., Van De Moortele, P. -F., Maraviglia, B., & Uğurbil, K. (2007). Sustained neuronal activation raises oxidative metabolism to a new steady-state level: evidence from 1H NMR spectroscopy in the human visual cortex. *Journal of Cerebral Blood Flow and Metabolism, 27*(5), 1055–1063.

Marjańska, M., Iltis, I., Shestov, A. A., & Deelchand, D. K. (2010). ScienceDirect.com-Journal of Magnetic Resonance-In vivo^{13}C spectroscopy in the rat brain using hyperpolarized [1-^{13}C]pyruvate and [2-^{13}C]pyruvate. *Journal of Magnetic Resonance, 206*(2), 210–218.

Marrett, S., & Gjedde, A. (1997). Changes of blood flow and oxygen consumption in visual cortex of living humans. *Advances in Experimental Medicine and Biology, 413*, 205–208.

Martin, W. R. W. (2007). MR spectroscopy in neurodegenerative disease. *Molecular Imaging And Biology, 9*(4), 196–203.

Mason, G. F., Gruetter, R., Rothman, D. L., Behar, K. L., Shulman, R. G., & Novotny, E. J. (1995). Simultaneous determination of the rates of the TCA cycle, glucose utilization, alpha-ketoglutarate/glutamate exchange, and glutamine synthesis in human brain by NMR. *Journal of Cerebral Blood Flow and Metabolism, 15*(1), 12–25.

Mason, G. F., Pan, J. W., Chu, W. J., Newcomer, B. R., Zhang, Y., Orr, R., et al. (1999). Measurement of the tricarboxylic acid cycle rate in human grey and white matter in vivo by ^{1}H-[^{13}C] magnetic resonance spectroscopy at 4.1 T. *Journal of Cerebral Blood Flow and Metabolism, 19*(11), 1179–1188.

Mason, G. F., Petersen, K. F., de Graaf, R. A., Kanamatsu, T., Otsuki, T., Shulman, G. I., et al. (2003). A comparison of ^{13}C NMR measurements of the rates of glutamine synthesis and the tricarboxylic acid cycle during oral and intravenous administration of [1-(13)C] glucose. *Brain Research Brain Research Protocols, 10*(3), 181–190.

Mason, G. F., Petersen, K. F., de Graaf, R. A., Shulman, G. I., & Rothman, D. L. (2007). Measurements of the anaplerotic rate in the human cerebral cortex using ^{13}C magnetic resonance spectroscopy and [1-^{13}C] and [2-^{13}C] glucose. *Journal of Neurochemistry, 100*(1), 73–86.

Mason, G. F., Petersen, K. F., Lebon, V., Rothman, D. L., & Shulman, G. I. (2006). Increased brain monocarboxylic acid transport and utilization in type 1 diabetes. *Diabetes, 55*(4), 929–934.

Mason, G. F., & Rothman, D. L. (2002). Graded image segmentation of brain tissue in the presence of inhomogeneous radio frequency fields. *Magnetic Resonance Imaging, 20*(5), 431–436.

Mason, G. F., & Rothman, D. L. (2004). Basic principles of metabolic modeling of NMR ^{13}C isotopic turnover to determine rates of brain metabolism in vivo. *Metabolic Engineering, 6*(1), 75–84.

Maycox, P. R., Hell, J. W., & Jahn, R. (1990). Amino acid neurotransmission: spotlight on synaptic vesicles. *Trends in Neurosciences, 13*(3), 83–87.

McKenna, M. C. (2007). The glutamate-glutamine cycle is not stoichiometric: fates of glutamate in brain. *Journal of Neuroscience Research, 85*(15), 3347–3358.

Moreno, A., Blüml, S., Hwang, J. H., & Ross, B. D. (2001). Alternative 1-^{13}C glucose infusion protocols for clinical ^{13}C MRS examinations of the brain. *Magnetic Resonance in Medicine, 46*(1), 39–48.

Nicholls, D., & Attwell, D. (1990). The release and uptake of excitatory amino acids. *Trends in Pharmacological Sciences, 11*(11), 462–468.

Novotny, E. J., Fulbright, R. K., Pearl, P. L., Gibson, K. M., & Rothman, D. L. (2003). Magnetic resonance spectroscopy of neurotransmitters in human brain. *Annals of Neurology, 54*(Suppl. 6), S25–S31.

Novotny, E. J., Hyder, F., Shevell, M., & Rothman, D. L. (1999). GABA changes with vigabatrin in the developing human brain. *Epilepsia, 40*(4), 462–466.

Novotny, E. J., Ogino, T., Rothman, D. L., Petroff, O. A., Prichard, J. W., & Shulman, R. G. (1990). Direct carbon versus proton heteronuclear editing of 2-13C ethanol in rabbit brain in vivo: a sensitivity comparison. *Magnetic Resonance in Medicine, 16*(3), 431–443.

Occhipinti, R., Somersalo, E., & Calvetti, D. (2009). Astrocytes as the glucose shunt for glutamatergic neurons at high activity: an in silico study. *Journal of Neurophysiology, 101*(5), 2528–2538.

Owen, O. E., Morgan, A. P., Kemp, H. G., Sullivan, J. M., Herrera, M. G., & Cahill, G. F. (1967). Brain metabolism during fasting. *Journal of Clinical Investigation, 46*(10), 1589–1595.

Oz, G., Berkich, D. A., Henry, P. -G., Xu, Y., LaNoue, K., Hutson, S. M., et al. (2004). Neuroglial metabolism in the awake rat brain: CO_2 fixation increases with brain activity. *Journal of Neuroscience, 24*(50), 11273–11279.

Pan, J. W., de Graaf, R. A., Petersen, K. F., Shulman, G. I., Hetherington, H. P., & Rothman, D. L. (2002). [2,4-13 C 2]-beta-Hydroxybutyrate metabolism in human brain. *Journal of Cerebral Blood Flow and Metabolism, 22*(7), 890–898.

Pan, J. W., Stein, D. T., Telang, F., Lee, J. H., Shen, J., Brown, P., et al. (2000). Spectroscopic imaging of glutamate C4 turnover in human brain. *Magnetic Resonance in Medicine, 44*(5), 673–679.

Pan, J. W., Williamson, A., Cavus, I., Hetherington, H. P., Zaveri, H., Petroff, O. A. C., et al. (2008). Neurometabolism in human epilepsy. *Epilepsia, 49*(Suppl. 3), 31–41.

Patel, A. B., Chowdhury, G. M. I., de Graaf, R. A., Rothman, D. L., Shulman, R. G., & Behar, K. L. (2005a). Cerebral pyruvate carboxylase flux is unaltered during bicuculline-seizures. *Journal of Neuroscience Research, 79*(1-2), 128–138.

Patel, A. B., de Graaf, R. A., Mason, G. F., Kanamatsu, T., Rothman, D. L., Shulman, R. G., et al. (2004). Glutamatergic neurotransmission and neuronal glucose oxidation are coupled during intense neuronal activation. *Journal of Cerebral Blood Flow and Metabolism, 24*(9), 972–985.

Patel, A. B., de Graaf, R. A., Mason, G. F., Rothman, D. L., Shulman, R. G., & Behar, K. L. (2005b). The contribution of GABA to glutamate/glutamine cycling and energy metabolism in the rat cortex in vivo. *Proceedings of the National Academy of Sciences of the USA, 102*(15), 5588–5593.

Patel, A. B., de Graaf, R. A., Rothman, D. L., Behar, K. L., & Mason, G. F. (2010). Evaluation of cerebral acetate transport and metabolic rates in the rat brain in vivo using ^{1}H-[^{13}C]-NMR. *Journal of Cerebral Blood Flow and Metabolism, 30*(6), 1200–1213.

Petroff, O. A., Graham, G. D., Blamire, A. M., al-Rayess, M., Rothman, D. L., Fayad, P. B., et al. (1992). Spectroscopic imaging of stroke in humans: histopathology correlates of spectral changes. *Neurology, 42*(7), 1349–1354.

Petroff, O. A., Mattson, R. H., & Rothman, D. L. (2000). Proton MRS: GABA and glutamate. *Advances in Neurology, 83*, 261–271.

Petroff, O. A. C., Errante, L. D., Rothman, D. L., Kim, J. H., & Spencer, D. D. (2002). Glutamate-glutamine cycling in the epileptic human hippocampus. *Epilepsia, 43*(7), 703–710.

Pfeuffer, J., Tkác, I., Choi, I. Y., Merkle, H., Ugurbil, K., Garwood, M., et al. (1999). Localized in vivo 1H NMR detection of neurotransmitter labeling in rat brain during infusion of [1-^{13}C] D-glucose. *Magnetic Resonance in Medicine, 41*(6), 1077–1083.

Prichard, J., Rothman, D., Novotny, E., Petroff, O., Kuwabara, T., Avison, M., et al. (1991). Lactate rise detected by 1H NMR in human visual cortex during physiologic stimulation. *Proceedings of the National Academy of Sciences of the USA, 88*(13), 5829–5831.

Raichle, M. E. (2009). A paradigm shift in functional brain imaging. *Journal of Neuroscience, 29*(41), 12729–12734.

Rapoport, S. I. (1999). Functional brain imaging in the resting state and during activation in Alzheimer's disease. Implications for disease mechanisms involving oxidative phosphorylation. *Annals of the New York Academy of Sciences, 893*, 138–153.

Ross, B., Lin, A., Harris, K., Bhattacharya, P., & Schweinsburg, B. (2003). Clinical experience with ^{13}C MRS in vivo. *NMR in Biomedicine, 16*(6-7), 358–369.

Ross, B. D., Jacobson, S., Villamil, F., Korula, J., Kreis, R., Ernst, T., et al. (1994). Subclinical hepatic encephalopathy: proton MR spectroscopic abnormalities. *Radiology, 193*(2), 457–463.

Rothman, D. L., Behar, K. L., Hetherington, H. P., den Hollander, J. A., Bendall, M. R., Petroff, O. A., et al. (1985). 1H-Observe/13C-decouple spectroscopic measurements of lactate and glutamate in the rat brain in vivo. *Proceedings of the National Academy of Sciences of the USA, 82*(6), 1633–1637.

Rothman, D. L., Behar, K. L., Hyder, F., & Shulman, R. G. (2003). In vivo NMR studies of the glutamate neurotransmitter flux and neuroenergetics: implications for brain function. *Annual Review of Physiology, 65*, 401–427.

Rothman, D. L., Howseman, A. M., Graham, G. D., Petroff, O. A., Lantos, G., Fayad, P. B., et al. (1991). Localized proton NMR observation of [3-^{13}C]lactate in stroke after [1-^{13}C]glucose infusion. *Magnetic Resonance in Medicine, 21*(2), 302–307.

Rothman, D. L., Novotny, E. J., Shulman, G. I., Howseman, A. M., Petroff, O. A., Mason, G., et al. (1992). ^{1}H-[^{13}C] NMR measurements of [4-^{13}C]glutamate turnover in human brain. *Proceedings of the National Academy of Sciences of the USA, 89*(20), 9603–9606.

Rothstein, J. D., Dykes-Hoberg, M., Pardo, C. A., Bristol, L. A., Jin, L., Kuncl, R. W., et al. (1996). Knockout of glutamate transporters reveals a major role for astroglial transport in excitotoxicity and clearance of glutamate. *Neuron, 16*(3), 675–686.

Sailasuta, N., Abulseoud, O., Harris, K. C., & Ross, B. D. (2010a). Glial dysfunction in abstinent methamphetamine abusers. *Journal of Cerebral Blood Flow and Metabolism, 30*(5), 950–960.

Sailasuta, N., Tran, T. T., Harris, K. C., & Ross, B. D. (2010b). Swift Acetate Glial Assay (SAGA): an accelerated human ^{13}C MRS brain exam for clinical diagnostic use. *Journal of Magnetic Resonance, 207*(2), 352–355.

Sanacora, G., Gueorguieva, R., Epperson, C. N., Wu, Y. -T., Appel, M., Rothman, D. L., et al. (2004). Subtype-specific alterations of gamma-aminobutyric acid and glutamate in patients with major depression. *Archives of General Psychiatry, 61*(7), 705–713.

Serres, S., Raffard, G., Franconi, J. -M., & Merle, M. (2008). Close coupling between astrocytic and neuronal metabolisms to fulfill anaplerotic and energy needs in the rat brain. *Journal of Cerebral Blood Flow and Metabolism, 28*(4), 712–724.

Shen, J., Petersen, K. F., Behar, K. L., Brown, P., Nixon, T. W., Mason, G. F., et al. (1999). Determination of the rate of the glutamate/glutamine cycle in the human brain by in vivo ^{13}C NMR. *Proceedings of the National Academy of Sciences of the USA, 96*(14), 8235–8240.

Shen, J., Rothman, D., Behar, K., & Xu, S. (2008). Determination of the glutamate-glutamine cycling flux using two-compartment dynamic metabolic modeling is sensitive to astroglial dilution. *Journal of Cerebral Blood Flow and Metabolism.*

Shen, J., Sibson, N. R., Cline, G., Behar, K. L., Rothman, D. L., & Shulman, R. G. (1998). ^{15}N-NMR spectroscopy studies of ammonia transport and glutamine synthesis in the hyperammonemic rat brain. *Developmental Neuroscience, 20*(4-5), 434–443.

Shephard, G. (1994). *The Synaptic Organization of the Brain.* Oxford, UK: Oxford University Press.

Shestov, A. A., Valette, J., Uğurbil, K., & Henry, P. -G. (2007). On the reliability of (13)C metabolic modeling with two-compartment neuronal-glial models. *Journal of Neuroscience Research, 85*(15), 3294–3303.

Shulman, R. G., Hyder, F., & Rothman, D. L. (2001). Cerebral energetics and the glycogen shunt: neurochemical basis of functional imaging. *Proceedings of the National Academy of Sciences of the USA, 98*(11), 6417–6422.

Shulman, R. G., & Rothman, D. L. (1998). Interpreting functional imaging studies in terms of neurotransmitter cycling. *Proceedings of the National Academy of Sciences of the USA, 95*(20), 11993–11998.

Sibson, N. R., Dhankhar, A., Mason, G. F., Behar, K. L., Rothman, D. L., & Shulman, R. G. (1997). In vivo ^{13}C NMR measurements of cerebral glutamine synthesis as evidence for glutamate-glutamine cycling. *Proceedings of the National Academy of Sciences of the USA, 94*(6), 2699–2704.

Sibson, N. R., Dhankhar, A., Mason, G. F., Rothman, D. L., Behar, K. L., & Shulman, R. G. (1998). Stoichiometric coupling of brain glucose metabolism and glutamatergic neuronal activity. *Proceedings of the National Academy of Sciences of the USA, 95*(1), 316–321.

Sibson, N. R., Mason, G. F., Shen, J., Cline, G. W., Herskovits, A. Z., Wall, J. E., et al. (2001). In vivo ^{13}C NMR measurement of neurotransmitter glutamate cycling, anaplerosis and TCA cycle flux in rat brain during. *Journal of Neurochemistry, 76*(4), 975–989.

Siesjö, B. K. (1978). *Brain Energy Metabolism.* New York: John Wiley & Sons.

Simpson, I. A., Carruthers, A., & Vannucci, S. J. (2007). Supply and demand in cerebral energy metabolism: the role of nutrient transporters. *Journal of Cerebral Blood Flow and Metabolism, 27*(11), 1766–1791.

Smith, D., Pernet, A., Hallett, W. A., Bingham, E., Marsden, P. K., & Amiel, S. A. (2003). Lactate: a preferred fuel for human brain metabolism in vivo. *Journal of Cerebral Blood Flow and Metabolism, 23*(6), 658–664.

Strelnikov, K. (2010). Neuroimaging and neuroenergetics: brain activations as information-driven reorganization of energy flows. *Brain and Cognition, 72*(3), 449–456.

Terpstra, M., Gruetter, R., High, W. B., Mescher, M., DelaBarre, L., Merkle, H., et al. (1998). Lactate turnover in rat glioma measured by in vivo nuclear magnetic resonance spectroscopy. *Cancer Research, 58*(22), 5083–5088.

van de Ven, K. C., Tack, C. J., Heerschap, A., van der Graaf, M., & de Galan, B. E. (2013). Patients with type 1 diabetes exhibit altered cerebral metabolism during hypoglycemia. *The Journal of Clinical Investigation, 123*(2), 623–629.

van de Ven, K. C., van der Graaf, M., Tack, C. J., Klomp, D. W., Heerschap, A., & de Galan, B. E. (2010). Optimized [1-^{13}C]glucose infusion protocol for ^{13}C magnetic resonance spectroscopy at 3 T of human brain glucose metabolism under euglycemic and hypoglycemic conditions. *Journal of Neuroscience Methods, 186*(1), 68–71.

Van den Berg, C. J., Krzalić, L., Mela, P., & Waelsch, H. (1969). Compartmentation of glutamate metabolism in brain. Evidence for the existence of two different tricarboxylic acid cycles in brain. *Biochemical Journal, 113*(2), 281–290.

van Eijsden, P., Behar, K. L., Mason, G. F., Braun, K. P. J., & de Graaf, R. A. (2010). In vivo neurochemical profiling of rat brain by ^{1}H-[^{13}C] NMR spectroscopy: cerebral energetics and glutamatergic/GABAergic neurotransmission. *Journal of Neurochemistry, 112*(1), 24–33.

van Hall, G., Strømstad, M., Rasmussen, P., Jans, O., Zaar, M., Gam, C., et al. (2009). Blood lactate is an important energy source for the human brain. *Journal of Cerebral Blood Flow and Metabolism, 29*(6), 1121–1129.

Wang, J., Jiang, L., Jiang, Y., Ma, X., Chowdhury, G. M. I., & Mason, G. F. (2010). Regional metabolite levels and turnover in the awake rat brain under the influence of nicotine. *Journal of Neurochemistry, 113*(6), 1447–1458.

Waniewski, R. A., & Martin, D. L. (1998). Preferential utilization of acetate by astrocytes is attributable to transport. *The Journal of Neuroscience, 18*(14), 5225–5233.

Wijnen, J. P., van der Graaf, M., Scheenen, T. W. J., Klomp, D. W. J., de Galan, B. E., Idema, A. J. S., et al. (2010). In vivo ^{13}C magnetic resonance spectroscopy of a human brain tumor after application of ^{13}C-1-enriched glucose. *Magnetic Resonance Imaging, 28*(5), 690–697.

Yang, J., & Shen, J. (2005). In vivo evidence for reduced cortical glutamate-glutamine cycling in rats treated with the antidepressant/antipanic drug phenelzine. *Neuroscience, 135*(3), 927–937.

Yang, J., Xu, S., & Shen, J. (2009). Fast isotopic exchange between mitochondria and cytosol in brain revealed by relayed ^{13}C magnetization transfer spectroscopy. *Journal of Cerebral Blood Flow and Metabolism, 29*(4), 661–669.

Yu, A. C., Drejer, J., Hertz, L., & Schousboe, A. (1983). Pyruvate carboxylase activity in primary cultures of astrocytes and neurons. *Journal of Neurochemistry, 41*(5), 1484–1487.

Hyperpolarized Magnetic Resonance Imaging and Spectroscopy of the Brain

Brian Ross

Director, Huntington Medical Research Institutes, Magnetic Resonance Spectroscopy Unit, Pasadena, CA, USA

INTRODUCTION

The emergence of hyperpolarization in biomedical magnetic resonance (MR) research is little more than 10 years old (note that the ambiguity of this terminology is unique to neuroscience, which previously applied the term "hyperpolarization" to the sodium—potassium electrogenic gradients established in excitable tissues including the nervous system). In the field of MR, hyperpolarization refers specifically to the ability to exceed the proportion of nuclei occupying higher or lower energy state ("P") as assigned in the Boltzmann equation. P is generally minute ($P < 10^{-5}$), little more than one part per million, and directly proportional to the ambient magnetic field, but could theoretically reach unity, $P = 1$, when the MR signal would be enhanced almost one million-fold. At that level, the sensitivity of MR imaging (MRI) for molecular detection would be equivalent to that obtained using positron emission tomography (PET) molecular imaging. Hyperpolarization, albeit transient and at enhancements of 50- to 250,000-fold, was known to NMR experts for several decades before its potential in biomedical imaging and spectroscopy was realized in practice. Once the potential was acknowledged, excitement was focused on a small number of topics: lung function in asthma and emphysema, cancer biology, vascular imaging and angiogenesis, and "heart attack" and ischemia more generally, where glycolysis may play an important role in recovery. Finally, and no less important was the possibility that the brain and neurological disorders, including neurodegenerative and psychiatric diseases, could all benefit from the "new look" apparently offered by hyperpolarized MR. For neuroscientists in particular, rapid *in vivo* imaging of heteronuclei held considerable added attraction;

significant new discoveries were the result of administering stable-isotope tracers to experimental animals and to man. Applying hyperpolarization techniques it was believed would accomplish *in vivo* stable-isotope ^{13}C and ^{15}N MR spectroscopy (MRS) in seconds rather than hours and would open the way to molecular neuroimaging, applications that are currently the exclusive province of (radioactive) PET. Next it was felt that hyperpolarized MRI, by delivering a complete examination in much shorter times and at lower magnetic fields, could reduce the spiraling costs of ultrahigh field MRI and MRS. Unfortunately, unlike some earlier medical discoveries, including x-ray and conventional MRI, which could be copied by any competent practitioner, hyperpolarized NMR techniques are very complex, demanding sophisticated new equipment and many modifications to existing MRI scanners. Individual techniques are also shrouded in patents and only a few privileged practitioners have had access. Last, even when accessible, hyperpolarization has generally been very costly in reagents: ^{13}C boutique molecules require hours of synthetic chemistry and cryogens needed in large volumes for one technique are becoming increasingly costly. Consequently, the strategies used to exploit hyperpolarized MR have been limited and preordained by blind guesswork as to likely medical priorities. Asthma and emphysema (COPD) have been the dominant favorites for noble-gas research. Prostate cancer was chosen for dynamic nuclear polarization (DNP) research and explored initially only with ^{13}C pyruvate, a single reagent that reproduced the Warburg effect and reflected the prior knowledge gained from fluorodeoxyglucose (FDG) PET studies of cancers elsewhere. Similar studies explored myocardial ischemia while other studies that did not depend upon further metabolism of the hyperpolarized imaging agent (angiography and tissue perfusion) were completed. In another broad category were *in vivo* studies that built directly upon the invention, after much trial and error, of double-bond ^{13}C substrates, which could be hyperpolarized from parahydrogen in uniquely catalyzed syntheses: Could [1-^{13}C]succinate, the first such biomolecule, perhaps, open the Krebs-tricarboxylic acid cycle (TCA) to inspection? While it is hard to criticize these pioneering studies, they did reveal just how hard it would be to handle, in a biological or a clinical environment, studies based upon the very short lived hyperpolarized state. Partly as a result, very few hyperpolarized MR studies have involved the brain (see Chapter 1.1). After more than a decade of effort it may be that hyperpolarization research is entering a "second generation" and new investigators have an opportunity to refocus on new goals.

Knowing a little more about the strengths and weaknesses of hyperpolarization per se, and with the successful resolution of many of the problems inherent in ultrafast signal decay, recasting conventionally proton-only imaging to encompass the heteronuclei, four broad areas of potential application suggest themselves. First, can "hyperpolarization" inject new life into clinical neurospectroscopy by its speed or its increased chemical specificity, thereby avoiding radioactivity and becoming the "poor man's PET"? Might hyperpolarization of ^{13}C designer reagents for molecular and receptor imaging in the brain supplant PET? The answer in part depends upon an unresolved question: Does hyperpolarization of ^{13}C within a small-molecule imaging reagent survive tight binding with a protein receptor? Third, can we make a "virtue of necessity," given the (generally) very brief survival time of all hyperpolarized reagents (the exception is silicon, discussed later), by inquiring whether imaging the first 1–100s of any biological event is more informative than the current norm? Traditional understanding of *in vivo* kinetics in biochemistry revolves around the limitations of many current medical diagnostic procedures applied at 30 min to 24 h. These technologies are therefore likely to record only stable genetic or molecular transformations—slower events that result from enzyme induction. It is highly likely that ultrafast MR imaging with hyperpolarizing techniques could be informative in several pathological settings, e.g., for hypoxic injury in brain and other tissues where we know that outcome is strongly dependent upon resupplying oxygen and substrates at the earliest possible moment. An example of new information provided by hyperpolarized MR is already available from the (isolated) ischemic heart (Merritt, et al. 2008). Using [1-^{13}C] pyruvate hyperpolarized by DNP to P > 10% investigators were able to monitor recovery of the isolated

perfused rat heart exposed to global hypoxia, with 1s time resolution. It took fully 20 min for the hypoxic injury to pyruvic dehydrogenase to be reversed. A similar pattern is to be expected in pathological hypoxic insults to the brain, from cardiac arrest to stroke and near-drowning. Conventional proton MRS, which has been widely used to explore this point, provides time resolutions of hours or days. An additional set of physiological questions relevant to modern neurology is whether subsecond ^{13}C MRS of the brain *in vivo* might throw light on the epilepsy syndromes. These are broadly understood to involve electrical events ("seizures") of approximately 10s to 2 min duration, but are in turn, subserved by events in the neuronal–axonal glutamine glutamate (GABA) cycle, which can currently only be observed using proton, direct, or indirect detection of administered ^{13}C, with time resolution of many minutes or hours. These few examples are offered in part as an argument that hyperpolarized NMR, if it is to be harnessed for biomedical research and clinical practice, needs a wider range of scientific and clinical medical input than it has received so far. Conventional MRI, first implemented in the mid-1970s, has had many thousands of exponents and is exposed to hundreds of relevant clinical questions every day to achieve its present dominance in medical imaging. *In vivo* spectroscopy using conventional (Boltzmann) MR, while less "popular" than anatomic and physiological MRI, nevertheless is practiced in hundreds, or even thousands of laboratories and hospitals worldwide and followed a similar trajectory over decades. The unfortunate term "killer app" describes the watershed event in every new technology before commercial and biomedical interests coincide to establish the field. We have not yet seen this for hyperpolarized MRI or MRS, and certainly not in neuroscience. The greatest advances have been seen elsewhere—cardiology, oncology, hepatology, and nephrology—in which several medical and scientific reviews have been made available. Literature in neurology and neuroscience is somewhat sparse. Perhaps summarizing the successes achieved by the handful of investigators currently involved will entice hundreds more to enter the field and apply their innovations. This chapter is designed to attract those still on the sidelines.

But, what is the way forward? Brain imaging, neurochemistry, and human neuroscience generally have been major beneficiaries of the NMR revolution. One needs to look no further than the Boltzmann and Bloch equations for inspiration in pulse sequence designs that have fueled these advances. Coupled with engineering advances, including higher and more homogeneous magnetic fields and speedier gradient rise times and radiofrequency electronics, conventional proton brain MRI contrast has evolved far beyond the initial concepts of proton density, T_1, and T_2 relaxation. Localized and "edited" proton, ^{13}C, and ^{15}N MRS and other multinuclear approaches have illuminated *in vivo* brain chemistry in laboratory animals and human subjects and broadly changed our perceptions with new knowledge in those fields (Ross & Bluml, 2001). The Achilles heel of MR remains its frustratingly low signal achieved at even the highest currently available magnetic fields in superconducting magnets (not to mention the attendant increase in purchase, operating, and maintenance costs associated with ultrahigh fields for human use). The delivered MR signal remains somewhat less than three orders of magnitude lower than that provided by PET, a competitive technology that dominates the field of "molecular neuroimaging." Thus, MR needs to be three orders of magnitude more sensitive in order to perform molecular imaging applications presently limited to PET. Hyperpolarization offers a potentially disruptive technology that can employ the existing installed base of 10,000 clinical low and mid-field MR scanners. Dramatically enhanced nuclear alignment has been observed for several of the techniques to be described and in practice reaches 30–40%, a signal enhancement of 30- to 40,000-fold.

Here we describe the first generation of *in vivo* brain imaging and spectroscopy studies utilizing such methods with an emphasis on new neuroscience thereby illuminated. Fig. 4.3.1 stratifies the approaches taken to date, and may be referred to as hypothesis-driven hyperpolarization. Hyperpolarization cannot be achieved directly *in vivo*. All of the known hyperpolarization techniques involve administration of a contrast agent, most of which have half-lives *in vivo* of 1 min or less. Usually referred to as T_1, this term is measured only approximately, even *in vitro*, and when incorporated into a complex *in vivo* MR study suffers from several additional approximations. Most hyperpolarized nuclei fall within the range of 20–60s T_1. If we allow that *in vivo* MR images and spectra might be acquired during $5 \times T_1$, current experimental studies must be completed within 5 min. The subject of prolongation of T_1 by introduction of the singlet state and other techniques (Tayler et al., 2012) is beyond the scope of this review. Largely as a consequence of the privileged status of brain and the blood–brain barrier (BBB), circulation time may exceed 20s during which much of the available enhanced MR signal has been consumed; neurological applications of *in vivo* hyperpolarized MR lag somewhat behind other fields. Based on circulation times *in vivo*, oncology, cardiology, and metabolic imaging of peripheral tissues and organs have been pursued with somewhat greater vigor. A description toward the end of this chapter of some of those non-neurological applications is provided as a "roadmap" of potential future work within the brain.

Physics and Chemistry of Hyperpolarized MR

Fig. 4.3.2 illustrates the leading methods available. Fig. 4.3.3 encapsulates, in simplified form, the chemistry and spin physics that underlies each of the methods of which complete details are available in several more exhaustive reviews.

Optical pumping for noble-gas MRI, DNP, and parahydrogen-induced polarization (PHIP; with its earlier more poetical acronyms PASADENA and ALTADENA, respectively, parahydrogen and synthesis) allow dramatically enhanced nuclear alignment or, adiabatic longitudinal alignment; Signal Amplification by Reversible Exchange (SABRE) is a more recent alternative parahydrogen technique whereby MR polarization is reported to reach 1000-fold and "brute-force" (Millikelvin Corporation) for which no *in vivo* data are currently available. Some understandable "spin-inflation" surrounds estimates of efficacy of polarization for each technique in available publications, but certainly 1–10% P are likely already achieved *in vitro*. Attempts at neuroimaging *in vivo* in smaller or larger animals have been published for each method, but human neuroimaging has been demonstrated effectively only with optical pumping of the noble gasses helium or xenon. Chronologically, DNP, the earliest biomedical technique, evolved from the initially controversial, eponymous observations of A. H. Overhauser (Overhauser, 1953) that nuclear spins can arise from interaction with the much higher spin difference associated with electrons. Known and employed for many years within solids, the crucial "breakthrough" by Ardenkjaer-Larsen et al. (2003) was a simple method of dissolution into aqueous environment while retaining a high proportion of "enhanced" spins. This has allowed exploitation of DNP *in vivo*. Two DNP technologies, Hypersense (Oxford Biotools) and SPINLab (GE Healthcare) were commercialized under a range of patents for *in vitro*, *in vivo* (small animals), and (ultimately) for human use. The almost universal ^{13}C-DNP biomolecule of interest has been [1-^{13}C]pyruvic acid, with more than 100 published accounts dominating the literature (Chen et al., 2012). Versatility of DNP has further been demonstrated across a much wider range of ^{13}C, ^{15}N-enriched precursors, and intrinsic ^{31}P, most of which await systematic evaluation.

Two DNP techniques for hyperpolarization have been described that are not dependent upon the method of rapid aqueous dissolution currently limited for use by subsequent patents (GE Healthcare). Hyperpolarization by DNP of water itself with *in vivo*

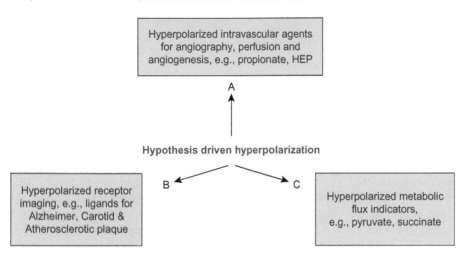

FIGURE 4.3.1 The three major arms of hyperpolarization research. A roadmap for introduction of hyperpolarization into *in vivo* biomedical research: the initial agenda included significant clinical utility.

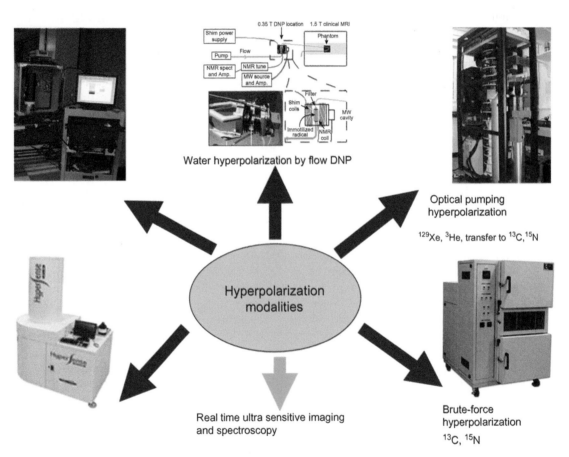

FIGURE 4.3.2 Different modalities of hyperpolarization. Several practical implementations of hyperpolarizing technologies are available to investigators engaged in exploring this novel advance in MRI and MRS.

brain imaging was recently reported (McCarney et al., 2007); *in vivo* imaging of hyperpolarized silicon particles and nanoparticles in noncerebral structures has also been achieved. The latter represents a major advance in confirming a technique for generating a hyperpolarized imaging reagent, which allows MR signal to persist *in vivo* for up to 1 h; at present all previous methods are limited to no more than a couple of minutes of *in vivo* imaging.

The special advantages of silicon nanoparticles for prolongation of hyperpolarization by DNP were realized only recently and confirmed by *in vivo* imaging by Cassidy et al. (2013). Parahydrogen-based techniques also have a long history, following the discovery in

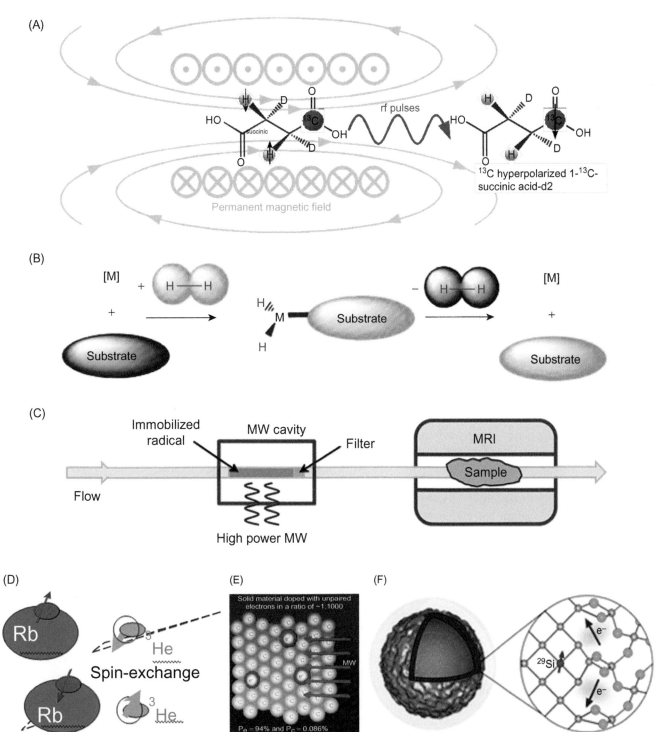

FIGURE 4.3.3 Mechanism of spin polarization in different hyperpolarization modalities. (A) Polarization transfer by radiofrequency from parahydrogen to ^{13}C nucleus in PHIP. (B) SABRE method of polarization transfer. (C) Continuous flow DNP method of hyperpolarizing (^1H) water by immobilized radicals. (D) Hyperpolarization of xenon gas. (E) DNP hyperpolarization of ^{13}C nucleus by free radical. (F) Radical free method of DNP hyperpolarization of ^{29}Si nuclear spins via unbonded electrons naturally occurring at the silicon−silicon dioxide interface.

1929 (Bonhoeffer & Harteck, 1929) that gaseous hydrogen exists in two forms with a huge difference in spin-distribution between ortho (low) and para (high) states. Initially harnessed by Bowers and Weitekamp (Abragam et al., 1976; Bowers & Weitekamp, 1986; Natterer & Bargon, 1997) (who baptized their two hyperpolarization paths with two California city names mentioned previously, now largely replaced by the general term PHIP introduced by Natterer). The technique initially described predicts the restrictive double- and triple-bond chemistry, specialized symmetrical hydrogenation reaction catalysis, and subtle ultralow-field NMR spin-physics required in this family of hyperpolarization techniques employed to transfer parahydrogen polarization to ^{13}C. These strict chemical requirements distinguish PHIP from DNP for which a wider range of ^{13}C or ^{15}N molecular targets was described earlier. Initially explored for surface chemistry and catalysis (Natterer & Bargon, 1997), it was many years before a practical device for transfer of the "spins" of parahydrogen, first to second nucleus, proton, and then to a third nucleus, ^{13}C, was encapsulated into a portable parahydrogen polarizer by investigators in the research laboratories of Nycomed-Amersham in Malmo, Sweden (Goldman, 2006). The first published *in vivo* MR image, a rat tail vein and inferior vena cava, using ^{13}C-parahydrogen was short lived (subsecond) not solely because reagent T_1 was necessarily short, but because toxic solvents and contrast agents were employed resulting in the speedy demise of the research subject. Subsequently parahydrogen-based hyperpolarized MR angiography became available, employing an aqueous, nontoxic but non-metabolizable reagent (Goldman, 2006), while Bhattacharya et al. (2005) demonstrated the first *in vivo* "survival" experiments with parahydrogen-hyperpolarized MR of a metabolizable, nontoxic, water-soluble biomolecule. These ingredients appeared to validate PHIP as a potentially disruptive addition to MRI. The "creative" catalysis and double-bond chemistry necessary to the discovery of useable biomolecules, and the absence of a commercial provider of parahydrogen generators, polarizers, and a nontoxic catalyst have restricted the scope of *in vivo* MR research with this technique to a small number of laboratories worldwide. SABRE, a parahydrogen technique that eliminates the catalytic step and has less rigorous chemical requirements, achieves less dramatic P values (Adams et al., 2009), but appears poised for transfer to *in vivo* use.

Nevertheless, the benefit of PHIP compared to DNP is the very short time required to generate the contrast reagent. Each polarization is achieved in seconds, compared to several hours for DNP, and at considerably lower cost of operation (millitesla magnetic field, close to ambient temperature, and no cryogens

are employed in the polarization process). For DNP, special equipment is required and while commercial equipment costs may ultimately fall, currently commercially available DNP polarizers are costly and the process, which must occur near zero temperature and at high magnetic field (the process requires two spectrometers), consumes large amounts of liquid helium, which is becoming increasingly expensive, for each "run." Optical pumping to hyperpolarize noble gases achieves its object of transferring spins from electrons to nuclei with laser-light irradiation of rubidium and commercial equipment (albeit at substantial cost) and is available to achieve this in quantities sufficient for human lung imaging *in vivo* to which may now be added applications in rodent and human brain. ^{129}Xe provides a variety of forms of contrast for this purpose but no direct metabolism. Transfer of the high spin-order achieved in a gas, to a more metabolically interesting biomolecule, [1-^{13}C]acetate has recently been achieved (Lisitza et al., 2009) so that wider metabolic imaging applications can be anticipated.

Brute-force is one of the underlying principles of DNP, in that at exceptionally high magnetic fields and near-absolute zero temperature many molecules become hyperpolarized. So, as long as this stringent condition is maintained, the increased spin states of ^{13}C-enriched compounds are thereby polarized. Transport and delivery to a biological imaging environment remains an unsolved challenge to this "simple" hyperpolarization technology. Indeed it should be noted that for all current hyperpolarization studies, the ultrashort life times add a challenge for *in vivo* and ultimately for clinical applications. Sterile laboratory facilities, already a feature of nuclear medicine and PET enterprises, would now be necessary for MR. This too from a practical standpoint raises the cost per study since more personnel need to be involved than in a standard MRI.

In summary, research to explore the biomedical uses of hyperpolarization is currently predominantly supported by DNP. PHIP is, however, much faster to achieve—seconds compared to several hours for completion of hyperpolarization using DNP and PHIP—and unlike DNP can be accomplished at close to room temperature and with a very low magnetic field. Overall this limits the equipment costs associated with a PHIP program probably one order of magnitude lower ($50,000 start-up vs. $500,000 for DNP or optical pumping of noble gases).

Harnessing hyperpolarization for translational animal and human *in vivo* MR initially stimulated enormous advances in ultrafast imaging and spectroscopy of ^{13}C, including selective excitation for unambiguous detection of the fast-decaying hyperpolarized agent and its principal metabolites. New ultrafast ^{13}C imaging methods now appear continuously in MR literature (for review, see Kurhanewicz et al., 2011; Mayer et al., 2011). Unresolved challenges include the extreme brevity of enhanced signal (30–60s), which is much shorter than conventional PET ligands, with the sole exception of silicon nanoparticles, which survive in a hyperpolarized state for at least 30 min *in vivo* (Cassidy et al., 2013). Spin physics and chemistry offer potential solutions to prolongation of T_1 decay. Deuteration of the imaging agent, addition of gadolinium (Gd) to the DNP mix during polarization, and substitution of ^{15}N for ^{13}C each offer marginal improvements (Bhattacharya et al., 2008). The current "holy grail" of the entire field of *in vivo* research is prolongation of a singlet state by a variety of novel methods, including chemical design. None can currently claim to be practical. Of greatest importance, however, for MRS is that hyperpolarized spins would be preserved through enzymatic processes as predicted by the magnetization transfer experiments of Forsen and Hoffman (1963) now confirmed in direct experiments with hyperpolarized molecules (Tyler, 2011). That the elevated spin state can be transmitted and preserved through single enzyme steps and then through multiple steps was verified early in practice and *in vivo* for DNP, using [1-^{13}C]pyruvate conversion to lactate, alanine, and bicarbonate and for parahydrogen, observing conversion of [1-^{13}C]succinate or [1-^{13}C]diethyl succinate to various Krebs cycle intermediates (Zacharias, et al., 2012).

Surprisingly, a high polarization state has been observed after lipid binding of specially designed hyperpolarized reagents *in vitro* and *in vivo*. This is most likely due to increased T_1 as a consequence of reduced mobility. The authors believe these reactions to be analogous to the binding of atheroma plaques (Bhattacharya et al., 2011). Since these biological reactions are, in turn, believed to involve tight binding equivalent to that involved in specific receptor binding of neurotransmitters, these results lead to the hope for hyperpolarized MRI of receptors in brain and other tissues, an application currently reserved for PET imaging. Biological test systems for hyperpolarization physiological science continue to expand, from isolated cells, spheroids in tissue culture, isolated perfused organs, particularly heart and liver, to whole living animals by various injection routes (intravenous, intra-arterial, intraperitoneal and oral), and explants of foreign and syngeneic tumor cell lines in normal and "nude" mice to larger rodents, porcine and canine patients, and up to and including humans. It must be admitted that hyperpolarized MR neuroscience has lagged and the number and variety of *in vivo* neurological applications is still small. This is partly as a result of the privileged position of the brain, behind an effective BBB, which the unusual chemicals developed cross with difficulty, if at all. This is an area ripe for innovation. In addition, despite its very high

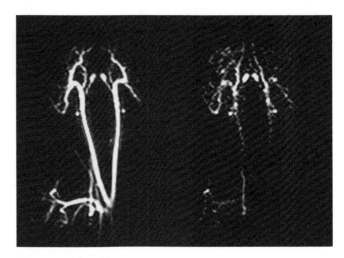

FIGURE 4.3.4 Real-time *in vivo* ^{13}C PHIP images of carotid artery and major blood vessels of a pig brain acquired at 1.5 T. Two images of a time-lapse series obtained subsequent to a single injection of aqueous hydroxyethyl propionate (1,^{13}C) with initial polarization P = 0.48. The scan time of each image was 0.7s.

blood flow, the transit time (2.8s in the rat, longer in man) across the brain exceeds the average T_1 of the currently available hyperpolarized contrast agents. In order to be useful in neurospectroscopic applications, further barriers and additional time is required for the agent to enter the appropriate brain cell or compartment and undergo further metabolism. Neurological studies were therefore initially focused on the vasculature and only more recently on metabolism and spectroscopy.

Hyperpolarized Cerebral Angiography and Perfusion

Excellent "real-time" ^{13}C angiography in rodents and in an anesthetized porcine (Fig. 4.3.4) was an early success, despite the lethal mixture of acetone solvent, toxic contrast agent, and rhodium-containing catalyst all of which militated against a long-term future for the method. The ultimate advantages in *in vivo* angiography with ^{13}C MRI over currently available methods are discussed in Golman et al., 2003. Hyperpolarized xenon, with more than a decade of safe human lung imaging (Albert et al., 1994), has also been an effective means of quantifying cerebral blood flow and perfusion. The recent application in humans (Killian et al., 2004; and see Fig. 4.3.5A) is a promising advance. Hyperpolarized xenon functional MRI in rats provided greater signal contrast in response to a prolonged pain stimulus than the equivalent blood oxygenation level-dependent proton MRI (Mazzanti et al., 2011; see Fig. 4.3.5B), an indication of new discoveries to come in clinical neurology when coupled with Killian et al.'s (2004) translation of hyperpolarized xenon imaging to human brain.

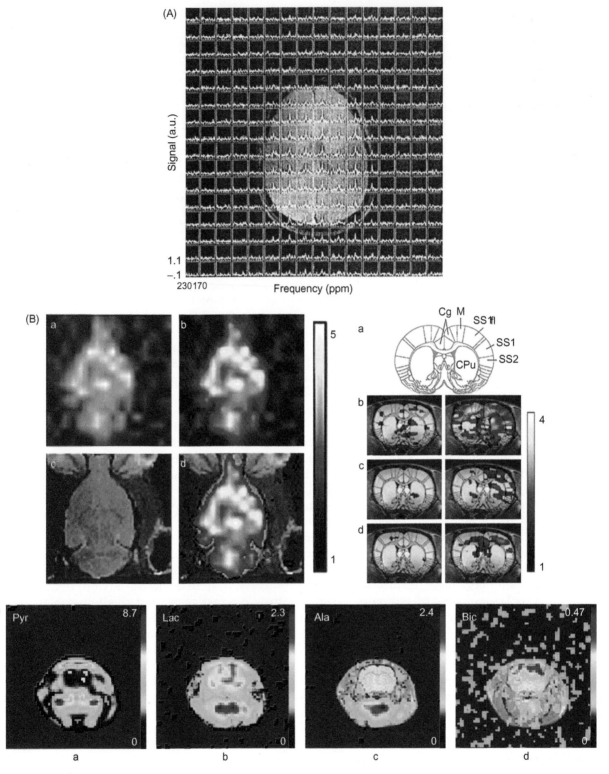

FIGURE 4.3.5 (A) Dynamic NMR spectroscopy of hyperpolarized ^{129}Xe in human brain. (Adapted from Kilian et al., 2004). (B) I. Hyperpolarized ^{129}Xe distribution in the rat brain. (a) Hyperpolarized ^{129}Xe chemical shift imaging (CSI) image acquired with a 2D CSI pulse sequence from rat head under normal breathing conditions (slice thickness 10 mm). (b) Same image with false color applied. Warmer colors indicate increased hyperpolarized ^{129}Xe signal intensity. (c) Proton MRI of a rat head showing a 1 mm coronal slice through the brain acquired with a RARE pulse sequence. (d) Proton image shown with overlay of hyperpolarized ^{129}Xe MRI, in which only hyperpolarized ^{129}Xe signal with a signal-to-noise ratio (SNR) >2 are shown. FOV was 25 mm. II. Hyperpolarized ^{129}Xe fMRI data from three animals. The ^{129}Xe signal is shown as a false color overlay on the corresponding 1 mm thick coronal proton reference image taken from the same animal. The left panel

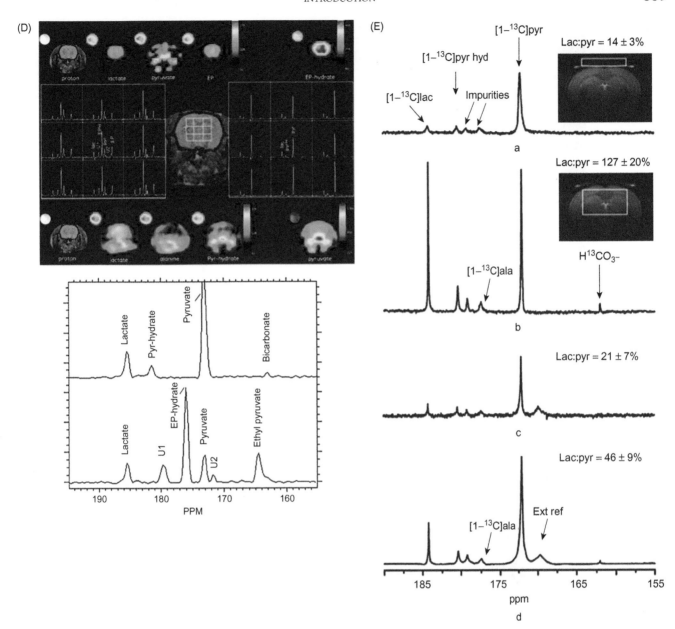

FIGURE 4.3.5 (*Continued*)

shows hyperpolarized ^{129}Xe signal intensity during baseline and the right panel shows hyperpolarized ^{129}Xe signal intensity after injection of capsaicin 20 µl (3 mg/mL) into the right forepaw. Color scale represents SNR and only signal with SNR >2 are shown. Superimposition of a rat brain atlas demarcates specific areas of the brain: Cg, cingulate cortex; M, motor cortex; SS1, SS1 fl, primary somatosensory cortex and SS1 forelimb region; SS2, secondary somatosensory cortex; CPu, striatum. (Adapted from Mazzanti et al. 2011.) (C) High-resolution brain metabolic maps acquired with three-shot spiral CSI (nominal FOV = 48 × 48 mm²) of (a) pyruvate, (b) lactate, (c) alanine, and (d) bicarbonate superimposed onto the corresponding ^{1}H-FSE image. The images were acquired 27s after the start of the injection of DNP hyperpolarized [1-^{13}C] pyruvate via tail vein. Data were averaged over four injections. (Adapted from Mayer et al., 2011.) (D) Metabolic images of [1-^{13}C]ethyl pyruvate and [1-^{13}C]pyruvate are compared at an image delay of 20s in a rat brain. Metabolite maps for the ethyl pyruvate (EP) injection are shown across the top, and maps for the pyruvate injection, across the bottom. Phased and baseline-corrected spectral array for a 3 × 3 grid of brain voxels is illustrated in the center, along with the voxel positions on a reference image. Left center shows an annotated spectral grid for the EP injection and right center shows an annotated spectral grid for the pyruvate injection. The figure also shows an expanded and annotated brain region of interest spectra from the EP run (bottom) and pyruvate run (top). (Adapted from Hurd et al., 2010.) (E) Hyperpolarized MRS in rat brain. Single-shot *in vivo* ^{1}H decoupled ^{13}C spectra acquired 9s after beginning of injection of hyperpolarized solution of [1-^{13}C] pyruvate via tail vein with (a) LASER sequence from 216 µL (9 × 1.6 × 16 mm³) voxel containing muscle and subcutaneous tissue (insert: RARE image of a rat brain showing the position and size of the localized volume), (b) LASER sequence from 405 µL (9 × 5 × 9 mm³) voxel

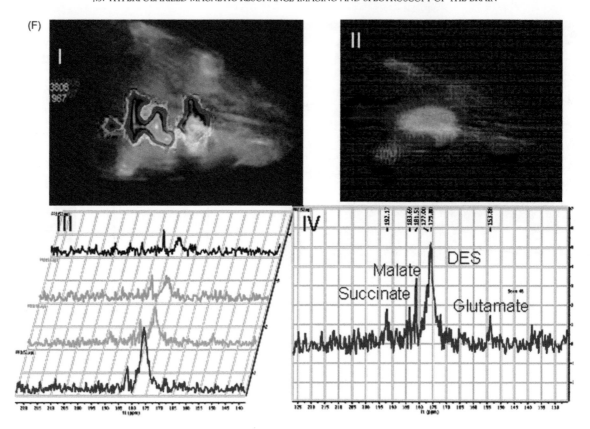

FIGURE 4.3.5   (*Continued*)

Direct Structural and Biochemical Imaging of Hyperpolarized ^{13}C and Other Heteronuclei in the Brain

Hyperpolarized heteronuclear imaging may appear to be a mere luxury compared to the high intrinsic hydrogen signal already provided at Boltzmann polarization by water-proton MRI. However, direct imaging of neurochemicals based on selective excitation of protons (e.g., *N*-acetylaspartate), ^{31}P (e.g., PCr and magnetization transfer of creatine kinase activity), has been useful, and understanding regional distribution of any ^{13}C imaging agent is a prerequisite of metabolic understanding. Single-shot ^{13}C images of injected intravenous hyperpolarized ^{13}C-maleate, [1-^{13}C]succinate, and [1-^{13}C]diethyl succinate as well as DNP-hyperpolarized [1-^{13}C]pyruvate and [1-^{13}C]acetate and its principal metabolites have been captured. While this has generally been a stepping stone to the primary purpose of real-time metabolic ^{13}C spectroscopy, it was an early claim among experts that hyperpolarization would eliminate the need for "spectra" since *in vivo* imaging would generate anatomically relevant maps of metabolism (for review, see Golman

containing only brain tissue (insert: RARE image of a rat brain showing the position and size of the localized volume), (c) small-flip angle pulse-acquire (4.5° at the center of the coil), and (d) 90° adiabatic BIR4 pulse-acquire. All spectra are shown with 2 Hz line broadening. The lactate to pyruvate ratio for each spectrum is reported on the right side. ala, alanine. (Adapted from Marjańska et al., 2010.) (F) Real-time biodistribution of the PHIP hyperpolarized diethyl succinate (DES) reveals that the compound is delivered to the brain of the rat by carotid arterial injection (I). The hyperpolarized succinate signal from the inflowing blood allowed for ^{13}C imaging and spectroscopy up to 1 min after injection. The majority of the hyperpolarized signal within the brain of the animal is also observed with ^{13}C CSI (II). ^{13}C MRS of the brain localized by the coil shows the formation of multiple downstream TCA cycle metabolic products from the injection of the hyperpolarized DES identified as succinate, malate, and glutamate (III and IV). (G) Representative anatomical images and the corresponding magnitude spectra from a hyperpolarized ^{13}C 2D MRSI study of a rat-implanted human glioblastoma (U-87 MG) xenograft, injected with [1-^{13}C] pyruvate. Axial T_1 post-Gd images within the MRSI slice show contrast-enhancing lesion inside the brain (a). These 1.2 mm thick axial images represent a fraction of volume that contributed to the ^{13}C signal acquired from a 10 mm slice. The white and black boxes represent the voxels around the brain and inside the brain, respectively. The corresponding magnitude spectra (b) and the zoomed-in spectra around the brain (c) clearly showed elevated ^{13}C lactate and pyruvate levels in the tumor (highlighted voxels in the black box in c) compared with the brain tissue in the contralateral hemisphere and, most important, the brain tissue from the normal rats. An axial T_1 pre-Gd image (d) and T_2 FSE images in axial, coronal, and sagittal planes (e–g) are also shown. (Adapted from Park et al., 2010.)

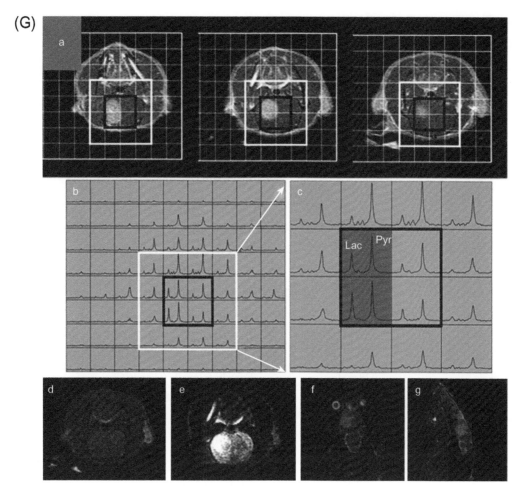

(G)

FIGURE 4.3.5 *(Continued)*

et al., 2003; Fig. 4.3.5C). An intensive investigation of the distribution of individual hyperpolarized reagents that cross the BBB and enter brain cells will be needed to define the possible role of such hyperpolarized ^{13}C imaging. An intermediate approach has already been explored, constructed on the properties of Xenon-129. This agent is widely distributed throughout the rodent (and human) brain, differentially so between white and gray matter. Readily demonstrated with Xenon-129 spectroscopy (Fig. 4.3.5A) there are four distinct resonance frequencies and two different T_1 times arising from brain, non-brain, blood, or gaseous compartments (Zhou et al., 2011).

Ultrafast ^{13}C MR Spectroscopy of Hyperpolarized Neurometabolites

Table 4.3.1 lists the brain concentration of likely identifiable target molecules. Table 4.3.2 lists those ^{13}C-enriched cerebral metabolites (more than 25) that have already been identified in a hyperpolarized state

in vivo, and Fig. 4.3.6 links these intermediates with their well-known metabolic pathways. The central hypothesis guiding research with hyperpolarized reagents is that the sensitivity limitation governing ^{13}C and ^{15}N MR neuroscience will be overcome once the 10,000-fold signal enhancement can be harnessed. A simple calculation explains that ^{13}C nuclei at ambient concentrations of 1–5 mM (e.g., glutamate and glutamine during human studies with precursors [1-^{13}C]glucose or [1-^{13}C]acetate) could be imaged with water proton sensitivity (40 M) when amplified 10- to 20,000-fold. Proof of principle in neuroimaging applications has been achieved in the intact rodent brain *in vivo* for [1-^{13}C]succinate (for parahydrogen methods) and [1-^{13}C]pyruvate (for DNP), with ample supporting evidence based on isolated glioma cells and explanted brain tumors. Selected *in vivo* brain studies are described here.

Hyperpolarized [1-^{13}C]ethyl pyruvate appears superior to [1-^{13}C]pyruvate, which preceded it as a metabolic neuroimaging agent, based upon higher

TABLE 4.3.1   Reported Tissue Concentrations of Important Brain Chemicals

Compound	Concentration
2-Oxoglutarate	0.2 mM*
Succinate	0.33/2.5 mM(hypoxia)*
Fumarate	0.075 mM*
Malate	0.25 mM
Malate mouse	0.44 mM
Oxaloacetate	0.004 mM
Citrate	0.25 mM
Isocitrate	0.015 mM
Pyruvate	0.1 mM
Lactate	2.0 mM
Glycogen (frog brain)	20 mM
Glucose	1–2 mM
Glucose-6-phosphate	0.15 mM
Glucose 1:6 diphosphate	0.075 mM
Fructose 1:6 diphosphate	0.10 mM
Fructose-6-phosphate	0.050 mM
Glycerol phosphate	0.04 mM
Phosphoenolpyruvate	0.005 mM
Amino acids etc.	
Alanine	0.5 mM*
Aspartate	2.5 mM
NAA	6 mM
Glutamine	5 mM*
Glutamate	10 mM*
Ammonia	0.4 mM
Coenzyme A	0.025 mM
Acetyl coenzyme A	0.01 mM
Acetylcarnitine	> 0.01 mM
Carnitine	0.25 mM
β-Hydroxybutyrate	?
Acetone	?
Bicarbonate	11 mM
Hydroxymethylglutaryl coenzyme A	0.025 mM (liver)

Indicates observed in brain in vivo.

TABLE 4.3.2   Hyperpolarized ^{13}C Molecules Observed in (Rodent) Brain In Vivo

Neurochemical	Method
[1-^{13}C]pyruvate	
[1-^{13}C]ethyl pyruvate	DNP
Alanine	DNP
HCO$_3$/CO$_2$/pH	DNP/PHIP
Lactate	DNP
Keto-isocaproic acid	DNP
Leucine	DNP
[2-^{13}C]pyruvate	DNP
Succinate	PHIP
Glutamate postmortem	PHIP
Glutamine postmortem	PHIP
Maleate	PHIP
Fumarate	DNP/PHIP
Malate	DNP/PHIP
Dehydroascorbate (vitamin C)	DNP
2-Oxoglutarate (C2 + C5)	DNP
[1-^{13}C]acetate	DNP
[2-^{13}C]acetate	DNP
Diethyl succinate	PHIP
Unidentified products	
Xenon and xenon products	Optical pumping

More than 25 hyperpolarized ^{13}C-labeled intermediates have been detected in the *in vivo* (rodent) brain.

lipophilicity and BBB transit (Fig. 4.3.5D; Hurd et al., 2010). Once within the brain, it is presumed that a nonspecific esterase releases pyruvate, because the ^{13}C-enriched intermediates alanine, lactate, and bicarbonate, which rapidly appear in ^{13}C spectra, are identical to those previously encountered in studies in which [1-^{13}C]pyruvate was the substrate (Fig. 4.3.5E). Each of the metabolic products confirms a well-established truth concerning brain metabolism: pyruvate transport into mitochondria where pyruvate dehydrogenase is located, an active alanine transaminase and ubiquitous lactic dehydrogenase in the cytosol of both neurons and astrocytes. ^{13}C-enriched TCA cycle intermediates have not been observed. However, as first demonstrated in practice for the isolated perfused rat heart (Tyler, 2011), substitution of [2-^{13}C] pyruvate results in the rapid enrichment of TCA cycle intermediates. This result was demonstrated in one of two published reports (Hurd et al, 2010); the other (Marjańska et al., 2010) is negative on this point indicating the need for careful confirmation of each "new" observation in this burgeoning field. Clear differentiation between TCA cycles of neuronal and glial metabolism of a hyperpolarized precursor has been obtained with both [1-^{13}C] and [2-^{13}C]-enriched hyperpolarized

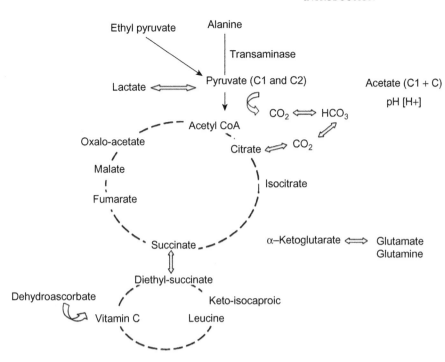

FIGURE 4.3.6 Metabolic pathways of brain illuminated by hyperpolarized MR techniques 2001–2012.

acetate. In each case the product is somewhat surprisingly 2-oxoglutarate, enriched appropriately at C5 or C2 positions (Mishkovsky et al., 2011). While in one sense the result is anticipated—an acetate transporter is available on glia but not on neurons—in another it is unexpected. Why 2-oxoglutarate but not glutamate or glutamine are detected, as in conventional ^{13}C acetate studies is unclear, but it may have something to do with the enormous and unphysiological concentrations of hyperpolarized acetate provided to the brain. The K_m of 2-oxoglutarate dehydrogenase for its substrate is 25 mM, whereas the ambient concentrations could well be much higher in the artificial conditions of the study. An even clearer demonstration of enrichment of TCA cycle intermediates with hyperpolarized ^{13}C was provided when the rodent brain was provided with excess hyperpolarized TCA cycle substrates succinate or diethyl succinate, hyperpolarized using parahydrogen. Zacharias and colleagues (2012) reported their study as follows (see Fig. 4.3.5F, I–IV):

> The goal of this research is to use hyperpolarized diethyl succinate to detect metabolism in a rat brain as well as to demonstrate that the compound crosses the blood-brain barrier. The main limitation for imaging agents to be used in the brain is their ability to cross the blood-brain barrier (BBB). We observed limited transport of the charged molecule succinate across the BBB in earlier studies. Neutral and hydrophobic compounds are known to have better transport through the BBB. The neutral compound hyperpolarized diethyl succinate has the potential of being an affective imaging agent for the brain. Diethyl 1-^{13}C 2,3-d$_2$ succinate is generated through the hydrogenation of diethyl 1-^{13}C 2,3-d$_2$ fumarate and hyperpolarized by PHIP (parahydrogen induced polarization) method, which increases the ^{13}C MR signal by 5000 fold. We have previously employed hyperpolarized diethyl succinate to image and observe real time metabolism in normal and tumor-bearing mice. Using ^{13}C MRS, metabolism of diethyl succinate in the Tricarboxylic Acid Cycle (TCA cycle) was observed in normal animals after a 10 micro-mol tail vein injection.
>
> We utilized PHIP to hyperpolarize diethyl 1-^{13}C 2,3-d$_2$ succinate in a custom-built polarizer and the hyperpolarized solution was injected via the carotid artery of normal male Sprague Dawley rat (N = 3) in near physiological concentrations (10-20 micromol). A ^{1}H/^{13}C dual resonance 4 cm ID solenoid volume coil was utilized for ^{13}C hyperpolarized in vivo imaging and spectroscopy. ^{13}C FISP sequence with a flip angle of 60o, FOV 6 or 7 cm, and slice thickness of 15.2 mm was used to observe the biodistribution of the compound. ^{13}C CSI with a 1 ms gauss pulse, 200 ms TR, 8 × 8 or 16 × 16 matrix, FOV ranging from 2.64 cm to 4 cm, slice thickness of 8 to 12 mm was used. CSI was processed using 3DiCSI software (Columbia University, Qui Zhao). The detection of the compound within the brain was determined using a simple pulse and acquire ^{13}C sequence. All ^{13}C imaging and spectroscopy was done on a horizontal bore Bruker Avance 4.7T animal scanner. Real time bio-distribution of the hyperpolarized compound reveals that diethyl succinate (DS) is delivered to the brain of the rat after carotid arterial injection. The hyperpolarized succinate signal from the inflowing blood allowed for ^{13}C imaging and spectroscopy up to 1 minute after injection. The hyperpolarized signal within the brain of the animal is also observed with ^{13}C CSI. ^{13}C MR spectroscopy of the brain localized by the coil shows the formation of multiple downstream TCA cycle metabolic products from the injection of the hyperpolarized diethylsuccinate (DS) identified as succinate, malate and glutamate.

That study confirmed that diethyl succinate crosses the BBB and, as a result, is a promising hyperpolarized metabolic imaging agent for studying the TCA cycle in brain.

Table 4.3.1, a summary of experimentally obtained cerebral metabolite concentrations, allows a formal comparison to be made with the early observations with hyperpolarized MR (Table 4.3.2; Fig. 4.3.6). This information may also govern which hyperpolarized metabolites will be observed in the future under experimental conditions *in vivo*, since by analogy with conventional ^{13}C and ^{15}N stable isotope studies, three factors—polarization, "P," fractional enrichment, and concentration—determine MR "visibility."

It is instructive to compare the preliminary PHIP study with more comprehensive studies of intermediary metabolism in the intact brain, employing [1-^{13}C] pyruvate or [1-^{13}C]ethyl pyruvate hyperpolarized by DNP (Hurd et al. 2010; Park et al., 2010). These latter studies are the first to have tackled the question of the origin, within the intact brain, of hyperpolarized metabolic signal. They concluded in the case of pyruvate that almost 100% remains within the vasculature, with undetectable ^{13}C pyruvate and only its metabolic product(s), principally ^{13}C lactate, providing intracerebral signal. The origin of ^{13}C diethyl succinate signal, on the other hand, remains unknown at this time. Nevertheless, it is reasonable to assume that its metabolic products, ^{13}C malate, glutamate, and succinate, are predominantly to be found within the brain. A second difference between these two seminal studies of neurological hyperpolarization concerns the concentrations of the precursor administered—only 10–20 μmol of ^{13}C diethyl succinate were given versus (perhaps) 160–240 μmol [1-^{13}C]pyruvic acid. Both numbers definitely "exceed" any physiologically meaningful stimulus; diethyl succinate is not a relevant physiological substrate, but even if totally converted to succinate as is probable, it would represent a 10-fold excess over the ambient brain concentration, reported (see Table 4.3.2) to be 0.5–2 mM, the higher number referring to the marked increase in ambient concentration of succinate in the brain exposed to hypoxia. The much higher concentrations of pyruvate administered must exceed any reasonable estimation of the measured intracerebral concentration 1000-fold, but, since as more recently established (see earlier), almost 100% the administered hyperpolarized ^{13}C pyruvate remains *outside* the brain. This may have less than the anticipated adverse effect on intracerebral redox state or lactate/pyruvate ratio. Indeed, as long as the rate of pyruvate entry is low relative to glycolysis it should not impact the redox state very much during time of measurement.

Thus, among other caveats in incorporating such "new knowledge" into neuroscience regards the almost universally unphysiological conditions applied in hyperpolarization research up to this time. As briefly illustrated earlier, the most important of these is the overwhelming concentration(s) of ^{13}C precursors

supplied to the animals, >100 mM in many cases and to our knowledge, never <10 mM at best. An abstract with the tempting title "How Low Can We Go?" (Bhattacharya et al., 2007b) explored the possibility of ultrafast imaging within physiologically meaningful conditions. Other limitations involve the inclusion in injected contrast agent solutions of ESR reagents (for DNP) and catalysts (for PHIP), some of which have highly toxic profiles. The obvious reason for an experimentalist to employ such high concentrations is the need to rapidly flood the system while the hyperpolarized state persists. This results in the second caveat, in this case probably a bonus in the longer term, that neurochemical changes in flux, when observed apply to approximately the first 100s of *in vivo* events. Previous biochemical studies are rarely available for comparison since incubations, infusions, and steady-state studies that dominate the ^{14}C (radioactive) and ^{13}C (NMR) literature record events over many minutes or hours. Initial attempts to redefine flux measurements suited to hyperpolarization research are discussed further in later sections. Another question which must be addressed is the relevance of tissue-loading studies when the substrate itself may be an exclusively mitochondrial or cytosolic component, arriving by unaccustomed routes after intravenous, intra-arterial, or intraperitoneal administration.

KINETIC ANALYSIS TO DERIVE IN VIVO METABOLIC RATE(S) FROM HYPERPOLARIZED MR STUDIES

The rapid accumulation of spectra possible in hyperpolarized MR studies spurred the search for a direct means of defining *in vivo* flux rates either through single enzymes or through entire metabolic pathways. Precedents include the detailed analyses conducted by Garfinkel and Hess, Chance, and others using radioactive ^{14}C and a succession of elegant studies performed by Mason, Gruetter, Rothman, Shulman, and others employing stable isotope ^{13}C or by Kanamori, employing ^{15}N; mathematical approaches are reviewed by (Rothman et al., 2003; see Chapter 4.2). Unfortunately, as investigators have discovered, hyperpolarized ^{13}C or ^{15}N signals are not as readily amenable to metabolic modeling analysis for rate determination. The challenge is at least threefold. First most prior studies, notably those concerning ^{13}C or ^{15}N flux in *in vivo* rodent and ^{13}C in human brain, have established steady-state conditions. Virtually all hyperpolarized MR studies have been in the form of bolus loading with no metabolic steady state. This is the result of the bulk preparation of reagents in DNP polarizers, at best repeated only every 3–4 h, so that continuous infusion is impractical. Parahydrogen methods may overcome this since new "batches" of hyperpolarized reagents can theoretically be prepared well within the lifetime of previously injected "spins." Bhattacharya and others (unpublished abstract) and Tang et al. (Tang, et al. 2011) propose such an approach but no *in vivo* applications have been described at this time. Second, the short T_1 of hyperpolarized precursors and their enriched metabolic products require special treatment to allow flux calculation, and finally, as is well recognized, the characteristic of conventional NMR whereby multiple excitations can be applied to the detection of ^{13}C, each excitation of hyperpolarized nuclei destroys signal, which is a fact that must be accounted for in any longitudinal timed study.

The most complete treatment of a neurochemical flux rate to date is that published by Hurd et al. (2010) where each of these challenges is addressed for the case of [1-^{13}C]pyruvate loading. After a 12s bolus of 80 mM pyruvate hyperpolarized to perhaps 20%, and administered via tail vein in an anesthetized rat, ^{13}C brain images of pyruvate and of lactate were separately acquired with 3s time resolution. The resulting quantifiable brain spectra were used to define K_d (the rate of transit of pyruvate across the BBB) and the cerebral blood volume (CBV). Both numbers approximated the known values from earlier studies, adding confidence to the subsequent mathematical treatment. Knowledge of the CBV and of the contemporaneous blood concentration of the substrate, ^{13}C pyruvate, permitted the proportion of pyruvate signal that arose from brain to be separated from that in the cerebral blood pool. The authors conclude that virtually 100% of pyruvate signal rose from blood, so that all ^{13}C from intracellular pyruvate had likely been converted instantaneously (i.e., within the 3s time window available through "real-time ^{13}C MRS"), to ^{13}C lactate. This result also appears likely since lactic dehydrogenase activity, which performs the latter process, exceeded the estimated pyruvate transport rate by 30- to 300-fold. This pioneering study offers an avenue whereby future *in vivo* metabolic flux rates might be assayed over very short time periods using hyperpolarization and "smart" imaging techniques. It is perhaps unreasonable to point out the remaining shortcomings of the study, since it was based on delivery of a huge excess of substrate, could not take into account the unphysiological lactate/pyruvate ratio, its impact on pyridine nucleotide redox state NADH/NAD, and other unwanted effects on brain metabolism. These issues require future work.

Other Metabolites and Cerebral Metabolic Pathways

Attempts to use hyperpolarization to probe cerebral metabolism beyond glycolysis and TCA include the use of hyperpolarized 2-keto- [1-^{13}C]isocaproate, which

is converted to [1-^{13}C]leucine by branched chain amino acid transferase (Butt et al., 2012).

Two different approaches have been used to determine intracerebral pH in *in vivo* rodent brain. Using hyperpolarized MR to illustrate how this very interesting physiological factor may be explored, Gallagher et al. (2008) hyperpolarized bicarbonate ($H^{13}CO_3$) with DNP and monitored intracranial distribution and metabolism over several minutes following intravenous administration to living rodents. As expected, $^{13}CO_2$ was a readily detected product: together with $H^{13}CO_3$ this permitted application of Henderson–Hasselbach calculations of intracerebral pH. An alternative approach used the novel parahydrogen hyperpolarized substrate, [1-^{13}C]succinate, the chemical shift of which is known to be pH dependent. After intra-arterial administration, [1-^{13}C]succinate was readily identified within the brain. In the stroke model employed for these studies, the chemical shift of [1-^{13}C]succinate differed between brain regions (Ross et al., 2010) leading the authors to speculate, and confirm in preliminary standard curves, that this was a possible result of differences in ambient pH. In 1973, Moon and Richards (1973) charted the 40 year future of conventional MRS in biomedicine with the observation that the chemical shift of intrinsic ^{31}P inorganic phosphate was sensitive to pH. Kanamori and Ross (1997) demonstrated compartmentation of intracerebral pH showing that proton-detected ^{15}N NMR could define intraglial pH during hyperammonemia in the intact rat brain. The concentration of natural abundance [bicarbonate] in ^{13}C MRS can be used to better define intracerebral pH in normal and fasting humans (Sailasuta et al, 2011). Prior direct measurements, for patient monitoring after trauma or hypoxia, have necessitated invasive in-patient procedures involving pCO$_2$ electrodes. It is not fanciful to envisage opportunities for a significant new contribution to the debate about physiological and pathological regulation of intracellular, extracellular, intraneuronal, and intraglial pH with hyperpolarized NMR biomarkers.

Hyperpolarized Neuro-Oncology

In keeping with the drive to use every new biomedical technology to unlock the metabolic profile of cancer, hyperpolarized MR has been applied to brain cancer (Fig. 4.3.5G). An early study addressed the question using an intracerebral glioma model; others have approached the question indirectly, exploring the metabolism of implanted brain tumor cells developing in a more accessible subcutaneous location. And yet other studies have explored the metabolism of isolated brain tumor cells in a bioreactor or as tumor spheroids. New knowledge is so far somewhat limited, since the initial goal has been to define imaging agents that can access the tumor. Here the absence of an intact BBB has proved an inducement for *in vivo* study. The first agent explored was a parahydrogen-hyperpolarized ^{13}C TCA-cycle intermediate, [1-^{13}C] succinate. The clue that such a reagent would be useful arose in an indirect way when the unmetabolized and even somewhat toxic precursor sodium maleate was administered to rats (Bhattacharya et al. 2005, 2007a). Hyperpolarized products nevertheless appeared *in vivo*, among which were [1-^{13}C]fumarate and [1-^{13}C]succinate. In the published study, ^{13}C metabolic products of administered hyperpolarized [1-^{13}C]succinate were reported. However, it is clear that the experiment in which brain and tumor were examined with ^{13}C NMR, delays were such that all "hyperpolarized spins" must have decayed and the spectra represent conventional Boltzmann products. Nevertheless, the potential for hyperpolarized *in vivo* imaging of a brain tumor was established. Subsequent studies with DNP-polarized [1-^{13}C]pyruvate administered to animals with implanted brain tumors confirmed that truly hyperpolarized metabolic products appear within tumors (Park et al., 2010). This more complete study investigated the accumulation of [1-^{13}C]pyruvate and its solitary metabolic product [1-^{13}C]lactate in normal brain of the rodent host, and within Gd-enhancing regions of two different glioblastoma models previously implanted and established within the living brain. As predicted by cancer theory of enhanced glycolytic activity in most if not all tumors, excess hyperpolarized ^{13}C lactate was quantified within the model glioblastomas compared to adjacent brain, with modest differences between the two tumor models. The difference in accumulation of both substrate and product is mainly attributable to the impaired BBB as already demonstrated for [1-^{13}C] succinate, However, drawing on other studies (see Hurd et al., 2010 and previous sections) involving compartmentation of hyperpolarized reagents delivered by the vascular route to the brain and more extensive studies already completed in extraneural tumors, specifically the prostate, is it likely that even this rather simple experiment has more to offer than the bald statements that tumors are glycolytic and lack an intact BBB. *In vitro* studies with hyperpolarized [1-^{13}C]pyruvate of brain tumor cells in culture allow for a more controlled environment and systematic exploration of the impact of abnormal glycolysis on the phosphatidylinositol-3-kinase pathway. Since this is a target of rapamycin and other novel drug therapy, the authors propose a role for hyperpolarized ^{13}C pyruvate to lactate imaging (Chaumiel et al.,

2012). Using hyperpolarized ^{13}C imaging reagents in the well-established cancer research model of subcutaneous implanted glioma cells has proved an efficient means of exploring both the potential of individual hyperpolarized imaging agents and the unique metabolic features of the explanted tumor. As proof of principle therefore we can assume a future for neuro-oncology employing biomarker contrast agents hyperpolarized by either parahydrogen or DNP methods.

It will be no surprise, however, to learn that purists in cancer research have severe reservations regarding "new knowledge" garnered from these models. While remaining confident that such knowledge will be crucial, we must await advances (as already achieved in TRAMP mouse and in human prostate cancer) that permit direct ^{13}C imaging of spontaneous brain tumors, either in canines where they occur frequently, or in human patients. A more comprehensive armamentarium of reagents designed to probe more current metabolic and genetic markers of neurological cancers will also be necessary if we are to escape the "futile cycle" of ever more sophisticated means of confirming Warburg's 75-year-old hypothesis, which focused solely on [1-^{13}C]pyruvate will inevitably be disappointing.

As an example, hyperpolarized neuroimaging appears poised to offer a new means of *in vivo* imaging of oncogenes. Succinic dehydrogenase, fumarase. and ultimately HIF-1 α, an important regulatory protein in many cancers, provide novel biomarkers of glioblastoma and other neural tumors. These modifications reflect a group of oncogenes that appear to result in differences in TCA cycle metabolism. This prediction has been confirmed in implanted non-neurological tumors studied with parahydrogen-hyperpolarized succinate or diethyl succinate (Bhattacharya et al., 2012). A number of investigators have identified a proton MRS biomarker of another prevalent (seen in 10% of glioblastomas) brain tumor oncogene, isocitric dehydrogenase, through its abnormal metabolite 2-hydroxyglutarate (Choi et al., 2012). It should be possible to devise a ^{13}C contrast agent to address this intriguing and potentially valuable biomarker.

SOME POINTERS TO FUTURE EXPLOITATION OF HYPERPOLARIZED MR IN NEUROSCIENCE AND NEUROLOGY

The editors of this volume particularly requested some forward thinking regarding what future might be anticipated for hyperpolarized MR in neuroscience. As we have indicated throughout this description, "horses-for courses" has ruled the first 10 years (or 20 years in the case of hyperpolarized noble-gas imaging) of exploration of this new technology. Finding a relevant and nontoxic biological agent, [1-^{13}C] pyruvate, was a master stroke, which we probably owe to Dr. Rolf Bunger (Bhattacharya et al., 2009) who had decades earlier explored in detail its impact on intermediary metabolism. Applying this imaging reagent to all "known" pathologies with abnormal glycolysis (or at least the final step to the enzyme-catalyzed conversion to lactate) has been extremely productive of publications and, more important, has fueled the much needed improvements in *in vivo* imaging of evanescent ^{13}C MR signal. Perhaps, by analogy with FDG-PET this will represent the defining role for hyperpolarized MR. Given the persistent inventiveness of the MR community this seems a highly unlikely scenario. More likely, among the 20 or so biologicals that have already shown significant hyperpolarization—using predominantly DNP, but also parahydrogen techniques, and polarization transfer methodologies harnessed to noble gases or silicon (Cassidy et al., 2013) to name only those we know at present—the second generation of *in vivo* hyperpolarization in brain that we are now entering will feature a high preponderance of hypothesis-driven research. It is likely that practicing neuroscientists already familiar with NMR will identify crucial questions for which the added signal or the sheer speed of hyperpolarized heteronuclear imaging offers an answer. Similarly, with the proliferation of practical polarizers for small animal and *in vitro*

research as well as the advent of the first "clinical" polarizers will entice neurologists to ask burning clinical questions in their specialty. A convenient starting point is to investigate the discoveries (and limitations) encountered when conventional (Boltzmann) heteronuclear MRS and imaging were applied to *in vivo* brain in rodents and, more recently, in humans (see Chapters 4.1 & 4.2). ^{13}C was detected directly, with and without proton decoupling and by inverse detection through attached protons, with great benefit. The contributions of ^{13}C to measuring and understanding glutamate and GABA neurotransmitter pathways and relation to energetics should be mentioned. Direct observation and quantification of TCA cycle flux, separate detection, and quantification of neuronal and glial TCA flux and of many associated reactions including glycogen synthesis and anaplerotic reactions previously little understood in intact brain were exhaustively studied. Pathological impact on these processes was defined for hepatic encephalopathy, schizophrenia, Alzheimer's disease, and perhaps most usefully, for a variety of inborn and acquired neurological disorders of childhood (see Chapter 4.2). ^{15}N MRS was pursued as a means of defining neurotransmitter pathways in rodent brain (no human ^{15}N NMR studies have been reported), and will perhaps define the principal limitations that may now be overcome through hyperpolarized ^{15}N neuroimaging. Thus, the concentration limit of conventional ^{15}N NMR appears to be around 1 mM (10^{-3} M); only the glutamate GABA transmitter systems are defined

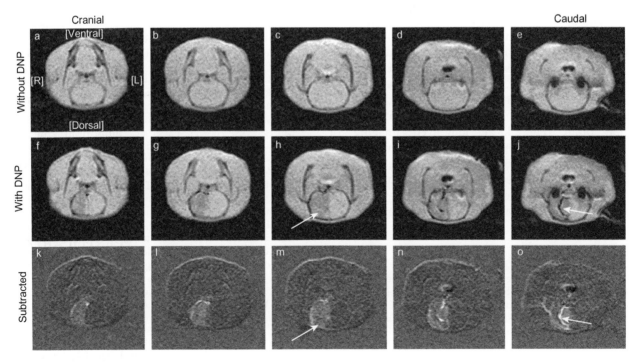

FIGURE 4.3.7   Hyperpolarized water image of rat brain *in vivo*. (*Adapted from McCarney, 2012.*)

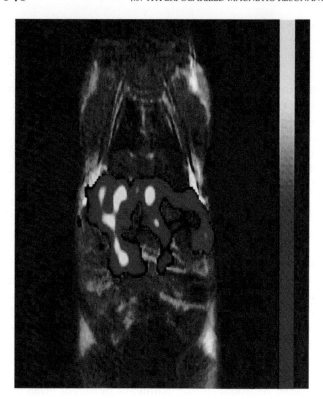

FIGURE 4.3.8 Only a matter of time. *In vivo* image of the bowel following administration of hyperpolarized silicon nanoparticles. (Image courtesy of Cassidy et al., 2012.)

since the multitude of nitrogen-based neurotransmitters are active in the concentration range 10^{-4} to 10^{-12} M. Here we can expect real progress from hyperpolarized neuroimaging in the future, in that the nitrogen gets incorporated into glutamine, glutamate, and other transmitters in one step. In contrast ^{13}C precursors like acetate take several steps to get to amino acid and other neurotransmitters. Last, we should not forget the extraordinary inventiveness of our parent disciplines, spin physics and NMR. Hyperpolarized water imaging of the brain (Fig. 4.3.7), long-lived imaging of reagents based on hyperpolarized silicon nanoparticles (Fig. 4.3.8, as yet no brain image is available), and…whatever happened to para-water? I am sure that readers of other chapters in this volume will come away with plenty of ideas.

Acknowledgments

Funding for work completed at Huntington Medical Research Institutes is made possible by the National Institutes of Health, National Cancer Institute, and Rudi Schulte Research Institute. This chapter was written with assistance from Dr. Pratip Bhattacharya, Associate Professor at M.D. Anderson, Division of Imaging Research; Cherise Charleswell; and Thao Tran. This chapter is dedicated to the late Rudolph Schulte of Altadena and Santa Barbara, philanthropist and enthusiast for MR neuroimaging.

References

Abragam, A., & Goldman, M. (1976). Principles of dynamic nuclear polarisation. *Reports on Progress in Physics, 41*(3), 395–467.

Adams, R. W., Aguilar, J. A., Atkinson, K. D., Cowley, M. J., Elliott, P. I., Duckett, S. B., et al. (2009). Reversible interactions with parahydrogen enhance NMR sensitivity by polarization transfer. *Science, 323,* 1708–1711.

Albert, M. S., Cates, G. D., Driehuys, B., Happer, W., Saam, B., Springer, C. S., Jr, et al. (1994). Biological magnetic resonance imaging using laser-polarized ^{129}Xe. *Nature, 370,* 199–201.

Ardenkjaer-Larsen, J. H., Fridlund, B., Gram, A., Hansson, G., Hansson, L., Lerche, M. H., et al. (2003). Increase in signal-to-noise ratio of > 10,000 times in liquid state NMR. *Proceedings of the National Academy of Sciences USA, 100*(18), 10158–10163.

Bhattacharya, P., Chekmenev, E. Y., Perman, W. H., Harris, K. C., Lin, A. P., Norton, V. A., et al. (2007a). Towards hyperpolarized ^{13}C-succinate imaging of brain cancer. *Journal of Magnetic Resonance, 186*(1), 150–155.

Bhattacharya, P., Chekmenev, E. Y., Reynolds, W. F., Wagner, S., Zacharias, N., Chan, H. R., et al. (2011). Parahydrogen-induced polarization (PHIP) hyperpolarized MR receptor imaging in vivo: a pilot study of ^{13}C imaging of atheroma in mice. *NMR in Biomedicine, 24*(8), 1023–1028.

Bhattacharya, P., Harris, K. C., Chekmenev, E. Y., Lin, A. P., Norton, V. A., Hovener, J., et al. (2007b). How low can we go? Limits of detection in PASADENA ^{13}C hyperpolarization. *Proceedings of the International Society of Magnetic Resonance Medicine, 15,* 1309.

Bhattacharya, P., Harris, K., Lin, A. P., Mansson, M., Norton, V. A., Perman, W. H., et al. (2005). Ultra-fast three dimensional imaging of hyperpolarized ^{13}C in vivo. *MAGMA, 18*(5), 245–256.

Bhattacharya, P., Ross, B. D., & Bunger, R. (2009). Cardiovascular applications of hyperpolarized contrast media and metabolic tracers. *Experimental Biology and Medicine, 234*(12), 1395–1416.

Bhattacharya, P., Wagner, S., Chan, H. R., Chekmenev, E. Y., Perman, W. H., & Ross, B. D. (2008). Hyperpolarized ^{15}N NMR: D^{15}NP and PASADE^{15}NA. *Proceedings of the International Congress of Magnetic Resonance Biological Systems, 13,* 158.

Bhattacharya, P., Zacharias, N. M., Sailasuta, N., Chan, H. R., Perman, W. H., Epstein, A. L., et al. (2012). *Proceedings of the International Society of Magnetic Resonance in Medicine, 20,* 4410.

Bonhoeffer, K. F., & Harteck, P. (1929). *Zeitschrift für Physikalische Chemie, Abt. B, 4,* 113.

Bowers, C. R., & Weitekamp, D. P. (1986). Transformation of symmetrization order to nuclear-spin magnetization by chemical reaction and nuclear magnetic resonance. *Physical Review Letters, 57,* 2645.

Butt, S. A., Søgaard, L. V., Magnusson, P. O., Lauritzen, M. H., Laustsen, C., Akeson, P., et al. (2012). Imaging cerebral 2-ketoisocaproate metabolism with hyperpolarized ^{13}C magnetic resonance spectroscopic imaging. *Journal of Cerebral Blood Flow and Metabolism, 32*(8), 1508–1514.

Cassidy, M., Chan, H. R., Ross, B. D., Bhattacharya, P., & Marcus, C. M. (2013). In-vivo magnetic resonance imaging of hyperpolarized silicon particles. *Nature Nanotechnology, 8*(5), 363–368.

Chaumeil, M. M., Gini, B., Yang, H., Iwanami, A., Sukumar, S., Ozawa, T., et al. (2012). Longitudinal evaluation of MPIO-labeled stem cell biodistribution in glioblastoma using high resolution and contrast-enhanced MR imaging at 14.1 Tesla. *Neuro-Oncology, 14*(8), 1050–1061.

Chen, A. P., Hurd, R. E., Schroeder, M. A., Lau, A. Z., Gu, Y. P., Lam, W. W., et al. (2012). Simultaneous investigation of cardiac pyruvate dehydrogenase flux, Krebs cycle metabolism and pH, using hyperpolarized [1,2-^{13}C2]pyruvate in vivo. *NMR in Biomedicine, 25*(2), 305–311.

Choi, C., Ganji, S. K., DeBerardinis, R. J., Hatanpaa, K. J., Rakheja, D., Kovacs, Z., et al. (2012). 2-hydroxyglutarate detection by magnetic resonance spectroscopy in IDH-mutated patients with gliomas. *Nature Medicine, 18*(4), 624–629.

Forsen, S., & Hoffman, R. A. (1963). Study of moderately rapid chemical exchange reactions by means of nuclear magnetic double resonance. *Journal of Chemistry and Physics, 39*, 2892.

Gallagher, F. A., Kettunen, M. I., Day, S. E., Hu, D. E., Ardenkjaer-Larsen, J. H., Zandt, R., et al. (2008). Magnetic resonance imaging of pH in vivo using hyperpolarized ^{13}C-labelled bicarbonate. *Nature, 453*, 940–943.

Goldman, M., Johannesson, H., Axelsson, O., & Karlsson, M. (2006). Design and implementation of ^{13}C hyper polarization from para-hydrogen, for new MRI contrast agents. *Comptes Rendus Chimie*357–363.

Golman, K., Olsson, L. E., Axelsson, O., Månsson, S., Karlsson, M., & Petersson, J. S. (2003). Molecular imaging using hyperpolarized ^{13}C. *British Journal of Radiology, 76*(Spec No 2), S118–S127.

Hurd, R. E., Yen, Y. F., Mayer, D., Chen, A., Wilson, D., Kohler, S., et al. (2010). Metabolic imaging in the anesthetized rat brain using hyperpolarized [1-^{13}C] pyruvate and [1-^{13}C] ethyl pyruvate. *Magnetic Resonance in Medicine, 63*(5), 1137–1143.

Kanamori, K., & Ross, B. D. (1997). Glial alkalinization detected in vivo by ^{1}H-^{15}N heteronuclear multiple-quantum coherence-transfer NMR in severely hyperammonemic rat. *Journal of Neurochemistry, 68*(3), 1209–1220.

Kilian, W., Seifert, F., & Rinneberg, H. (2004). Dynamic NMR spectroscopy of hyperpolarized ^{129}Xe in human brain analyzed by an uptake model. *Magnetic Resonance in Medicine, 51*, 843–847.

Kurhanewicz, J., Vigneron, D. B., Brindle, K., Chekmenev, E. Y., Comment, A., Cunningham, C. H., et al. (2011). Analysis of cancer metabolism by imaging hyperpolarized nuclei: prospects for translation to clinical research. *Neoplasia, 13*(2), 81–97.

Lisitza, N., Muradian, I., Frederick, E., Patz, S., Hatabu, H., & Chekmenev, E. Y. (2009). Toward ^{13}C hyperpolarized biomarkers produced by thermal mixing with hyperpolarized ^{129}Xe. *Journal of Chemistry and Physics, 131*(4), 044508.

Marjańska, M., Iltis, I., Shestov, A. A., Deelchand, D. K., Nelson, C., Ugurbil, K., et al. (2010). In Vivo ^{13}C spectroscopy in the rat brain using hyperpolarized [1-^{13}C]pyruvate and [2-^{13}C]pyruvate. *Journal of Magnetic Resonance, 206*(2), 210–218.

Mayer, D., Yen, Y. F., Takahashi, A., Josan, S., Tropp, J., Rutt, B. K., et al. (2011). Dynamic and high-resolution metabolic imaging of hyperpolarized [1-^{13}C]-pyruvate in the rate brain using high-performance gradient insert. *Magnetic Resonance in Medicine, 65*(5), 1228–1233.

Mazzanti, M. L., Walvick, R. P., Zhou, X., Sun, Y., Shah, N., Mansour, J., et al. (2011). Distribution of hyperpolarized xenon in the brain following sensory stimulation: preliminary MRI findings. *PLoS One, 6*(7), e21607.

McCarney, E. R., Armstrong, B. D., Lingwood, M. D., & Han, S. (2007). Hyperpolarized water as an MRI contrast agent.

Proceedings of the National Academy of Sciences USA, 104(6), 1754–1759.

Merritt, M. E., Harrison, C., Storey, C., Sherry, A. D., & Malloy, C. R. (2008). Inhibition of carbohydrate oxidation during the first minute of reperfusion after brief ischemia: NMR detection of hyperpolarized ^{13}CO$_2$ and H^{13}CO$_3$. *Magnetic Resonance in Medicine, 60*, 1029–1036.

Mishkovsky, M., Comment, A., & Gruetter, R. (2011). In vivo detection of brain Krebs cycle intermediate by hyperpolarized MR. *Proceedings of the International Society of Magnetic Resonance Medicine, 19*, 660 Montreal, Quebec, Canada.

Moon, R. B., & Richards, J. H. (1973). Determination of Intracellular pH by ^{31}P magnetic resonance. *Journal of Biological Chemistry, 248*, 7276–7278.

Natterer, J., & Bargon, J. (1997). Parahydrogen induced polarization. *Progress in Nuclear Magnetic Resonance Spectroscopy, 31*, 293–315.

Overhauser, A. W. (1953). Polarization of nuclei in metals. *Physical Review, 92*(2), 411–415.

Park, I., Larson, P. E., Zierhut, M. L., Hu, S., Bok, R., Ozawa, T., et al. (2010). Hyperpolarized ^{13}C magnetic resonance imaging: application to brain tumors. *Neuro-Oncology, 12*, 133–144.

Ross, B. D., & Bluml, S. (2001). Magnetic resonance spectroscopy of the human brain. *Anatomical Record, 265*(2), 54–84.

Ross, B. D., Bhattacharya, P., Wagner, S., Tran, T., & Sailasuta, N. (2010). Hyperpolarized MR imaging: neurologic applications of hyperpolarized metabolism. *American Journal of Neuroradiology, 31*(1), 24–33.

Rothman, D. L., Behar, K. L., Hyder, F., & Shulman, R. G. (2003). In vivo NMR studies of the glutamate neurotransmitter flux and neuroenergetics: implications for brain function. *Annual Review of Physiology, 65*, 401–427.

Sailasuta, N., Harris, K. C., Tran, T., & Ross, B. D. (2011). Define impact of fasting on human brain acid-base homeostasis using natural abundance ^{13}C and ^{31}P MRS. *J. Magn, Reson. Imaging*, doi:10.1002/jmri.24166.

Tang, J. A., Gruppi, F., Fleysher, R., Sodickson, D. K., Canary, J. W., & Jerschow, A. (2011). Extended para-hydrogenation monitored by NMR spectroscopy. *Chemical Communications, 47*, 958–960.

Tayler, M. C., Marco-Rius, I., Kettunen, M. I., Brindle, K. M., Levitt, M. H., & Pileio, G. (2012). Direct enhancement of nuclear singlet order by dynamic nuclear polarization. *Journal of America Chemical Society, 134*(18), 7668–7671.

Tyler, D. J. (2011). Cardiovascular Applications of Hyperpolarized MRI. *Current Cardiovascular Imaging Reports, 4*, 108–115.

Zacharias, N. M., Chan, H. R., Sailasuta, N., Ross, B. D., & Bhattacharya, P. (2012). Real-time molecular imaging of tricarboxylic acid cycle metabolism in vivo by hyperpolarized 1-^{13}C diethyl succinate. *Journal of the American Chemical Society, 134*(2), 934–943.

Zhou, X., et al. (2011). MRI of stroke using hyperpolarized ^{129}Xe. *NMR in Biomedicine, 24*, 170–175.

Index

351

Printed and bound by CPI Group (UK) Ltd, Croydon, CR0 4YY

08/05/2025

01865034-0002